Essentials of Maternal-Newborn Nursing

Essentials of Maternal-Newborn Nursing

Patricia A. Ladewig, RNC, MSN, NP
Associate Professor
Loretto Heights College
Denver, Colorado,
and Doctoral Candidate
University of Denver
Denver, Colorado

Marcia L. London, RNC, MSN, NNP
Assistant Professor
Beth-el College of Nursing
Colorado Springs, Colorado

Sally B. Olds, RNC, MS
Assistant Professor
Beth-el College of Nursing
Colorado Springs, Colorado

Deborah Gale, Developmental Editor

Addison-Wesley Publishing Company, Inc.
Health Sciences Division, Menlo Park, California
Reading, Massachusetts • Don Mills, Ontario • Wokingham, UK
Amsterdam • Sydney • Singapore • Tokyo • Mexico City
Bogota • Santiago • San Juan

Sponsoring Editor: *Nancy Evans*
Developmental and Production Editor: *Deborah Gale*
Copyeditor: *Antonio Padial*
Book Design: *John Edeen*
Cover Design: *Michael A. Rogondino, John Edeen*
Artist: *Jack Tandy*
Unit and Chapter Opening Photographs: *Suzanne Arms*
Color Plates: *William Thompson*
Color Plate Opening Photograph: *Suzanne Arms*

In-text Photographs: *Suzanne Arms, George Fry III,
    William Thompson*

Library of Congress Cataloging in Publication Data

Ladewig, Patricia A.
    Essentials of maternal-newborn nursing.

    Includes bibliographies and index.
    1. Obstetrical nursing. 2. Infants (Newborn)—
Diseases—Diagnosis. 3. Infants (Newborn)—Family
relationships. 4. Pediatric nursing. I. London,
Marcia L. II. Olds, Sally B., 1940–   . III. Gale,
Deborah. IV. Title. [DNLM: 1. Neonatology—nurses'
instruction. 2. Obstetrical Nursing. WY 157.3 L154e]
RG951.L33   1986   610.73'678   85-13334
ISBN 0-201-12680-X

EFGHIJ-RN-898

The authors and publishers have exerted every effort to ensure that
drug selection, dosage, and composition of formulas set forth in
this text are in accord with current formulations, recommendations,
and practice at the time of publication. However, in view of
ongoing research, changes in government regulations, the
reformulation of nutritional products, and the constant flow of
information relating to drug therapy and drug reactions, the reader
is urged to check product information or composition on the
package insert for each drug for any change in indications of
dosage and for added warnings and precautions. This is particularly
important where the recommended agent is a new and/or
infrequently employed drug.

Addison-Wesley Publishing Company
Health Sciences Division
2725 Sand Hill Road
Menlo Park, California 94025

We dedicate this book to our parents—

To Warren and Alice Wieland

Together they have given me values, and education, and a desire to be all that I can be. They are a constant source of encouragement. They taught me the meaning of love.

> *With love,*
> *Your daughter, Pat*

To Kenneth and Edna Brown

To my father who gave me an understanding of life and how it works—I wish he could share in my joys. To my mother who always knew I could be who I am.

> *Lovingly,*
> *Your daughter, Marcia*

To Randall and Naomi Brookens

To my father who always saw me as more than I thought I was—I wish he could see who I have become. To my mother who is the embodiment of all a woman can be and who believes in me.

> *Love,*
> *Your daughter, Sally*

Preface

In today's varied nursing curricula, the course in maternal-newborn nursing can range from 4–13 weeks, depending on the type of program, availability of clinical facilities, and other factors. Such variability means that no one text can effectively meet the needs of all students and faculty. While the acceptance of *Maternal-Newborn Nursing: A Family-Centered Approach* has been most gratifying, a number of educators have expressed the need for a smaller textbook focusing on the essentials of safe, thoughtful, family-centered nursing care. This book has been developed to meet that need.

Essentials of Maternal-Newborn Nursing retains the same warmth, sensitivity, and phil osophical approach as the larger text, with the nursing process as the framework for care and the family as co-participants in childbirth. Throughout the presentation of essential theoretical content, pregnancy and childbirth are viewed as normal life processes. However, because the student must be aware of potential complications to provide safe, effective care, the more common complications have been presented in separate high-risk chapters.

Development of this text involved much more than the deletion of selected content. Based on extensive market research and comments from reviewers and other faculty, much of the content has been streamlined and rewritten for enhanced clarity and readability. All content has been thoroughly updated to maintain the state-of-the-art quality of the larger book. New art and photographs have been added, and the entire text has been redesigned in a slightly smaller trim size. A new two-color format enhances student appeal and learning effectiveness.

Organization

Essentials of Maternal-Newborn Nursing comprises five units:

- Basic Concepts in Maternal-Newborn Nursing
- Pregnancy
- Labor and Delivery
- The Newborn
- The Puerperium

Within each unit the chapter sequence moves logically from normal to abnormal. As in the larger text, content on the adolescent and on cultural variations is integrated appropriately throughout. To provide greater focus, new chapters on "Maternal Nutrition" and "Preparation for Childbirth" have been included.

Learning Aids

This book includes many of the popular learning aids from *Maternal-Newborn Nursing*, plus some new features. Each chapter begins with a **content outline**, **learning objectives**, and a new feature, a list of **key terms**. These terms are bold-faced when they first appear in the text to quickly identify their importance to the student. All key terms are defined in the comprehensive **glossary** at the end of the text.

Within the chapters, information is readily accessible in **tables**, **nursing assessment guides**, **nursing care plans**, **procedures**, and **drug guides**. Many chapters include a new feature, **Essential Facts to Remember**, which helps students focus on key information necessary when caring for the childbearing family.

The chapters conclude with a summary, updated references, and additional readings. Certain chapters list national resource groups that can provide information and support to childbearing families.

In addition, several of the chapters contain **case studies**. These case studies help the student undestand more clearly how nursing care may be individualized.

Photography

To enhance student interest and involvement, photographs by Suzanne Arms, noted photojournalist and childbirth educator, were commissioned to open each unit and chapter of this book. Eloquent expressions of the drama and poignancy inherent in family-centered childbirth, these pictures underscore the emphasis on the family as co-participants in this experience.

In addition to these original black and white photographs, the text includes four pages of **full-color photographs**. A popular feature of the larger text, these photographs depict some common and some not-so-common clinical conditions related to pregnancy and birth.

Supplements

Essentials of Maternal-Newborn Nursing offers a complete package of supplementary teaching-learning aids. The *Instructor's Manual* that accompanied *Maternal-Newborn Nursing* has been modified by Virginia Kinnick to coincide with the shorter text. *Maternal-Newborn Nursing Care: A Workbook* can be used effectively with this text or with the larger text, as can the *Transparency Resource Kit*. In addition, a 500-item *Test Bank* is available to adopters as computerized software or a test booklet.

The fine reception given our first text and the valuable comments it evoked have inspired us to develop this second book. Although in a sense an offspring of the larger book, *Essentials of Maternal-Newborn Nursing* has a character all its own, shaped by the audience it is intended to serve. We hope that faculty and students using this text will continue to offer their suggestions for shaping future editions.

Acknowledgments

During the course of our writing together, we have been challenged and stimulated by many people, but especially by our students. Their questions, their insights, their enthusiasm have helped make our writing exciting and even, at times, fun! For this we thank them.

We are also grateful for the encouragement and support of our friends and colleagues. They are always willing to lend words of encouragement or to share new knowledge. Through the course of our writing, we have come in contact with many nurse educators and practicing nurses, and we have been enriched because of it.

We are also grateful to the contributors to the second edition of the larger text. Their work formed the nucleus of this text. They include: Joan Edelstein, Ann Havenhill, Louise Westberg Hedstrom, Linda Andrist Hereford, E. JoAnne Jones, Joy M. Khader, Virginia Gramzow Kinnick, Nancy Ellen Krauss, Joy Kub, Mary Ann Leppink, Anne L. Matthews, Nancy McCluggage, Cynthia A. McMahon, Anne Garrard McMath, Donna Rae Meirath Moriarity, Karen Rooks Nauer, Sally J. Phillips, Lovena L. Porter, Joanne F. Ruth, M. Carole Schoffstall, Constance Lawrenz Slaughter, Mari Lou Steffen, Elvira Szigeti, Janel N. Timmins, and Bette Blome Winyall.

We are grateful to all the nurses who reviewed and critiqued this manuscript as it evolved. Their perceptions of what is truly essential for a maternity nurse to know helped us keep this text well-focused and "tight." They include: Bonnie Anderson, Napa Community College, Napa, California; LuAnn Beavers, Owens Technical College, Toledo, Ohio; Joea Bierchen, St. Petersburg Jr. College, St. Petersburg, Florida; Gary Boyce, University of Florida, Gainesville; Barbara Byrd, Hocking Technical College, Nelsonville, Ohio; Sharon Carlson, Prince George's Community College, Largo, Maryland; Mary Lou Cook, Walters State Community College, Morristown, Tennessee; Jean Cuppet, Conemaugh Valley Memorial Hospital, Johnstown, Pennsylvania; Patricia Jansson, Williamsport Hospital, Williamsport, Pennsylvania; Mary Norville, Essex Community College, Baltimore County, Maryland; Rita Tracy, Washburn University, Topeka, Kansas; Susan Trippett and

Enid Zwirn, Indiana University/Purdue University at Indianapolis; Jan Twiss, University of Nebraska, Omaha; Lynn Wohler, Lamar University, Beaumont, Texas; Betty Zaring, Oscar Rose Jr. College, Midwest City, Oklahoma.

A project of this scope requires the support and cooperation of many people. We would like to personally thank the following individuals for their special contributions:

- *Deborah Gale* revised three chapters and served as developmental editor and production coordinator. Throughout our eight-year association, Deborah has been our "catalyst." When we work with her, we become more creative and, somehow, better. She is a very special friend.
- *Nancy Evans* is our sponsoring editor. She has been consistently caring, supportive, and helpful. We look forward with pleasure to many years of close working ties with her. She understands the pains and the joys of writing.
- *Suzanne Arms* is justly renowned for her concern for the childbearing family. It has been an honor to have her support on this project. She captures on film the essence of the nurse and the childbearing family.

- *Nick Keefe*, General Manager of the Nursing Division, is always ready to offer a word of encouragement and support.
- *Jack Tandy*, another old friend, rendered some fine new art for this text.
- *Antonio Padial* worked as copyeditor on this text. His awareness of inconsistencies and his eye for detail helped us produce a sharper book.
- *Ginny Mickelson* modified some existing art. Her work enabled us to add color to the figures.
- *Judith Hibbard* served as the in-house production coordinator. She helped bring the project to completion.

We would also like to thank the families who agreed to be photographed. Their sharing of a part of themselves has given the text special warmth.

As always, we would be lost without our families. How can you adequately thank people who so lovingly tolerate inconvenience, late nights, numerous phone calls, and the sound of typing, and who are always ready to lend a hand or simply a word of encouragement and support. They are our strength and we love them.

Patricia A. Ladewig
Marcia L. London
Sally B. Olds

Contents
in Brief

Contents
in Detail

A listing of special features follows on p. xx.

Essentials of
Maternal-Newborn
Nursing

The sudden workings of nine months of pregnancy, culminating in an event that never seems less than miraculous, changes us in more ways than the simple addition of a child to our lives. It puts us in touch with the past and the future. . . .

NANCY CALDWELL SOREL

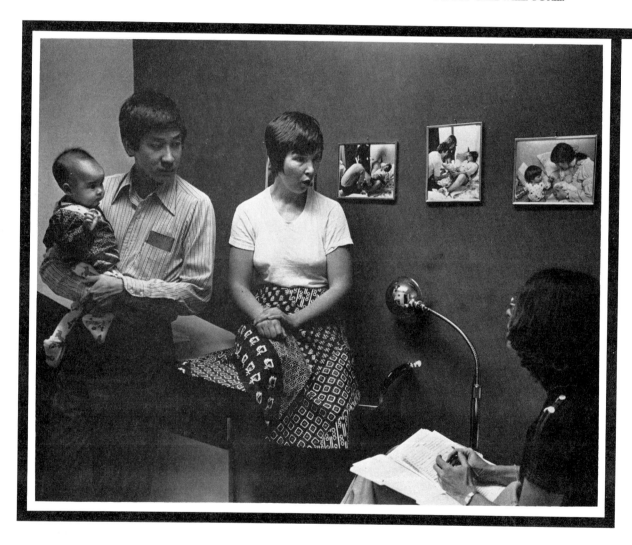

I

Basic Concepts in Maternal-Newborn Nursing

1
Contemporary Maternal-Newborn Care

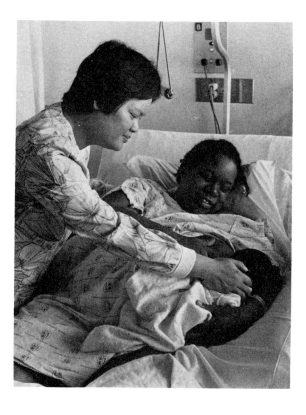

Chapter Contents

Childbearing in the Twentieth Century

Maternal-Newborn Government Programs

Maternal-Newborn Nursing
  Roles and Settings
  Nurse-Midwifery
  The Nurse and the Family
  Legal Considerations
  Professional Issues

Issues in Maternal-Newborn Care
  Biomedical Technology
  Changes in Health Care Relationships
  Ethical Issues

Tools for Maternal-Newborn Nursing Practice
  Knowledge Base
  Nursing Process
  Nursing Diagnosis
  Communication
  Statistics
  Nursing Research
  Application of Tools for Nursing Practice

Objectives

* Describe changes in childbirth practice in the twentieth century.

* Discuss the various nursing roles in maternity care.

* Describe some nursing strategies for caring for the family.

- Briefly discuss selected state-of-the-art advances in the care of the childbearing family.

- Contrast the arguments advanced for specific ethical issues affecting maternity care.

- Discuss selected tools used in maternity nursing practice.

- Contrast descriptive and inferential statistics.

Key Terms

biopsychosocial	maternal mortality
birth rate	neonatal mortality
client	neonatology
client advocate	nurse-midwife
descriptive statistics	nursing diagnosis
family-centered care	nursing process
fertility rate	perinatal mortality
fetal death	perinatology
inferential statistics	problem-oriented
informed consent	record system

At the moment a child is born, the quality of his or her future depends on many genetic and environmental factors. Some of these factors are present at the time of conception; others become apparent as the child develops.

The actions and decisions of parents and health professionals have great impact on children's lives. Health professionals can improve a child's chances for a healthy future by providing expert care to the expectant family. Parents can provide a positive family environment for their children by living as healthfully as possible and seeking help from professionals when a family member's physical or psychologic condition is threatened.

This textbook is about the contribution of maternity nurses to the quality of a child's life. Since the psychologic and physical health of parents has a marked effect on their offspring, our focus is the childbearing family and the responsibilities of the nurse caring for that family. This chapter is an introduction to childbearing and maternity nursing in North America.

Childbearing in the Twentieth Century

Before 1900, few infants were delivered in hospitals. Only very poor or unwed women went to a hospital for childbirth. As the scope of medical practice increased, hospital deliveries gained acceptance from more affluent clients. By the middle of the twentieth century, most women were hospitalized for childbirth.

Until early in this century, newborns remained with their mothers after a hospital delivery. Outbreaks of diarrhea, scarlet fever, diphtheria, and other communicable diseases, however, caused a large number of infant and maternal deaths. Physicians emphasized the need for separate care for mother and infant to prevent the spread of infection. Newborn nurseries became firmly entrenched, and an era of rigid management of pregnancy, labor, and delivery began.

Labor and delivery were treated as a medical problem, controlled by the obstetrician and hospital staff. Many types of analgesic agents were administered during labor, and general anesthetics were given for delivery. Some of these agents were harmful to the fetus. During labor and delivery, the father sat in the waiting room. After the delivery, the father saw his child through the window of the nursery.

Frequently, the mother was separated from her infant for hours after the delivery. During the remainder of the hospital stay, maternal-infant contact depended on hospital routine. Strict asepsis and scheduled formula feedings were accepted practices. Postpartal stays for mother and child usually lasted about 10 days, and infant care classes were unknown. Little thought was given to the psychologic effects of these policies on the childbearing family.

In the early 1940s, social scientists and health care professionals began analyzing the effects of this rigid management of childbirth on family relationships and on individual members. Studies showed that the psychologic and social well-being of family members was affected by impersonal, rigid hospital practices.

By the early 1950s, it became clear to some that more personalized and family-oriented maternity care was essential. They began advocating changes in the care given during childbearing. These advocates included Grantly Dick-Read, who introduced the concept of preparing the mother and father for childbirth and allowing the father to participate in labor and delivery; Arnold Gesell, who supported the practice of rooming-in so that newborns could remain in the hospital rooms with their mothers; and John Bowlby, who described the tragic effects of maternal deprivation on children.

The movement toward **family-centered care** during childbirth was advanced in the late 1950s by the Family-Centered Maternity Care Program established at St. Mary's Hospital in Evansville, Indiana. This program was based on the concept that a hospital could provide professional services to mothers, fathers, and infants in a homelike environment that would enhance the integrity of the family unit.

The movement toward family-centered care received added impetus from families themselves. In the 1960s, when many people began questioning long-held beliefs about many areas of life, those pertaining to traditional medical practices and philosophies also came under scrutiny. The consumer, feminist, and self-help movements made people take a new look at childbearing and its medical management. Couples began demanding assistance, not control, from physicians and nurses. Women began realizing that the successful outcome of their pregnancy had more to do with their role and activities than those of the obstetrician. People began asking for complete information about medical practices—what, why, and how much—so that they could make their own decisions. Childbearing couples began seeking alternatives to traditional obstetric management, including home birth and midwives as birth attendants.

The health care system has responded to the demands of health care consumers and professionals. Hospital policies and practices have been modified, and alternatives to conventional institutional childbirth are being offered to women considered at low risk for complications.

Today's typical childbearing experience is characterized by its focus on the family. Fathers are participants during the birth, not passive bystanders. Even when cesarean delivery is necessary, the father usually can remain with the woman. Analgesic and anesthetic agents for pain relief are carefully monitored and used minimally, and special breathing patterns and other methods are used to relieve discomfort.

Unless the newborn is at risk and requires immediate care, he or she remains with the parents so that they can become acquainted. The newborn is usually fed on demand instead of on a schedule. The mother may have the infant in her room as much as she desires. The hospital stay for a healthy mother and newborn may be as brief as 12 hours.

Many hospitals offer alternative birth facilities to childbearing couples. Labor and delivery rooms have been remodeled to convey a homelike atmosphere. Some hospitals have established outpatient birth centers as well as birthing rooms within the hospital. In birthing rooms and birth centers, the father and others important to the mother are allowed to participate in the birth. Some birth facilities allow siblings to be present during delivery.

Occasionally, the birth center is established and managed by nurse-midwives, who are also in attendance during labor and delivery. If a complication arises, clients are transferred to a health care facility that is equipped to handle the situation.

The goal of the maternity staff in birth facilities is to promote a meaningful experience for the childbearing family as well as to ensure the health of mother and child. Most couples come away from their childbearing experience feeling satisfied with their maternity care.

Maternal-Newborn Government Programs

More than 60 years ago, the United States government became involved in improving the quality of maternity care. The Sheppard-Towner Act of 1921 was the first federal legislation to provide funds for state programs in maternal and child care; this act was in force until 1929. In 1935, the Social Security Act was passed, which provides federal grants for health and welfare programs, with many services in the maternal-child health area.

In 1964, the Maternity and Infant (M&I) Care Projects were begun by the Public Health Service of the Department of Health, Education, and Welfare. These projects were started in 56 geographic areas where maternal and infant mortality rates were much higher than the national average. The states now manage these projects, although they are still federally funded.

The purpose of these projects is to provide high-risk women safe, effective maternity care with the goals of reducing maternal and infant mortality and preventing prematurity, birth trauma, and mental retardation. Services range from medical and dental care to infant care. These projects have been very effective.

A supplemental food program for Women, Infants, and Children (WIC) was established in 1975 to provide food and nutrition counseling to low-income families. WIC has been important in promoting the nutritional well-being of women and small children.

Maternal-Newborn Nursing

Nurses who want to care for childbearing families can choose from a variety of career positions and settings. Depending on the nurse's qualifications, the nurse may *assist* the primary caregiver or *be* the primary caregiver during the pregnancy and birth. This section explores professional options for nurses as well as other issues arising from the expansion of nursing practice.

Underlying all maternity nursing care, no matter what the nurse's position, is a family-centered approach. A major goal of family-centered maternity care is to help each member of the expectant family become or stay healthy. The nurse who wants to care for childbearing families must understand family structures, roles of family members, and family processes. An in-depth discussion of the family unit is beyond the scope of this book, but there are many excellent books and articles on the subject. Later in this section, some general principles of nursing care for the family are provided.

Roles and Settings

Maternity nurses are found in the obstetric departments of acute care facilities, physician's offices, public health department clinics, and any other setting where women seek maternity care. The depth of care provided by the nurse depends on her or his qualifications and scope of practice. A *professional nurse* has graduated from an accredited basic program in nursing, has successfully completed the nursing licensure examination, is currently licensed as a registered nurse, and is qualified to provide basic nursing care. The *nurse practitioner* (NP) has received specialized education in a master's degree program or a continuing education program and thus can function in an expanded role. Nurse practitioners often provide ambulatory care services to the expectant family, performing physical and psychosocial assessments and certain diagnostic tests and procedures. Nurse practitioners also work in normal or high-risk neonatal nurseries.

The *clinical nurse specialist* has a master's degree and specialized knowledge and competence in a specific clinical area. The *certified nurse-midwife* (CNM) is educated in the two disciplines of nursing and midwifery and possesses evidence of certification according to the requirements of the American College of Nurse-Midwives. The nurse-midwife is trained to manage independently the care of women at low risk for complications during pregnancy and birth and the care of normal newborns.

Nurse-Midwifery

Throughout history, birth attendants or midwives have had an important place in most societies. Midwifery is an honored profession that has developed throughout the ages. Even today, eight of ten women in the world are attended in childbirth by a midwife.

Midwifery and nursing are distinct disciplines; in fact, the education, regulation, and practice of the professional midwife were instituted before organized professional nursing came into existence in 1871. They are complementary disciplines, however, and this has led to the development of the **nurse-midwife**.

The nurse-midwife practices within the framework of a medically directed health service in accord with the guidelines specified by the American College of Nurse-Midwives (1979). The basic beliefs and commitments of nurse-midwives are reflected in the following statement:

Every childbearing family has a right to a safe, satisfying experience with respect for human dignity and worth; for variety in cultural forms; and for the parents' right to self-determination.

Comprehensive maternity care, including educational and emotional support as well as management of physical care throughout the childbearing years, is a major means of intercession into, and improvement and maintenance of, the health of the nation's families. Comprehensive maternity care is most effectively and efficiently delivered by interdependent health disciplines.

Nurse-midwifery is an interdependent health discipline focusing on the family and exhibiting responsibility for insuring that its practitioners are provided with excellence in preparation and that those practitioners demonstrate professional behavior in keeping with these stated beliefs (American College of Nurse-Midwives, 1972).

Nurse-midwifery made a major advance in 1981, when Congress authorized Medicaid payments for the services of nurse-midwives.

The Nurse and the Family

Because each person develops as a member of a family unit, the nurse must acquire understanding of the family to understand the individual. This is especially important in the maternity setting because the nurse is directly responsible for the well-being of two members of the same family—mother and child.

The family unit has been identified as critical for the success of health care services for the following reasons (Friedman, 1981):

1. In a family unit, a dysfunction of one or more family members generally affects each individual as well as the family unit. If the nurse considers only the individual, nursing care is fragmented rather than complete and holistic.

2. Assessing the family aids the nurse's understanding of the individual functioning within his or her own primary social context. With the childbearing family, the nurse is able to assist the prospective parents to prepare for the new family member.

3. There is a strong interrelationship between the health status of the family as a whole and that of its members. The nurse can have a positive effect not only on individuals but also on their families.

4. In considering the family as a whole, the nurse can identify potential risk factors and thereby prevent illness.

5. When illness occurs, the family is instrumental in seeking medical assistance and in determining their attitude and that of the sick person toward the illness.

In family-centered maternity nursing, the nurse generally focuses on health promotion and maintenance and prevention of illness. The nurse uses a **biopsychosocial** approach, which recognizes the influence of the prenatal environment and the quality of parenting on the growth and development of the child. Principles of management of the childbearing family include the following:

• The nurse should keep in mind the intimate relationships among family members. The woman receiving maternity care assumes a unique role within the family group, a role that must be acknowledged if the family is to function optimally.

• An ailing family member becomes dependent on others in the family, thereby increasing stress and perhaps temporarily or permanently impeding the ability of the family to perform its tasks. A pregnant woman or a woman who has just come home with a newborn baby may not be ill, but she may need to rely on others in her family to perform activities that she previously performed. The nurse can help the other family members devise methods of taking on added responsibilities and finding outside resources to support family functioning.

• The nurse must consider how variables such as cultural beliefs, community resources, and health beliefs affect the family's response to health care.

To be effective, nurses must be aware of their own cultural beliefs and values and recognize their biases and beliefs about other cultures. The nurse must avoid generalizations and assumptions about families from a particular culture because there is diversity within every culture.

Legal Considerations

Nurses are legally responsible for performing their duties according to the scope of nursing function, specified standards of care, and their recognized level of skill and training. The scope of nursing function is basically spelled out in the nurse practice act of each state. Although these acts vary somewhat from state to state, they usually offer broad descriptions of the actions the nurse may perform and identify functions and actions beyond the scope of nursing. Many current nurse practice acts also address the issues of qualifications and scope of practice of nurses in expanded roles, especially nurse practitioners, certified nurse-midwives, and nurse anesthetists.

Nurses in expanded roles often find it necessary to make decisions formerly in the realm of medicine. These nurses generally work under *protocols*, or accepted guidelines for practice, and make judgments about care using these guidelines. According to Bille (1980), "If the professional nurse has been educated to make this type of judgment (even though the education came from the institution's staff development department, rather than from formal academic institutions), the nurse is legally capable of making such *medical* decisions." This also protects nurses working in highly technical areas such as neonatal or adult intensive care units.

Specified or accepted standards of care form another basis on which all nurses are held legally accountable. Standards of care may be specified by the employing agency in its policies and procedures manual, by the standards of the Joint Commission on Accreditation of Hospitals (JCAH), and by accepted community practices and policies. Negligence may exist if it can be

established that the nurse "is doing something or failing to do something contrary to what a reasonable, prudent nurse would do under all the facts and circumstances, in accordance with prevailing professional standards in the community or in similar communities under like circumstances" (Southwick, 1978).

Nurses who are careless, who do not meet the acceptable standards of care in performing their duties, or who behave unprofessionally place their clients at risk. If a person suffers loss or damage that can be proven to result from faulty action or failure to act by the nurse, the nurse and employing institution can be held liable in a civil action.

Informed consent is a legal concept that has great significance for nurses. Basically, the policy protects a person's right to autonomy and self-determination by specifying that no action may be taken without that person's prior understanding and freely given consent. While this policy is usually enforced for such major procedures as surgery or regional anesthesia, it pertains to *any* nursing, medical, or surgical intervention. To touch a person without consent (except in an emergency) constitutes battery. In a normal, uncomplicated labor, when the woman has time to give consent, consent must be obtained. Consent is not informed unless the woman understands the usual procedures, their rationales, and any associated risks. To be a truly active participant in decision making about her care, she should also understand possible alternatives.

Just as the physician must, under the doctrine of informed consent, explain associated risks and benefits of any diagnostic or treatment activities performed (Cushing, 1984), the nurse is responsible for education about any nursing care provided. Prior to each nursing intervention, the nurse lets the woman know what to expect, thus ensuring her cooperation and obtaining her consent. Afterward, the nurse documents the teaching and the learning outcomes in the woman's record.

The importance of clear, concise, and complete nursing records cannot be overemphasized. These records are evidence that the nurse obtained consent, performed prescribed treatments, reported important observations to the appropriate staff, and adhered to acceptable standards of care.

Professional Issues

The maternity nurse faces the same job-related issues confronting other nurses, including the following:

Diagnostic Related Groups prospective reimbursement plan   The federal Diagnostic Related Groups (DRGs) reimbursement plan requires that hospitals change their per diem fee system in an attempt to control costs for hospital care. Under the DRG plan, illnesses, injuries, and surgical procedures are divided into diagnostic classifications. The cost of the care given to patients with a specific diagnosis is established prior to hospitalization; this cost represents the average cost of care given to patients with the same diagnosis. The DRG plan has important implications for nurses because it forces hospitals and nurses to quantify nursing services by time and cost. Proposed amendments to the DRG plan include a system tying nursing services to patient outcomes (Curtin, 1983).

Nurses and physicians   Nurse-midwives and nurse practitioners are becoming major providers of health services to childbearing families. These nursing professionals are establishing and operating family planning clinics, general health clinics, and birth centers. Such facilities are often independent of physician control, although women are referred to physicians when necessary.

The response of physicians to this trend has been mixed. Some physicians support independent nursing practice wholeheartedly, while others have attempted to block moves by nurses for autonomy. The reason physicians usually give for their negative reaction is that these alternatives pose a threat to the safety of the childbearing woman. Other reasons for the negative reaction of physicians may exist, however. Some suggest that physicians may feel their professional status and financial well-being are being threatened by the potential loss of clients who choose the services of other health care professionals (Tomich, 1978; Lubic, 1981).

Issues in Maternal-Newborn Care

Biomedical Technology

Tremendous strides have been made in maternal and newborn health care. These advances include the development of clinical and research specialties that focus on various aspects of fetal development, childbearing, and newborn care. **Perinatology** is the medical specialty concerned with the diagnosis and treatment of high-risk conditions of the pregnant woman and her fetus. **Neonatology** is the specialty that focuses on the management of high-risk conditions of the newborn.

New diagnostic and treatment methods have been developed that enhance a woman's chances for having a healthy baby. Some of these developments are listed here:

1. *Ultrasound.* Ultrasound examination is used to assess fetal status. High-frequency sound waves are directed into the maternal abdomen to identify fetal and maternal structures.

2. *Amniocentesis.* In an amniocentesis, amniotic fluid is removed from the amniotic sac for analysis. Amniotic fluid analysis provides information about the fetus's genetic makeup, well-being, sex, and maturity.

3. *Electronic fetal monitoring.* Electronic monitoring equipment can be attached to the pregnant woman or the fetus to measure the fetal heart rate (FHR). In conjunction with other procedures, electronic fetal monitoring can be used to determine fetal well-being and the fetus's ability to withstand the stress of labor before labor begins.

4. *Intrauterine surgery.* Intrauterine surgery is the surgical attempt to correct fetal problems while the fetus is still in the uterus.

5. *Infertility procedures.* Artificial insemination, in vitro fertilization, and embryo transplants are techniques used to treat infertility. *Artificial insemination* is the introduction of sperm into the vagina by artificial means. The sperm may be from the woman's partner or a donor. In *in vitro fertilization*, a mature ovum is collected from a woman whose ovaries are functioning but whose fallopian tubes are blocked. The ovum is fertilized in a petri dish by sperm collected from her partner. The embryo is then implanted in the woman's uterus. The *embryo transplant* procedure is used when the woman's ovaries are not functioning. An ovum from another woman is fertilized by sperm collected from the partner. The embryo is then transplanted into the infertile woman's uterus.

The benefits of these technologic advances are clear. Because of these advances, a healthy baby was delivered in a San Francisco hospital from a brain-dead mother whose body was kept functioning for over 2 months until the fetus was viable. Because of these advances, previously childless couples are having children. Yet concern is growing that the reliance on technology in maternal-newborn care is excessive and that in some cases the risks of certain procedures outweigh their advantages.

The controversy about electronic fetal monitoring is representative of the issue of technologic excess in obstetrics. Initially, electronic fetal monitoring was used to monitor high-risk labors. In the past few years, however, its use in low-risk pregnancies has increased. Electronic monitoring has gained widespread acceptance in some birth facilities because it can detect fetal distress in cases prenatally categorized as low risk.

But electronic fetal monitoring can have adverse effects on the laboring woman and fetus. For example, the increasing incidence of cesarean births has been attributed to the routine use of fetal monitoring. Cesarean delivery is performed when fetal distress, indicated by abnormal FHR patterns, is diagnosed. The data from the monitoring equipment, however, may be misleading, and the fetus may not be in distress at all. The woman is then subjected to an unnecessary surgical procedure.

Do intrapartal fetal monitoring and similar procedures in cases of low-risk labor and delivery constitute excessive medical intervention? Some argue that every pregnancy and delivery pose potential medical problems and that maternity clients should be managed intensively to prevent complications. To that end, the use of any medical intervention is justified. Others argue that pregnancy and childbirth are natural, normal processes and should not be managed in the same rigorous way as diseases

or high-risk conditions. Medical intervention is perceived as unnecessary and costly interference in low-risk cases.

Opinion is growing that clients receiving certain services should be more carefully screened. Because of the high cost and, as in the case of ultrasound, unknown risks, consumers and insurance companies are questioning the necessity of certain procedures.

Implications The idea that medical and nursing actions should depend on the pregnant woman's level of risk is gaining support from consumers and health professionals. To evaluate a woman's level of risk properly, nurses are being encouraged to develop their assessment skills. Each woman's physical and psychologic status should be monitored throughout pregnancy, labor, and delivery to detect changes indicating increased risk. The unnecessary use of assessment and diagnostic procedures, however, should be avoided. For example, the use of ultrasound for a pregnant woman at low risk is usually unnecessary, but its use is increasing. Although the woman may find "seeing" her baby exciting, ultrasound should be used only when necessary since its long-term effects are still unknown.

Advances in technology have affected the educational requirements for nurses. The knowledge needed by nurses who provide general health maintenance services to maternity clients is growing. Nurses must take continuing education courses and read more professional literature to keep up with the expanding and changing knowledge base.

The professional opportunities for nurses in maternal-newborn care have also grown as a result of biomedical advances. Nurses are specializing in perinatology and neonatology. Other nurses are entering the field of research.

Changes in Health Care Relationships

For many years, the term *patient* was applied to the person receiving health care services. The relationship between the patient and health professional was one of dependence; the patient depended on the professional to make decisions about matters of health and sickness.

The patient placed trust and faith in the professional's expertise, and the professional "took care" of the passive patient.

Over the past two decades, attitudes of those using health care services have changed radically. The patients of traditional medicine have become "consumers." The consumer and health professional are in a buyer-seller relationship. Satisfaction with services rendered determines the continuation of this relationship.

Health care professionals have recognized that the traditional patient–health professional relationship is no longer acceptable or desirable. The two parties should be in a collaborative relationship, not a dependent or even a buyer-seller relationship.

Many health professionals refer to those seeking and receiving services as **clients.** The term *client* implies an active role, not a passive one. In the client–health professional relationship, the client assumes responsibility for decisions about his or her health. The client seeks advice and assistance from individuals who have special skills and knowledge. It is understood that the client can choose not to accept the professional's advice and that the health professional cannot proceed with a plan of action without the client's consent.

Implications   The nursing profession has been at the forefront in recognizing that people should take an active role in their own health care. Nurses involved in a maternity client–health care professional relationship must understand that it is their professional expertise that is being sought. They should not make decisions for their clients.

An important role for nurses is that of **client advocate** (Kohnke, 1982). The maternity nurse advocate informs clients by clearly identifying all available options and the benefits and risks of each one, by explaining the nursing actions simply but completely, and by answering all questions with facts and not personal opinions. The maternity nurse advocate then supports the client's decision by adhering to it and ensuring that others do the same.

The nursing profession is meeting consumer and client demands in maternal-newborn care in important ways. Nurses are usually the instructors of prenatal and postpartal education classes. Nurse practitioners and nurse-midwives are the primary caregivers in many clinics and birth centers that emphasize family-centered health. Maternity clients and their families are finding that nursing's orientation toward education, self-care, and health maintenance meshes with their desire to participate in and make decisions about their birth experience.

Ethical Issues

Although ethical dilemmas confront nurses in all areas, those involving pregnancy, birth, and the newborn seem especially difficult to resolve. These dilemmas result from conflicting social, cultural, and religious values and beliefs held by individuals.

Most of the ethical questions in maternity care are aimed at delineating and protecting the rights of the pregnant woman or couple, the fetus, and the newborn. Ethical issues related to childbearing include the following:

Abortion   Induced abortion is the purposeful termination of a pregnancy. In 1973, a decision by the United States Supreme Court made obtaining and performing abortions legal. Despite its legality, abortion continues to spur ethical and moral debate. Opponents of abortion, the "pro-life" group, support one moral principle: The unborn fetus is a human being with an undeniable right to life. For supporters of abortion, the "pro-choice" group, the primary consideration is the right of a woman to control her own body and reproductive activity.

Passive euthanasia   Passive euthanasia occurs when someone is allowed to die because of inaction or lack of treatment. Some believe that a person's life should be preserved by any and all means, regardless of the wishes of that person or the quality of that person's life. Others believe that the quality of life is more important than the sanctity of life and that one has the right to refuse extraordinary medical measures if he or she believes a meaningful life is not possible after treatment.

Maternity nurses are confronted with the issue of passive euthanasia when the decision is made to allow a severely handicapped newborn to die by withholding life-sustaining treatment, including nutritional support (Curtin,

1984). The decision is usually made by the parents of the infant, in consultation with medical and religious authorities, who must determine whether their child's life will be improved or merely prolonged by extraordinary medical intervention. The President's Commission for the Study of Ethical Problems in Medicine and Biomedical and Behavioral Research (1983) has provided guidelines for making such decisions. In some cases, however, it is not always clear whether a medical intervention would be futile or beneficial, and the decision to provide or forego treatment can have legal consequences (Hubbard, 1984).

Intrauterine surgery   Intrauterine surgery has many ethical ramifications. Does the fetus have the absolute right to treatment? Is the fetus a patient? What are the rights of the fetus versus the rights of the pregnant woman? Can a woman be required to undergo surgery to ensure a better quality of life for her fetus? If the fetus dies or is injured during surgery, what are the legal implications for those performing the surgery?

In vitro fertilization, embryo transplants, and surrogate childbearing   In vitro fertilization and embryo transplants were described on pp. 8–9. Surrogate childbearing occurs when a woman agrees to become pregnant for a childless couple. She is artificially inseminated with the male partner's sperm. If fertilization occurs, the woman carries the fetus to term and then releases the infant to the couple after delivery. These three methods of resolving infertility raise many ethical questions, including the problem of religious objections to artificial conception, the question of who will assume financial and moral responsibility for a child born with a congenital defect, the issue of candidate selection, and the threat of genetic engineering. With surrogate childbearing and embryo transplants, the rights of the surrogate mother and the woman donating the embryo must be considered.

Implications   The complex ethical issues facing maternity nurses have many social, legal, and professional ramifications. Nurses must learn to anticipate ethical dilemmas and to develop some basic beliefs about the issues. To

do so, they may read about bioethical issues or attend courses and workshops on ethical topics pertinent to their areas of practice. Further, nurses need to develop skills in logical thinking and critical analysis.

Nurses must thoughtfully assess their values and identify any clinical situations in which they feel they could not function. It may be difficult to help a client make decisions based on the client's needs when the nurse's values are in conflict with the client's. Nurses must remember that they are to act in the client's best interests, and not their own. This means "helping them [clients] clarify values and beliefs, to develop their understanding of self and of the situation, and to make decisions based on their own goals and wishes" (Benoliel, 1983).

A nurse may be caring for a client who is faced with a problem with many ethical ramifications. The client may ask for assistance in resolving the dilemma. In the case of a severely deformed newborn, for example, the parents who are considering passive euthanasia may request information from the nurse about their child's chances for recovery and the quality of life their child can expect after treatment. The nurse can clarify her or his own ethical position as well as help the parents make their decision by using these guidelines (Kozier and Erb, 1983):

1. *Establish a complete data base.* Find out all the information about the situation, including data about those involved; their physical, psychologic, financial, and support resources; the proposed action and the reason behind it; and the possible results of the proposed action.

2. *Identify the ethical conflicts created by the problem.* Determine what the ethical problems are for the clients, the health care agency, and the various health professionals involved.

3. *Outline various courses of action.* Present alternative solutions to the problem.

4. *Determine possible outcomes of the suggested actions.* What are the consequences of the various courses of action as well as the proposed action?

5. *Determine who "owns" the problem and who should make the decision.* The following factors must be considered: who will be affected by the decision, who is the decision being made for, whose moral principles or legal responsibilities are being affected, and what degree of consent is needed from those involved.

6. *Define the obligations of the nurse.* In situations requiring ethical decision making, nurses must determine their obligations both to the client and to themselves.

Tools for Maternal-Newborn Nursing Practice

Professional maternity nurses use a variety of "tools" in everyday practice that enable them to deliver high-quality nursing care. These tools are:

• Knowledge
• Nursing process
• Nursing diagnosis
• Communication
• Statistics
• Nursing research

This section is not designed to give a complete explanation of nursing tools but to highlight them and explore ways in which the maternity nurse may use them in practice.

Knowledge Base

Current knowledge and theories from a variety of disciplines form the basis for nursing actions. The nursing knowledge base is subject to change as new discoveries are made, statistical analysis reveals new trends, and new technology is developed. The nursing knowledge base is continually expanding, presenting a challenge to nurses to keep current.

Nursing Process

The **nursing process**, which serves as a framework for nursing, is a logical approach to problem identification and resolution. It consists of five overlapping steps, described here:

• *Assessment* is the accumulation of both subjective and objective data about the health status of a client.

• *Analysis* is the interpretation of data to identify problem areas and probable causes in order to formulate a nursing diagnosis.

• *Planning* is the identification of priorities of care, nursing interventions, and expected outcomes of those interventions.

• *Implementation* is the performance of the nursing interventions outlined in the plan of care.

• *Evaluation* is the determination of the client's progress or lack of progress toward the identified expected outcomes.

Although the problems of clients vary, as do the settings in which maternity care is required, the nursing process is a reliable tool for problem solving.

Nursing Diagnosis

Nursing diagnosis is both a process and an outcome. The process represents problem solving and consists of analyzing, assimilating, and categorizing data gathered during assessment. The categories may be defined as medical problems or nursing problems. Medical problems can be treated by physicians, and nursing problems can be treated by nurses.

Nursing diagnosis as an outcome refers to a classification system of diagnostic labels (Carpenito, 1983). The nursing diagnosis is a two-part statement that includes the health problem and related etiology (Kim, McFarland, and Mclane, 1984). The North American Nursing Diagnosis Association (NANDA) has developed a list of acceptable nursing diagnoses.

In the nursing care plans in this book, examples of possible nursing diagnoses are included not only to show the format of nursing diagnoses but also to provide a more complete picture of the place of nursing diagnosis in the nursing process.

Communication

Information about the client and care provided must be shared with all members of the health care team. The most reliable method of communication is written records.

The **problem-oriented record (POR) system** allows for the documentation and retrieval of information about a client's care and progress. POR is a system of charting observations and interventions using the SOAP format. The acronym SOAP stands for the four components of each charting entry: **S**ubjective data, **O**bjective data, **A**nalysis (sometimes called **A**ssessment), and **P**lan. Each nursing diagnosis or problem is listed numerically on a problem sheet kept on the chart. The subjective and objective data, which come from the nursing assessment, are recorded under the appropriate problem number. The analysis entry represents the nurse's conclusions, based on the data collected, about the client's progress. Finally, the plan of care is continued or changed in accordance with the data analysis.

The importance of the POR system for nursing is twofold: (a) the SOAP format provides readily accessible data in a systematic way as well as a basis for ongoing evaluation of the effects of nursing care and (b) the other members of the health team are kept informed in writing about the client.

Statistics

Nurses often overlook or underestimate the usefulness of statistics. Health-related statistics, however, provide an objective basis for projecting client needs, planning for use of resources, and determining the effectiveness of treatment.

There are two major types of statistics—descriptive and inferential. **Descriptive statistics** describe or summarize a set of data. They report the facts—what is—in a concise and easily retrievable way. Although no conclusion may be drawn from these statistics about *why* some phenomenon has occurred, certain trends and high-risk "target groups" can be identified and possible research questions generated. **Inferential statistics** allow the investigator to draw conclusions or inferences about what is happening between two or more variables in a population and to establish or refute causal relationships between them.

Descriptive statistics are the starting point for the formation of research questions. Inferential statistics answer specific questions and generate theories to explain relationships between variables. These theories can be applied in nursing practice to help change the specific variables that may be causing or contributing to certain health problems.

In this section, descriptive statistics that are particularly important to maternal-newborn health care are discussed. Inferential considerations are addressed as possible research questions that may assist in identifying relevant variables.

Birth rate   **Birth rate** refers to the number of live births per 1000 population. A related statistic, the **fertility rate,** is the number of births per 1000 women aged 15–44 years in a given population.

Table 1-1 compares live births, birth rates, and fertility rates by race for 1970–1983 in the United States. After reaching a peak of 25.0 for all races in 1955, the birth rate declined, reaching a low in 1975 and 1976 of 14.6 live births per 1000 population. The birth rate began increasing in 1977, except for slight drops in 1978 and 1983.

Live births, birth rate, and general fertility for Canada are presented in Table 1-2. The birth rate there is similar to that in the United States; however, the fertility rate is lower.

Research questions that can be posed about the birth rates include the following:

• Is there an association between birth rates and changing societal values?

• Is the difference in birth rate between various age groups reflective of education? Or does it represent availability of contraceptive information?

• What factors might contribute to the differences in fertility rates between Canada and the United States?

Age of mother   In 1980, women 20–24 years of age had the highest birth rate for a first child (115.1 births per 1000 women of that age) in the United States (National Center for Health Statistics, 1982). Women 25–29 years of age had the next highest rate for first births (112.9 births per 1000 women of that age). Teenagers in the 15–19 age group had a birth rate of 53 per 1000 females of that age for first births.

Of all age groups, the smallest increase, less than 1%, occurred in teenage girls 15–17 years

Table 1-1
Live Births, Birth Rates, and Fertility Rates, by Race of Child, United States, 1970–1983*

| | Number | | Birth rate[†] | | | | Fertility rate[†] | | | |
| | | | | | All other | | | | All other | |
Year	All races	All races	White	Total	Black	All races	White	Total	Black
1983	3,614,000	15.5	—[‡]	—	—	—	65.4	—	—
1982	3,704,000	16.0	—	—	—	—	67.8	—	—
1981	3,646,000	15.8	—	—	—	—	—	—	—
1980	3,612,258	15.9	14.9	22.5	22.1	68.4	64.7	88.6	88.1
1979..........	3,494,398	15.6	14.5	22.2	22.0	67.2	63.4	88.5	88.3
1978	3,333,279	15.0	14.0	21.6	21.3	65.5	61.7	87.0	86.7
1977..........	3,326,632	15.1	14.1	21.6	21.4	66.8	63.2	87.7	88.1
1976	3,167,788	14.6	13.6	20.8	20.5	65.0	61.5	85.8	85.8
1975..........	3,144,198	14.6	13.6	21.0	20.7	66.0	62.5	87.7	87.9
1974	3,159,958	14.8	13.9	21.2	20.8	67.8	64.2	89.8	89.7
1973..........	3,136,965	14.8	13.8	21.7	21.4	68.8	64.9	93.4	93.6
1972	3,258,411	15.6	14.5	22.8	22.5	73.1	68.9	99.5	99.9
1971..........	3,555,970	17.2	16.1	24.6	24.4	81.6	77.3	109.1	109.7
1970	3,731,386	18.4	17.4	25.1	25.3	87.9	84.1	113.0	115.4

*Data from the National Center for Health Statistics. *Monthly Vital Statistics Report*, Vol. 31, No. 8, 1983, and Vol. 32, No. 13, 1984. Public Health Service, Hyattsville, Md.
[†]Birth rates per 1000 population. Fertility rates per 1000 women aged 15–44 years.
[‡]— indicates data not available.

Table 1-2
Canada: Live Births, Birth Rates, and General Fertility*

Year	Live births[†]	Birth rate[‡]	General fertility[§]
1980	370,709	15.5	57.9
1979	366,064	15.5	58.2

*Modified from *Vital statistics*. Vol. 1. Births and deaths. 1980. Canada Health Division Vital Statistics and Disease Registry. Cat. 84–204. Minister of Supply and Services. May 1982. Table 1, p. 2.
[†]Live births = per 1000 population
[‡]Live birth rate = per 1000 population
[§]General fertility rate = birth rate per 1000 women 15–49 years

of age. Women 30–34 years old had a birth rate of 61.9 in 1980. The largest increase in births occurred in this age group—a 60% increase in 1980 from 1975.

The variables that affect the birth rate of different age groups may be identified by investigating the following research questions:

- Is there an association with changing societal values? With changing roles of women? With changing national economic conditions and financial status?

- Is there a correlation with years of education? With availability of contraceptive information for different age groups?

Infant mortality   The *infant death rate* is the number of deaths of infants under 1 year of age per 1000 live births in a given population. **Neonatal mortality** is the number of deaths of infants less than 28 days of age per 1000 live births. **Perinatal mortality** includes both neonatal deaths and fetal deaths per 1000 live births. (**Fetal death** is death in utero after 20 weeks or more of gestation.)

Table 1-3
Infant Mortality by Age: United States, Selected Years 1950–1982*

Year	Under 1 year	Under 28 days	28 days–11 months
1982	11	7.6	3.6
1980	12.6	8.5	4.1
1979	13.1	8.7	4.2
1978	13.8	9.5	4.3
1977	14.1	9.9	4.2
1976	15.2	10.9	4.3
1975	16.1	11.6	4.5
1974	16.7	12.3	4.4
1973	17.7	13.0	4.8
1972	18.5	13.6	4.8
1971	19.1	14.2	4.9
1970	20.0	15.1	4.9
1965	24.7	17.7	7.0
1960	26.0	18.7	7.3
1950	29.2	20.5	8.7

*Data from National Center for Health Statistics: *Vital Statistics of the United States*. Vol. 3. US Government Printing Office, Washington, DC: 1982; and *Monthly Vital Statistics*. Vol. 31, No. 13. Public Health Service, Hyattsville, Md.: 1983.

Table 1-4
Canada: Infant Mortality (Total Infant Death Rate per 1000 Live Births)*

Year	Under 1 year	Under 28 days	28 days–11 months
1980	10.4	6.7	3.8
1979	10.9	7.2	3.7

*Modified from *Vital statistics*. Vol. 1. Births and deaths. 1980. Canada Health Division Vital Statistics and Disease Registry. Cat. 84–204 Minister of Supply and Services. May 1982. Table 1, p. 2.

Table 1-5
U.S. Maternal Mortality per 100,000 Live Births*

Year	Rate	Year	Rate
1980	9.2	1969	22.5
1979	9.6	1968	24.5
1978	9.6	1967	28.0
1977	11.2	1966	29.1
1976	12.3	1965	31.6
1975	12.8	1964	33.3
1974	14.6	1963	35.8
1973	15.2	1962	35.2
1972	18.8	1961	36.9
1971	18.8	1960	37.1
1970	21.5	1950	83.3

*From National Center for Health Statistics: *Vital Statistics of the United States*. US Government Printing Office, Washington, DC: 1981, 1983.

Table 1-3 presents infant mortality rates in the United States for selected years, and Table 1-4 presents infant mortality rates in Canada for 1979 and 1980. Comparison of these statistics shows that Canada has a lower infant mortality. The United States ranked fifteenth highest among nations in infant deaths in 1980. With few exceptions, however, neonatal and post-neonatal deaths have declined steadily in the United States since 1940.

Among the principal causes of infant death are congenital anomalies; sudden infant death syndrome (SIDS), respiratory distress syndrome, and disorders related to preterm infants and those with low birth weights.

Some research questions raised by the infant mortality statistics include the following:

• Does infant mortality correlate with a specific maternal age?

• Is it associated with the time during pregnancy that the woman seeks prenatal care? With the number of prenatal visits?

• Is there a difference among racial groups? If so, is it associated with educational level? Availability of prenatal care?

Maternal mortality Maternal mortality is the number of deaths from any cause during the pregnancy cycle (including the 42-day post-partal period) per 100,000 live births.

The maternal death rate in the United States has decreased steadily in the last 30 years (Table 1-5). In 1980, 250 women died of causes listed as complications of pregnancy, childbirth, and puerperium. In Canada, 8 women died of similar causes in 1980.

Factors influencing the decrease in maternal mortality include the increased use of hospitals and specialized health care personnel by antepartal, intrapartal, and postpartal maternity clients; the establishment of care centers for high-risk mothers and infants; the prevention and control of infection with antibiotics; the availability of blood and blood products for transfusions; and the lowered rates of anesthesia-related deaths. Additional factors may be identified by asking the following research questions:

- Is there a correlation between maternal mortality and age?
- Is there a correlation with availability of health care? Economic status?

Implications   Nurses can use statistics to:

- Determine populations at risk
- Assess the relationship between specific factors
- Help establish a data base for different client populations
- Determine the levels of care needed by particular client populations
- Evaluate the success of specific nursing interventions
- Determine priorities in case loads
- Estimate staffing and equipment needs of hospital units and clinics
- Determine whether a problem exists

Statistical information is available through many sources, including professional literature; state and city health departments; vital statistics sections of private, county, state, and federal agencies; and special programs of family planning and similar agencies. Nurses who use this information will be better prepared to promote the health needs of maternity clients and their families.

Nursing Research

Research is a vital step toward establishing a science of nursing as well as establishing nursing as a true profession with its own unique knowledge base. Research is also a means to improve client care by translating research findings into clinical practice.

Research by nurses can help clarify the relationships between the health professional and the client. Nursing research also can help determine the psychosocial and physical risks and benefits of nursing and medical interventions.

The gap between research and practice is being narrowed by the publication of research findings in popular nursing journals, the establishment of departments of nursing research in hospitals, and collaborative research efforts by nurse researchers and clinical practitioners. In addition, numerous journal articles giving "how-to" information for translating research into practice have been published in the last few years.

Application of Tools for Nursing Practice

Each of the tools—knowledge, nursing process, communication, statistics, and nursing research—can exist separately, but in practice they overlap and complement each other. The maternity nurse can put each of these tools to use in a variety of ways. An example of just one possible situation is presented in the following case study.

—————— CASE STUDY ——————

Two labor and delivery nurses express concerns to each other about the number of adolescents who have been delivering in their unit. At the next staff meeting, they voice their concerns and raise questions about whether the number of teenage mothers seen in their unit is larger than normal. After discussion, the nurses decide they need to formulate a plan to gather more information. Each nurse volunteers to pursue a particular aspect of the plan of action.

Their plan includes the following activities:

- Contacting the local public health department for local and national statistics on this age group
- Investigating the availability of health care for adolescents in their community

- Checking the availability of prenatal education groups for adolescents
- Finding out whether their community has school health programs and what the program content is
- Looking at national statistics that identify when adolescents seek prenatal care
- Talking with community nurse-midwives, physicians, and prenatal clinic personnel to see if the national statistics apply to their community
- Collecting information about legislative issues affecting adolescent health care
- Seeking further information about the needs of adolescents during pregnancy and delivery by doing library research
- Looking for continuing education programs dealing with the pregnant adolescent client

At subsequent staff meetings, each nurse shares information, and other areas are investigated as the need is identified. How they evaluate the data and apply them will depend on the requirements of their maternity unit and the needs of their community.

Possible outcomes may include developing a research study, doing volunteer work in local adolescent clinics, developing and teaching prenatal classes for adolescents, volunteering to teach in community school health programs, organizing a continuing education program on the adolescent mother for community hospitals, and forming a network within their professional nursing organizations to stay informed about legislative issues pertaining to adolescents.

As the case study demonstrates, the application of tools for nursing practice helps define a problem, guides the collection of data, and provides a framework for intervention.

Summary

The experience of childbearing has changed dramatically for families during this century. The rigid, hospital- and physician-controlled labor and delivery of the first two-thirds of this century have been replaced by a family-oriented, collaborative experience.

Many of the improvements in health care services to maternity clients are a result of scientific and medical advances. Other changes are due to the efforts of health care professionals, social scientists, and clients to keep the focus on the family.

The role of the maternity nurse also has changed over the years. Maternity nurses can choose among many professional avenues. They can give general care to maternity clients, or they can specialize in neonatology, perinatology, nurse-midwifery, or other areas.

Various tools for nursing practice are available to maternity nurses. They can use these tools to provide the childbearing family with the highest quality care possible.

The changes in the health care system as well as in nursing have been positive. These changes, however, have also brought controversy and conflict. The advances in medical technology have led to exciting developments but have created complex ethical and moral dilemmas. The demands of clients and changes in their attitudes about health care professionals and services have created a relationship different from the traditional patient–health professional relationship. The expanded role of nurses has affected the relationship between physicians and nurses as well.

The health care system and nursing in particular will continue to change. The maternity nurse can contribute positively to that change by being a competent, assertive, and actively functioning member of the health care team.

Resource Groups

The Clearing House for Nursing Diagnosis (St. Louis University School of Nursing, 3525 Caroline Street, St. Louis, MO 63104)   The clearing house has three functions: (a) to collect material on nursing diagnosis; (b) to publish a newsletter; and (c) to coordinate the national conference held every two years.

American Nurses' Association (ANA) (1101 14th Street N.W., Washington, D.C. 20005)   The ANA works toward improving education and training of nurses, increasing access to health care, and improving the professional role of nurses.

References

American College of Nurse-Midwives: *Statement of Philosophy.* Washington, D.C.: 1972.

American College of Nurse-Midwives: *What Is a Nurse-Midwife?* Washington, D.C.: 1979.

Benoliel JQ: Ethics in nursing practice and education. *Nurs Outlook* July/August 1983; 31:210.

Bille DA: Legal considerations in nursing service. *Nurs Admin Q* Fall 1980; 5:73–82.

Carpenito LJ: *Nursing Diagnosis: Application to Clinical Practice.* New York: Lippincott, 1983.

Curtin L: Determining costs of nursing services per DRG. *Nurs Management* April 1983; 14:16.

Curtin L: Should we feed Baby Doe? *Nurs Management* August 1984; 15:22.

Cushing M: Informed consent: An MD's responsibility? *Am J Nurs* 1984; 84:437.

Friedman MM: *Family Nursing Theory and Assessment.* New York: Appleton-Century-Crofts, 1981.

Hubbard R: Caring for Baby Doe. *Ms* May 1984; p. 84.

Kim MJ, McFarland GK, Mclane AM (editors): *Classification of Nursing Diagnoses: Proceedings of the Fifth National Conference.* St. Louis: Mosby, 1984.

Kohnke MF: *Advocacy; Risk and Reality.* St. Louis: Mosby, 1982.

Kozier B, Erb G: *Fundamentals of Nursing,* 2nd ed. Menlo Park, Calif: Addison-Wesley, 1983.

Lubic RW: Alternative maternity care: Resistance and change. In: *Childbirth: Alternatives to Medical Control.* Romalis S (editor). Austin: University of Texas Press, 1981.

National Center for Health Statistics: *Monthly Vital Statistics Report.* Vol. 31, No. 8, Supp. DHHS Pub. No. (PHS) 83-1120. Public Health Service, Hyattsville, Md., November 1982.

President's Commission for the Study of Ethical Problems in Medicine and Biomedical and Behavioral Research: *Deciding to Forego Life-Sustaining Treatment.* Washington, D.C.: Government Printing Office, 1983.

Southwick AF: *The Law of Hospital and Health Care Administration.* Ann Arbor, Mich.: Health Administration Press, 1978.

Tomich JH: The expanded role of the nurse: Current status and future prospects. In: *The Nursing Profession: Views Through the Mist.* Chaska NL (editor). New York: McGraw-Hill, 1978.

Additional Readings

Arras J, Hunt R: *Ethical Issues in Modern Medicine,* 2nd ed. Palo Alto, Calif. Mayfield Publishing Co, 1983.

Dickenson S: The nursing process and the professional status of nursing. *Nurs Times* June 1982; 8:61.

Duvall EM: *Marriage and Family Development,* 5th ed. New York: Lippincott, 1977.

Fagerhaugh S, Strauss A, Suczek B, et al: The impact of technology on patients, providers, and care patterns. *Nurs Outlook* November 1980; 28:666.

Fletcher JC: The fetus as patient: Ethical issues. *JAMA* August 1981; 246:772.

Luker K: *Abortion and the Politics of Motherhood.* Berkeley: University of California Press, 1984.

Marsh FH, Self DJ: In vitro fertilization: Moving from theory to therapy. *Hastings Center Report* June 1980; 10:5.

Nursing Life poll report: The right to die. *Nursing Life* March/April 1984; 4:45.

Sandelowski M: Perinatal nursing: Whose specialty is it anyway? *MCN* September/October 1983; 8:317.

The new origins of life. *Time* September 10, 1984; p. 46.

2

Reproductive and Sexual Anatomy and Physiology

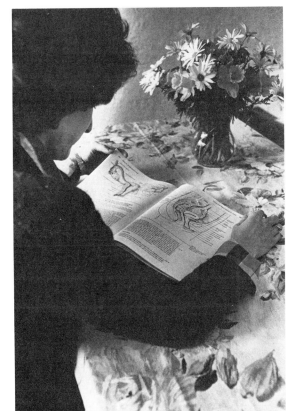

Chapter Contents

Early Development of Reproductive Structures and Processes

Puberty
  Major Physical Changes
  Physiology of Onset

Female Reproductive System
  External Genitals
  Internal Genitals
  Bony Pelvis
  Breasts

Female Reproductive Cycle
  Neurohumoral Basis of the Female
    Reproductive Cycle
  Ovarian Cycle
  Uterine Cycle

Male Reproductive System
  External Genitals
  Internal Genitals

Sexual Intercourse
  Psychosocial Aspects
  Physiology of Sexual Response

The Nurse as Counselor on Sexuality and Reproduction

Objectives

- Describe the major changes that occur during puberty.

- Identify the structures and functions of the female and male reproductive systems.

- Discuss the significance of specific structures of the female reproductive system during childbirth.

- Identify the hormones affecting reproductive and sexual development and functioning and discuss their specific actions.

- Explain the physical and psychologic aspects of the female reproductive cycle.

- Describe the nurse's role as teacher and counselor in the areas of reproduction and sexuality.

Key Terms

ampulla	nipple
areola	obstetric conjugate
breasts	oogenesis
broad ligament	ovarian ligaments
cardinal ligaments	ovary
cervix	ovulation
conjugate vera	ovum
cornua	pelvic cavity
corpus	pelvic diaphragm
corpus luteum	pelvic floor
diagonal conjugate	pelvic inlet
endometrium	pelvic outlet
estrogens	perimetrium
external os	perineal body
fallopian tubes	perineum
false pelvis	polar body
female reproductive cycle (FRC)	progesterone
	pubis
fimbria	round ligaments
follicle-stimulating hormone (FSH)	rugae
	sacral promontory
fundus	spermatogenesis
graafian follicle	spermatozoa
infundibulopelvic ligament	symphysis pubis
	testis
innominate bones	transverse diameter
internal os	true pelvis
ischial spines	uterosacral ligaments
isthmus	uterus
luteinizing hormone (LH)	vagina
	vulva
myometrium	zona pellucida

Understanding childbearing requires more than understanding sexual intercourse or the process by which the male and female sex cells unite. One must also become familiar with the structures and functions that make childbearing possible. In this chapter, the anatomic, physiologic, and sexual aspects of the male and female reproductive systems will be considered.

The male and female reproductive organs are *homologous*; that is, they are fundamentally similar in structure and function. The primary functions of both the male and female reproductive systems are to produce sex cells and to transport the sex cells to locations where their union can occur. The sex cells, called *gametes*, are produced by specialized organs called *gonads*. A series of ducts and glands within both the male and female reproductive systems contribute to the production and transport of the gametes.

Early Development of Reproductive Structures and Processes

Although the genetic sex of the embryo is determined at fertilization, sexual differentiation does not occur until the eighth week of pregnancy. The male gonad, the **testis,** develops between the seventh and eighth week. The female gonad, the **ovary**, is recognizable about the tenth week of fetal development.

The testis produces the male gametes, called **spermatozoa** or *sperm*, by a process called **spermatogenesis**, which is described later in the chapter. Spermatogenesis of mature sperm does not occur until the onset of puberty.

Every egg available for maturation in a woman's reproductive life is present at her birth. During fetal life, the ovary produces *oogonia*, cells that become primitive ovarian eggs, called *oocytes*, by the process of **oogenesis**. No oocytes are formed after fetal development. About 400,000 oocytes are contained in the ovary at birth. Each oocyte is contained in a small ovarian cavity called a *primordial* or *primitive follicle*.

During a female's reproductive years, every month one of the oocytes undergoes a process of cellular division and maturation that transforms it into a fertilizable egg, or **ovum**. At **ovulation**, the ovum is released from its follicle. Only about 400 ova are released during the reproductive years. The remaining follicles and oocytes degenerate over time.

Puberty

The term *puberty* refers to the developmental period between childhood and attainment of adult sexual characteristics and functioning. Its onset is never sudden, although it may appear so to parents or to the young person who is not prepared for the physical and emotional changes of puberty. Generally, boys mature physically about 2 years later than girls. In boys, the age of onset of puberty ranges from 10–19 years; 14 years is the average age of onset. In girls, the age of onset ranges from 9–17 years; 12 years is the average age of onset.

Puberty occurs over a period lasting 1½–5 years and involves profound physical, psychologic, and emotional changes. These changes result from the interaction of the central nervous system and the endocrine organs.

Closely associated with puberty is the period of adolescence. Early adolescence begins 1–2 years before the onset of puberty.

Major Physical Changes

In both boys and girls, puberty is preceded by an accelerated growth rate called *adolescent spurt* (Gold and Josimovich, 1980). Widespread body system changes occur, including maturation of the reproductive organs.

Although the pattern of physical changes varies among individuals, usually boys first note such changes as an increase in the size of the external genitals; the appearance of pubic, axillary, and facial hair; the deepening of the voice; and nocturnal seminal emissions without sexual stimulation. Girls experience a broadening of the hips, then budding of the breasts, the appearance of the pubic and axillary hair, and the onset of menstruation, called *menarche*.

Physiology of Onset

Puberty is initiated by the maturation of the hypothalamic-pituitary-gonad complex, referred to as the *gonadostat*, and input from the central nervous system. The process, which begins in fetal life, is sequential and complex.

The central nervous system releases a neurotransmitter that stimulates the hypothalamus to synthesize and release *gonadotrophin-releasing factor* (GnRF). GnRF is transmitted to the anterior pituitary, where it causes the synthesis and secretion of the gonadotrophins, **follicle-stimulating hormone (FSH)** and **luteinizing hormone (LH)**.

Although the gonads do produce small amounts of *androgens* (male sex hormones) and *estrogens* (female sex hormones) before the onset of puberty, FSH and LH stimulate increased secretion of these hormones. Androgens and estrogens influence the development of secondary sex characteristics (Figure 2-1). FSH and LH stimulate the processes of spermatogenesis and maturation of ova.

Other hormones are involved in the onset of puberty. Their action, although less direct, is essential. Abnormally high or low levels of adrenocorticotrophic hormone (ACTH), thyroid hormone, or somatotrophic (growth) hormone (STH) can disrupt the onset of normal puberty.

Female Reproductive System

The female reproductive system consists of the external and internal genitals and the accessory organs of the breasts. Also discussed in this chapter are the bony pelvis and its structure because of their importance to childbearing.

External Genitals

All the external reproductive organs, except the glandular structures, can be directly inspected. The size, color, and shape of these structures vary extensively among races and individuals.

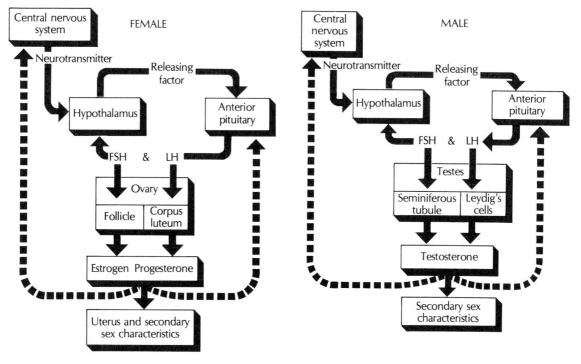

Figure 2-1

Solid lines indicate positive feedback, and broken lines indicate negative feedback. Through a neurotransmitter, the central nervous system stimulates the hypothalamus, which in turn produces a gonadotrophin-releasing factor that causes the anterior pituitary to produce gonadotrophins (FSH or LH). These hormones stimulate specific structures in the gonads to secrete steroid hormones (estrogen, progesterone, or testosterone). The rise in pituitary hormone production increases hypothalamus activity in a positive feedback relationship. Elevated steroid hormone levels stimulate the central nervous system and pituitary to inhibit hormone production in a negative feedback relationship.

The female external genitals, referred to as the **vulva** or *pudendum*, include the following structures (Figure 2-2):

- Mons pubis
- Labia majora
- Labia minora
- Clitoris
- Urethral meatus and paraurethral (Skene's) glands
- Vaginal vestibule (vaginal orifice, vulvovaginal glands, hymen, and fossa navicularis)
- Perineal body

Although not true parts of the female reproductive system, the urethral meatus and perineal body are considered here because of their proximity and relationship to the vulva.

The vulva has a generous supply of blood and nerves. As a woman ages, hormonal activity decreases, causing the vulvar organs to atrophy and become subject to a variety of lesions.

Mons pubis   The *mons pubis* is a softly rounded mound of subcutaneous fatty tissue beginning at the lowest portion of the anterior abdominal wall. Also known as the *mons veneris*, this structure covers the front portion of the symphysis pubis. The mons pubis is covered with pubic hair, typically with the hairline forming a transverse line across the lower abdomen. The hair is short and varies from sparse and fine in the Oriental woman to heavy, coarse, and curly in the Black woman.

The mons pubis has two functions:

- To protect the pelvic bones, especially during coitus
- To enhance sexual arousal

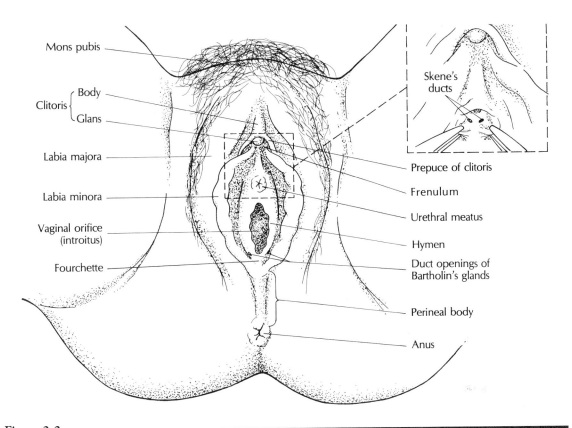

Figure 2-2
Female external genitals.

Labia majora   The *labia majora* are longitudinal, raised folds of pigmented skin, one on either side of the vulvar cleft. As the pair descend, they narrow, enclosing the vulvar cleft, and merge to form the *posterior commissure* of the perineal skin.

The vascular supply is extensive. Because of the extensive venous network in the labia majora, varicosities may occur during pregnancy, and obstetric or sexual trauma may cause hematomas.

The labia majora share an extensive and diffuse lymphatic supply with the other structures of the vulva. Understanding this supply is important in understanding malignancies of the female reproductive organs.

The labia majora have an extensive network of nerve endings that make the labia extremely sensitive to touch, pressure, pain, and temperature.

The chief functions of the labia majora are:

• To protect the components of the vulvar cleft

• To enhance sexual arousal

Labia minora   The *labia minora* are soft folds of skin within the labia majora that converge near the anus, forming the *fourchette*. Each labium minus has the appearance of shiny mucous membrane, moist and devoid of hair follicles. The labia minora are rich in sebaceous glands. Because the sebaceous glands do not open into hair follicles but directly onto the surface of the skin, sebaceous cysts commonly occur in this area. Vulvovaginitis in this area is very irritating because the labia minora have many tactile nerve endings.

The functions of the labia minora are as follows:

• To lubricate and waterproof the vulvar skin

• To provide bactericidal secretions

• To heighten sexual arousal and pleasure

Clitoris   The *clitoris* is the most erotically sensitive part of the female genital tract and is a common site of masturbation. The clitoris, located between the labia minora, is about 5–6 mm long and 6–8 mm across. Its tissue is essentially erectile.

The clitoris consists of the *glans*, the *corpus* or *body*, and two *crura*. The glans is partially covered by a fold of skin called the *prepuce*. This area often appears as an opening to an orifice, and, on visualization, may be confused with the urethral meatus. Attempts to insert a catheter here produce extreme discomfort.

The clitoris has very rich blood and nerve supplies. Overall, the clitoris has a richer nerve supply than the penis.

The clitoris exists primarily for female sexual enjoyment. In addition, it secretes *smegma*, whose odor may be sexually stimulating to the male.

Urethral meatus   Beneath the clitoris in the midline of the vestibule, the *urethral meatus* often appears as a puckered and slitlike opening. Urine passes out of the body from this orifice.

Paraurethral glands   The paraurethral glands, or *Skene's ducts*, open into the wall of the urethra close to its orifice. Their secretions lubricate the vaginal vestibule, facilitating sexual intercourse.

Vaginal vestibule   The vaginal vestibule is a boat-shaped depression enclosed by the labia majora and visible when they are separated. The vestibule contains the vaginal opening, or *introitus*, which is the border between the external and internal genitals.

The *hymen* is a thin, elastic membrane that partially closes the vaginal opening. Its strength, shape, and size vary greatly among women. The hymen is essentially avascular. The belief that the intact hymen is a sign of virginity and that it is broken at first sexual intercourse with resultant bleeding is not valid. The hymen can be broken through strenuous physical activity, masturbation, menstruation, or the use of tampons.

At the base of the vestibule are the ducts of the *vulvovaginal* or *Bartholin's glands*. They secrete a clear, sticky, alkaline mucus. These properties enhance the viability and motility of sperm deposited in the vaginal vestibule.

The vaginal vestibule generally is not sensitive to touch. The hymen, however, contains many free nerve endings.

Perineal body   The **perineal body** is a wedge-shaped mass of fibromuscular tissue found between the lower part of the vagina and anal canal. This area is also referred to as the **perineum**.

The muscles that meet at the perineal body are the external sphincter ani, both levator ani, the superficial and deep transverse perineal, and the bulbocavernosus. These muscles mingle with elastic fibers and connective tissue in an arrangement that allows a remarkable amount of stretching.

The perineal body is much larger in the female than in the male and is subject to laceration during childbirth. It is the site of episiotomy during delivery.

Internal Genitals

The female internal reproductive organs are the vagina, uterus, fallopian tubes, and ovaries. These are the target organs for estrogenic hormones, and each organ plays a unique role in the reproductive cycle. They are shown in Figure 2-3. These organs can be palpated during vaginal examination.

Ovaries   The ovaries are two almond-shaped structures just below the pelvic brim. One ovary is located on either side of the pelvic cavity. Their size varies among women and within individuals. Each ovary weighs approximately 6–10 g and is 1.5–3 cm wide, 2–5 cm long, and 1–1.5 cm thick. The ovaries of girls are small but become larger after puberty. They also change in appearance from a dull white, smooth-surfaced organ to a pitted gray organ. The pitting is caused by scarring due to ovulation.

The ovaries are held in place by the broad, ovarian, and infundibulopelvic ligaments. These ligaments are discussed in greater detail later in the chapter.

The ovaries are composed of three layers: the tunica albuginea, cortex, and medulla. The *tunica albuginea*, which is dense and dull white, serves as a protective layer. The *cortex* is the main functional part because it contains all the ova-containing follicles, the degenerated follicles, corpora lutea, and the degenerated corpora lutea. The *medulla* is completely surrounded by the cortex and contains the

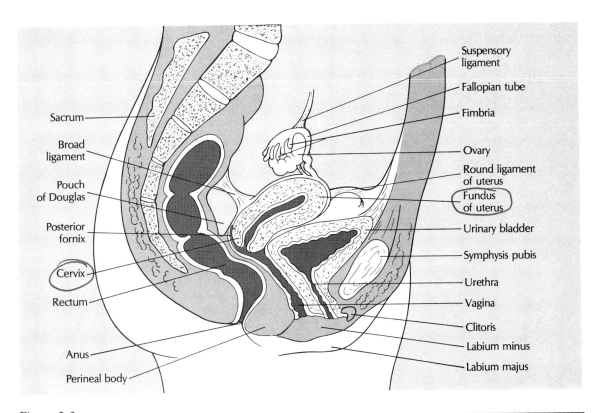

Figure 2-3
Female internal reproductive organs.

nerves, the blood vessels, and the lymphatic vessels (Figure 2-4).

The ovaries are the primary source of two important hormones: the estrogens and progesterone. **Estrogens** are associated with those characteristics contributing to femaleness. Although there are six natural estrogens, the major estrogenic effects are due primarily to three: estrone, β-estradiol, and estriol. β-estradiol is the major estrogen. In nonpregnant women, the ovaries secrete large amounts of estrogen; the adrenal cortex secretes minute amounts.

Progesterone is often called the *hormone of pregnancy* because its effects on the uterus allow pregnancy to be maintained. This hormone also prepares the breasts for lactation.

The interplay between the ovarian hormones and other hormones such as FSH and LH is responsible for the cyclic changes that allow pregnancy. Later in this chapter, the hormonal and physical changes that occur during the female reproductive cycle are discussed in depth.

The unique and vital function of the ovaries is to release a mature ovum monthly for fertilization. When a woman reaches the age of 45–55 years, the ovary no longer secretes estrogen. Ovulatory activity ceases and menopause occurs.

Fallopian tubes The **fallopian tubes**, also known as the *oviducts*, arise from each side of the uterus and reach almost to the sides of the pelvis, where they turn toward the ovaries (Figure 2-5). Each tube is approximately 8–13.5 cm long. A short section of each fallopian tube is inside the uterus.

Each tube may be divided into three parts: the isthmus, the ampulla, and the infundibulum or fimbria. The **isthmus** is straight and narrow, with a thick muscular wall and an opening (lumen) 2–3 mm in diameter. It is the site of tubal ligation, a surgical procedure to prevent pregnancy (Chapter 24).

Next to the isthmus is the curved **ampulla**, which comprises the outer two-thirds of the tube. Fertilization of the ovum by a spermato-

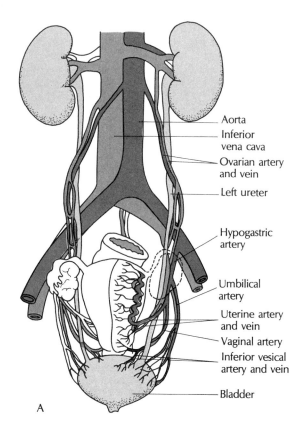

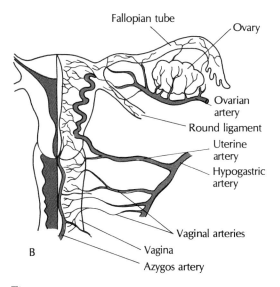

Figure 2-4 ▬▬▬▬

Blood supply to internal reproductive organs. **A**, Pelvic blood supply. **B**, Blood supply to vagina, ovary, uterus, and fallopian tube.

zoon usually occurs here. The ampulla ends at the **fimbria**, which is a funnel-like enlargement with many projections, called *fimbriae*, reaching out to the ovary. The longest of these, the *fimbria ovarica*, is attached to the ovary to increase the chances of intercepting the ovum as it is released. The fimbriae are dynamic and restless, constantly seeking the ovum to be released from the ovary.

The wall of the fallopian tube is made up of four layers: peritoneal (serous), subserous (adventitial), muscular, and mucosal. The peritoneal layer covers the tubes. The subserous layer contains the blood and nerve supply. The muscular layer is responsible for the wavelike, contracting (peristaltic) movements of the tube. The mucosal layer contains cilia and nonciliated cells. The cilia propel the ovum toward the uterus. The nonciliated cells secrete a protein-rich, serous fluid that nourishes the ovum.

A rich blood supply serves each fallopian tube (Figure 2-4). Thus, the tubes have an unusual ability to recover from an inflammatory process.

The lymphatic and nerve supplies to the fallopian tubes are extensive.

The functions of the fallopian tubes are as follows:

- To provide transport for the ovum from the ovary to the uterus
- To provide a site for fertilization
- To serve as a warm, moist, nourishing environment for the ovum or zygote

Uterus   The **uterus** is a hollow, muscular, thick-walled, pear-shaped organ lying in the center of the pelvic cavity. It is between the base of the bladder and the rectum and above the vagina (Figure 2-3). The mature organ weighs about 60 g and is approximately 7.5 cm long, 5 cm wide, and 1–2.5 cm thick.

The position of the uterus can vary, depending on a woman's posture, number of children borne, bladder and rectal fullness, and even normal respiratory patterns. Only the cervix is anchored laterally. The body of the uterus can move freely forward or backward. The axis also varies. Generally, the uterus bends forward, forming a sharp angle with the vagina. There is a bend in the area of the isthmus of the uterus;

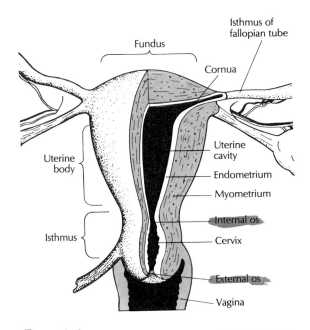

Figure 2-5
Structures of the uterus.

from there the cervix points downward. The uterus is said to be *anteverted* when it is in this position. The anteverted position is considered normal.

The uterus is kept in place by three sets of supports. The upper supports are the broad and round ligaments. The middle supports are the cardinal, pubocervical, and uterosacral ligaments. The lower supports are those structures considered to be the pelvic muscular floor.

The isthmus, referred to earlier in this section, is a slight constriction in the uterus that divides it into two unequal parts. The upper two-thirds of the uterus is the **corpus**, or *body*, composed mainly of myometrium. The lower third is the **cervix**, or *neck*. The rounded uppermost portion of the corpus that extends above the points of attachment of the fallopian tubes is called the **fundus**. The elongated portion of the uterus where the fallopian tubes open is called the **cornua**.

The cervix is about 2.5 cm in both length and diameter. It is canal-like; its exit into the vagina is called the **external os**, and its entrance into the corpus is called the **internal os** (Figure 2-5).

The cervix is a protective portal for the body of the uterus as well as the connection between the vagina and the uterus. The cervix appears pink, and its canal is rosy red and lined with ciliated epithelium containing mucus-secreting glands.

Elasticity is the chief characteristic of the cervix. Its ability to stretch is due to the high fibrous and collagenous content of the supportive tissues and also to the vast number of folds in the cervical lining.

The cervical mucosa has three functions:

- To provide lubrication for the vaginal canal
- To act as a bacteriostatic agent
- To provide an alkaline environment to shelter deposited sperm from the acidic vagina.

At ovulation, cervical mucus is clearer, thinner, and more alkaline than at other times.

The isthmus is about 6 mm above the internal os, and it is in this area that the uterine endometrium changes into the mucous membrane of the cervix. The isthmus takes on importance during pregnancy because it becomes the lower uterine segment. At delivery this segment is the site for lower-segment cesarean deliveries (Chapter 18).

The corpus of the uterus is made up of three layers. The outermost layer is the *serosal layer* or **perimetrium**, which is composed of peritoneum. The middle layer is the *muscular uterine layer* or **myometrium**. This muscle layer is continuous with the muscle layer of the fallopian tubes and with that of the vagina. This helps these organs present a unified reaction to various stimuli—ovulation, orgasm, or the deposit of sperm in the vagina. The myometrium has three indistinct layers of involuntary muscle fibers (Figure 2-6). The outer layer is made up of longitudinal muscle fibers, which expel the fetus during birth. The muscle fibers of the middle layer surround large blood vessels, and their contraction produces a hemostatic action. The inner muscle layer forms sphincters at the fallopian tube attachment sites and at the internal os. The sphincters at the fallopian tubes prevent the menstrual blood from flowing backward from the uterus into the fallopian tubes. The internal os sphincter inhibits the expulsion of the uterine contents during pregnancy.

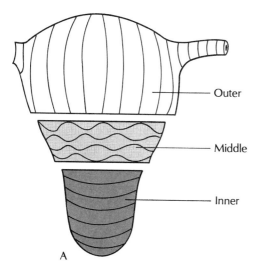

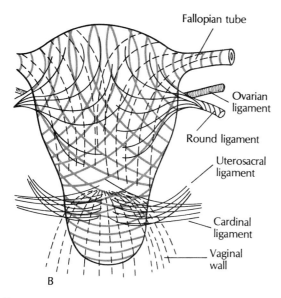

Figure 2-6

Uterine muscle layers. **A**, Muscle fiber placement. **B**, Interlacing of uterine muscle layers.

The innermost layer of the corpus is the *mucosal layer* or **endometrium**. This layer is composed of a single layer of columnar epithelium, glands, and stroma. From menarche to menopause, the endometrium undergoes monthly degeneration and renewal in the absence of pregnancy. As it responds to a governing hormonal cycle, the endometrium varies in thickness from 0.5–5 mm.

The glands of the endometrium are simple and tubular and produce a thin, watery, alkaline

secretion that keeps the uterine cavity moist. This "endometrial milk" not only helps the sperm travel to the fallopian tubes, but also nourishes the fertilized ovum before it lodges in the endometrium.

The blood supply to the endometrium is unique. Some of the blood vessels are not sensitive to cyclic hormonal control, and others are extremely sensitive to cyclic hormonal control. These differing responses allow part of the endometrium to remain intact, while other endometrial tissue is shed during menstruation.

Pregnancy changes both the corpus and the cervix permanently. The corpus never returns to its original size, and the external os changes from a circular opening of about 3 mm to a transverse slit with irregular edges.

The blood and lymphatic supplies to the uterus are extensive (Figure 2-4). Innervation of the uterus is entirely by the autonomic nervous system and seems to be more regulatory than primary in nature. Even without an intact nerve supply, the uterus can contract adequately for delivery as illustrated by the fact that hemiplegic patients have adequate uterine contractions (Beller et al., 1980).

The function of the uterus is to provide a safe environment for fetal development. The uterine lining is cyclically prepared by hormones for implantation of the embryo. Once the embryo is implanted, the developing fetus is protected until it is expelled.

Uterine ligaments   The uterine ligaments support and stabilize the various reproductive organs. The ligaments shown in Figures 2-6 and 2-7 are described in this section.

1. The **broad ligament** keeps the uterus centrally placed and provides stability within the pelvic cavity. It is a double mesenteric layer that is continuous with the abdominal peritoneum. The broad ligament covers the uterus anteriorly and posteriorly and extends outward from the uterus to enfold the fallopian tubes. The round and ovarian ligaments are at the upper border of the broad ligament. At its lower border, it forms the cardinal ligaments. Between the folds of the broad ligament are connective tissue, involuntary muscle, blood and lymph vessels, and nerves.

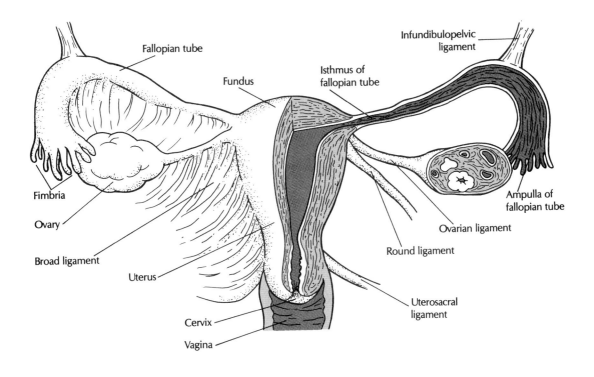

Figure 2-7

Uterine ligaments (uterosacral and cardinal ligaments not shown). (Modified from Spence AP and Mason EB: Human Anatomy and Physiology, 2nd ed. Menlo Park, Calif.: Benjamin/Cummings, 1983, p. 742.)

2. The **round ligaments** help the broad ligament keep the uterus in place. Each of the round ligaments arises from the sides of the uterus near the fallopian tube insertion. They course outward between the folds of the broad ligament, passing through the inguinal ring and canals and eventually fusing with the connective tissue of the labia majora. Made up of longitudinal muscle, the round ligaments enlarge during pregnancy. During labor the round ligaments steady the uterus, pulling downward and forward so that the presenting part is forced into the cervix.

3. The **ovarian ligaments** anchor the lower pole of the ovary to the cornua of the uterus. They are composed of muscle fibers, which allow the ligaments to contract. This contractile ability influences the position of the ovary to some extent, thus helping the fimbriae of the fallopian tubes to "catch" the ovum as it is released each month.

4. The **cardinal ligaments** are the chief uterine supports, suspending the uterus from the side walls of the true pelvis (Figure 2-6). These ligaments, also known as *Mackenrodt's* or the *transverse cervical ligaments*, arise from the sides of the pelvic walls and attach to the cervix in the upper vagina. These ligaments prevent uterine prolapse and also support the upper vagina.

5. The **infundibulopelvic ligament** suspends and supports the ovaries (Figure 2-7). Arising from the outer third of the broad ligament, the infundibulopelvic ligament contains the ovarian vessels and nerves.

6. The **uterosacral ligaments** provide support for the uterus and cervix at the level of the ischial spines (Figure 2-6). Arising on each side of the pelvis from the posterior wall of the uterus, the uterosacral ligaments sweep back around the rectum and insert on the sides of the first and second sacral vertebras. These ligaments contain smooth muscle fibers, connective tissue, blood and lymph vessels, and nerves.

Vagina   The **vagina** is a muscular and membranous tube that connects the external genitals with the center of the pelvis (Figure 2-3). It passes from the vulva to the uterus in a position nearly parallel to the plane of the pelvic brim. The vagina is often referred to as the *birth canal* because it forms the lower part of the axis through which the presenting part of the fetus must pass during birth.

Because the cervix of the uterus projects into the upper part of the anterior wall of the vagina, the anterior wall is approximately 2.5 cm shorter than the posterior wall. Measurements range from 6–8 cm for the anterior wall and 7–10 cm for the posterior wall.

In the upper part of the vagina, which is called the vaginal *vault*, there is a recess or hollow around the cervix. This area is referred to as the vaginal *fornix*. Generally, the anterior and posterior vaginal walls meet; thus, on transverse section, the vagina in repose is shaped like an H.

The walls of the vaginal vault are very thin. This structure facilitates pelvic examination. Various structures can be palpated through the walls and fornix of the vaginal vault, including the uterus, a distended bladder, the ovaries, the appendix, the cecum, the colon, and the ureters.

When a woman lies on her back, the space in the fornix permits the pooling of semen after intercourse. The collection of a large number of sperm near the cervix in a favorable environment increase the chances of impregnation.

The walls of the vagina are covered with ridges, or **rugae**, crisscrossing each other. These rugae allow the vagina to stretch during the descent of the fetal head.

During a woman's reproductive life, an acidic vaginal environment is normal (pH 4–5). Secretion from the vaginal epithelium provides a moist environment. The acidic environment is maintained by a symbiotic relationship between lactic acid–producing bacilli (Döderlein bacillus or lactobacillus) and the vaginal epithelial cells. These cells contain glycogen, which is broken down by the bacilli into lactic acid. The amount of glycogen is regulated by the ovarian hormones. Any interruption of this process can destroy the normal self-cleansing action of the vagina. Such interruption may be caused by antibiotic therapy, douching, or use of vaginal sprays or deodorants.

The acidic vaginal environment is normal only during the mature reproductive years and in the first days of life when maternal hormones are operating in the infant. A relatively neutral pH of 7.5 is normal from infancy until puberty and after menopause.

The vagina's blood and lymphatic supplies are extensive (Figure 2-4). The nerve supply is meager, causing it to be a relatively insensitive organ. Pain during labor is less than if innervation were greater.

The functions of the vagina are as follows:

- To serve as the passage for sperm and for the fetus during delivery
- To provide passage for the menstrual products from the uterine endometrium to the outside of the body
- To protect against trauma from sexual intercourse and infection from pathogenic organisms

Bony Pelvis

The female bony *pelvis* has two unique functions:

- To support and protect the pelvic contents
- To form the relatively fixed axis of the birth passage

Because the pelvis is so important to childbearing, its structure must be understood clearly.

Bony structure   The pelvis is made up of four bones: two innominate bones, the sacrum, and the coccyx. The pelvis resembles a bowl or basin; its sides are the innominate bones, and its back is the sacrum and coccyx. Lined with fibrocartilage and held tightly together by ligaments, the four bones join at the symphysis pubis, the two sacroiliac joints, and the sacrococcygeal joints (Figure 2-8).

The **innominate bones**, also known as the *hip bones* or *os coxae*, are made up of three separate bones: the ilium, ischium, and pubis.

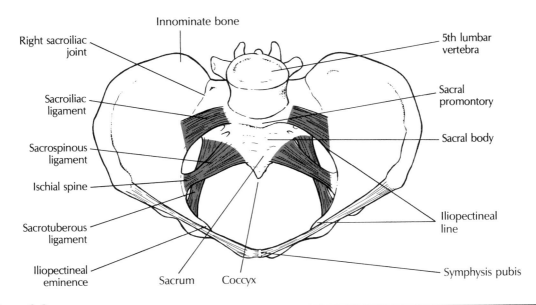

Figure 2-8
Bony pelvis with its supporting ligaments.

These bones fuse to form a circular cavity, the *acetabulum,* which articulates with the femur.

The *ilium* is the broad, upper prominence of the hip. The *iliac crest* is the margin of the ilium. The *iliac spine,* the foremost projection nearest the groin, is the site of attachment for ligaments and muscles.

The *ischium,* the strongest bone, is under the ilium and below the acetabulum. The L-shaped ischium ends in a marked protuberance, the *ischial tuberosity,* on which the weight of a seated body rests. The **ischial spines** arise near the junction of the ilium and ischium and jut into the pelvic cavity. The shortest diameter of the pelvic cavity is between the ischial spines. The ischial spines can serve as a reference point during labor to evaluate the descent of the fetal head into the birth canal.

The **pubis** forms the slightly bowed front portion of the innominate bone. Extending medially from the acetabulum to the midpoint of the bony pelvis, the pubis meets the other pubis to form a joint, the **symphysis pubis**. The triangular space below this junction is known as the *pubic arch.* The fetal head passes under this arch during birth. The symphysis pubis is formed by heavy fibrocartilage and the superior and inferior pubic ligaments. The mobility of the inferior ligament, also known as

the *arcuate pubic ligament,* increases during pregnancy.

The *sacrum* is a wedge-shaped bone formed by the fusion of five vertebras. On the anterior upper portion of the sacrum is a projection into the pelvic cavity known as the **sacral promontory**. This projection is another obstetric guide in determining pelvic measurements.

The small triangular bone last on the vertebral column is the *coccyx.* It articulates with the sacrum at the sacrococcygeal joint. The coccyx usually moves backward during labor to provide more room for the fetus.

The sacroiliac joints also are more relaxed and thus more mobile during pregnancy. This relaxation is caused by the hormones of pregnancy.

Pelvic floor   The muscular **pelvic floor** of the bony pelvis is designed to overcome the force of gravity exerted on the pelvic organs. It acts as a buttress to the irregularly shaped pelvic outlet, thereby providing stability and support for surrounding structures.

Deep fascia and the levator ani and coccygeal muscles form the part of the pelvic floor known as the **pelvic diaphragm**. Above it is the pelvic cavity; below and behind it is the perineum.

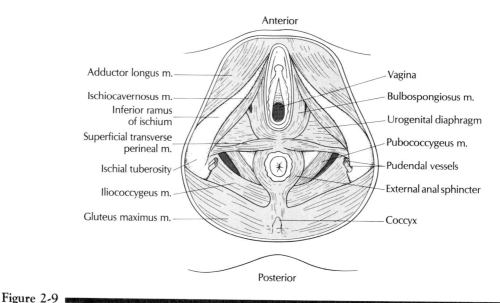

Figure 2-9

Muscles of the pelvic floor. The puborectalis, pubovaginalis, and coccygeal muscles cannot be seen from this view.

The levator ani muscle makes up the major portion of the pelvic diaphragm and consists of four muscles: ileococcygeus, pubococcygeus, puborectalis, and pubovaginalis. The coccygeal muscle, a thin muscular sheet underlying the sacrospinous ligament, helps the levator ani support the pelvic organs. Muscles of the pelvic floor are shown in Figure 2-9.

Pelvic division The pelvic cavity is divided into the false pelvis and the true pelvis (Figure 2-10,*A*). The **false pelvis** is the portion above the linea terminalis. Its primary function is to support the weight of the enlarged pregnant uterus.

The **true pelvis** is the portion that lies below the linea terminalis. The bony circumference of the true pelvis is made up of the sacrum, coccyx, and innominate bones. The true pelvis is important in childbearing because its size and shape must be adequate for the fetus to pass through during labor and delivery. The true pelvis has three parts: the inlet, cavity, and outlet (Figure 2-10,*B*).

The **pelvic inlet** is the upper border of the true pelvis. The size and shape of the pelvic inlet are determined by assessing three anteroposterior diameters. The **diagonal conjugate** extends from the subpubic angle to the middle

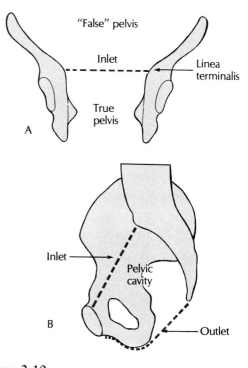

Figure 2-10

Female pelvis. **A**, False and true pelves. **B**, Pelvic cavity.

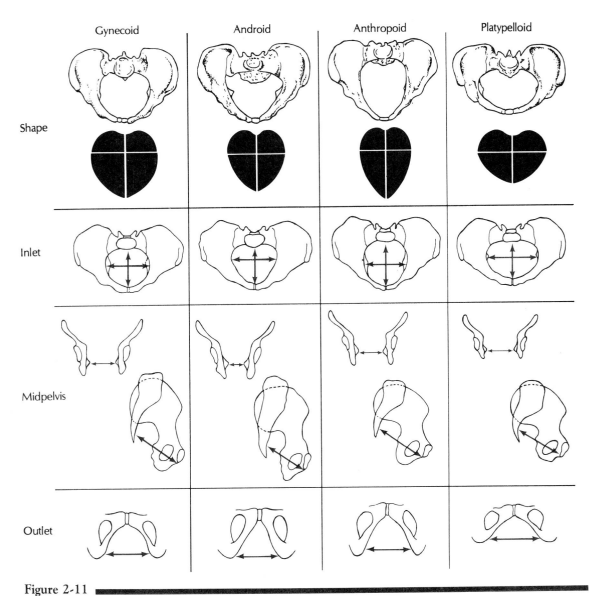

	Gynecoid	Android	Anthropoid	Platypelloid
Shape				
Inlet				
Midpelvis				
Outlet				

Figure 2-11

Comparison of Caldwell-Moloy pelvic types.

of the sacral promontory. The diagonal conjugate can be measured manually during a pelvic examination. The **obstetric conjugate** extends from the middle of the sacral promontory to an area approximately 1 cm below the pubic crest. Its length is estimated by subtracting 1.5 cm from the diagonal conjugate. The fetus passes through the obstetric conjugate, and the size of this diameter determines whether the fetus can move down into the birth canal. The true (anatomic) conjugate, or **conjugate vera**, extends from the middle of the sacral promontory to the middle of the pubic crest (superior surface of

the symphysis). One additional measurement, the **transverse diameter**, helps determine the shape of the inlet. The transverse diameter is the largest diameter of the inlet and is measured using the linea terminalis as the point of reference. The female pelvic inlet is typically round.

The **pelvic cavity** is a curved canal with a longer posterior than anterior wall. The curvature of the lumbar spine influences the shape and tilt (inclination) of the pelvic cavity.

The **pelvic outlet** is at the lower border of the true pelvis. The size of the pelvic outlet can be determined by assessing the *transverse diameter,* which is also called the *bi-ischial* or *intertuberous diameter*. This diameter extends from the inner surface of one ischial tuberosity to the other. The pubic arch is also a part of the pelvic cavity. The pubic arch has great importance because the fetus must pass under it during delivery. If it is narrow, the baby's head may be pushed backward toward the coccyx, making extension of the head difficult. The clinical assessment of each of these diameters is discussed further in Chapter 6.

Pelvic types   The Caldwell-Moloy classification of pelves is widely used to differentiate bony pelvic types (Caldwell and Moloy, 1933). The four basic types are *gynecoid, android, anthropoid*, and *platypelloid* (Figure 2-11). The type of pelvis is determined by assessing the posterior segment of the pelvic inlet. Each type has a characteristic shape, and each shape has implications for labor and delivery. See Chapter 12 for further discussion.

Breasts

The **breasts**, or *mammary glands,* considered accessories of the reproductive system, are specialized sebaceous glands. They are conical and symmetrically placed on the sides of the chest. The greater pectoral and anterior serratus muscles underlie each breast. Suspending the breasts are fibrous tissues, called *Cooper's ligaments*, that extend from the deep fascia in the chest outward to just under the skin covering the breast. Frequently, the left breast is larger than the right.

In the center of each mature breast is the **nipple**, a protrusion about 0.5–1.3 cm in diameter. The nipple is composed mainly of erectile tissue, which becomes more rigid and prominent during the menstrual cycle, sexual excitement, pregnancy, and lactation. The nipple is surrounded by the heavily pigmented **areola**, 2.5–10 cm in diameter. Both the nipple and areola are roughened by small papillae called *tubercles of Montgomery*. As an infant suckles, these tubercles secrete a fatty substance that helps lubricate and protect the breasts.

The breasts are composed of glandular, fibrous, and adipose tissue. The glandular tissue is arranged in a series of 15 to 24 lobes separated by fibrous and adipose tissue. Each lobe is made up of several lobules composed of many alveoli clustered around tiny ducts. The lining of these ducts secretes the various components of milk. The ducts from several lobules merge to form the larger ducts, called the *lactiferous ducts*, which open on the surface of the nipple (Figure 2-12).

The biologic function of the breasts is to provide nourishment and protective maternal antibodies to infants. They also are a source of pleasurable sexual sensation.

Female Reproductive Cycle _____

The monthly rhythmic changes in sexually mature females is usually called the *menstrual cycle*. A more accurate term is the **female reproductive cycle (FRC)**. The FRC is composed of the ovarian cycle, during which ovulation occurs, and the uterine cycle, during which menstruation occurs. These two cycles take place simultaneously (Figure 2-13).

Menstruation is cyclic uterine bleeding in response to cyclic hormonal changes. Menstruation occurs when the ovum is not fertilized and begins about 14 days after ovulation. The menstrual discharge, also referred to as the *menses* or *menstrual flow*, is composed of blood mixed with fluid, cervical and vaginal secretions, bacteria, mucus, leukocytes, and other cellular debris. The menstrual discharge is dark red and has a distinctive odor. It results from physiologic tissue death caused by lack of blood and oxygen to the endometrium.

Menarche—the onset of menstruation—usually occurs when the girl is about 12–13 years of age. Frequently, ovulation does not occur in early cycles; these are called *anovulatory cycles*. Early cycles also are often irregular in frequency, amount of flow, and duration. Within several months to 2–3 years, a regular cycle becomes established.

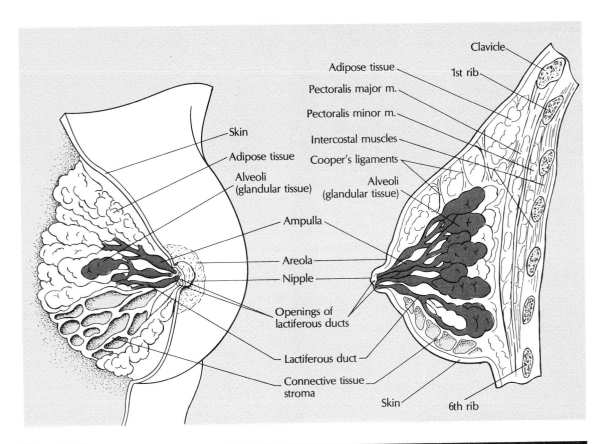

Figure 2-12

Anatomy of the breast. **A,** Anterior view of partially dissected left breast. **B,** Sagittal view. (Modified from Spence AP, and Mason EB: *Human Anatomy and Physiology*, 2nd ed. Menlo Park, Calif.: Benjamin/Cummings, 1983, p. 747.)

Menstrual parameters vary greatly among individuals. Generally, menstruation occurs every 28 days, plus or minus 5–10 days. Emotional and physical factors such as illness, excessive fatigue, and stress or anxiety can alter the cycle interval. In addition, certain environmental factors such as temperature and altitude may affect the cycle.

The duration of menses is from 2–8 days, with the blood loss averaging 30–100 mL and the loss of iron averaging 0.5–1 mg daily.

Menopause, the cessation of menstruation, usually occurs when the woman is 45–52 years of age. The age of onset may be influenced by nutritional, cultural, or genetic factors. The physiologic mechanisms initiating its onset are not known exactly.

Neurohumoral Basis of the Female Reproductive Cycle

The FRC is controlled by complex interactions between the nervous and endocrine systems and their target tissues. These interactions involve the hypothalamus, anterior pituitary, and ovaries; their functions are reciprocal.

The hypothalamus controls anterior pituitary hormone production by secretion of gonadotrophin-releasing hormone (GnRH). This releasing hormone is often called both luteinizing hormone–releasing hormone (LHRH) and follicle-stimulating hormone–releasing hormone (FSHRH).

In response to GnRH, the anterior pituitary secretes the gonadotrophic hormones FSH and LH. FSH primarily is responsible for the matu-

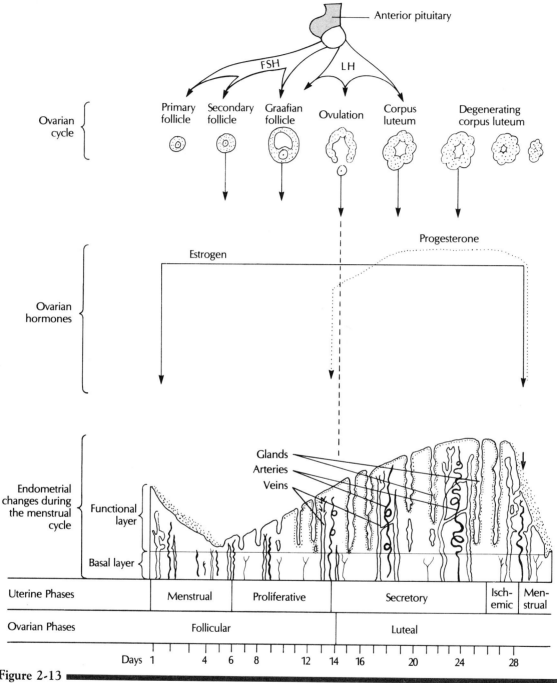

Figure 2-13

Female reproductive cycle: Interrelationships of hormones and the four phases of the uterine cycle and the two phases of the ovarian cycle.

ration of the primordial ovarian follicle. As the follicle matures, it secretes increasing amounts of estrogen, which enhance the development of the follicle. (This estrogen also is responsible for the rebuilding of the endometrium after it is shed during menstruation.)

Final maturation of the follicle will not come about without the action of LH. The anterior pituitary's production of LH increases sixfold to tenfold as the follicle matures. About 18 hours after the peak production of LH, ovulation occurs.

Estrogen levels fall the day before ovulation, and progesterone levels begin to increase. Estrogen causes the vaginal epithelium to proliferate and the cervix to secrete thin, watery, clear mucus. Breast glandular tissue increases in size and complexity. After ovulation, the ruptured follicle undergoes rapid change. The mass of cells becomes the corpus luteum. The lutein cells secrete large amounts of progesterone with smaller amounts of estrogen. Seven or eight days after ovulation, the corpus luteum begins to regress, losing its secretory function. The production of both progesterone and estrogen is severely diminished. The anterior pituitary responds with increasing amounts of FSH; a few days later, LH production begins. As a result, new follicles become responsive and begin maturing.

Prostaglandins have an important role in the female reproductive cycle. These complex lipid compounds are tissue hormones rather than humoral hormones, and only very small amounts circulate (Lackritz, 1981).

Although the precise mechanisms by which prostaglandins control or mediate ovulation are not known, release of the ovum is thought to be caused by prostaglandins. Significant amounts of prostaglandins are found in and around the follicle at the time of ovulation. Prostaglandins may act as intracellular regulators in hormone action (Little and Billiar, 1981). Prostaglandins also are postulated to induce progesterone withdrawal, which causes the corpus luteum to regress, resulting in the onset of menses.

Endometrium and menstrual fluid are rich sources of prostaglandins. It is thought that estrogen acts on the uterus, primed by progesterone, to produce prostaglandins.

Ovarian Cycle

The ovarian cycle has two phases: the follicular phase (days 1–14) and the luteal phase (days 15–28). During the *follicular phase*, the primordial follicle matures as a result of FSH. Within the follicle, the oocyte grows. A mature **graafian follicle** appears about the fourteenth day. It is a large structure, measuring about 5–10 mm. In the mature graafian follicle, the oocyte is surrounded by fluid and enclosed in a thick elastic capsule called the **zona pellucida**.

Just before ovulation, the mature oocyte completes its first meiotic division (see Chapter 4 for a description of meiosis). As a result of this division, two cells are formed: a small cell called a **polar body** and a larger cell called the *secondary oocyte*. The secondary oocyte matures into the ovum. The second meiotic division does not occur until the sperm penetrates the ovum.

As the graafian follicle matures and enlarges, it comes close to the surface of the ovary. The ovary surface forms a blisterlike protrusion, and the follicle walls become thin. The secondary oocyte, polar body, and the follicular fluid are pushed out. Discharged near the fimbria of the fallopian tube, the ovum is pulled into the tube and begins its journey through it.

Occasionally, ovulation is accompanied by midcycle pain, known as *mittelschmerz*. This pain may be caused by a thick tunica albuginea or by a local peritoneal reaction to the expelling of the follicular contents. Vaginal discharge may increase during ovulation, and a small amount of blood (midcycle spotting) may be discharged as well.

The body temperature increases about 0.3–0.6C (0.5–1.0F) at the time of ovulation or shortly thereafter. It remains elevated until the second or third day after ovulation. These temperature changes are useful clinically to determine the approximate time of ovulation.

Generally, the ovum takes several minutes to travel through the ruptured follicle to the fallopian tube opening. The contractions of the tube's smooth muscle and ciliary action propel the ovum through the tube. The ovum remains in the ampulla, where it may be fertilized and cleavage can begin. The ovum is thought to be fertile for only 6–24 hours. It reaches the uterus 72–96 hours after its release from the ovary.

The *luteal phase* begins when the ovum leaves its follicle. Under the influence of LH, the **corpus luteum** develops from the ruptured follicle. Within 2 or 3 days, the corpus luteum becomes yellowish and spherical and increases in vascularity. If the ovum is fertilized and implants in the endometrium, the fertilized egg begins to secrete human chorionic gonadotrophin (hCG), which is needed to maintain the corpus luteum. If fertilization does not occur, within about a week after ovulation, the corpus luteum begins to degenerate, eventually becoming a connective tissue scar called the *corpus albicans.* Approximately 14 days after ovulation (in a 28-day cycle), in the absence of pregnancy, menstruation begins. Figure 2-14 depicts the changes that the follicle undergoes during the ovarian cycle.

Uterine Cycle

The uterine cycle has four phases: the menstrual phase (days 1–5), proliferative phase (days 6–14), secretory phase (days 15–16), and ischemic phase (days 27–28). During the *menstrual phase,* menstruation occurs. Some endometrial areas are shed, while others remain. Some of the remaining tips of the endometrial glands begin to regenerate. Following menstruation, the endometrium is in a resting state. Estrogen levels are low, and the endometrium is 1–2 mm deep. The cervical mucosa during this part of the cycle is scanty, viscous, and opaque.

The *proliferative phase* begins when the endometrial glands enlarge, becoming tortuous and longer, in response to increasing amounts of estrogen. The blood vessels become prominent and dilated, and the endometrium increases in thickness sixfold to eightfold. This gradual process reaches its peak just before ovulation. The cervical mucosa becomes thin, clear, watery, and more alkaline, making the mucosa more favorable to spermatozoa. As ovulation nears, the cervical mucosa shows increased elasticity, called *spinnbarkeit*. At ovulation, the mucosa will stretch more than 5 cm. On microscopic examination, the mucosa shows a characteristic *ferning* pattern (see Figure 3-3). The signs of ovulation are summarized in Essential Facts to Remember.

The *secretory phase* follows ovulation. The endometrium, under estrogenic influence, undergoes slight cellular growth. Progesterone, however, causes such marked swelling and growth that the epithelium is warped into folds. The amount of tissue glycogen increases. The glandular epithelial cells begin to fill with cellular debris, become tortuous, and dilate. The glands secrete small quantities of endometrial fluid in preparation for a fertilized ovum. The vascularity of the entire uterus increases greatly, providing a nourishing bed for implantation. If

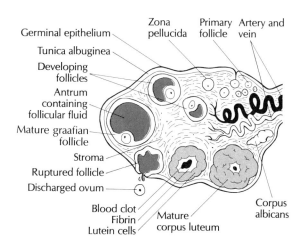

Figure 2-14
Various stages of development of the ovarian follicles.

Labels on figure: Germinal epithelium; Tunica albuginea; Developing follicles; Antrum containing follicular fluid; Mature graafian follicle; Stroma; Ruptured follicle; Discharged ovum; Blood clot; Fibrin; Lutein cells; Mature corpus luteum; Zona pellucida; Primary follicle; Artery and vein; Corpus albicans

✸ ESSENTIAL FACTS TO REMEMBER

Signs of Ovulation

The cervical mucosa changes in the following ways:

- The amount of mucus increases.
- It appears thin, watery, and clear.
- Spinnbarkeit greater than 5 cm is present.
- A ferning pattern appears on microscopic examination.

Body temperature increases 0.3 to 0.6C.
Mittelschmerz may be present.
Midcycle spotting may occur.

implantation occurs, the endometrium, under the influence of progesterone, continues to develop and become even thicker. (See Chapter 4 for an in-depth discussion of implantation.)

If fertilization does not occur, the *ischemic phase* begins. The corpus luteum begins to degenerate, and as a result both estrogen and progesterone levels fall. Areas of necrosis appear under the epithelial lining. Extensive vascular changes occur also. Small blood vessels rupture, and the spiral arteries constrict and retract, causing a deficiency of blood in the endometrium. The endometrium becomes pale. This ischemic phase is characterized by the escape of blood into the stromal cells of the uterus. The menstrual flow begins, thus beginning the uterine cycle again.

Male Reproductive System

The primary reproductive functions of the male genitals are to produce and transport its sex cells, sperm, through and eventually out of the genital tract into the female genital tract. The male reproductive system consists of the external and internal genitals (Figure 2-15).

External Genitals

The two external reproductive organs are the penis and scrotum. The *penis* is an elongated, cylindrical structure consisting of a body, termed the *shaft*, and a cone-shaped end called the *glans*. The penis lies in front of the scrotum.

The shaft of the penis is made up of three longitudinal columns of erectile tissue: the paired *corpora cavernosa* and a third, the *corpus spongiosum*. These columns are covered by dense fibrous connective tissue and then enclosed by elastic tissue. The penis is covered by a thin outer layer of skin.

The corpus spongiosum contains the urethra. The urethra terminates in a slitlike opening, located in the tip of the glans, called the *urethral meatus*. A circular fold of skin arises just behind the glans and covers it. Known as the *prepuce*, or *foreskin*, it is frequently removed by the surgical procedure of circumcision (Chapter 21).

Sexual stimulation causes the penis to elongate, thicken, and stiffen, a process called *erection*. The penis becomes erect when its blood vessels become engorged, a consequence of parasympathetic nerve stimulation. If stimulation is intense enough, the forceful and sudden expulsion of semen occurs through the rhythmic contractions of the penile muscles. This phenomenon is called *ejaculation*.

The penis serves both the urinary and reproductive systems. Urine is expelled through

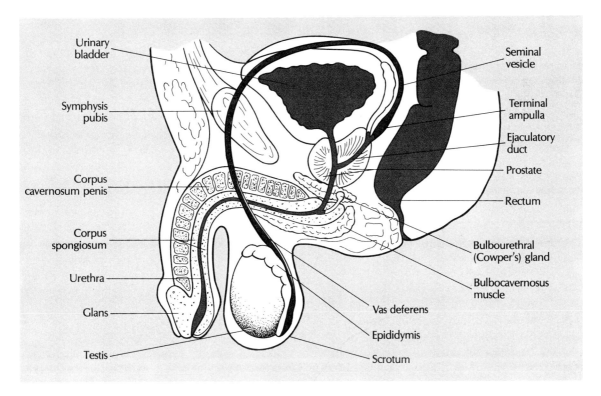

Figure 2-15

Male reproductive system.

the urethral meatus. The reproductive function of the penis is to deposit sperm in the vagina so that fertilization of the ovum can occur.

The *scrotum* is a pouchlike structure that hangs in front of the anus and behind the penis. Composed of skin and muscle, the scrotum appears rough and wrinkled.

Inside the scrotum are two lateral compartments, each containing a testis with its related structures. The left testis and its scrotal sac usually hang lower than the right.

The function of the scrotum is to protect the testes and the sperm by maintaining a temperature lower than that of the body. The scrotum's sensitivity to touch, pressure, temperature, and pain contributes to its protective function.

Internal Genitals

The male internal reproductive organs include the gonads (testes or testicles), a system of ducts (epididymides, vas deferens, ejaculatory duct, and urethra), and accessory glands (seminal vesicles, prostate gland, bulbourethral glands, and urethral glands).

Testes   The *testes* are a pair of oval glandular organs contained in the scrotum. In the sexually mature male, they are the site of spermatozoa production and the secretion of several male sex hormones.

Each testis is 4–6 cm long, 2–3 cm wide, and 3–4 cm thick. Each weighs about 10–15 g. It is covered by an outer serous membrane and an inner capsule composed of tough fibrous connective tissue. The connective tissue sends projections inward, dividing the testis into 250–400 lobules. Each lobule contains one to three tightly packed, convoluted *seminiferous tubules*. These tubules contain sperm cells in all stages of development, arranged in layers.

The seminiferous tubules are surrounded by loose connective tissue, which houses abundant blood and lymph vessels and *interstitial (Leydig's) cells*. The interstitial cells produce testosterone, the primary male sex hormone.

The many seminiferous tubules come together to form 20–30 straight tubules, which in turn form an anastomotic network of thin-walled spaces, the *rete testis*. The rete testis forms 10–15 ducts that empty into the duct of the epididymis.

Most of the cells lining the seminiferous tubules undergo spermatogenesis, a process of maturation in which spermatocytes become spermatozoa. (Chapter 4 discusses this process also.) Sperm production varies among and within the tubules, with cells in different areas of the same tubule undergoing different stages of spermatogenesis. The tubules also contain *Sertoli's cells*, which nourish and protect the spermatocytes. The sperm are eventually released from the tubules into the epididymis, where they mature further.

Like the female reproductive cycle, the process of spermatogenesis and other functions of the testes are the result of complex neural and hormonal controls. The hypothalamus secretes releasing factors, which stimulate the anterior pituitary to release the gonadotrophins—FSH and LH. These hormones cause the testes to produce *testosterone,* which maintains spermatogenesis, increases sperm production by the seminiferous tubules, and stimulates production of seminal fluid.

Testosterone is the most prevalent and potent of the testicular hormones. Its target organs are the testes, prostate, and seminal vesicles. In addition to being essential for spermatogenesis, testosterone is responsible for the development of secondary male characteristics and certain behavioral patterns. The effects of testosterone include structural and functional development of the male genital tract, emission and ejaculation of seminal fluid, distribution of body hair, promotion of growth and strength of long bones, increased muscle mass, and enlargement of the vocal cords. The action of testosterone on the central nervous system is thought to produce aggressiveness and sexual drive. The action of testosterone is constant, not cyclic like that of the female hormones, and is not limited to a certain number of years.

In summary, the primary functions of the testes are to serve as the site of spermatogenesis and to produce testosterone.

Epididymides   The *epididymis* is a duct about 5.6 m long, although it is convoluted into a compact structure about 3.75 cm long. An epididymis lies behind each testis. It arises from the top of the testis, courses downward, and then passes upward, where it becomes the vas deferens.

The epididymis provides a reservoir where spermatozoa can survive for a long period. When discharged from the seminiferous tubules into the epididymis, the sperm are immotile and incapable of fertilizing an ovum. The spermatozoa remain in the epididymis for 2–10 days, until maturation is complete.

Vas deferens and ejaculatory ducts   The *vas deferens*, also known as the *ductus deferens*, is about 40 cm long and connects the epididymis with the prostate. One vas deferens arises from the posterior border of each testis. It joins the spermatic cord and weaves over and between several pelvic structures until it meets the vas deferens from the opposite side. Each vas deferens then unites with a seminal vesicle duct to form the *ejaculatory ducts*, which enter the prostate gland, terminating in the prostatic urethra.

Prior to its entrance into the prostate, the vas deferens enlarges. This enlargement is called the *terminal ampulla* and serves as the primary storehouse for spermatozoa, which are still relatively immotile, and tubule secretions. The ejaculatory ducts serve as passageways for semen and fluid secreted by the seminal vesicles.

Urethra   The male *urethra* is the passageway for both urine and semen. The urethra begins in the bladder and passes through the prostate gland, where it is called the *prostatic urethra*. The urethra emerges from the prostate gland to become the membranous urethra. It terminates in the penis, where it is called the *penile urethra*.

Accessory glands   The male accessory glands are specialized structures under endocrine and neural control. Each secretes a unique and essential component of the total seminal fluid in an ordered sequence.

The *seminal vesicles* are two glands composed of many lobes. Each vesicle is about 7.5 cm long. They are situated between the bladder and rectum and immediately above the base of the prostate. The epithelium lining the seminal vesicles secretes an alkaline, viscid, clear fluid rich in high-energy fructose, prostaglandins, fibrinogen, and proteins. During ejaculation, this fluid empties into the ejaculatory ducts and mixes with the sperm. This fluid helps provide an environment favorable to sperm motility and metabolism.

The *prostate gland* surrounds the upper part of the urethra and lies below the neck of the urinary bladder. Made up of several lobes, it measures about 4 cm in diameter and weighs 20–30 g. The prostate is made up of both glandular and muscular tissue. It secretes a thin, milky, slightly acidic fluid (pH 6.5) containing high levels of zinc, calcium, citric acid, and acid phosphatase. This fluid protects the sperm from the acidic environment of the vagina and the male urethra (Vick, 1984).

The *bulbourethral* or *Cowper's glands* are a pair of small round structures on either side of the membranous urethra. The glands secrete a clear, viscous, alkaline fluid rich in mucoproteins that becomes part of the semen. This secretion also lubricates the penile urethra during sexual excitement as well as neutralizes the acid in the male urethra and vagina, thereby enhancing sperm motility.

The *urethral* or *Littre's glands* are tiny mucous-secreting glands found throughout the membranous lining of the penile urethra. Their secretions add to those of the bulbourethral glands.

Semen   The male ejaculate, *semen* or *seminal fluid*, is made up of spermatozoa and the secretions of the bulbourethral glands, urethral glands, prostate, epididymides, and seminal vesicles. The seminal fluid transports viable and motile sperm to the female reproductive tract. Effective transportation of sperm requires adequate nutrients, an adequate pH (about 7.5), a specific concentration of sperm to fluid, and an optimal osmolarity.

A spermatozoon is made up of a *head* and a *tail*. The tail is divided into the middle piece and end piece (Figure 2-16). The head's main components are the *acrosome, nucleus,* and *nuclear vacuoles.* The head carries the haploid number of chromosomes (23), and it is the part that enters the ovum at fertilization (Chapter 4). The tail, or *flagellum,* is specialized for motility.

Sperm may be stored in the male genital system for a period of several to 42 days, depending primarily on the frequency of ejaculations. The average volume of ejaculate following abstinence for several days is 2–5 mL

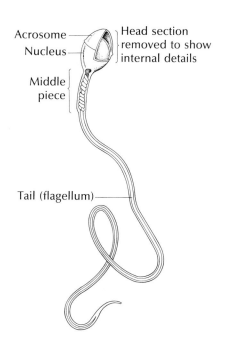

Figure 2-16 ■
Schematic representation of a mature spermatozoon.

but may vary from 1–10 mL. Repeated ejaculation results in decreased volume. Once ejaculated, sperm can live only 2 or 3 days in the female genital tract.

Sexual Intercourse

Many terms are used to describe the sexual mating of a sexually mature male and female. These include coitus, sexual intercourse, copulation, making love, and the sex act. Coitus is defined as the insertion of the erect penis into the vagina. After repeated thrusting movements of the penis, the man experiences ejaculation of semen concurrent with orgasm. *Orgasm* is the involuntary climax of the sexual experience, involving a series of muscular contractions, profound physiologic bodily response, and intense sensual pleasure. Orgasm may be achieved by other methods of sexual stimulation besides sexual intercourse, such as masturbation and oral stimulation.

Although the basic events of coitus are the same for all couples, wide variation exists in sexual positions, technique, duration, intent, meaning, and reactions among individuals.

Psychosocial Aspects

Coitus is a personal act between two consenting adults. It can signify a variety of feelings, beliefs, and attitudes.

The traditional purpose of coitus is procreation. However, with the availability of contraceptive methods and with changing social mores, sexual intercourse has become accepted as a pleasurable and personally gratifying experience in itself. The sexual union of two individuals may reflect their mutual commitment and caring, or it may be a more immediate interaction for the purpose of personal pleasure or merely temporary companionship. In our society, sexual intercourse ideally is the sharing by two persons of their emotions and bodies in the context of the larger sharing of their lives. Such sexual interactions are the result of mutual caring and love.

Physiology of Sexual Response

Masters and Johnson (1966) have identified and described the physiology of the sexual response in both males and females. All the responses can be classified as either vasocongestive or myotonic. *Vasocongestion* involves the congestion or engorgement of blood vessels and is the most common physiologic response to sexual arousal. *Myotonia,* a secondary physiologic response, is increased muscular tonus, which produces tension.

Sexual response occurs in four phases: excitement, plateau, orgasm, and resolution. Essentially, the sexual response of males and females is the same, involves the total body, and is continuous. Individual variations do occur.

The male physical response is relatively constant, resulting in orgasm if erection and sexual stimulation are maintained. Female sexual response varies considerably. Not all women experience orgasm consistently; they are influenced by their psychologic state, health, current sexual motivation, and environmental distractions. A woman may not experience orgasm during a particular act of coitus, or she may experience one or multiple orgasms of varying intensity. Such variation is usual in a woman of "normal" sexual activity, interest, and response.

Men and women exhibit several identical responses. The *sex flush* is a maculopapular rash that usually begins in the epigastric area and spreads quickly to the breasts. Less than half of men exhibit the sex flush, whereas more than half of women do. Heart rate and blood pressure increase in proportion to the degree of sexual excitement. Muscles tense beginning in the excitement phase. This tension increases during the plateau phase. Hyperventilation occurs just before and during orgasm. At orgasm, muscle tension is extreme. The face may contort, while muscles of the neck, extremities, abdomen, and buttocks contract tightly. Individuals may moan, murmur, or cry out and will experience a total surrender to bodily responses, accompanied by acute pleasure and relief.

The Nurse as Counselor on Sexuality and Reproduction

On occasion, most of us experience concern and even anxiety about some aspect of our sexuality. Societal standards and pressures cause us to evaluate and compare with others our sexual attractiveness, our technical abilities, the frequency of sexual interaction, and so on. Appearance and sexual behavior are not the only causes for concern; the reproductive implications of sexual intercourse must be considered as well. Some people desire conception; others wish to avoid it at all costs.

Because sexuality and its reproductive implications are such an intrinsic and emotion-laden part of life, people have many problems, needs, and questions about sex roles, sexual behaviors, family planning, sex education, sexual inhibitions, and other related areas. Clients frequently voice these concerns to the nurse, who may need to assume the role of counselor on sexual and reproductive matters.

Nurses who assume this role must be secure about their own sexuality. They also need to know about the structures and functions of male and female reproductive systems.

Continuing education for the practicing nurse and appropriate courses in undergraduate and graduate nursing education programs may help nurses achieve this sense of self-security and the knowledge about aspects of sexuality. These courses can teach nurses about sexual values, attitudes, alternative life-styles, cultural factors, and misconceptions and myths about sex and reproduction.

As nurses extend their expertise in the area of sexuality, taking a sexual history will become a standard procedure in the assessment phase of the nursing process. Although Mims and Swenson (1980) warn against the gathering of personal information for which there is no use, they urge the nurse to make logical assessments appropriate to each client's developmental level, educational level, and cultural background.

The adolescent clinic is one area in which discussion about sexuality and pregnancy risk is important. Assessing each adolescent's adjustment to the difficult teenage period naturally includes sexual assessments. The nurse can promote self-esteem, correct misconceptions, and even give the adolescent permission to say no to sexual intercourse.

Although there is no consensus about the level of counseling the professional nurse can give without additional preparation in the areas of sex education, family planning, and counseling, the nurse needs some judgment to make appropriate referrals. Most authorities agree that the higher the level of intervention, the greater the professional skill needed (Watts, 1979).

Rather than judging sexual behavior by predetermined standards of so-called normal behavior, the nurse should allow each individual or couple to evaluate their own sexual activities and reproductive choices. If nurses are to meet the needs of their clients satisfactorily, they must acknowledge personal differences in sexual behaviors and family planning measures and provide support or information whenever requested.

Summary

The miracle of life begins with the fusion of the egg and sperm in the woman's body. The structures and processes that make this miracle possible have been described in this chapter. The female and male reproductive systems are also involved in the expression of sexuality.

Both the development and continuing function of the reproductive organs are under neural and hormonal control. The roles of the hypothalamus and anterior pituitary are significant. These organs produce hormones necessary for the development of male and female characteristics as well as for the processes of spermatogenesis and oogenesis.

Understanding the development and processes of the reproductive organs enables nurses to counsel clients about reproduction as well as sexuality. Although the expression of sexuality is largely learned, nurses who understand the biologic and physical factors of sexuality can better answer clients' questions and help them make choices about sex and reproduction.

Resource Groups

Center for Population Options (2031 Florida Avenue N.W., Suite 301, Washington, D.C. 20009) The center develops program materials designed to encourage teens to be sexually responsible and works with youth-serving agencies to help develop sexuality education programs.

Institute for Family Research and Education (Syracuse University, 760 Ostrom Avenue, Syracuse, NY 13210) The institute sponsors National Family Sex Education Week and supports research and programs in sex and parent education.

Planned Parenthood Federation of America (810 Seventh Avenue, New York, NY 10019) The federation publishes family planning pamphlets for teenagers. Community educators in some localities visit classrooms and community groups.

References

Beller FK et al: *Gynecology: A Textbook for Students*, 3rd ed. New York: Springer-Verlag, 1980.

Caldwell WE, Moloy HC: Anatomical variations in the female pelvis and their effect on labor with a suggested classification. *Am J Obstet Gynecol* 1933; 26:479.

Gold JJ, Josimovich JB (editors): *Gynecologic Endocrinology*, 3rd ed. Hagerstown, Md.: Harper & Row, 1980.

Lackritz RM: Prostaglandins in pregnancy. In: *Gynecology and Obstetrics*. Vol 5. Sciarra JJ et al (editors). Hagerstown, Md.: Harper & Row, 1981.

Little AB, Billiar RB: Endocrinology. In: *Gynecology and Obstetrics: The Health Care of Women*, 2nd ed. Romney SL et al (editors). New York: McGraw-Hill, 1980.

Masters WH, Johnson VE: *Human Sexual Response*. Boston: Little, Brown, 1966.

Mims FH, Swenson M: *Sexuality: A Nursing Perspective*. New York: McGraw-Hill, 1980.

Vick RL: *Contemporary Medical Physiology*. Menlo Park, Calif.: Addison-Wesley, 1984.

Watts RJ: Dimensions of sexual health. *Am J Nurs* 1979; 77:1568.

Additional Readings

Crooks R, Baur K: *Our Sexuality*, 2nd ed. Menlo Park, Calif.: Benjamin/Cummings, 1983.

Fogel CI, Woods NF: *Health Care of Women: A Nursing Perspective*. St. Louis: Mosby, 1981.

Fromer MJ: *Ethical Issues in Sexuality and Reproduction*. St. Louis: Mosby, 1983.

Leach AM: Threat to nurses' sexual identity. In: *Comprehensive Psychiatric Nursing*, 2nd ed. Haber J et al (editors). New York: McGraw-Hill, 1982.

Spence AP, Mason EB: *Human Anatomy and Physiology*, 2nd ed. Menlo Park, Calif.: Benjamin/Cummings, 1983.

Woods NF: *Human Sexuality in Health and Illness*, 3rd ed. St. Louis: Mosby, 1984.

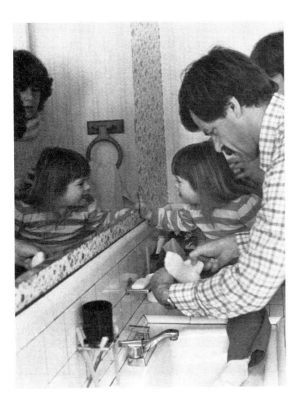

3

Families with Special Reproductive Problems

Chapter Contents

Infertility
Essential Components of Fertility
Preliminary Investigations
Tests for Infertility
Methods of Infertility Management
The Nurse's Role

Genetic Abnormalities
Chromosomes and Chromosomal Aberrations
Patterns of Inheritance
Prenatal Diagnosis
Postnatal Diagnosis
Genetic Counseling: The Nurse's Role

Objectives

- Discuss infertility and its effect on couples.

- Identify the various tests done in an infertility workup.

- Identify indications for chromosomal analysis.

- Discuss the significance of the Barr body in identifying sex chromosome abnormalities.

- Identify general characteristics of an autosomal dominant disorder.

- Compare autosomal recessive disorders with X-linked (sex-linked) recessive disorders.

- Compare prenatal and postnatal diagnostic procedures that may be used to determine the presence of genetic disease.

- Explain the nurse's responsibility in genetic counseling.

Key Terms ▬▬▬▬▬▬▬

autosomes
Barr body
basal body temperature (BBT)
chromosomes
ferning
heterozygous
homozygous

infertility
karyotype
Mendelian (single-gene) inheritance
sex chromosomes
spinnbarkeit
sterility
trisomies

Most couples who want children are able to have them with little trouble. Pregnancy and childbirth usually take their normal course, and a healthy child is born. But a few couples are not so fortunate and are unable to fulfill their dream to have healthy children because of special reproductive problems.

In this chapter, we examine two particularly troubling reproductive problems facing some couples—the inability to conceive and the risk of bearing children with genetic abnormalities.

Infertility ▬▬▬▬▬▬▬

For many couples, having children is an important and desired goal. But for some of these couples, conception is either impossible or difficult. These couples are identified as infertile.

Infertility is the inability of a couple to produce a living child either because they cannot conceive or because the woman cannot carry a fetus to a viable state. The term *primary infertility* is applied to those women who have never conceived. *Secondary infertility* describes the client who has formerly been pregnant but has not conceived during 1 or more years of unprotected intercourse (Coulam, 1982). The term **sterility** is applied when there is an absolute factor preventing pregnancy.

The incidence of infertility appears to be increasing, which may be related to the following factors:

1. More couples are delaying marriage and postponing childbearing until they have passed the age of optimal fertility (20–25 years of age).

2. Anovulation may be prolonged after using birth control pills.

3. Infections associated with intrauterine devices or following abortions can affect fertility.

4. Sexually transmitted diseases may cause obstructive disease of the male and female reproductive systems.

Essential Components of Fertility

Understanding the elements essential for normal fertility can help the nurse identify the many factors that may cause infertility. In Table 3-1, the essential components of normal fertility are correlated with possible causes for deviations. In addition to these necessary elements, certain general physiologic and psychologic conditions must be present to support conception. With intricacies of timing and environment playing such a crucial role, it is amazing that approximately 85% of couples in the United States are able to conceive. Of the remaining 15%, 40 in 100 couples will have a male deficiency; 10–15 in 100, a female hormonal defect; 20–30, a female tubal disorder; 5, a cervical defect; and 10–20, no discernible cause of infertility (Coulam, 1982). In 35 of 100 couples, multiple etiologies will be identified. Professional intervention can help approximately 30% of infertile couples to achieve pregnancy.

Couples usually are concerned about their fertility. Couples are considered infertile following their inability to conceive after at least 1 year of attempting to achieve pregnancy.

Preliminary Investigation

Evaluation and preliminary investigations should be available for couples seeking help for infertility. Extensive testing is avoided until data confirm that the timing of intercourse and length of coital exposure have been adequate. Figure 3-1 shows the sequence of health care interventions for couples seeking treatment for infertility.

During the first visit for preliminary investigation, the basic infertility investigation is explained. The basic investigation includes assessment of ovulatory function, cervical

Table 3-1
Possible Causes of Infertility

Necessary normal elements	Causes of deviations from normal
MALE	
Normal semen analysis	Congenital defect in testicular development, mumps after adolescence, cryptorchidism, varicocele, infections, gonadal exposure to x-rays, smoking, alcohol abuse, malnutrition, chronic or acute metabolic disease, medications (for example, morphine and cocaine), constrictive underclothing
Unobstructed genital tract	Infections, tumors, congenital anomalies, vasectomy
Normal genital tract secretions	Infections, autoimmunity to semen, tumors
Ejaculate deposited at the cervix	Premature ejaculation, hypospadias, retrograde ejaculation (for example, if diabetic), neurologic cord lesions
FEMALE	
Favorable cervical mucus for spermatozoa	Cervicitis, immunologic response ("hostile" mucus), use of coital lubricants
Clear passage between cervix and tubes	Myomas, adhesions, adenomyosis, polyps, endometritis, cervical stenosis, endometriosis, congenital anomalies (for example, septate uterus)
Patent tubes with normal motility	Pelvic inflammatory disease, peritubal adhesions, endometriosis, intrauterine device (IUD), salpingitis (for example, tuberculosis), neoplasm, ectopic pregnancy, tubal ligation
Ovulation and release of ova	Primary ovarian failure, polycystic ovarian disease, hypothyroidism, pituitary tumor, lactation, periovarian adhesions, endometriosis, medications (for example, oral contraceptives), premature ovarian failure
No obstruction between ovary and fimbria	Adhesions, endometriosis, pelvic inflammatory disease
Endometrial preparation for implantation	Anovulation, luteal phase defect, IUD

mucus, sperm, tubal patency, and pelvic organs. The foundation for a trusting relationship is established between the health professionals and the couple during this first visit. The couple is informed that a comprehensive history (including detailed sexual history) will be taken and that a physical examination is performed to identify any obvious causes of infertility before a costly, time-consuming, and emotionally trying investigation is undertaken. Infertility is a deeply personal, emotion-laden problem for the couple. The self-esteem of one or both partners may be threatened if the inability to conceive is perceived as a lack of virility or femininity. The nurse can comfort the client by offering a sympathetic ear, a nonjudgmental atmosphere, and appropriate information and instructions.

Tests for Infertility

Four general areas of function are investigated during a fertility evaluation: ovulatory function, cervical mucosal adequacy/receptivity to sperm, sperm adequacy, and tubal patency. The general condition of the pelvic organs is assessed as well. The tests to investigate these functions are designed to evaluate the anatomy, physiology, and sexual compatibility of the couple.

Ovulatory function   Ovulatory function tests include basal body temperature assessment, hormonal assays, endometrial biopsy, and ultrasound. The woman records her **basal body temperature (BBT)** daily using a special thermometer that measures temperature in tenths of a degree between 96F and 100F. This

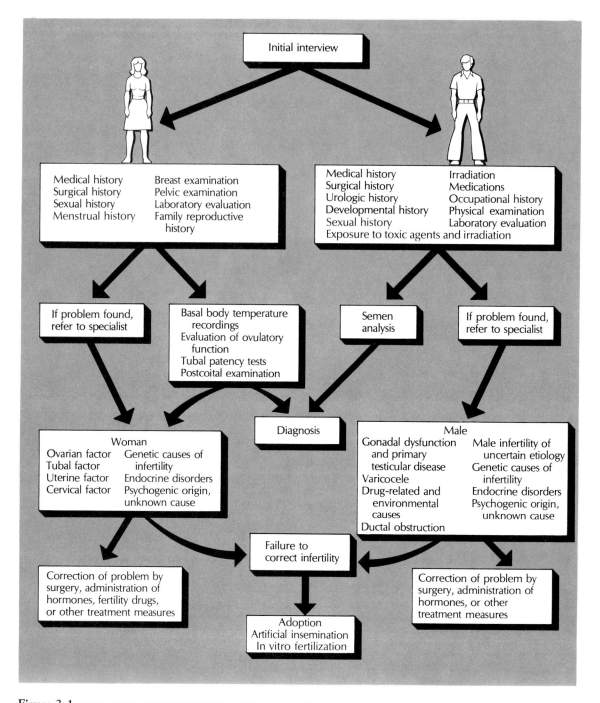

Figure 3-1

Flow chart for management of the infertile couple.

thermometer makes it easier to detect slight temperature changes. The thermometer should be kept beside the bed, and the woman should take her temperature upon awakening before any activity. Daily variations should be recorded on a temperature graph. The temperature graph and the readings are used for detecting ovulation and for timing intercourse.

BBT of females in the preovulatory phase is usually below 98F (36.7C). As ovulation approaches, production of estrogen increases and at its peak may cause a drop in the BBT. Then, when ovulation occurs, progesterone is produced by the corpus luteum, causing a 0.5–1.0F (0.3–0.6C) rise in basal temperature. Figure 3-2 shows a BBT chart. The rise in BBT is associated with increased progesterone production by the ovaries.

With the additional documentation of coitus, serial BBT charts can be used to indicate if, and approximately when, the client is ovulating and whether intercourse is occurring at the proper time to achieve conception.

Hormonal assessments of ovulatory function tests are available but used infrequently because they are too expensive and time-consuming. These tests fall into three categories:

1. *LH assays.* Daily samplings of serum LH at midcycle can detect the LH surge. The day of the LH surge is believed to be the day of maximum fertility. LH assay tests are still being refined.

2. *Estrogen assay.* Serum estradiol measurement at midcycle can be used to estimate the time of ovulation. Estrogen peaks approximately 1 day before the LH surge and 37 hours before ovulation.

3. *Progesterone assays.* Progesterone levels furnish the best evidence of ovulation and corpus luteum functioning. Plasma progesterone levels begin to rise with the LH surge and peak about 8 days after the LH surge.

Biopsy of the endometrium provides information regarding the effects of progesterone produced after ovulation by the corpus luteum. The biopsy is usually performed 2–6 days before menstruation, since this is the time of the greatest luteal function.

Ultrasound is now also being used to detect ovulation and changes in follicular development to determine the best time for artificial insemination or in vitro fertilization.

Cervical mucosal tests The postcoital examination (Sims-Huhner test) is performed 1 or 2 days prior to the expected date of ovulation. The couple is asked to have intercourse 2–4 hours before the examination. The evaluation consists of examining the cervical mucus and the number and motility of sperm present at the endocervix.

Changes in the cervical mucus can be used to evaluate hormonal influences. As described in Chapter 2, **spinnbarkeit** is assessed by stretching cervical mucus between two glass slides (Figure 3-3, A), by grasping some mucus at the external os and stretching it in the vagina

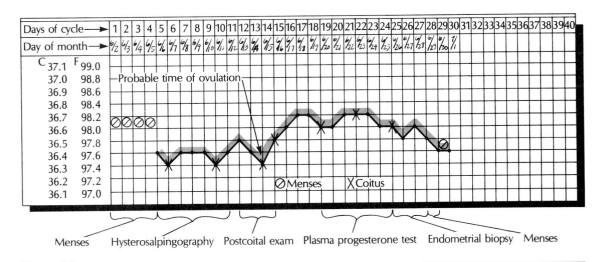

Figure 3-2

Basal body temperature chart with different types of testing and the time in the cycle that each would be performed.

toward the introitus, or by stretching the mucus between two fingers. Spinnbarkeit is most pronounced at the time of ovulation.

Crystallization of the cervical mucus, known as **ferning** (Figure 3-3, *B*), also increases as ovulation approaches. Ferning is caused by increased levels of salt and water interacting with the glycoproteins in the mucus during the ovulatory period. This mucosal change is an indirect indication of estrogen production. Mucus is obtained from the cervical os, spread on a glass slide, allowed to air dry, and examined under the microscope to detect ferning.

Sperm adequacy tests   Sperm analysis is the most important diagnostic study of the male.

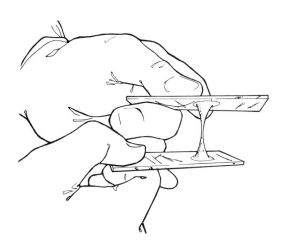

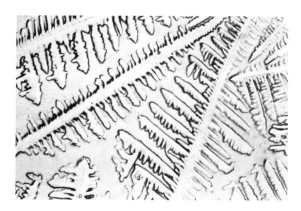

Figure 3-3
A, Spinnbarkeit (viscosity). **B**, Ferning. (Courtesy of Lovena L. Porter.)

Sperm may be obtained from a postcoital examination of the woman or from a semen specimen provided by the male. Optimum results are obtained when a specimen is collected after 2 days of abstinence.

Sperm analysis can provide information about sperm motility, morphology, and absolute number of sperm. Analysis of normal semen shows at least 50 million sperm per milliliter, semen volume of 2–5 mL, pH level of 7.2–7.8, sperm motility of greater than 60% (within 2 hours of collection) with normal progression, and at least 70% normal sperm forms. The chance to impregnate is remote if the semen analysis reveals less than 10 million sperm per milliliter, less than 50%–60% active sperm, or less than 70% normal sperm forms.

Recent studies document the occurrence of autoimmunity to sperm. Spermatozoa have been shown to possess intrinsic antigens that may provoke immunologic infertility. Therapy has been attempted with immunosuppressive agents and insemination techniques (Dondero et al., 1979).

Tubal patency tests   Tubal patency is confirmed with either tubal insufflation with carbon dioxide gas (Rubin's test) or hysterosalpingography.

Tubal insufflation gives only presumptive evidence of tubal patency, but its advantages are otherwise limited.

Hysterosalpingography, or a hysterogram, is an instillation of a radiopaque substance into the uterine cavity. It can reveal tubal patency and any distortions of the endometrial cavity. In addition, pregnancy has been frequently achieved within the first three cycles following the test.

Culdoscopy is used to assess tubular function. The fallopian tubes can be directly visualized with a culdoscope.

Laparoscopy is replacing culdoscopy as a favored means of viewing the pelvic organs directly. Women are usually given a general anesthetic before this procedure. An incision is made in the area of the umbilicus, and the peritoneal cavity is distended with carbon dioxide gas. With the laparoscope, the clinician can visualize the pelvic organs directly through the incision and tubular function can be assessed. Evaluation for endometriosis, adhesions, organ fixations, pelvic inflammatory disease, tumors, and cysts is done by instillation of a dye into the uterine cavity from below. Visualization is best when the procedure is performed in the early follicular stage of the cycle (Valle, 1984).

Routine preanesthesia instructions should be given. The client is told she may have some discomfort from organ displacement and shoulder and chest pain caused by carbon dioxide gas in the abdomen. This pain lasts 24–48 hours after the procedure. She should be informed that after resting for about 2 days she can resume normal activities.

Methods of Infertility Management

Pharmacologic methods   The treatment for a defect in ovulation depends on the specific etiology of the problem. In the presence of normal ovaries and an intact pituitary gland, clomiphene citrate (Clomid) is often used. This medication induces ovulation in 70%–80% of women. Supplemental low-dose estrogen may be needed to ensure appropriate quality and quantity of cervical mucus because clomiphene citrate may inhibit production of mucus.

Human menopausal gonadotrophin (hMG), a combination of FSH and LH obtained from postmenopausal women's urine, can be given during the first half of the cycle to stimulate follicular development. To effect ovulation, hCG must also be given. This method of treatment can cause severe reactions.

When endometriosis is determined to be the cause of the infertility, danazol (Danocrine) may be given. This medication suppresses ovulation and menstruation and causes the ectopic endometrial tissue to atrophy. It has an antigonadotrophin effect and suppresses both FSH and LH. Temporary suppression has been shown to result in healing of the endometrium. The return of menstrual function and fertility is prompt after discontinuation of danazol, with the first menstrual period occurring within 4–6 weeks.

Artificial insemination   *Artificial insemination* is the depositing of semen at the cervical os by mechanical means. The semen may be the husband's (AIH) or that of a donor (AID). The conception rates are approximately 30% for AID and 15% for AIH. AIH is used in cases of too small or large a semen volume, too few or too many sperm, low levels of spermatozoal motility, anatomic defects accompanied by inadequate deposition or penetration of semen, or retrograde ejaculation.

AID is considered in cases of total lack of sperm motility or combination of inadequate motility and viability of sperm, or inherited disorders affecting only males (pp. 58–59). AID is not appropriate therapy in cases of women with antibodies, since they have antibodies against antigens common to all human sperm cells, not just to their husband's sperm (Wallach et al., 1984).

In vitro fertilization   When tubal factors are the cause of infertility, *in vitro fertilization* is sometimes attempted. Human oocytes are collected by aspiration during laparotomy or laparoscopy for in vitro (outside the body) fertilization, then implanted in the uterus after early cell division has occurred (Machol, 1984). The first successful in vitro fertilization was reported in Great Britain in 1978. Since then, the number of births resulting from this method has increased (see Chapter 1 for a discussion of related ethical issues).

Adoption   The adoption of an infant is not as trouble free today as it was in the past. A waiting period of as long as 5–7 years to even begin the adoption process is not uncommon. Many out-of-wedlock infants are being reared by their mothers instead of surrendered for adoption as in the past, and many unwanted pregnancies are being terminated by elective abortion. Some couples seek international adoptions or consider adopting older children, those with handicaps, or children of mixed parentage because the adoption process is quicker.

The Nurse's Role

Approximately 4–5 million Americans are unable to conceive or carry a pregnancy to term, even after years of medical evaluation and treatment. The physical, emotional, and financial costs to a couple may be tremendous. Correction of infertility may require surgery, administration of hormones, or other treatment. The role of the nurse is to provide information and emotional support to the infertile couple throughout the procedures.

The nurse must be constantly aware of the emotional needs and sometimes irrational thoughts and fears of the couple with a fertility problem. Constant attention to temperature charts and instructions about their sex life from a person outside the relationship naturally affects the spontaneity of a couple's interactions. Their relationship will be stressed by these and other intrusive but necessary measures. The tests may heighten feelings of frustration or anger between the partners. It is in this emotionally laden atmosphere that infertility evaluation and management must take place.

Infertility may be perceived as a loss by one or both partners. Like the death of a loved one, this situation is attended by feelings of grief and mourning. Each couple passes through several stages of feelings, not unlike those identified by Kübler-Ross: surprise, denial, anger, isolation, guilt, grief, and resolution (Menning, 1980). Nonjudgmental acceptance and a professional caring attitude on the nurse's part can go far to reduce the negative emotions the couple may experience while going through this process. This is also a time when the nurse can assess the quality of the couple's relationship: Are they able and willing to communicate verbally and share feelings? Are they mutually supportive? The answers to such questions help the nurse identify areas of strength and weakness that will assist in counseling and developing an appropriate plan of care. At times, individual or group counseling with other infertile couples may help the couple resolve feelings brought about by their own difficult situation.

Genetic Abnormalities _____

The desired and expected outcome of any pregnancy is the birth of a healthy, "perfect" baby. Unfortunately, a small but significant number of parents experience grief, fear, and anger at this moment, when they discover that their baby has been born with a defect or a genetic disease. Such an abnormality may be evident at birth or may not appear for some time. The child may have inherited a disease from one parent, creating more guilt and strife within the family.

Regardless of the type or scope of the problem, parents will have many questions: "What did I do?" "What caused it?" "Will it happen again?" The nurse must anticipate the parents' questions and concerns and guide, direct, and support the family. To do so, the nurse must have a basic knowledge of genetics and genetic counseling. Many congenital malformations and diseases are genetic or have a strong genetic component. Others are not genetic at all. The genetic counselor attempts to categorize the problem and answer the family's questions. Professional nurses can help expedite this process if they already have an understanding of the principles involved and are able to direct the family to the appropriate resources.

Chromosomes and Chromosomal Aberrations

All hereditary material is carried on tightly coiled strands of DNA known as **chromosomes**. The chromosomes carry the genes, the smallest unit of inheritance.

All somatic (body) cells contain 46 chromosomes, which is the *diploid* number, while the sperm and egg contain 23 chromosomes, or the *haploid* number (see Chapter 4). There are 23 pairs of *homologous* chromosomes (a matched pair of chromosomes, one inherited from each parent). Twenty-two of the pairs are known as **autosomes** (nonsex chromosomes), and one pair are the **sex chromosomes**, X and Y. A normal male has a 46,XY chromosome constitution; the normal female, 46,XX (Figures 3-4 and 3-5).

The **karyotype**, or pictorial analysis of these chromosomes, is usually obtained from specially treated and stained peripheral blood lymphocytes. Although the use of peripheral blood is an easy, convenient method of obtaining chromosomes, almost any tissue can be examined to get this information.

Chromosome abnormalities can occur in either the autosomes or the sex chromosomes and can be divided into two categories: abnormalities of number and abnormalities of struc-

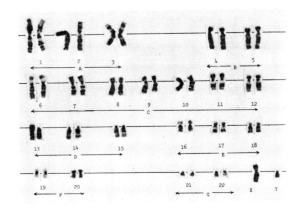

Figure 3-4

Normal male karyotype. (Courtesy Dr. Arthur Robinson, National Jewish Hospital and Research Center.)

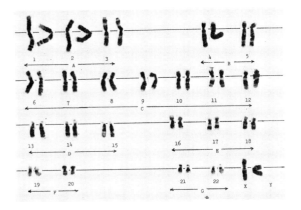

Figure 3-5

Normal female karyotype. (Courtesy Dr. Arthur Robinson, National Jewish Hospital and Research Center.)

ture. Even small alterations in chromosomes can cause problems, especially those associated with slow growth and development or with mental retardation. The child need not have obvious major malformations to be affected. In addition, some of these abnormalities can be passed on to other offspring. Thus, in some cases chromosomal analysis is appropriate even if clinical manifestations are mild.

Indications for chromosomal analysis include:

- Chromosome syndrome suspected (or clients with a clinical diagnosis of Down syndrome)
- Mental retardation and congenital malformations

- Abnormal sexual development (primary amenorrhea and lack of secondary sex characteristics)
- Ambiguous genitals
- Multiple miscarriages
- Possible balanced translocation carrier

Autosome abnormalities

Abnormalities of chromosome number Abnormalities of chromosome number are most commonly seen as trisomies, monosomies, and as mosaicism.

Trisomies are the product of the union of a normal gamete (egg or sperm) with a gamete that contains an extra chromosome. The individual will have 47 chromosomes and is trisomic (has three chromosomes the same) for whichever chromosome is extra. Down syndrome, or mongolism, is the most common trisomy abnormality seen in children. The presence of the extra chromosome 21 produces distinctive clinical features (see Table 3-2 and Figure 3-6).

Trisomies can occur among other autosomes, the two most common being trisomy 18 and trisomy 13 (see Table 3-2 and Figures 3-7 and 3-8). The prognosis for both trisomy 13 and 18 is extremely poor. Most children (70%) die within the first 3 months of life.

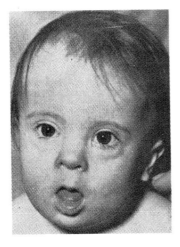

Figure 3-6

A child with Down syndrome. (From Smith, D. W. *Recognizable Patterns of Human Malformations.* © 1982 by the W. B. Saunders Company, Philadelphia, Pa.)

Table 3-2
Chromosomal Syndromes

Altered chromosome	Genetic defect and incidence	Characteristics	
21	Trisomy 21 (Down syndrome) (2° nondisjunction or 14/21 unbalanced translocation) 1 in 700 live births (Figure 3-6)	CNS:	Mental retardation Hypotonia at birth
		Head:	Flattened occiput Depressed nasal bridge Mongoloid slant of eyes Epicanthal folds White speckling of the iris (Brushfield's spots) Protrusion of the tongue High, arched palate Low-set ears Broad, short fingers
		Hands:	Short fingers Abnormalities of finger and foot dermal ridge patterns (dermatoglyphics) Transverse palmar crease (simian line)
		Other:	Congenital heart disease
21	2° mosaicism (Down syndrome)	Classic symptoms as described in trisomy 21 except that the child has normal intelligence	
18	Trisomy 18 1 in 3000 live births (Figure 3-7)	CNS:	Mental retardation Severe hypertonia
		Head:	Prominent occiput Low-set ears Corneal opacities Ptosis (drooping of eyelids)
		Hands:	Third and fourth fingers overlapped by second and fifth fingers Abnormal dermatoglyphics Syndactyly (webbing of fingers)
		Other:	Congenital heart defects Renal abnormalities Single umbilical artery Gastrointestinal tract abnormalities Rocker-bottom feet Cryptorchidism Various malformations of other organs
18	Deletion of long arm of chromosome 18	CNS:	Severe psychomotor retardation
		Head:	Microcephaly Stenotic ear canals with conductive hearing loss
		Other:	Various other organ malformations

Table 3-2
Chromosomal Syndromes (continued)

Altered chromosome	Genetic defect and incidence	Characteristics	
13	Trisomy 13 1 in 5000 live births (Figure 3-8)	CNS:	Mental retardation Severe hypertonia Seizures
		Head:	Microcephaly Microphthalmia and/or coloboma Malformed ears Aplasia of external auditory canal Micrognathia Cleft lip and palate
		Hands:	Polydactyly (extra digits) Abnormal posturing of fingers Abnormal dermatoglyphics
		Other:	Congenital heart defects Hemangiomas Gastrointestinal tract defects Various malformations of other organs
5	Deletion of short arm of chromosome 5 (cri du chat—cat cry syndrome) 1 in 20,000 live births	CNS:	Severe mental retardation A catlike cry in infancy
		Head:	Microcephaly Hypertelorism Epicanthal folds Low-set ears
		Other:	Failure to thrive Various organ malformation
X (sex chromosome)	Only one X chromosome in female (Turner syndrome) 1 in 300 to 7000 live female births	CNS:	No intellectual impairment Some perceptual difficulties
		Head:	Low hairline Webbed neck
		Trunk:	Short stature Cubitus valgus (increased carrying angle of arm) Excessive nevi Broad shieldlike chest with widely spaced nipples
		Other:	Fibrous streaks in ovaries Underdeveloped secondary sex characteristics Primary amenorrhea Usually infertile Renal anomalies Coarctation of the aorta
X	Extra X in male (Klinefelter syndrome) 1 in 1000 live male births, approx. 1%–2% of institutionalized males	CNS:	Mild mental retardation
		Trunk:	Occasional gynecomastia Eunuchoid body proportions
		Other:	Small, soft testes Underdeveloped secondary sex characteristics Usually sterile

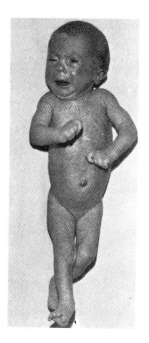

Figure 3-7 ▬▬▬▬▬▬

Infant with trisomy 18. (From Smith, D. W. *Recognizable Patterns of Human Malformations.* © 1982 by the W. B. Saunders Company, Philadelphia, Pa.)

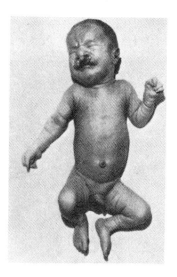

Figure 3-8 ▬▬▬▬▬▬

Infant with trisomy 13. (From Smith, D. W. *Recognizable Patterns of Human Malformations.* © 1982 by the W. B. Saunders Company, Philadelphia, Pa.)

Monosomies occur when a normal gamete unites with a gamete that is missing a chromosome. In this case, the individual will have only 45 chromosomes and is said to be monosomic. Monosomy of an entire autosomal chromosome is incompatible with life. The only exception is in the sex chromosomes. A female can survive with only one X chromosome; this condition is known as *Turner syndrome* (Table 3-2).

Mosaicism occurs after fertilization and results in an individual who has two different cell lines, each with a different chromosomal number. Mosaicism tends to be more common in the sex chromosomes, but when it does occur in the autosomes, it is most common in Down syndrome.

Clinical signs and symptoms may vary if mosaicism is present. In Down syndrome, the clinical signs may be classic, minimal, or non-apparent, depending on the number and location of the abnormal cells. An individual with many classic signs of Down syndrome but with normal or near normal intelligence should be investigated for the possibility of mosaicism.

Abnormalities of chromosome structure Abnormalities of chromosome structure involving only parts of the chromosome generally occur in two forms: translocation, and deletions and/or additions. Over 100 such abnormalities have been described in the literature. Again, Down syndrome is one of the most common syndromes described.

Not all children born with Down syndrome have trisomy 21. Instead, they may have an abnormal rearrangement of chromosomal material known as a *translocation*. Clinically, the two types of Down syndrome are indistinguishable. What is of major importance to the family is that the two different types have significantly different risks of recurrence. The only way to distinguish the two is to do a chromosome analysis.

The translocation occurs when the carrier parent has 45 chromosomes, usually with one of the number 21 chromosomes fused to one of the number 14 chromosomes. The parent has one normal 14, one normal 21, and one 14/21 chromosome. Since all the chromosomal material is present and functioning normally, the parent is clinically normal. This individual is known as a *balanced translocation carrier*. When this person has a child with a person who has a structurally normal chromosome constitution, there are several possible outcomes. The off-spring can receive the carrier parent's normal number 21 and normal number 14 chromosomes in combination with the noncarrier parent's normal chromosomes 21 and 14. In this case the offspring is chromosomally normal. Or the child may receive one of the balanced translocations, thus becoming a carrier like the carrier parent—chromosomally abnormal but clinically normal. If, however, the offspring receives the carrier parent's normal number 21 chromosome and the 14/21 chromosome and the noncarrier parent's normal chromosomes, the offspring receives two functioning number 14 chromosomes and three functioning number 21 chromosomes. At first glance, the child seems to have 46 chromosomes but actually has an extra chromosome 21. Thus the child has an *unbalanced translocation* and has Down syndrome. Other types of translocations can occur. But regardless of the chromosome involved, any person having a balanced chromosome rearrangement (translocation) has the potential of having a child with an unbalanced chromosome constitution. This usually means a substantial negative effect on normal growth and development.

The other type of structure abnormality seen is caused by *additions and/or deletions* of chromosomal material. Any portion of a chromosome may be lost or added, generally leading to some adverse effect. Depending on how much chromosomal material is involved, the clinical effects may be mild or severe. Many types of additions and deletions have been described, such as the deletion of the short arm of chromosome 5 (cri du chat syndrome) or the deletion of the long arm of chromosome 18 (see Table 3-2).

Sex chromosome abnormalities   To better understand normal X chromosome function and thus abnormalities of the sex chromosomes, the nurse should know that in females, at an early embryonic stage, one of the two normal X chromosomes becomes inactive. The inactive X chromosome forms a dark staining area known as the **Barr body**, or *sex chromatin body* (Figure 3-9).

The Barr body may be seen by examining the cells scraped from the inside of a client's mouth. This procedure, the *buccal smear*, will show the number of inactivated X chromosomes or Barr bodies present. The normal female has one Barr body, since one of her two X chromosomes has been inactivated. The normal male has no Barr bodies, since he has only one X chromosome to begin with. The number of Barr bodies seen on the buccal smear *is always* one less than the number of X chromosomes present in the client's cells.

When Y cells are stained and viewed, the Y chromosome appears as a bright body within the nucleus. The number of Y bodies present is equal to the number of Y chromosomes present. Males should have one Y body, and females should have none.

The most common sex chromosome abnormalities are *Turner syndrome* in females (45,X with no Barr bodies present) and *Klinefelter syndrome* in males (47,XXY with one Barr body present). See Table 3-2 for clinical description of these abnormalities.

Patterns of Inheritance

Many inherited diseases are produced by an abnormality in a single gene or pair of genes. In such instances, the chromosomes are grossly normal: The defect is at the gene level and cannot be detected by present laboratory techniques.

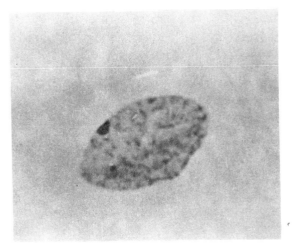

Figure 3-9 ▬▬▬▬▬
Nucleus with one Barr body; the patient is sex chromatin positive. (Courtesy Dr. Arthur Robinson, National Jewish Hospital and Research Center.)

There are two major categories of inheritance: **Mendelian** or **single gene inheritance**, and *non-Mendelian*, or *polygenic inheritance*. Each single-gene trait is determined by a pair of genes working together. These genes are responsible for the observable expression of the trait, referred to as the *phenotype*. The total genetic makeup of an individual is referred to as the *genotype*. One of the genes for a trait is inherited from the mother; the other, from the father. An individual who has two identical genes at a given locus is considered to be **homozygous** for that trait. An individual is considered to be **heterozygous** for a particular trait when he or she has two different *alleles* (alternate forms of the same gene) at a given locus on a pair of homologous chromosomes.

The well-known modes of single-gene inheritance are autosomal dominant, autosomal recessive, and X-linked (sex-linked) recessive. There is also an X-linked dominant mode of inheritance that is less common.

Autosomal dominant inheritance   An individual is said to have an autosomal dominantly inherited disorder if the disease trait is heterozygous. That is, the abnormal gene overshadows the normal gene of the pair. It is essential to remember that in autosomal dominant inheritance:

1. An affected individual generally has an affected parent. Thus, the family pedigree (graphic representation of a family tree) usually shows multiple generations having the disorder.

2. The affected individual has a 50% chance of passing on the abnormal gene to each of his or her offspring.

3. Both males and females are equally affected, and a father can pass the abnormal gene on to his son. This is an important principle when distinguishing autosomal dominant disorders from X-linked disorders.

4. An unaffected individual in most cases cannot transmit the disorder to his or her children.

5. Dominantly inherited disorders may have varying degrees of severity. A parent may have a mild form of the disease, whereas his or her child may have a severe form.

Some common autosomal dominantly inherited disorders are Huntington's chorea, polycystic kidney disease, neurofibromatosis (von Recklinghausen disease), and achondroplastic dwarfism.

Autosomal recessive inheritance   An individual has an autosomal recessively inherited disorder if the disease manifests itself only as a homozygous trait. That is, because the normal gene overshadows the abnormal one, the individual must have two abnormal genes to be affected. The notion of a *carrier state* is appropriate here. An individual who is heterozygous for the abnormal gene is clinically normal. It is not until two individuals mate and pass on the same abnormal gene that affected offspring may appear. It is essential to remember that in autosomal recessive inheritance:

1. An affected individual has clinically normal parents, but they are both carriers of the abnormal gene (Figure 3-10).

2. Parents who are both carriers of the same abnormal gene have a 25% chance of both passing the abnormal gene on to any of their offspring (Figure 3-10).

3. If the offspring of two carrier parents is clinically normal, there is a 50% chance that he or she is a carrier of the gene (Figure 3-10).

4. Both males and females are equally affected.

5. Parents who are closely related are more likely to have the same genes in common than two parents who are unrelated.

Some common autosomal recessive inherited disorders are cystic fibrosis, phenylketonuria (PKU), galactosemia, sickle cell anemia, Tay-Sachs disease, and most metabolic disorders.

X-linked recessive inheritance   X-linked or sex-linked disorders are those for which the abnormal gene is carried on the X chromosome. A female may be heterozygous or homozygous for a trait carried on the X chromosome, since she has two X chromosomes. A male, however, has only one X chromosome, and there are some traits for which no comparable genes are

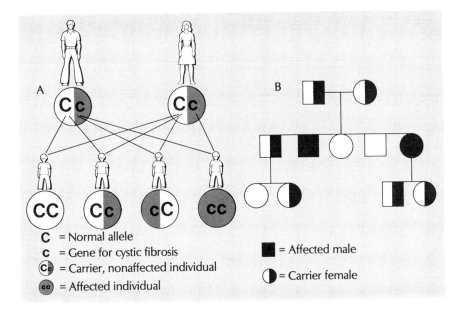

C = Normal allele
c = Gene for cystic fibrosis
Cc = Carrier, nonaffected individual
cc = Affected individual

■ = Affected male
◖ = Carrier female

Figure 3-10
A, Autosomal recessive inheritance. Both parents are carriers. Statistically, 25% of offspring are affected, regardless of sex. **B**, Autosomal recessive pedigree.

located on the Y chromosome. The male in this case is considered to be *hemizygous*, having only one allele instead of a pair for a given trait or disorder. Thus an X-linked disorder is manifested in a male who carries the abnormal gene on his X chromosome. His mother is considered to be a carrier when the normal gene on one X chromosome overshadows the abnormal gene on the other X chromosome. It is essential to remember that in X-linked recessive inheritance:

1. There is no male-to-male transmission. Fathers pass only their Y chromosomes to their sons and their X chromosomes to their daughters. Daughters receive one X chromosome from the mother and one from the father.

2. Affected males are related through the female line.

3. There is a 50% chance that a carrier mother will pass the abnormal gene to each of her sons, who will thus be affected. There is a 50% chance that a carrier mother will pass the normal gene to each of her sons, who will thus be unaffected. Finally, there is a 50% chance that a carrier mother will pass the abnormal gene to each of her daughters, who become carriers like their mother (Figure 3-11).

4. Fathers affected with an X-linked disorder cannot pass the disorder to their sons, but *all* their daughters become carriers of the disorder.

5. Occasionally, a female carrier may show some symptoms of an X-linked disorder. This situation is probably due to random inactivation of the X chromosome carrying the normal allele. Thus, a heterozygous female may show some manifestation of an X-linked disorder.

Common X-linked recessive disorders are hemophilia, Duchenne's muscular dystrophy, and color blindness.

X-linked dominant inheritance   X-linked dominant disorders are extremely rare, the most common being vitamin D–resistant rickets. When X-linked dominance does occur, the pattern is similar to X-linked recessive inheritance except that heterozygous females are affected. It is essential to remember that in X-linked dominant inheritance:

1. The abnormal gene is dominant and overshadows the normal gene.

2. There is no male-to-male transmission. An affected father will have affected daughters, but no affected sons.

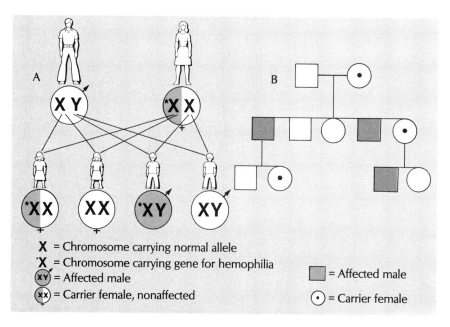

X = Chromosome carrying normal allele
˙X = Chromosome carrying gene for hemophilia
(XY) = Affected male
(XX) = Carrier female, nonaffected

▦ = Affected male

⊙ = Carrier female

Figure 3-11

A, X-linked recessive inheritance. The mother is the carrier. Statistically, 50% of male offspring are affected, and 50% of female offspring are carriers. **B**, X-linked pedigree.

Polygenic inheritance Many common congenital malformations, such as cleft palate, heart defects, spina bifida, dislocated hips, clubfoot, and pyloric stenosis are caused by an interaction of many genes and an environmental influence on those genes. They are, therefore, polygenic in origin. It is essential to remember that in polygenic inheritance:

1. The malformations may vary from mild to severe. For example, spina bifida may range in severity from mild, as spina bifida occulta, to more severe, as a myelomeningocele. It is believed that the more severe the defect, the greater the number of genes present for that defect.

2. There is often a bias of sex. Clubfoot is more commonly seen in males, whereas cleft palate is more common among females.

3. In the presence of environmental influence (such as seasonal changes, altitude, irradiation, chemicals in the environment, or exposure to toxic substances), it may take fewer genes to manifest the disease in the offspring.

Although most congenital malformations are polygenic traits, a careful family history should always be taken, since occasionally cleft lip and palate, certain congenital heart defects, and other malformations can be inherited as autosomal dominant or recessive traits. Other disorders thought to be within the polygenic inheritance group are diabetes, hypertension, some heart diseases, and mental illness.

Nongenetic conditions Not all disorders or congenital malformations are inherited or have an inherited component. Malformations present at birth may represent an environmental insult during pregnancy, such as exposure to a drug or an infectious agent (see Chapter 10). Some malformations, however, cannot be explained by genetic mechanisms or teratogens. These disorders are considered to have a developmental cause. Thus, a couple who has a child with phocomelia (abnormality of the limbs), in the absence of any other problems or family history, may be reassured that the problem is developmental in etiology and the risk for future pregnancies is low. Such reassurance is also appropriate for families concerned about a child's seizures or developmental delays, if they can be attributed to an acquired problem. For example, if the child was hypoxic during a difficult labor and delivery or had spinal meningitis, the resulting developmental delays can be attributed to the postnatal insult and not to a genetic mechanism.

Prenatal Diagnosis

Parent-child and family planning counseling have become a major responsibility of professional nurses. To be effective counselors, nurses must have the most current knowledge available concerning prenatal diagnosis.

The ability to diagnose certain genetic diseases by various diagnostic tools has enormous implications for the practice of preventive health care. Several methods are available for prenatal diagnosis, although some are still being used on an experimental basis. *Ultrasound* examination involves directing sound waves over the abdomen. With ultrasound, one can visualize the fetal head (from which fetal size and gestation can be approximated); locate the placenta; and determine the size of the uterus, the presence of twins, and structural abnormalities. Craniospinal defects (anencephaly, microcephaly, hydrocephalus), gastrointestinal malformations (omphalocele, gastroschisis), renal malformations (dysplasias or obstruction), and skeletal malformations are only some of the disorders that have been diagnosed in utero by ultrasound (Sabbagha et al., 1981). To date, there has been no evidence of harmful effects to either mother or fetus from exposure to ultrasound.

Amniography (the instillation of dye into the amniotic cavity to outline the fetus) and *amnioscopy* (direct visualization of the fetus through a scope) are two methods of prenatal diagnosis that are not yet available for general clinical use. These methods are used primarily to observe the fetus for major structural abnormalities or to obtain fetal blood and tissue.

The major method of prenatal diagnosis is genetic amniocentesis. The procedure is described in Chapter 11. The indications for genetic amniocentesis include:

- Previous child born with a chromosomal abnormality
- Parent carrying a chromosomal abnormality (balanced translocation)
- Increased maternal age (age 37 and over)
- Mother carrying an X-linked disease
- Parents carrying an inborn error of metabolism that can be diagnosed in utero
- Family history of neural tube defects (anencephaly or spina bifida)

One of the major indications for genetic amniocentesis is increased maternal age, since any woman 37 or older is at greater risk for having children with chromosome abnormalities. This maternal age effect is most pronounced for trisomy 21. For women between 35 and 40, the risk for having children with Down syndrome is 1%–3%; between 40 and 45 years, the risk is 4%–12%; after 45 years, it is 12% or greater.

Another fairly common indication for genetic amniocentesis is the risk of an autosomal recessive disorder, usually one of the biochemical inborn errors of metabolism. Presently, over 70 inherited metabolic disorders have been diagnosed in utero. Diagnosis is made by testing the cultured amniotic fluid cells (either enzyme level, substrate level, or product level) or the fluid itself.

Recently, genetic amniocentesis has been made available to those couples who have had a child with neural tube defects or who have a family history of these conditions, which include anencephaly, spina bifida, and myelomeningocele. Neural tube defects are usually polygenic traits.

Regardless of the statistical risk for a given family, whether for an isolated neural tube defect or a disorder in which a neural tube defect is a constant feature, the risk of recurrence can be reduced (possibly by as much as 90%) through α-fetoprotein (AFP) determination of the amniotic fluid. Normally α-fetoprotein is a substance found in high levels in a developing fetus and in low levels in maternal serum and in amniotic fluid. In pregnancies in which the fetus has an open neural tube defect, α-fetoprotein leaks into the amniotic fluid and levels are elevated. α-fetoprotein may also be elevated in cases of fetal distress, imminent or actual fetal death, and several other disorders. Thus, genetic amniocentesis allows those families for whom the risk of a neural tube defect is increased the opportunity to choose whether to have a child affected with such a disorder.

To date, most research has been in the prenatal diagnosis of hemoglobinopathies. Both sickle cell anemia and β-thalassemia have been diagnosed using fetal blood samples obtained by amnioscopy. Hemophilia A has also been diagnosed in fetal blood by measuring the ratio of factor VIII coagulant to factor VIII-related antigen (Frishein et al., 1979).

Perhaps one of the most promising breakthroughs is the prenatal diagnosis of cystic fibrosis. Walsh and Nadler (1980) report reduced amounts of 4-methylumbelliferyl quanidinobenzoate (MUGB) reactive proteases in amniotic fluid samples from fetuses with cystic fibrosis. If these findings continue to be confirmed, the prenatal diagnosis of cystic fibrosis may become a reality.

With the advent of diagnostic techniques such as amniocentesis, couples at risk, who would not otherwise have additional children, can decide to conceive. The percentage of therapeutic abortions after amniocentesis is small; most couples find peace of mind throughout the remainder of the pregnancy after prenatal diagnosis.

After prenatal diagnosis, a couple can decide not to have a child with a genetic disease. For many couples, prenatal diagnosis is not a solution, since the only method of preventing a genetic disease is preventing the birth by aborting the affected fetus. This decision can only be made by the family.

Prenatal diagnosis cannot guarantee the birth of a normal child. It can only determine the presence or absence of specific disorders (within the limits of laboratory error). Nonspecific mental retardation, cleft lip and palate, and PKU are a few of the disorders that cannot be determined by intrauterine diagnosis.

In the future, cure or treatment of diagnosable disorders may be possible. Prenatal diagnosis may allow for treatment to begin during the pregnancy, thus possibly preventing irreversible damage. For other disorders, effective postnatal treatment may make prenatal diagnosis unnecessary. The ability to diagnose many diseases in utero is proved every day. In light of the philosophy of preventive health care, this information should be made available to all couples who are expecting a child or who are contemplating pregnancy.

Postnatal Diagnosis

Questions concerning genetic disorders, cause, treatment, and prognosis are most often first discussed in the newborn nursery or during the infant's first few months of life. When a child is born with anomalies, has a stormy neonatal period, or does not progress as expected, a genetic evaluation may well be warranted. Before the primary health care provider can make an accurate diagnosis and direct appropriate care for the child, data from the following sources must be collected and evaluated.

- Complete and detailed histories to determine if the problem is prenatal (congenital), postnatal, or familial in origin
- Thorough physical examination, including dermatoglyphic analysis (Figure 3-12)
- Laboratory analysis, which includes chromosome analysis; enzyme assay for inborn errors of metabolism (see Chapter 21 for further discussion on these specific tests); and antibody titers for infectious teratogens, such as toxoplasmosis, rubella, cytomegalovirus, and herpes virus (TORCH)
- Consultation with other specialists
- Review of the current literature

This permits the geneticist to evaluate all the available information before arriving at a diagnosis and a plan of action.

Genetic Counseling: The Nurse's Role

Genetic counseling is a communication process in which the family is provided with the most complete and accurate information on the occurrence or the risk of recurrence of a genetic disease in that family. The goals are threefold:

1. Genetic counseling allows families to make informed decisions about reproduction.

2. It helps families assess the available treatments, consider appropriate alternatives to decrease the risk, learn about the usual course and outcome of the genetic disease or abnormality, and deal with other psychologic and social implications that often accompany such problems.

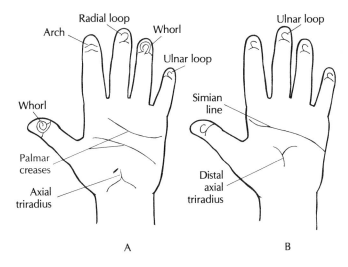

Arch · Radial loop · Whorl · Ulnar loop · Whorl · Palmar creases · Axial triradius · Ulnar loop · Simian line · Distal axial triradius

A   B

Figure 3-12

Dermatoglyphic patterns of the hands in **A**, a normal individual and **B**, in a child with Down syndrome.

Note the simian line, distally placed axial triradius, and increased number of ulnar loops.

3. Genetic counseling may help decrease the incidence and impact of genetic disease.

What can families expect?   The process of genetic counseling usually begins after the birth of a child diagnosed as having a congenital abnormality or genetic disease. After the parents have been referred to the genetics clinic, they are sent a form requesting information on the health status of various family members. At this time, the nurse can help by discussing the form with the family or clarifying the information needed to complete it.

At the initial genetic counseling visit, an extensive family history is taken in the form of a pedigree. The counselor gathers additional information about the pregnancy, the affected child's growth and development, and the family's understanding of the problem. Generally, the child is given a physical examination. Other family members may also be examined. If any laboratory tests, such as chromosomal analysis, metabolic studies, or viral titers, are indicated, they are performed at this time. The genetic counselor may then give the family some preliminary information based on the data in hand.

When all the data have been carefully examined and analyzed, the family returns for a follow-up visit. At this time, the parents are given all the information available, including the medical facts, diagnosis, probable course of the disorder, and any available management; the

inheritance pattern for this particular family and their risk of recurrence; and the options or alternatives for dealing with the risk of recurrence. The remainder of the counseling session is spent discussing the course of action that seems appropriate to the family in view of their risk and family goals.

The family may return a number of times to air their questions and concerns. It is most desirable for the nurse working with the family to attend many or all of these counseling sessions. Since the nurse has already established a rapport with the family, the nurse can act as a liaison between the family and the genetic counselor. Hearing directly what the genetic counselor says helps the nurse clarify issues for the family, which in turn helps them formulate questions.

When the parents have completed the counseling sessions, the counselor sends them and their physician a letter detailing the contents of the sessions. The family keeps this document for reference.

Appropriate referrals   Genetic counseling is an appropriate course of action for any family wondering "Will it happen again?" Nurses who are aware of families at an increased risk are in an ideal position to make the referral.

Following are the major categories of indications that help the nurse decide whether referral for genetic counseling is appropriate:

1. *Congenital abnormalities, including mental retardation.* Any couple who has a child or a relative with a congenital malformation may be at an increased risk and should be so informed. Also, if mental retardation of unidentified cause has occurred in a family, there may be an increased risk of recurrence.

In many cases, the genetic counselor will identify the cause of a malformation as a teratogen (see Chapter 10). The family should be aware of teratogenic substances so they can avoid exposure during any subsequent pregnancy.

2. *Familial disorders.* Families should be told that certain diseases may have a genetic component and that the risk of their occurrence in a particular family may be higher than that for the general population. Such disorders as diabetes, heart disease, cancer, and mental illness fall into this category.

3. *Known inherited diseases.* Families may know that a disease is inherited but not know the mechanism or the specific risk for them. An important point to remember is that family members who are not at risk for passing on a disorder should be as well informed as those family members who are at an increased risk.

4. *Metabolic disorders.* Any families at risk for having a child with a metabolic disorder or biochemical defect should be referred. Because most inborn errors of metabolism are autosomal recessively inherited ones, a family may not be identified as at risk until the birth of an affected child.

Carriers of the sickle cell trait can be identified before pregnancy is begun, and the risk of having an affected child can be determined. Prenatal diagnosis of an affected fetus is available on an experimental basis only.

5. *Chromosomal abnormalities.* As discussed previously, any couple who has had a child with a chromosomal abnormality may be at an increased risk of having another child similarly affected. This group would include families in which there is concern for a possible translocation.

Alternatives to increased risk   An important part of the genetic counseling session is discussion of the alternatives for a family at increased risk. Depending on the family history, the inheritance pattern of the disease, and the disease process, none, one, or several alternatives may be appropriate for the family to consider. Among those options are adoption, artificial insemination, delayed childbearing, prenatal diagnosis, and early detection and treatment.

Follow-up counseling   Perhaps one of the most important and crucial aspects of genetic counseling in which the nurse is involved is follow-up counseling. The nurse with the appropriate knowledge of genetics is in an ideal position to help families review what has been discussed during the counseling sessions and to answer any additional questions they might have. As the family returns to the daily aspects of living, the nurse can provide helpful information on the day-to-day aspects of caring for the child, answer questions as they arise, support parents in their decisions, and refer the family to other health and community agencies.

If the couple is considering having more children or if siblings want information concerning their affected brother or sister, the nurse should recommend that the family return for another follow-up visit with the genetic counselor. At this time, appropriate options can again be defined and discussed, and any new information available can be given to the family. Many genetic centers have found the public health nurse to be the ideal health professional to provide such follow-up care.

Summary

Understanding a couple's desire to have children is important for the health care provider. The nurse can help couples identify and correct causes of infertility and achieve their goal.

For families at risk of genetic problems, the nurse serves as the vital link between the genetic counseling team and the family. The nurse may be involved in case finding, referral, and preparation of the family for counseling. The nurse acts as a liaison during the counseling sessions and as a resource person after the sessions. Thus, it is imperative that nurses have a sound understanding of genetic principles and genetic counseling to provide families with the benefits of this aspect of preventive health care.

Resource Groups

Cystic Fibrosis Foundation (3379 Peachtree Road N.E., Atlanta, GA 30326)

Down's Syndrome Congress (P.O. Box 1527, Brownwood, TX 76801)

March of Dimes Birth Defects Foundation (1275 Mammoneck Avenue, White Plains, NY 10605)

National Association of Sickle Cell Disease, Inc. (945 South Western Avenue, Los Angeles, CA 90006)

National Genetics Foundation (250 West 57th Street, New York, NY 10019)

National Self-Help Clearinghouse (184 5th Avenue, New York, NY 10010)

Planned Parenthood, a national group with offices throughout the United States, offers contraceptive information and counseling services.

RESOLVE, Inc., a national organization with chapters throughout the United States, offers counseling, referral, and support for the infertile couple.

In addition, there are support groups for most disease conditions. Information about them often may be obtained from the family physician. The National Self-Help Clearinghouse can generally refer people to an appropriate support group.

References

Coulam CB: The diagnosis and management of infertility. In: *Gynecology and Obstetrics*. Vol 5. Sciarra JJ et al (editors). Hagerstown, Md.: Harper & Row, 1982.

Dondero F et al: Treatment and follow up of patients with infertility due to spermagglutinins. *Fertil Steril* 1979; 31:48.

Frishein SI, Joyer LW, Lazarchick J, et al: Prenatal diagnosis of classic hemophilia. *N Engl J Med* 1979; 300:937.

Machol L: Referring your patient for in vitro fertilization. *Contemp Ob/Gyn* 1984; 23:127.

Menning BE: The emotional needs of the infertile couple. *Fertil Steril* 1980; 34(4): 313.

Sabbagha R, Tamura RK, Dal Compo S: Antenatal ultrasonic diagnosis of genetic defects: Present status. *Clin Obstet Gynecol* 1981; 24:1103.

Valle RF: How endoscopy aids the infertility workup. *Contemp Ob/Gyn* 1984; 23:191.

Wallach EE, Beck WW, Eisenberg E, Hammond CB: Ethical Considerations in treating infertility. *Contemp Ob/Gyn* 1980; 23:226.

Walsh MMJ, Nadler HL: Methylumbelliferyl quanidinobenzoate-reactive proteases in human amniotic fluid: Promising market for the intrauterine detection in cystic fibrosis. *Am J Obstet Gynecol* 1984; 137:978.

Additional Readings

Grimes EM: For infertile couples: A holistic approach. *Contemp Ob/Gyn* 1984; 23:179.

Riccardi VM: *The Genetic Approach to Human Disease*. New York: Oxford University Press, 1977.

McKusick VA: *Mendelian Inheritance in Man*, 6th ed. Baltimore: Johns Hopkins University Press, 1982.

Shane JM, Schiff I, Wilson EA: The infertile couple. *Clin Symp* 1976; 28(5):2.

Smith DW: *Recognizable Patterns of Human Malformations*, 3rd ed. Philadelphia: Saunders, 1982.

Stanbury J et al: *The Metabolic Basis of Inherited Disease*, 5th ed. New York: McGraw Hill, 1982.

Stenchever MA: How to use the sperm penetration assay. *Contemp Ob/Gyn* 1984; 23:219.

Strickland OL: In vitro fertilization: Dilemma or opportunity? *ANS* January 1981; 3(2):41.

Whaley L: *Understanding Inherited Disorders*. St. Louis: Mosby, 1974.

Wiehe VR: Psychological reaction to infertility: Implications for nursing in resolving feelings of disappointment and inadequacy. *J Obstet Gynecol Neonatal Nurs* July/August 1976; 5:28.

These first kicks seemed timid, so light I wasn't certain expectation had not created them, but then as the weeks passed and they grew stronger. . . . I grew more confident. . . . It was not an illusion.

ANNE ROIPHE

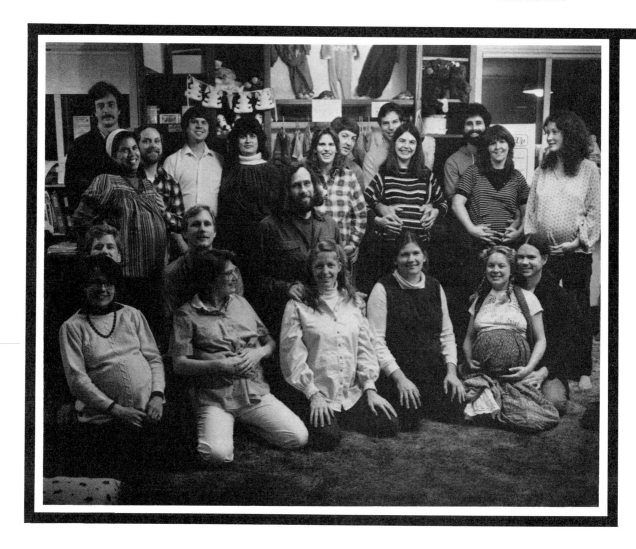

II

Pregnancy

4
Conception and Fetal Development

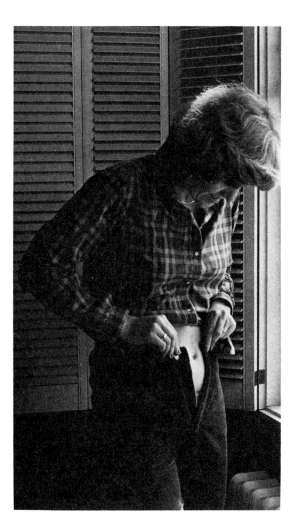

Chapter Contents

Cellular Division
   Mitosis
   Meiosis

Gametogenesis
   Ovum
   Sperm

Sex Determination

Fertilization

Intrauterine Development
   Cellular Multiplication
   Implantation
   Cellular Differentiation
   Intrauterine Organ Systems
   Embryonic and Fetal Development and
     Organ Formation
   Twins

Objectives

- Discuss the differences between meiotic cellular division and mitotic cellular division.

- Describe the structure and functions of the umbilical cord and placenta during intrauterine life.

- Identify the significant changes in growth and development of the fetus in utero at 4, 8, 12, 20, 24, 28, 36 and 40 weeks' gestation.

- Identify the vulnerable periods during which malformations of various organ systems may occur and describe the resulting congenital malformations.

Key Terms

amnion
amniotic fluid
blastocyst
chorion
cleavage
cotyledon
decidua basalis
decidua capsularis
decidua vera
  (parietalis)
diploid number of
  chromosomes
ductus arteriosus
ductus venosus
ectoderm
embryo
endoderm

fertilization
fetus
foramen ovale
gametogenesis
haploid number of
  chromosomes
lanugo
meiosis
mesoderm
mitosis
morula
trophoblast
umbilical cord
vernix caseosa
Wharton's jelly
zygote

Every person is unique. What is interesting about this uniqueness is that all of us have most if not all the same "parts," and these parts usually function similarly. Even our chromosomes, those determiners of the structure and function of our organ systems and traits, are made of the same biochemical substances. How do we become unique, then? The answer lies in the physiologic mechanisms of heredity, the processes of cellular division, and the environmental factors that influence our development from the moment we are conceived. This chapter explores the processes involved in conception and fetal development—the basis of uniqueness.

Cellular Division

All humans begin life as a single cell. This single cell reproduces itself, and in turn each new cell also reproduces itself in a continuing process. The new cells must be basically similar to the cells from which they came.

Cells are reproduced either by **mitosis** or **meiosis**, two different but related processes. Mitosis results in the production of additional body (somatic) cells. Mitosis makes growth and development possible, and in mature individuals it is the process by which our body cells continue to divide and replace themselves. Meiosis, by contrast, leads to the development of a new organism.

Mitosis

During mitosis, the cell undergoes several changes, ending in cell division. Before cell division occurs, the deoxyribonucleic acid (DNA) within the chromosomes replicates itself. The chromosomes then reproduce themselves, and the nuclear membrane and cell nucleus disappear. The duplicated chromosomes separate in pairs to opposite sides of the cell. A furrow develops in the cytoplasm at the midline of the cell, dividing it into two *daughter cells*, each with its own nucleus. Daughter cells have the same **diploid number of chromosomes** (46) and same genetic makeup as the cell from which they came. In other words, after a cell with 46 chromosomes undergoes mitosis, two identical (or daughter) cells, each with 46 chromosomes, result.

Meiosis

Meiosis consists of two successive cell divisions. In the first division, the chromosomes replicate. Instead of separating immediately as in mitosis, the similar chromosomes become closely intertwined. An exchange of parts between chromatids (the arms of the chromosomes) often takes place. At each point of contact, there is also a physical exchange of genetic material between the chromatids. New combinations are provided by the newly formed chromosomes; these combinations account for the wide variation of traits in people. The chromosome pairs then separate, each member of a pair moving to opposite sides of the cell. The cell divides, forming two daughter cells, each with half (23) of the usual number of chromosomes. In the second division, the chromatids of each chromosome separate and move to opposite poles of each of the daughter cells. Cell division occurs, resulting in the formation of four cells, each containing 23 chromosomes (the **haploid number of chromosomes**).

Gametogenesis

Meiosis occurs during **gametogenesis**, the process by which germ cells, or *gametes*, are produced. The gametes must have a haploid number (23) of chromosomes so that when the female gamete (ovum) and the male gamete (spermatozoon) unite to form the **zygote**, the normal human diploid number of chromosomes (46) is reestablished.

Ovum

As discussed in Chapter 3, the ovaries begin to develop early in the fetal life of the female. All the ova that the female will produce are formed by the sixth month of fetal life. The ovary gives rise to oogonial cells, which develop into oocytes. Meiosis begins in all oocytes before the female infant is born but stops before the first division is complete and remains in this arrested phase until puberty. During puberty, the mature primary oocyte proceeds (by oogenesis) through the first meiotic division in the graafian follicle of the ovary.

The first meiotic division produces two cells of unequal size with unequal amounts of cytoplasm but with the same number of chromosomes. These two cells are the *secondary oocyte* and a minute *polar body*. Both the secondary oocyte and the first polar body contain 22 autosomal chromosomes and one sex chromosome (X). At the time of ovulation, second meiotic division begins. Division is again not equal. An oocyte with the haploid number of chromosomes and another (second) polar body are formed from the secondary oocyte. Only when fertilized by the sperm does the secondary oocyte complete the second meiotic division, becoming a mature ovum. The first polar body has now also divided, producing two additional polar bodies. Thus, when meiosis is completed, four haploid cells have been produced: three small polar bodies, which eventually disintegrate, and one ovum (Figure 4-1).

Sperm

During puberty, the germinal epithelium in the seminiferous tubules of the testes begins the process of spermatogenesis, which produces the male gamete (sperm). As the diploid spermatogonium enters the first meiotic division, it is called the *primary spermatocyte*. During this first meiotic division, the spermatogonium forms two haploid cells termed *secondary spermatocytes*, each of which contains 22 autosomal chromosomes and either an X sex chromosome or a Y sex chromosome. During the second meiotic division, they divide to form four spermatids, each with the haploid number of chromosomes (Figure 4-1). The spermatids undergo a series of changes during which they lose most of their cytoplasm. The nucleus becomes compacted into the head of the sperm. (see Figure 2-17).

Sex Determination

The two chromosomes of the twenty-third pair (either XX or XY) are called *sex chromosomes*. The larger of the sex chromosomes is designated X, and the smaller sex chromosome is called Y. Females have two X chromosomes, and males have an X and a Y chromosome. Because male cells contain both an X and a Y chromosome, meiosis in the male produces two gametes with an X chromosome and two gametes with a Y chromosome from each primary spermatocyte. The sex chromosomes in oocytes are both X, and thus the mature ovum can have only one type of sex chromosome. To produce a female child, each parent must contribute an X chromosome. To produce a male, the mother must contribute an X chromosome and the father a Y chromosome.

The Y chromosomes contain mainly genes for maleness. The X chromosomes carry several genes other than those for sexual traits. As discussed in Chapter 3, these other traits are termed *sex linked* because they are controlled by the genes on the X sex chromosome. Two examples of sex-linked traits are color blindness and hemophilia.

Fertilization

The process of **fertilization** takes place in the ampulla (or outer third) of the fallopian

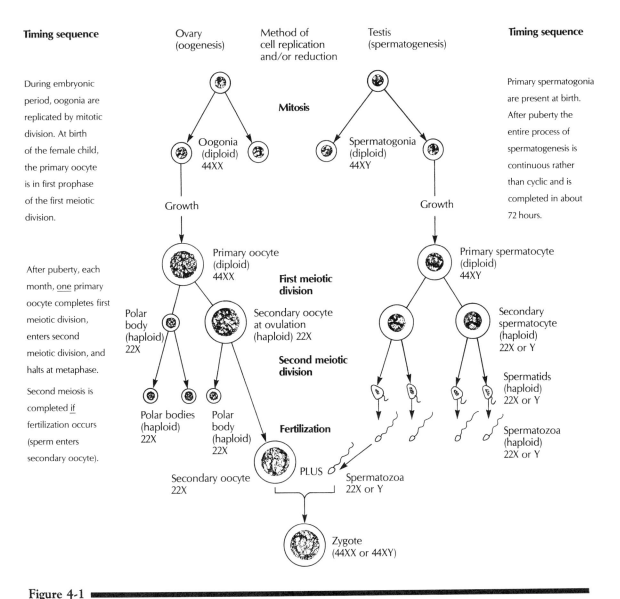

Timing sequence

During embryonic period, oogonia are replicated by mitotic division. At birth of the female child, the primary oocyte is in first prophase of the first meiotic division.

After puberty, each month, <u>one</u> primary oocyte completes first meiotic division, enters second meiotic division, and halts at metaphase.

Second meiosis is completed <u>if</u> fertilization occurs (sperm enters secondary oocyte).

Ovary (oogenesis)

Method of cell replication and/or reduction

Testis (spermatogenesis)

Timing sequence

Primary spermatogonia are present at birth. After puberty the entire process of spermatogenesis is continuous rather than cyclic and is completed in about 72 hours.

Mitosis

Oogonia (diploid) 44XX

Spermatogonia (diploid) 44XY

Growth

Growth

Primary oocyte (diploid) 44XX

First meiotic division

Primary spermatocyte (diploid) 44XY

Polar body (haploid) 22X

Secondary oocyte at ovulation (haploid) 22X

Secondary spermatocyte (haploid) 22X or Y

Second meiotic division

Polar bodies (haploid) 22X

Polar body (haploid) 22X

Spermatids (haploid) 22X or Y

Fertilization

Spermatozoa (haploid) 22X or Y

Secondary oocyte 22X

PLUS

Spermatozoa 22X or Y

Zygote (44XX or 44XY)

Figure 4-1

Gametogenesis involves meiosis within the ovary and testis. Note that during meiosis, each oogonium produces a single haploid ovum, whereas each spermatogonium produces four haploid spermatozoa.

(Modified from Spence, A. P., and Mason, E. B. 1983. *Human anatomy and physiology*. 2nd ed. Menlo Park, Calif.: Benjamin/Cummings Publishing Co., pp. 739, 748.)

tube. High estrogen levels during ovulation increase the ability of the fallopian tubes to contract, which helps move the ovum down the tube. The high estrogen levels also cause a thinning of the cervical mucus, facilitating penetration by the sperm.

The mature ovum and spermatozoa have only a brief time to unite. Ova are considered fertile for about a 24-hour period after ovula-

tion. Sperm can survive in the female reproductive tract for up to 72 hours but are believed to be healthy and highly fertile for only about 24 hours (Silverstein, 1980).

In a single ejaculation, the male deposits approximately 200–400 million spermatozoa in the vagina. The spermatozoa move up the female tract by the flagellar movement of their tails. Prostaglandins in the semen may increase uterine smooth muscle contractions, which help transport the sperm (Spence, 1982). The fallopian tubes have a dual ciliary action that facilitates movement of the ovum toward the uterus and movement of the sperm from the uterus toward the ovary.

The sperm must undergo two processes before fertilization can happen; they are *capacitation and the acrosomal reaction.* Capacitation is the removal of the plasma membrane overlying the spermatozoa's acrosomal area. Capacitation must occur in the female reproductive tract and is thought to take about 7 hours.

The acrosomal reaction follows capacitation. The acrosomal covering of the head of the sperm is believed to contain the enzyme hyaluronidase. As millions of sperm surround the ovum, they deposit minute amounts of hyaluronidase in the *corona radiata*, the outer layer of the ovum. This activity is the acrosomal reaction. The hyaluronidase breaks down enough hyaluronic acid in the outer layer of the ovum for one spermatozoon to penetrate the ovum (Figure 4-2). At the moment of penetration, a cellular change occurs in the ovum that renders it inpenetrable by other spermatozoa; thus only one spermatozoon enters a single ovum.

At the moment of penetration, the second meiotic division is completed in the nucleus of the oocyte, and the second polar body is produced. At the union of the gametes, each containing a haploid number of chromosomes (23), the diploid number (46) is restored. Also at this time, the sex of the new individual is established. Within the cell, the nuclei of the spermatozoon and oocyte unite, and their individual nuclear membranes disappear. Their chromosomes pair up, and a new cell, the zygote, is created. The zygote contains a new combination of genetic material, resulting in an individual different from either parent and from anyone else.

Intrauterine Development

Intrauterine development after fertilization can be divided into three phases: cellular multiplication, cellular (embryonic membrane) dif-

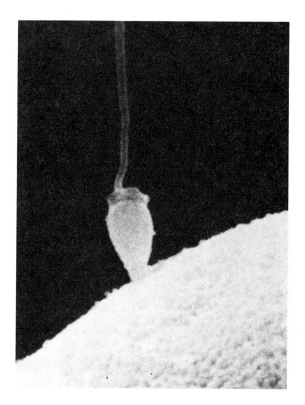

Figure 4-2
Electron micrograph of a sperm about to penetrate the surface of an ovum. (From Bloom, W., and Fawcett, D. W. 1975. *A textbook of histology.* 10th ed. Philadelphia: W. B. Saunders Co.)

ferentiation, and development of organ systems. These phases, intrauterine organ systems, and the process of implantation will be discussed next.

Cellular Multiplication

Cellular multiplication begins as the zygote moves through the fallopian tube into the cavity of the uterus. This transport takes 3 days or more (Pritchard, MacDonald, Gant, 1985).

The zygote now enters a period of rapid mitotic divisions called **cleavage**, in which it divides into two cells, four cells, eight cells, and so on. These cells, called *blastomeres*, are so small that the developing cell mass is only slightly larger than the original zygote. The blastomeres are held together by the *zona pellucida*, a layer of cells under the corona radiata. The blastomeres will eventually form a solid ball of cells called the **morula**. Upon reaching the uterus, the morula floats freely for a day, and then a cavity forms within the cell mass. The inner solid mass of cells is called the **blastocyst**. The outer layer of cells that surround the cavity and have replaced the zona pellucida is the **trophoblast**. Eventually, the trophoblast develops into one of the embryonic membranes, the **chorion**. The blastocyst develops into the embryo and the other embryonic membrane (the **amnion**). The journey of the fertilized ovum to its destination in the uterus is illustrated in Figure 4-3.

Implantation

While floating in the uterine cavity, the blastocyst is nourished by the uterine glands, which secrete a mixture of lipids, mucopolysaccharides, and glycogen. The trophoblast attaches itself to the surface of the endometrium for further nourishment. The most frequent site of attachment is the upper part of the posterior uterine wall (Figure 4-3). Between days 7 to 9 after fertilization, the blastocyst implants itself by burrowing into the uterine lining until it is completely covered. The lining of the uterus

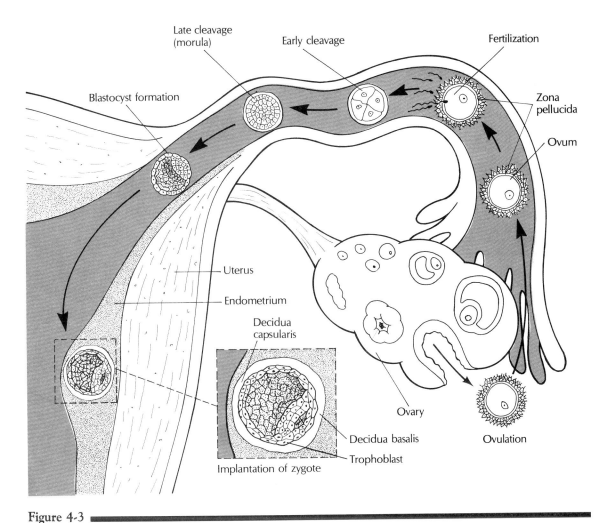

Figure 4-3

During ovulation, the ovum leaves the ovary and enters the fallopian tubes. Fertilization generally occurs in the outer third of the fallopian tubes. Subsequent changes in the zygote from conception to implantation are depicted.

thickens below the implanted blastocyst, and the cells of the trophoblast grow down into the thickened lining, forming processes called *villi*.

The endometrium, under the influence of progesterone, increases in thickness and vascularity in preparation for implantation and nutrition of the ovum. After implantation, the endometrium is called the *decidua*. The portion of the decidua that covers the blastocyst is called the **decidua capsularis**; the portion directly under the implanted blastocyst is the **decidua basalis**; and the portion that lines the rest of the uterine cavity is the **decidua vera** (*parietalis*). The maternal part of the placenta develops from the decidua basalis, which contains large numbers of blood vessels.

Cellular Differentiation

Embryonic membranes   The embryonic membranes begin to form at the time of implantation (Figure 4-4). These membranes protect and support the embryo as it grows and develops inside the uterus. The first membrane to form is the **chorion**, the outermost embryonic membrane that encloses the amnion, embryo, and yolk sac. The chorion is a thick membrane that develops from the trophoblast and has many fingerlike projections, called *chorionic villi*, on its surface. The villi begin to degenerate, except for those just under the embryo, which grow and branch into depressions in the uterine wall. By the fourth month of pregnancy, the surface of the chorion is smooth except at the place of attachment to the uterine wall.

The second membrane, the **amnion**, originates from the ectoderm, a primary germ layer, during the early stages of embryonic development. The amnion is a thin protective membrane that contains amniotic fluid. The space between the membrane and the embryo is the *amniotic cavity*. This cavity surrounds the embryo and yolk sac, except where the developing embryo (germ layer disk) attaches to the trophoblast via the umbilical cord. As the embryo grows, the amnion expands until it comes in contact with the chorion. These two slightly adherent membranes form the fluid-filled sac that protects the floating embryo.

Amniotic fluid   **Amniotic fluid** functions as a cushion to protect against mechanical injury. It also helps control the embryo's temperature, prevents adherence of the amnion, and allows freedom of movement so that the embryo-fetus can change position. The amount of amniotic fluid at 10 weeks is about 30 mL and increases to 350 mL at 20 weeks. After 20 weeks, the volume ranges from 500–1000 mL. The amniotic fluid volume is constantly changing as the fluid moves back and forth across the placental membrane. As the pregnancy continues, the fetus contributes to the volume of amniotic fluid by excreting urine. The fetus also swallows up to 400 mL every 24 hours. Amniotic fluid is slightly alkaline and contains albumin, uric acid, creatinine, lecithin, sphingomyelin, bilirubin, fat, epithelial cells, enzymes, and lanugo hair.

Yolk sac   In humans, the yolk sac is small and only functions early in embryonic life. It develops about the eighth or ninth day after conception and forms primitive red blood cells during the first 6 weeks of development until the embryo's liver takes over the process.

Primary germ layers   About the tenth to fourteenth day after conception, the homogenous mass of blastocyst cells differentiate into the primary germ layers. These layers, the **ectoderm**, **mesoderm**, and **endoderm** (Figure 4-5), are formed at the same time as the embryonic membranes. From these primary germ cell layers, all tissues, organs, and organ systems will develop (Table 4-1).

Intrauterine Organ Systems

Placenta   The placenta is the means of metabolic and nutrient exchange between the embryonic and maternal circulations. Placental development and circulation does not begin until the third week of development. The placenta develops at the site where the developing embryo attaches to the uterine wall. Expansion of the placenta continues until about the twentieth week, when it covers about one-half of the internal surface of the uterus. After 20 weeks' gestation, the placenta becomes thicker but not wider. At 40 weeks' gestation, the placenta is

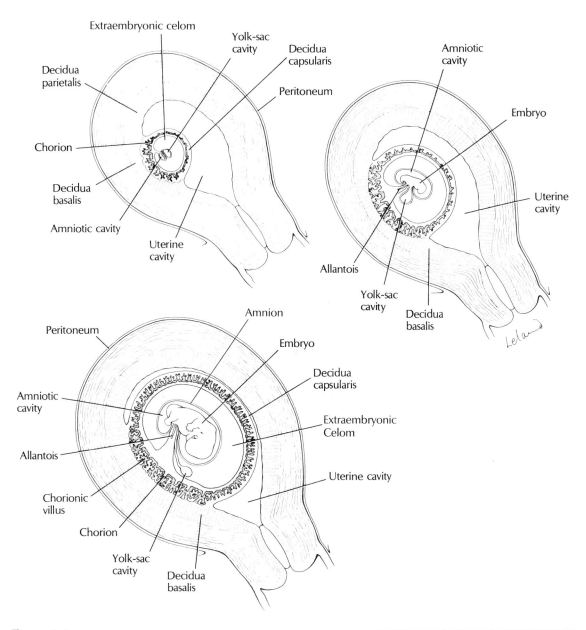

Figure 4-4

Early development of the embryonic membranes. Starting at the top left and moving clockwise, the early development of selected structures is depicted. The time sequence is from the 10th to the 14th day after conception to approximately the eighth week of pregnancy. (From Spence, A. P., and Mason, E. B. 1983. *Human anatomy and physiology.* 2nd ed. Menlo Park, Calif.: Benjamin/Cummings Publishing Co., p. 767.)

about 15–20 cm (5.9–7.9 in) in diameter and 2.5–3.0 cm (1.0–1.2 in) in thickness. At that time, it weighs about 400–600 g (14–21 oz).

The placenta has two parts: the maternal and fetal portions. The maternal portion consists of the decidua basalis and its circulation. Its surface is red and fleshlike. The fetal portion consists of the chorionic villi and their circulation. The fetal surface of the placenta is covered by the amnion, which gives it a shiny, gray appearance.

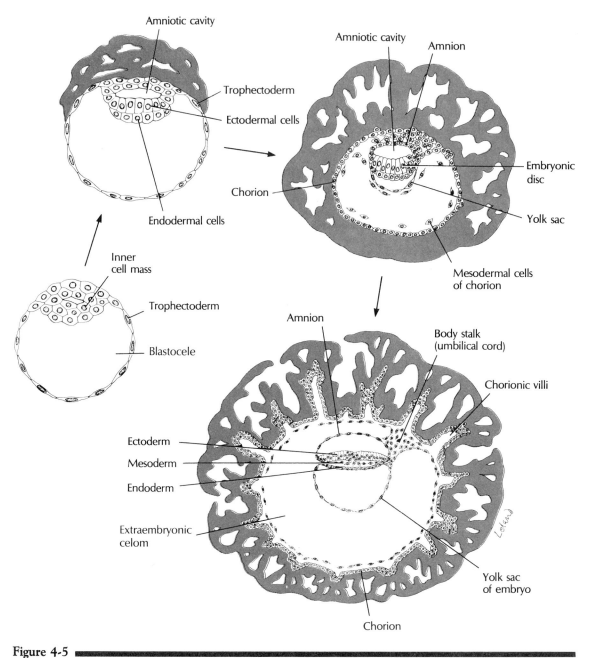

Figure 4-5

Formation of primary germ layers. (From Spence, A. P., and Mason, E. B. 1983. *Human anatomy and physiology*. 2nd ed. Menlo Park, Calif.: Benjamin/Cummings Publishing Co., p. 766.)

Development of the placenta begins with the chorionic villi. The trophoblast cells of the chorionic villi form spaces in the tissue of the decidua basalis. These spaces fill with maternal blood, and the chorionic villi grow into these spaces. As the chorionic villi differentiate, two trophoblastic layers appear: an outer layer, called the *syncytium* (consisting of syncytiotrophoblasts) and an inner layer, known as the *cytotrophoblast*. The cytotrophoblast thins out and disappears about the fifth month, leaving only a single layer of syncytium covering the chorionic villi. The syncytium is in direct contact with the maternal blood in the intervillous

Table 4-1
Derivation of Body Structures from Primary Cell Layers

Ectoderm	Mesoderm	Endoderm
Epidermis	Dermis	Respiratory tract epithelium
Sweat glands	Wall of digestive tract	Epithelium (except nasal), including
Sebaceous glands	Kidneys and ureter (suprarenal cortex)	pharynx, tongue, tonsils, thyroid,
Nails	Reproductive organs (gonads, genital	parathyroid, thymus, tympanic cavity
Hair follicles	ducts)	Lining of digestive tract
Lens of eye	Connective tissue (cartilage, bone, joint	Primary tissue of liver and pancreas
Sensory epithelium of internal and	cavities)	Urethra and associated glands
external ear, nasal cavity, sinuses,	Skeleton	Urinary bladder (except trigone)
mouth, anal canal	Muscles (all types)	Vagina (parts)
Central and peripheral nervous systems	Cardiovascular system (heart, arteries,	
Nasal cavity	veins, blood, bone marrow)	
Oral glands and tooth enamel	Pleura	
Pituitary glands	Lymphatic tissue and cells	
Mammary glands	Spleen	

spaces. It is the functional layer of the placenta and secretes the placental hormones of pregnancy.

A third, inner layer of connective mesoderm develops in the chorionic villi, forming *anchoring villi*. These anchoring villi eventually form the *septa* (partitions) of the placenta. These septa divide the mature placenta into 15–20 segments called **cotyledons**. In each cotyledon, the *branching villi* form a highly complex vascular system that allows compartmentalization of the uteroplacental circulation. The exchange of gases and nutrients takes place across these vascular systems.

In the fully developed placenta, fetal blood in the villi and maternal blood in the intervillous spaces are separated by three to four thin layers of tissue. The capillaries of the villi are lined with an extremely thin endothelium and are surrounded by a layer of connective tissue covered by chorionic syncytium (Figure 4-6).

Exchange of substances across the placenta is minimal during the early months of development. The villous membrane has not been reduced to its minimum thickness. Placental permeability increases until about the last month of pregnancy, when it begins to decrease as the placenta ages.

As the placenta is developing, the **umbilical cord** is also being formed from the amnion. The *body stalk*, which attaches the embryo to the yolk sac, contains blood vessels that extend into the chorionic villi. The body stalk fuses with the embryonic portion of the placenta to pro-

vide a circulatory pathway from the chorionic villi to the embryo. As the body stalk elongates to become the umbilical cord, the vessels in the cord decrease to one large vein and two smaller arteries. About 1% of umbilical cords have only two vessels, an artery and a vein; this condition is associated with congenital malformations. A specialized connective tissue known as **Wharton's jelly** surrounds the blood vessels. This tissue, plus the high blood volume pulsating through the vessels, prevents compression of the umbilical cord in utero. At term, the average cord is 2 cm (0.8 in) across and about 55 cm (22 in) long. The cord can attach itself to the placenta in various sites. Central insertion into the placenta is considered normal. (See Chapter 17 for a discussion of the various attachment sites.)

In the fully developed placenta, fetal blood flows through the two umbilical arteries to the capillaries of the villi and back through the umbilical vein into the fetus. Late in pregnancy, a soft blowing sound (*funic souffle*) can be heard over the area of the umbilical cord of the fetus. The sound is synchronous with the fetal heartbeat and the flow of fetal blood through the umbilical arteries.

Maternal blood, rich in oxygen and nutrients, spurts from the uterine spiral arteries into the intervillous spaces. These spurts are produced by the maternal blood pressure. The blood is then drained through the uterine and other pelvic veins. A uterine souffle, timed precisely with the mother's pulse, is also heard just

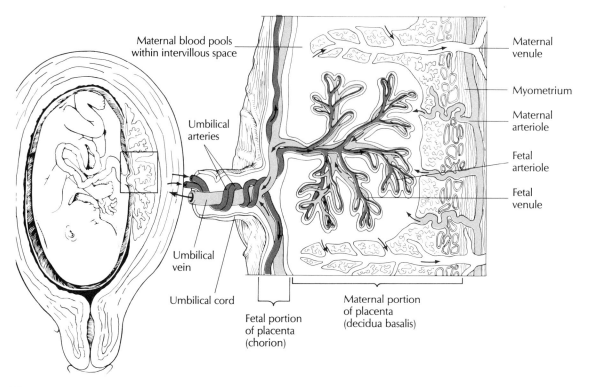

Maternal blood pools
within intervillous space

Umbilical
arteries

Umbilical
vein

Umbilical cord

Fetal portion
of placenta
(chorion)

Maternal portion
of placenta
(decidua basalis)

Maternal
venule

Myometrium

Maternal
arteriole

Fetal
arteriole

Fetal
venule

Figure 4-6

Vascular arrangement of the placenta. Arrows indicate the direction of blood flow. Maternal blood flows through the uterine arteries to the intervillous spaces of the placenta and returns through the uterine veins to maternal circulation. Fetal blood flows through the umbilical arteries into the villous capillaries of the placenta and returns through the umbilical veins to the fetal circulation. (From Spence, A. P., and Mason, E. B. 1983. *Human anatomy and physiology.* 2nd ed. Menlo Park, Calif.: Benjamin/Cummings Publishing Co., p. 764.)

above the mother's symphysis pubis during the last months of pregnancy. This souffle is caused by the augmented blood flow entering the dilated uterine arteries.

The functions of the placenta include fetal respiration, nutrition, excretion, endocrine functions, and special immunologic functions. Placental exchange functions can occur only in those fetal vessels that are in direct contact with the covering syncytial membrane. The syncytium villi have brush borders containing many microvilli, which greatly increase the exchange rate between the maternal and fetal circulation (Langman, 1981).

Endocrine functions The placenta produces hormones that are vital to the survival of the fetus. These include hCG; human placental lactogen (hPL); and two steroid hormones, estrogen and progesterone.

The hormone hCG is similar to LH and prevents the normal involution of the corpus luteum. If the corpus luteum stops functioning before the eleventh week of pregnancy, spontaneous abortion occurs. The hCG also causes the corpus luteum to secrete increased amounts of estrogen and progesterone. In the male fetus, hCG stimulates the fetal testes to produce small amounts of testosterone, which causes the male sex organs to grow.

The hormone hPL (sometimes referred to as human chorionic somatomammotrophin or hCS) is similar to human pituitary growth hormone; hPL stimulates certain changes in the mother's metabolic processes, which ensure that more protein, glucose, and minerals are available for the fetus.

After the tenth week of pregnancy, the placenta takes over the production of progesterone, which decreases the contractility of the uterus and thus prevents one cause of spontaneous abortions. By the seventh week of pregnancy, the placenta produces more than 50% of the estrogens in the maternal circulation. The primary estrogen secreted by the placenta is estriol, a different estrogen than that produced by the ovaries (estradiol). The placenta cannot synthesize estriol by itself. The fetal adrenal glands must provide estriol precursors. Measurement of estriol, therefore, can be a test of both fetal well-being and placental functioning.

Immunologic properties   The placenta and embryo are transplants of living tissue within the same species and are therefore considered *homografts.* Unlike other homografts, the placenta and embryo appear exempt from immunologic reaction by the host. Most recent data suggest that there is a suppression of cellular immunity by the placental hormones (progesterone and hCG) during pregnancy (Gudson and Sain, 1981).

Metabolic activities   The placenta produces glycogen, cholesterol, and fatty acids continuously for fetal use and hormone production. The placenta also produces numerous enzymes required for fetoplacental transfer, and it breaks down certain substances, such as epinephrine and histamine. In addition, it stores glycogen and iron.

Transport function   The placental membranes actively control the transfer of a wide range of substances by five major mechanisms:

1. *Simple diffusion* moves substances such as water, oxygen, carbon dioxide, electrolytes (sodium and chloride), anesthetic gases, and drugs across the placenta from an area of higher concentration to an area of lower concentration.

2. *Facilitated transport* involves a carrier system to move molecules from an area of greater concentration to an area of lower concentration. Molecules such as glucose, galactose, and some oxygen are transported by this method.

3. *Active transport* can work against a concentration gradient and allows molecules to move from areas of lower concentration to areas of higher concentration. Amino acids, calcium, iron, iodine, water-soluble vitamins, and glucose are transferred across the placenta this way.

4. *Pinocytosis* is important for transferring large molecules, such as albumin and gamma-globulin. Materials are engulfed by amebalike cells forming plasma droplets.

5. *Bulk flow of water* and some solutes result from hydrostatic and osmotic pressures.

Other modes of transfer exist. For example, fetal red blood cells pass into the maternal circulation through breaks in the placental membrane, particularly during delivery. Certain cells, such as maternal leukocytes, and microorganisms, such as viruses and *Treponema pallidum* (which causes syphilis) also cross the placenta, but the exact transport mechanism is not known. Some bacteria and protozoa cause lesions in the placenta and then enter the fetal blood system.

Reduction of the placental surface area, as with abruptio placentae, lessens the area that is available for exchange. Placental diffusion distance also affects exchange. In conditions such as diabetes and placental infection, edema of the villi increases the diffusion distance, thus increasing the distance the substance has to be transferred. Blood flow alteration changes the transfer rate of substances. Decreased blood flow in the intervillous space is seen in labor and with certain maternal diseases such as hypertension. Mild fetal hypoxia increases the umbilical blood flow, and severe hypoxia results in decreased blood flow.

Fetal circulatory system   Because the fetus must maintain the blood flow to the placenta to obtain oxygen and nutrients and to remove carbon dioxide and other waste products, the circulatory system of the fetus has several unique features.

Most of the blood supply bypasses the fetal lungs since they do not carry out respiratory gas exchange. The placenta assumes the function of the fetal lungs by supplying oxygen and allowing the fetus to excrete carbon dioxide into the maternal bloodstream. The blood from the placenta flows through the umbilical vein, which penetrates the abdominal wall of the fetus. It divides into two branches, one of which circulates a small amount of blood through the fetal liver and empties into the inferior vena cava through the hepatic vein. The second and larger branch, called the **ductus venosus**, empties directly into the fetal vena cava. This blood then enters the right atrium, passes through the **foramen ovale** into the left atrium, and pours into the left ventricle, which pumps it into the aorta. Some blood returning from the head and upper extremities by way of the superior vena cava is emptied into the right atrium and passes through the tricuspid valve into the right ventricle. This blood is pumped into the pulmonary artery, and a small amount passes to the lungs, to provide nourishment only. The larger portion of blood passes from the pulmonary artery through the **ductus arteriosus** into the descending aorta, bypassing the lungs. Finally, blood returns to the placenta through the two umbilical arteries, and the process is repeated (Figure 4-7).

The fetus receives oxygen via diffusion from the maternal circulation. The fetus is able to obtain sufficient oxygen from the maternal circulation (even though the Po$_2$ is 30 mm Hg) due to special fetal hemoglobin, which carries as much as 20%–30% more oxygen than adult hemoglobin. Also, the fetal hemoglobin concentration is about 50% greater than that of the mother. For further discussion, see Chapter 19. Fetal circulation delivers the highest available oxygen concentration to the head, neck, brain, and heart and a lesser amount of oxygenated blood to the abdominal organs and the lower body. This circulatory pattern leads to *cephalocaudal* (head-to-tail) development.

Embryonic and Fetal Development and Organ Formation

Pregnancy is calculated to last about 280 days (40 weeks). This period of 280 days is calculated from the beginning of the last menstrual period to the time of delivery. The gestational age of the fetus is calculated to be about 2 weeks less, or 266 days (38 weeks). The latter measurement is more accurate because it measures time from the fertilization of the ovum, or conception. The basic events of organ development in the embryo and fetus are outlined in Table 4-2. The time periods in the table are gestational age periods (postconception development).

Preembryonic stage   The first 14 days of human development, starting on the day the ovum is fertilized, are referred to as the *preembryonic stage* or the *stage of the ovum*. This period is characterized by rapid cellular multiplication and differentiation and the establishment of the embryonic membranes and primary germ layers, discussed earlier.

Embryonic stage   The stage of the **embryo** starts on the fifteenth day (the beginning of the third week after conception) and continues until approximately the eighth week or until the embryo reaches a crown-to-rump (C-R) length of 3 cm or 1.2 in. This length is usually reached about 49 days after fertilization (the end of the eighth gestational week). During the embryonic stage, tissues differentiate into essential organs, and the main external features develop.

Third week   In the third week the embryonic disk becomes elongated and pear-shaped with a broad cephalic end and a narrow caudal end (Figure 4-8). The ectoderm has formed a long cylindrical tube for brain and spinal cord development. The gastrointestinal tract, created from the endoderm, appears as another tubelike structure communicating with the yolk sac. The most advanced organ is the heart. At 3 weeks, a single tubular heart forms just outside the body cavity of the embryo.

Fourth to fifth weeks   During days 21 to 32, *somites*, a series of mesodermal blocks, form on either side of the embryo's midline. The vertebras that form the spinal column will develop from these somites. Prior to 28 days, arm and leg buds are not visible, but the tail bud is present. The pharyngeal arches—which will form the lower jaw, hyoid bone, and larynx—develop at this time. The pharyngeal pouches appear now; these pouches will form the eustachian tube and cavity of the middle ear, the tonsils, and the parathyroid and thymus glands. The primordia of the ear and eye are also present. By the end of 28 days, the tubular heart is beating at a regular rhythm and pushing its own primitive blood cells through the main blood vessels. By day 35, the arm and leg buds are well developed, with paddle-shaped hand and foot plates. The brain has differentiated, and ten cranial nerve pairs are recognizable.

Text continued on p. 86.

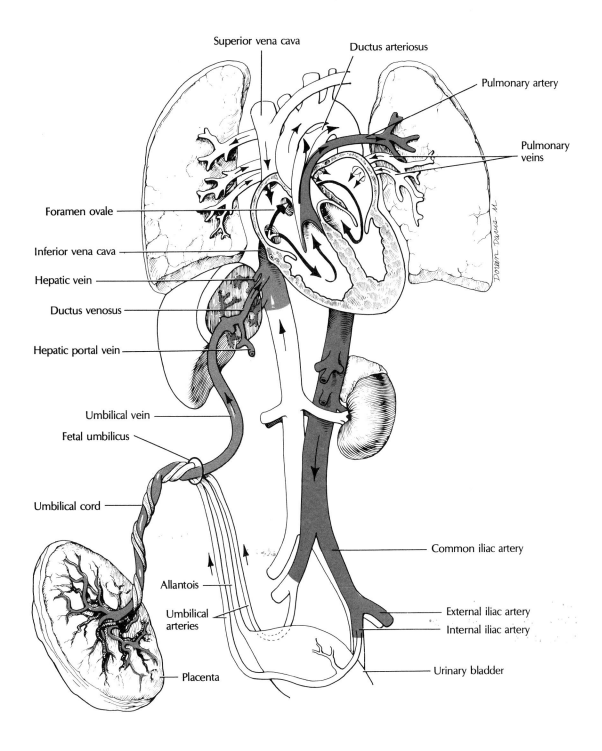

Figure 4-7

Fetal circulation. Blood leaves the placenta and enters the fetus through the umbilical vein. After circulating through the fetus, the blood returns to the placenta through the umbilical arteries. The ductus venosus, the foramen ovale, and the ductus arteriosus allow the blood to bypass the fetal liver and lungs. (From Spence, A. P., and Mason, E. B. 1983. *Human anatomy and physiology*. 2nd ed. Menlo Park, Calif.: Benjamin/Cummings Publishing Co., p. 776.)

Table 4-2
Classification of Organ System Development*

Gestational age[†]	Length[‡]	Weight	Nervous system	Musculoskeletal system	Cardiovascular system	Gastrointestinal system
Conception						
2–3 weeks	2 mm C–R		Groove is formed along middle of back as cells thicken; neural tube formed from closure of neural groove		Beginning of blood circulation; heart begins to form during third week	
4 weeks	4–5 mm C–R	0.4 g	Anterior portion of neural tube closes to form brain; closure of posterior end forms spinal cord	Noticeable limb buds	Tubular heart is beating at 24 days and primitive red blood cells are circulating through fetus and chorionic villi	Mouth: formation of oral cavity; primitive jaws present; esophagotracheal septum begins division of esophagus and trachea Digestive tract: stomach forms; esophagus and intestine become tubular; ducts of pancreas and liver forming
5 weeks	8 mm C–R	Only 0.5% of total body weight is fat (to 20 weeks)	Brain has differentiated and cranial nerves are present	Developing muscles have innervation	Atrial division has occurred	
6 weeks	12 mm C–R			Bone rudiments present; primitive skeletal shape forming; muscle mass begins to develop; ossification of skull and jaws begins	Chambers present in heart; groups of blood cells can be identified	Oral and nasal cavities and upper lip formed
7 weeks	18 mm C–R				Fetal heartbeats can be detected	Mouth: tongue separates; palate folds Digestive tract: stomach attains final form

*Adapted from Langman, J. 1981. *Medical embryology*. 4th ed. Baltimore: Williams & Wilkins; and Moore, K. L. 1977. *The developing human*. 2nd ed. Philadelphia: W. B. Saunders.
[†]Refers to gestational age of fetus/conceptus; postconception age.
[‡]C-R = crown-rump; C-H = crown-heel

Table 4-2
Classification of Organ System Development (continued)

Genitourinary system	Respiratory system	Skin	Specific organ systems	Sexual development
Formation of kidneys beginning	Nasal pits forming		Endocrine system: thyroid tissue appears Eyes: optic cup and lens pit have formed; pigment in eyes Ear: auditory pit is now enclosed structure Liver function begins	
	Trachea, bronchi, and lung buds present		Ear: formation of external, middle, and inner ear continues Liver begins to form red blood cells	Embryonic sex glands appear
Separation of bladder and urethra from rectum	Diaphragm separates abdominal and thoracic cavities		Eyes: optic nerve formed; eyelids appear; thickening of lens	Differentiation of sex glands into ovaries and testes begins

Table 4-2
Classification of Organ System Development (continued)

Gestational age[†]	Length[‡]	Weight	Nervous system	Musculoskeletal system	Cardiovascular system	Gastrointestinal system
8 weeks	2.5–3 cm C–R	2 g		Digits formed; further differentiation of cells in primitive skeleton; cartilaginous bones show first signs of ossification; development of muscles in trunk, limbs, and head; some movement of fetus is now possible	Development of heart is essentially complete; fetal circulation follows two circuits — four extraembryonic and two intraembryonic	Mouth: completion of lip fusion Digestive tract: rotation in midgut; anal membrane has perforated
10 weeks	5–6 cm C–H	14 g	Neurons appear at caudal end of spinal cord; basic divisions of the brain present	Fingers and toes begin nail growth		Mouth: separation of lips from jaw; fusion of palate folds Digestive tract: developing intestines enclosed in abdomen
12 weeks	8 cm C–R, 11.5 cm C–H	45 g		Clear outlining of miniature bones (12–20 weeks); process of ossification is established throughout fetal body; appearance of involuntary muscles in viscera		Mouth: completion of fusion of palate Digestive tract: appearance of muscles in gut; bile secretion begins; liver is major producer of red blood cells
16 weeks	13.5 cm C–R, 15 cm C–H	200 g		Teeth: beginning formation of hard tissue that will become central incisors.		Mouth: differentiation of hard and soft palate Digestive tract: development of gastric and intestinal glands; intestines begin to collect meconium
18 weeks				Teeth: beginning formation of hard tissue (enamel and dentine) that will become lateral incisors	Fetal heart tones audible with fetoscope at 16–20 weeks	
20 weeks	19 cm C–R, 25 cm C–H	435 g (6% of total body weight is fat)	Myelination of spinal cord begins	Teeth: beginning formation of hard tissue that will become canine and first molar Lower limbs are of final relative proportions		Fetus actively sucks and swallows amniotic fluid; peristaltic movements begin

Table 4-2

Classification of Organ System Development (continued)

Genitourinary system	Respiratory system	Skin	Specific organ systems	Sexual development
			Ear: external, middle, and inner ear assuming final structure forms Eyelids fusing closed	Male and female external genitals appear similar until end of ninth week
Bladder sac formed Urine formed			Endocrine system: islets of Langerhans differentiated Eyes: development of lacrimal duct	
	Lungs acquire definitive shape	Skin pink, delicate	Endocrine system: hormonal secretion from thyroid Immunologic system: appearance of lymphoid tissue in fetal thymus gland	
Kidneys assume typical shape and organization		Appearance of scalp hair; lanugo present on body; transparent skin with visible blood vessels	Eye, ear, and nose formed Sweat glands developing	Sex determination possible
		Lanugo covers entire body; brown fat begins to form; vernix caseosa begins to form	Immunologic system: detectable levels of fetal antibodies (IgG type) Blood formation: iron is stored and bone marrow is increasingly important	

Table 4-2
Classification of Organ System Development (continued)

Gestational age[†]	Length[‡]	Weight	Nervous system	Musculoskeletal system	Cardiovascular system	Gastrointestinal system
24 weeks	23 cm C-R, 30 cm C-H	780 g	Structure of brain; looks like mature brain	Teeth: beginning formation of hard tissue that will become second molar		
28 weeks	27 cm C-R, 35 cm C-H	1250 g	Nervous system begins regulation of some body functions			
32 weeks	31 cm C-R, 40 cm C-H	2000 g	More reflexes present			
36 weeks	35 cm C-R, 45 cm C-H	2750 g		Distal femoral ossification centers present		
40 weeks	40 cm C-R, 50 cm C-H	3200+ g (16% of total body weight is fat)				

Sixth week At 6 weeks, the trunk is straighter (Figure 4-9). The upper and lower jaw are visible, and the external nares are well formed. The trachea has developed, and its caudal end is bifurcated for beginning lung formation. The upper lip has formed, and the palate is developing. Both arms and legs have digits, although they may still be webbed, and the arms are more developed than the legs. Beginning at this stage, the prominent tail recedes. The heart now has most of its definitive characteristics, and fetal circulation begins to be established. The liver begins to produce blood cells.

Eighth week At the eighth week, the embryo is approximately 3 cm (1.2 in) long (C-R) and clearly resembles a human being (Figure 4-10). Facial features continue to develop. The eyelids, which fuse by the end of the eighth week, will not open until 28 weeks. External genitals appear but are not discernible, and the rectal passage opens with the perforation of the

Table 4-2
Classification of Organ System Development (continued)

Genitourinary system	Respiratory system	Skin	Specific organ systems	Sexual development
	Respiratory movements may occur (24–40 weeks) Nostrils reopen Alveoli appear in lungs and begin production of surfactant; gas exchange possible	Skin reddish and wrinkled, vernix caseosa present	Immunologic system: IgG levels reach maternal levels Eyes structurally complete	
		Adipose tissue accumulates rapidly; nails appear; eyebrows and eyelashes present	Eyes: eyelids open (28–32 weeks)	Testes descend into inguinal canal and upper scrotum
		Skin pale; body rounded; lanugo disappearing; hair fuzzy or woolly; few sole creases; sebaceous glands active and helping to produce vernix caseosa (36–40 weeks)	Ear lobes soft with little cartilage	Scrotum small and few rugae present; descent of testes into upper scrotum to stay (36–40 weeks)
At 38 weeks, lecithin-sphingomyelin (L/S) ratio approaches 2:1		Skin smooth and pink; vernix present in skinfolds; moderate to profuse silky hair; lanugo hair on shoulders and upper back; nails extend over tips of digits; creases cover sole	Ear lobes stiffened by thick cartilage	Males: rugous scrotum Females: labia majora well developed

anal membrane. The circulatory system through the umbilical cord is well established. Long bones are beginning to form, and the large muscles are now capable of contracting.

Fetal stage   By the end of the eighth week, the embryo is sufficiently developed to be called a **fetus**. Every organ system and external structure that will be found in the full-term newborn is present. The remainder of gestation is devoted to refining structures and perfecting function.

Twelfth week   The fetus reaches a 8 cm (3.2 in) C-R length and weighs about 45 g (1.6 oz). The large head comprises almost half of the fetus's size. The face is well formed, the nose protrudes, the chin is small and receding, and the ear acquires an adult shape. Some reflex lip movements suggestive of the sucking reflex have been observed at 3 months. Tooth buds now appear for all 20 baby teeth. The limbs are long and slender with well-formed digits. The genitourinary tract completes its development,

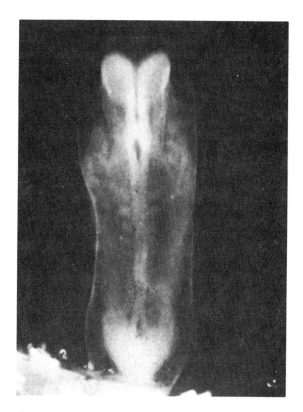

Figure 4-8
Third week. (Courtesy Drs. Roberts Pugh and Landrum B. Shettles.)

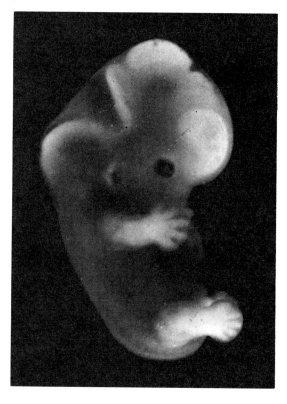

Figure 4-9
Sixth week. (Courtesy Drs. Roberts Pugh and Landrum B. Shettles.)

well-differentiated genitals appear, and the kidneys begin to produce urine.

Twentieth week The fetus doubles its C-R length and now measures 19 cm or 8 in, and fetal weight is between 435 and 465 g. **Lanugo**, a fine, downy hair, covers the entire body and is especially prominent on the shoulders. Subcutaneous deposits of brown fat, which has a rich blood supply, make the skin less transparent. Nipples now appear over the mammary glands. The head is covered with fine, "wooly" hair, and the eyebrows and eyelashes are beginning to form. Nails are present on both fingers and toes. Muscles are well developed, and the fetus is active. The mother feels fetal movement, known as *quickening*. The fetal heartbeat is audible through a stethoscope. Quickening and fetal heartbeat can help confirm the estimated delivery date.

Twenty-fourth week The fetus reaches a crown-to-heel (C-H) length of 28 cm (11.2 in). It weighs about 780 g (1 lb 10 oz). The eyes are

structurally complete and the eyelids will soon open. The fetus has a reflex hand grip (grasp reflex) and, by the end of the sixth month, a startle reflex. Skin covering the body is reddish and wrinkled, with little subcutaneous fat. Skin ridges on palms and soles form distinct footprints and fingerprints. The skin over the entire body is covered with a protective cheeselike, fatty substance called **vernix caseosa**. The alveoli in the lungs are beginning to form.

Twenty-eighth week The fetus looks like a little old man; the skin is still red, wrinkled and covered with vernix. The brain develops rapidly, and the nervous system can regulate body functions to some degree. If the fetus is male, the testes begin to descend into the scrotal sac. Respiratory and circulatory systems have developed sufficiently to initiate extrauterine functioning. If born at this time, the fetus requires intensive specialized care to survive. The fetus at 28 weeks (Figure 4-11) is about 35–38 cm (14–15 in) long (C-H) and weighs about 1200–1250 g (2 lbs 10.5 oz–2 lbs 12 oz).

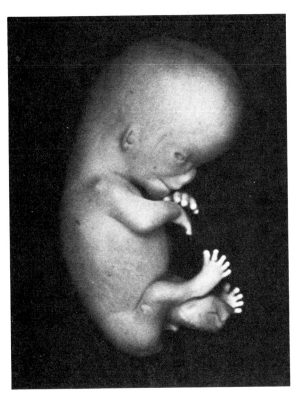

Figure 4-10 ▰▰▰
Eighth week. (Courtesy Drs. Roberts Pugh and Landrum B. Shettles.)

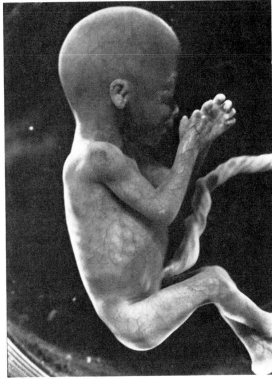

Figure 4-11 ▰▰▰
Twenty-eighth week. (Courtesy Drs. Robert Pugh and Landrum B. Shettles.)

Thirty-sixth week   The fetus begins to get plump, with less wrinkled skin covering the deposits of subcutaneous fat. Lanugo hair begins to disappear, and the nails now reach the edge of the fingertips. By 36 weeks, the fetus weighs 2500–2750 g (5 lb 12 oz–6 lb 11.5 oz) and measures about 42–48 cm (16–19 in) C-H. If born at this time, the infant has a good chance of surviving but may require some special care.

Thirty-eighth to fortieth weeks   The fetus is considered full term 38 weeks after conception. Length varies from 48–52 cm C-H (19–21 in), with males usually longer than females. Males also generally weigh more than females. The weight at term is about 3000–3600 g (6 lb 10 oz–7 lb 15 oz). The skin is pink and has a smooth, polished look. The only lanugo left is on the upper arms and shoulders. The hair is now coarse and about an inch long. Vernix is more apparent in the creases and folds of the skin. The body and extremities are plump, and the fingernails extend beyond the fingertips. The chest is prominent but still a little smaller than the head. In males, the testes are in the scrotum or palpable in the inguinal canal. The amniotic fluid decreases to about 500 mL or less as the fetal body mass fills the uterine cavity. The fetus assumes what is called its *position of comfort* or *lie* and generally follows the shape of the uterus, with the head pointed downward. After the fifth month, feeding, sleeping, and activity patterns become established so that at term the fetus has its own body rhythms and individual style of response.

The Essential Facts to Remember box lists some important developmental milestones.

Factors influencing embryonic and fetal development   Among the factors that may affect embryonic development are the quality of the sperm and ovum from which the zygote was formed and the genetic code established at fertilization. In addition, the adequacy of the intrauterine environment is important for optimal growth. If the environment is unfavorable before cellular differentiation occurs, all cells will be affected and either spontaneous abortion

ESSENTIAL FACTS TO REMEMBER

Fetal Development

- 4 weeks: The fetal heart begins to beat.
- 6 weeks: The fetal circulation is established.
- 16 weeks: Sex can be determined visually.
- 20 weeks: Lanugo covers the entire body. The fetal heartbeat can be auscultated with fetoscope. The mother feels movement (quickening).
- 24 weeks: Vernix caseosa covers the entire body.
- 26–28 weeks: The eyes reopen after being closed since 8 weeks.
- 36 weeks: Fingernails are to the end of fingers.
- 40 weeks: Lanugo remains on upper arms and shoulders only. Vernix is apparent only in creases and folds of skin. Fingernails extend beyond fingertips.

Table 4-3
Developmental Vulnerability Timetable*

Weeks since conception	Potential teratogen-induced malformation
3	Ectromelia (congenital absence of one or more limbs) Ectopedia cordis (heart lies outside thoracic cavity)
4	Omphalocele Tracheoesophageal fistula (4–5† weeks) Hemivertebra (4–5† weeks)
5	Nuclear cataract Microphthalmia (abnormally small eyeballs; 5–6† weeks) Facial clefts Carpal or pedal ablation (5–6† weeks)
6	Gross septal or aortic abnormalities Cleft lip, agnathia (absence of the lower jaw)
7	Interventricular septal defects Pulmonary stenosis Cleft palate, micrognathia (smallness of the jaw) Epicanthus Brachycephalism (shortness of the head; 7–8† weeks) Mixed sexual characteristics
8	Persistent ostium primum (persistent opening in atrial septum) Digital stunting (shortening of fingers and toes)

*Modified from Danforth, D. N. 1982. *Obstetrics and gynecology.* 4th ed. Philadelphia: Harper & Row, p. 265.
†May occur in several different time periods after conception.

or slowed growth results. When differentiation is complete and the fetal membranes have been formed, an injurious agent has the greatest effect on those cells undergoing the most rapid growth. Thus the time of injury or insult is critical in the development of abnormalities. Because organs are formed primarily in the early weeks of gestation, the growing organism is considered most vulnerable at this time. Table 4-3 relates malformations to the time of the insult. Chapter 8 discusses the effects of specific teratogenic agents on the developing fetus. A *teratogen* is any agent, such as a drug or virus, that can cause abnormalities in an embryo.

Adequacy of the maternal environment is also important during the periods of rapid embryonic and fetal development. The period of maximum brain growth begins at the twentieth week of gestation and continues during the first 6 months after birth. Amino acids, glucose, and fatty acids are considered the primary dietary factors in brain growth. A subtle type of damage that affects associative learning may be caused by nutritional deficiency at this stage. Maternal nutrition during pregnancy is discussed in Chapter 8.

Twins

Twins may be either fraternal or identical. If they are fraternal, the are *dizygotic*; that is, they arise from two separate ova fertilized by two separate spermatozoa. They have two placentas, two chorions, and two amnions. The placentas sometimes fuse and appear to be one. Fraternal twins are no more similar than ordinary siblings. The sex of fraternal twins may be the same or different.

Identical, or *monozygotic*, twins develop from a single fertilized ovum. They have the same sex and appearance. Division of the single fertilized ovum into two units occurs only after the embryo consists of thousands of cells. Complete separation of the cellular mass into two parts is necessary for twin formation. Identical twins have a common placenta and a single chorion but always two separate amnions (Figure 4-12).

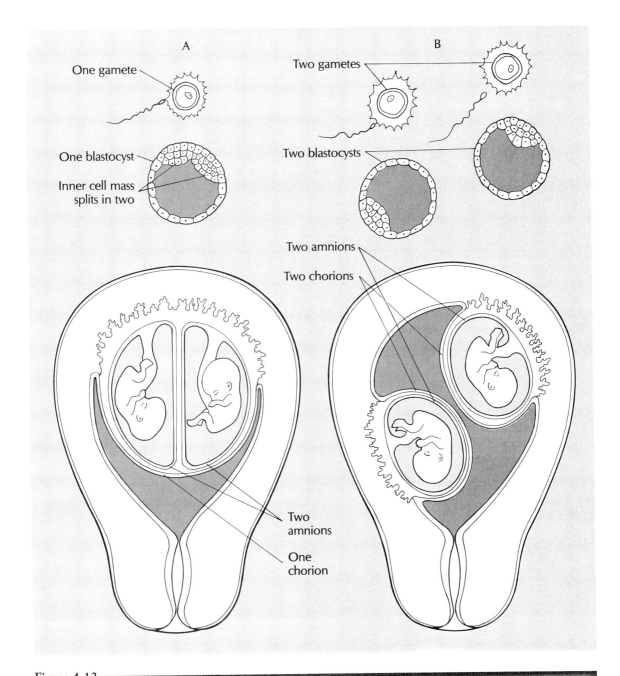

Figure 4-12
A, Formation of identical twins. **B**, Formation of fraternal twins.

Summary

From a single fertilized cell, through an orderly series of events, a complex human being develops and begins his or her existence. This process is one of the most dynamic events in nature. The period of embryonic and fetal development is characterized by rapid cellular division, multiplication, and differentiation and by the formation of the placenta, fetal membranes, and umbilical cord.

To be effective caregivers and teachers, nurses must understand the processes and mechanisms of embryonic, fetal, and placental development. This knowledge is essential to appreciate the various critical influences that timing of cellular division and environment have on the successful completion of fetal development.

References

Danforth DN: *Obstetrics and Gynecology*, 4th ed. Philadelphia: Harper & Row, 1982.

Gudson JP, Sain LE: Uterine and peripheral blood concentrations and human chorionic gonadotropin and human placental lactogen. *Am J Obstet Gynecol* March 1981; 39(2):705.

Langman J: *Medical Embryology*, 4th ed. Baltimore: Williams & Wilkins, 1981.

Moore KL: *The Developing Human: Clinically Oriented Embryology*, 2nd ed. Philadelphia: Saunders, 1977.

Pritchard JA, MacDonald PC, Gant NF: *Williams Obstetrics*, 17th ed. New York: Appleton-Century-Crofts, 1985.

Silverstein A: *Human Anatomy and Physiology*. New York: John Wiley, 1980.

Spence AP: *Basic Human Anatomy*. Menlo Park, Calif.: Benjamin/Cummings, 1982.

Additional Readings

Aladjem S, Lueck J: Placental physiology. In: *Gynecology and Obstetrics*. Vol 3. Sciarra JJ et al (editors). Hagerstown, Md.: Harper & Row, 1982.

Battaglia FC, Meschia G: Fetal and placental metabolism: Their interrelationship and impact upon maternal metabolism. *Proc Nutr Soc* 1981; 40 (1):99.

Dilts PV: Placental transfer. *Clin Obstet Gynecol* June 1981; 24(2):555.

Jaffe RB: Fetoplacental endocrine and metabolic physiology. *Clin Perinatol* October 1983; 10(3):669.

Koffler H: Fetal and neonatal physiology. *Clin Obstet Gynecol* June 1981; 24(2):545.

Naeye RL: Maternal blood pressure and fetal growth. *Am J Obstet Gynecol* December 1981; 141(7):780.

Vorherr H: Factors influencing fetal growth. *Am J Obstet Gynecol* March 1982; 142(5):577.

Whaley LF: *Understanding Inherited Disorders*. St. Louis: Mosby, 1974.

5
Physical and Psychologic Responses to Pregnancy

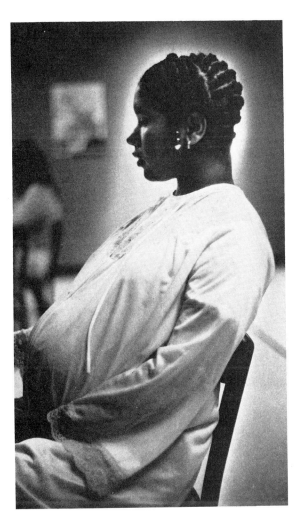

Chapter Contents

Objectives

- Compare subjective (presumptive) and objective (probable) changes of pregnancy.

- Describe the various tests used to determine pregnancy.

- List the diagnostic (positive) changes of pregnancy.

- Relate the physiologic changes that occur in the body systems as a result of pregnancy to the signs and symptoms that develop.

- Discuss the emotional and psychologic changes that women commonly undergo during pregnancy.

- Identify cultural factors that may influence a family's response to pregnancy.

Key Terms

Braxton Hicks contractions	Hegar's sign
Chadwick's sign	last menstrual period (LMP)
chloasma	mitleiden
couvade	striae
Goodell's sign	vena caval syndrome

During pregnancy, a woman undergoes numerous physical and psychologic changes; her family, too, experiences change. Typically, a pregnancy lasts about 9 calendar months, 10 lunar months, 40 weeks, or 280 days. This time allows the fetus to develop and also gives the expectant family time to plan for a new member.

Pregnancy is traditionally divided into three trimesters of 3 months each. Each trimester brings predictable changes for both the mother and the fetus. This chapter identifies the physical and psychologic changes that accompany each trimester. In subsequent chapters, the nurse will use this knowledge to plan and provide effective nursing care.

Subjective (Presumptive) Changes

Many of the changes the pregnant woman experiences during pregnancy are used to diagnose the pregnancy itself. They are called the *subjective* or *presumptive* changes, the *objective* or *probable* changes, and the *diagnostic* or *positive* changes of pregnancy. The guidelines for differentiating among these three are identified in the Essential Facts to Remember box, p. 97.

The subjective changes of pregnancy are the symptoms the woman experiences and reports. Because they can be caused by other conditions, they cannot be considered proof of pregnancy (Table 5-1). The following subjective signs can be diagnostic clues when other signs and symptoms of pregnancy are also present.

Amenorrhea, or the absence of menses, is the earliest symptom of pregnancy. The missing of more than one menstrual period, especially in a woman whose cycle is ordinarily regular, is an especially useful diagnostic clue.

Table 5-1
Differential Diagnosis of Pregnancy— Subjective Changes

Subjective changes	Possible causes
Amenorrhea	Endocrine factors: early menopause; lactation; thyroid, pituitary, adrenal, ovarian dysfunction Metabolic factors: malnutrition, anemia, climatic changes, diabetes mellitus, degenerative disorders Psychologic factors: emotional shock, fear of pregnancy or venereal disease, intense desire for pregnancy (pseudocyesis) Obliteration of endometrial cavity by infection or curettage Systemic disease (acute or chronic), such as tuberculosis or malignancy
Nausea and vomiting	Gastrointestinal disorders Acute infections such as encephalitis Emotional disorders such as pseudocyesis or anorexia nervosa
Urinary frequency	Urinary tract infection Cystocele Pelvic tumors Urethral diverticula Emotional tension
Breast tenderness	Premenstrual tension Chronic cystic mastitis Pseudocyesis Elevated estrogen levels
Quickening	Increased peristalsis Flatus (``gas'') Abdominal muscle contractions Shifting of abdominal contents

Nausea and vomiting occur frequently during the first 3 months of pregnancy. Because these symptoms often occur in the early part of the day, they are commonly referred to as *morning sickness*. In reality, the symptoms may occur at any time and can range from merely a distaste for food to severe vomiting.

Excessive fatigue may be noted within a few weeks after the first missed menstrual period and may persist throughout the first trimester.

Urinary frequency is experienced during the first trimester as the enlarging fetus presses on the bladder.

Changes in the breasts are frequently noted in early pregnancy. These changes include tenderness and tingling sensations, increased pigmentation of the areola and nipple, and changes in Montgomery's glands.

Quickening, or the mother's perception of fetal movement, occurs about 18–20 weeks after the **last menstrual period (LMP)**. Quickening is a fluttering sensation in the abdomen that gradually increases in intensity and frequency.

Objective (Probable) Changes

An examiner can perceive the objective changes that occur in pregnancy. However, since these changes also can have other causes, they do not confirm pregnancy (see Table 5-2).

Changes in the pelvic organs—the only physical changes detectable during the first 3 months of pregnancy—are caused by increased vascular congestion. These changes are noted on pelvic examination. There is a softening of the cervix called **Goodell's sign**. **Chadwick's sign** is a bluish or deep red discoloration of the mucous membranes of the cervix, vagina, and vulva (some sources consider this a presumptive sign). **Hegar's sign** is a softening of the isthmus of the uterus, the area between the cervix and the body of the uterus (Figure 5-1).

General enlargement and softening of the body of the uterus can be noted after the eighth week of pregnancy. The fundus of the uterus is palpable just above the symphysis pubis at about 10–12 weeks' gestation and at the level of the umbilicus at 20–22 weeks' gestation (Figure 5-2).

Table 5-2
Differential Diagnosis of Pregnancy—Objective Changes

Objective changes	Possible causes
Changes in pelvic organs	Increased vascular congestion
Goodell's sign	Estrogen-progestin oral contraceptives
Chadwick's sign	Vulvar, vaginal, cervical hyperemia
Hegar's sign	Excessively soft walls of nonpregnant uterus
Uterine enlargement	Uterine tumors
Enlargement of abdomen	Obesity, ascites, pelvic tumors
Braxton Hicks contractions	Hematometra; pedunculated, submucous, and soft myomas
Uterine souffle	Large uterine myomas, large ovarian tumors or any condition with greatly increased uterine blood flow
Pigmentation of skin	Estrogen-progestin oral contraceptives
Chloasma	
Linea nigra	Melanocyte hormonal stimulation
Nipples/areola	
Abdominal striae	Obesity, pelvic tumor
Ballottement	Uterine tumors/polyps, ascites
Pregnancy tests	Increased pituitary gonadotrophins at menopause, choriocarcinoma, hydatidiform mole
Palpation for fetal outline	Uterine myomas

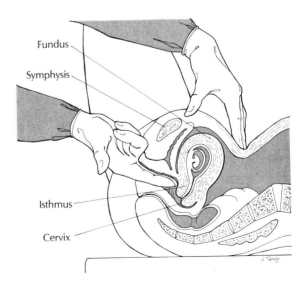

Figure 5-1
Hegar's sign.

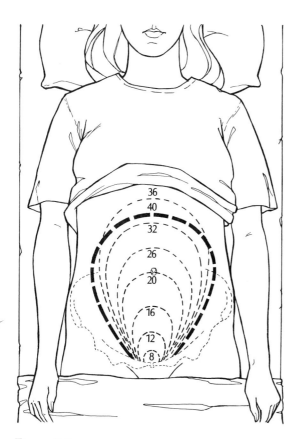

Figure 5-2
Approximate height of the fundus at various weeks of pregnancy.

Enlargement of the abdomen during the childbearing years is usually regarded as evidence of pregnancy especially if it is continuous and accompanied by amenorrhea.

Braxton Hicks contractions are painless uterine contractions that occur at irregular intervals throughout pregnancy but can be felt most commonly after the twenty-eighth week.

Uterine souffle may be heard when the examiner auscultates the abdomen over the uterus. This souffle is a soft, blowing sound that occurs at the same rate as the maternal pulse and is due to the increased uterine blood flow and blood pulsating through the placenta.

Changes in pigmentation of the skin are common in pregnancy. The nipples and areola may darken, and the skin in the middle of the abdomen may develop a pigmented line, the *linea nigra*.

Facial **chloasma** (also known as the *mask of pregnancy*) is a darkening of the skin over the forehead and around the eyes that may occur in varying degrees after week 16.

As the uterus enlarges, reddish, irregular, wavy streaks known as **striae** appear on the abdomen and buttocks as the underlying connective tissue breaks down.

The *fetal outline* may be identified by palpation in many pregnant women after 24 weeks' gestation.

Ballottement is the fetal movement elicited when the examiner taps the cervix with two fingers. This pushes the fetal body up, and a rebound is felt as it falls back.

Pregnancy tests detect the presence of hCG in the maternal blood or urine. These are not considered a positive sign of pregnancy because other conditions can cause elevated hCG levels.

Pregnancy Tests

Historically, most pregnancy tests were bioassays that used laboratory animals. These tests were time consuming and subject to error. Consequently, they are seldom used and have been replaced by immunoassays and radioreceptor assay tests.

Immunoassay tests are based on the antigenic properties of hCG. Two of these tests are done on the first early morning urine specimen of the woman because it is adequately concentrated. The tests become positive 10–14 days after the first missed menstrual period. In the *hemagglutination-inhibition test (Pregnosticon R)* no clumping of cells occurs when the urine of a pregnant woman is added to the hCG-sensitized red blood cells of sheep. In the *latex agglutination tests (Gravidex and Pregnosticon Slide tests)*, latex particle agglutination is inhibited in the presence of urine containing hCG.

Radioimmune assay   *Radioimmune assay* (RIA) for the β subunit of hCG is the most accurate pregnancy test. It is done on maternal serum and will show positive results within 8–9 days after ovulation. Thus, it is useful in diagnosing pregnancy even before the woman misses a period.

Radioreceptor assay   Radioreceptor assay is a sensitive test that can be quickly performed on maternal blood. It utilizes radioiodine-labeled hCG. Because the test fails to distinguish between hCG and LH, however, cross reactions may occur. This limitation may be overcome by setting the test sensitivity at 200 mIU/mL serum. Because this level is higher than the midcycle peak of LH (175 mIU/mL serum) confusion is avoided (Danforth, 1982). This setting, however, makes the radioreceptor assay somewhat less sensitive than the RIA.

Over-the-counter pregnancy tests   Over-the-counter pregnancy tests are available for a nominal fee. These tests, performed on urine, use the hemagglutination-inhibition principle. False results may occur if a test is performed too soon after a missed period or if the specimen used was not the first morning urine. Other factors that may contribute to a false reading include using a dirty kit or a kit containing traces of soap or detergent, exposing the sample to heat or sunlight, allowing the sample to stand longer than the specified time, or moving the test-tube sample during the timing period.

Diagnostic (Positive) Changes

A sign of pregnancy is positive if it proves conclusively that a woman is pregnant, but such signs are usually not present until after the fourth month of gestation.

 ESSENTIAL FACTS TO REMEMBER

Differentiating the Signs of Pregnancy

These guidelines help differentiate among the presumptive, probable, and positive changes of pregnancy:

Subjective (presumptive) changes

- Symptoms the woman experiences and reports
- May have causes other than pregnancy

Objective (probable) changes

- Signs perceived by the examiner
- May have causes other than pregnancy

Diagnostic (positive) changes

- Signs perceived by the examiner
- Can be caused *only* by pregnancy

The *fetal heartbeat* can be detected with a fetoscope by approximately weeks 17–20 of pregnancy. The electronic Doppler device allows the examiner to detect the fetal heartbeat as early as weeks 10–12 of pregnancy.

Fetal movement is actively palpable by a trained examiner after the eighteenth week of pregnancy.

Visualization of the fetus by ultrasound or x-ray examination confirms a pregnancy. Ultrasound may be used as early as the sixth week of pregnancy for a positive diagnosis. Fetal movement can be detected with real-time ultrasound methods by 12 weeks' gestation. Radiologic examination can show a fetal skeleton by week 16 of gestation but is not used to diagnose pregnancy because of the possibility of causing gonadal damage and genetic abnormalities. See Chapter 11 for further discussion of ultrasound.

Anatomy and Physiology of Pregnancy

Reproductive System

Uterus   The changes in the uterus during pregnancy are phenomenal. Before pregnancy, the uterus is a small, semisolid, pear-shaped organ measuring approximately 7.5 × 5 × 2.5 cm and weighing about 60 g (2 oz). At the end of pregnancy it measures about 28 × 24 × 21 cm and weighs approximately 1000 g; its capacity has also increased from about 10 mL to 5 L or more (Pritchard, MacDonald, Gant, 1985).

The enlargement of the uterus is primarily due to enlargement of the preexisting myometrial cells. These cells increase greatly in size as a result of the stimulating influence of estrogen and the distention caused by the growing fetus. The fibrous tissue between the muscle bands increases markedly, which adds to the strength and elasticity of the muscle wall.

The enlarging uterus, developing placenta, and growing fetus require additional blood flow to the uterus. By the end of pregnancy, one-sixth the total maternal blood volume is contained within the vascular system of the uterus.

Irregular, painless Braxton Hicks contractions of the uterus occur throughout pregnancy. They may be felt through the abdominal wall beginning about the fourth month of pregnancy.

In later pregnancy, these contractions become uncomfortable and may be confused with true labor contractions.

Cervix   Estrogen stimulates the glandular tissue of the cervix, which increases in cell number and becomes hyperactive. The endocervical glands secrete a thick, sticky mucus that accumulates and forms a plug, which seals the endocervical canal and prevents the ascent of organisms into the uterus. This mucous plug is expelled when cervical dilatation begins. The hyperactivity of the glandular tissue also increases the normal physiologic mucorrhea, at times resulting in profuse discharge. Increased cervical vascularity also causes both the softening of the cervix and its bluish discoloration (Chadwick's sign).

Ovaries   The ovaries stop producing ova during pregnancy. The corpus luteum continues to produce hormones until about weeks 10–12 of pregnancy. The progesterone it secretes maintains the endometrium until the placenta assumes this task. The corpus luteum begins to regress and is almost completely obliterated by the middle of pregnancy.

Vagina   Estrogen causes a thickening of the vaginal mucosa, a loosening of the connective tissue, and an increase in vaginal secretions. These secretions are thick, white, and acidic (pH 3.5–6.0). The acidity helps prevent bacterial infection but favors the growth of yeast organisms. Thus, the pregnant woman is more susceptible to monilial infection than usual.

The supportive connective tissue of the vagina loosens throughout pregnancy. By the time of delivery, the vagina and perineal body are sufficiently relaxed to permit passage of the infant.

Breasts

Estrogen and progesterone cause many changes in the mammary glands. The breasts enlarge and become more nodular as the glands increase in size and number in preparation for lactation. Superficial veins become more prominent, the nipples become more erectile, and the areolas darken. Montogomery's follicles enlarge, and striae may develop.

Colostrum, an antibody-rich, yellow secretion, may leak or be expressed from the breasts during the last trimester. Colostrum gradually converts to mature milk during the first few days after delivery.

Respiratory System

Many respiratory changes occur to meet the increased oxygen requirements of a pregnant woman. Progesterone decreases airway resistance, permitting a 15%–20% increase in oxygen consumption and a 30%–40% increase in the volume of air breathed each minute.

As the uterus enlarges, it presses upward and the diaphragm is elevated. The substernal angle increases so that the rib cage flares. The anteroposterior diameter increases, and the chest circumference expands by as much as 6 cm; for this reason, there is no significant loss of intrathoracic volume. Breathing changes from abdominal to thoracic as pregnancy progresses, and descent of the diaphragm on inspiration becomes less possible. The respiratory rate may increase slightly, and some hyperventilation may occur.

Cardiovascular System

During pregnancy, the blood flow increases to those organ systems with an increased work load. Thus, blood flow to the uterus and kidneys is increased, while hepatic and cerebral flow remains unchanged.

The pulse may increase by as many as 10–15 beats/min at term. The blood pressure may be slightly lower during the second trimester and highest during the last weeks of pregnancy.

The enlarged uterus may press on pelvic and femoral vessels, interfering with the returning blood flow and causing stagnation of blood in the lower extremities. This condition may lead to dependent edema and varicosity of the veins in the legs, vulva, and rectum (hemorrhoids) in late pregnancy. This increased blood volume in the lower legs may also make the pregnant woman more prone to postural hypotension.

The enlarging uterus may press on the vena cava when the pregnant woman lies supine, lowering blood pressure and causing dizziness, pallor, and clamminess. This is called the *supine hypotensive syndrome* (Figure 5-3) or the **vena caval syndrome**.

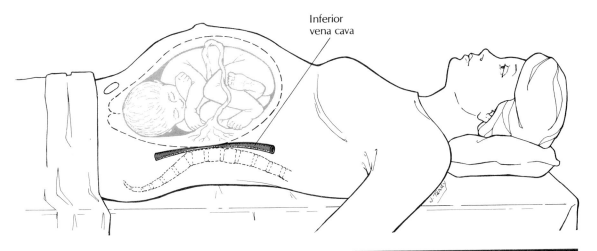

Inferior
vena cava

Figure 5-3

Vena caval syndrome. Gravid uterus compresses vena cava when the woman is supine. The blood flow returning to the heart is reduced, and maternal hypotension may result.

Blood volume progressively increases beginning in the first trimester, increasing rapidly in the second trimester, and slowing in the third. At term, blood volume is 30%–50% above the prepregnant level.

The red blood cell count and hemoglobin levels increase during pregnancy. However, because the plasma volume increases more, the hematocrit decreases an average of 7%. This results in the *physiologic anemia of pregnancy* (*pseudoanemia*).

Leukocyte production increases slightly to an average of 10,000–11,000/mm³. During labor, these levels may reach 25,000/mm³.

Both the fibrin and plasma fibrinogen levels increase during pregnancy. Although the blood-clotting time of the pregnant woman does not differ significantly from that of the nonpregnant woman, clotting factors VII, IX, and X increase; thus, pregnancy is a somewhat hypercoagulable state. These changes, coupled with venous stasis in late pregnancy, increase the pregnant woman's risk of developing venous thrombosis.

Gastrointestinal System

Nausea and vomiting are common during the first trimester because of elevated hCG levels and changed carbohydrate metabolism. Gum tissue may soften and bleed easily. The secretion of saliva may increase and even become excessive (*ptyalism*). Gastric acidity also decreases.

Elevated progesterone levels cause smooth muscle relaxation, resulting in delayed gastric emptying and decreased peristalsis. As a result, the pregnant woman may complain of bloating and constipation. These symptoms are aggravated as the enlarging uterus displaces the stomach superiorly and the intestines laterally and posteriorly. The cardiac sphincter also relaxes, and heartburn (*pyrosis*) may occur due to reflux of acidic secretions into the lower esophagus.

Hemorrhoids frequently develop in late pregnancy from pressure on vessels below the level of the uterus.

Urinary Tract

During the first trimester, the enlarging uterus is still a pelvic organ and presses against the bladder, producing urinary frequency. This symptom decreases during the second trimester when the uterus is an abdominal organ. Frequency reappears during the third trimester, when the presenting part descends into the pelvis and again presses on the bladder, reducing bladder capacity and irritating the bladder.

The ureters (especially the right ureter) elongate and dilate above the pelvic brim. The glomerular filtration rate (GFR) rises by as much as 50% beginning in the second trimester and remains elevated until delivery. To compensate for this, renal tubular reabsorption also increases. However, glycosuria is sometimes seen during pregnancy because of the kidney's inability to reabsorb all the glucose filtered by the glomeruli. This may be normal or may indicate gestational diabetes, so glycosuria always warrants further testing.

Skin

Elevated hormone levels may cause darkening of the nipples and areolas, a linea nigra on the abdomen, and facial chloasma. Chloasma is more prominent in dark-haired women and is aggravated by exposure to the sun. Fortunately, chloasma fades or becomes less prominent soon after delivery when the hormonal influence of pregnancy subsides. Striae may appear on the breasts and abdomen because elevated adrenal steroid levels reduce connective tissue strength. In addition, the sweat and sebaceous glands are often hyperactive during pregnancy.

Skeletal System

No demonstrable changes occur in the teeth of pregnant women. The dental caries that sometimes accompany pregnancy are probably caused by the fact that saliva is slightly more acidic during pregnancy and by inadequate oral hygiene, especially if the woman has problems with bleeding gums.

The joints of the pelvis relax somewhat due to hormonal influences. The result is often a waddling gait. As the pregnant woman's center of gravity gradually changes, the lumbar spinal curve is accentuated, and the posture changes (see Figure 5-4). This posture change compensates for the increased weight of the uterus anteriorly and frequently results in low backache.

Metabolism

Most metabolic functions increase during pregnancy because of the increased demands of the growing fetus and its support system. The expectant mother must meet her own tissue replacement needs and those of her unborn child. In addition, her body must anticipate the needs of labor and lactation.

For a detailed discussion of nutrient, vitamin, and mineral metabolism, see Chapter 8.

Weight gain   The average weight gain during a normal pregnancy is 25–30 lb (11–13.6 kg). An average increase of 3, 12, and 12 lb (1.4, 5.5, and 5.5 kg) occurs in the first, second, and third trimesters, respectively. The total weight gain may be accounted for as follows: fetus, 7.5 lb (3.4 kg); placenta and membranes, 1.5 lb (0.7 kg); amniotic fluid, 2 lb (0.9 kg); uterus, 2.5 lb (1.1 kg); breasts, 3 lb (1.4 kg); and increased

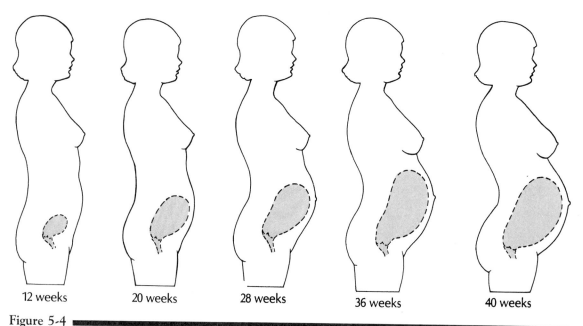

12 weeks   20 weeks   28 weeks   36 weeks   40 weeks

Figure 5-4

Postural changes during pregnancy.

blood volume, 2–4 lb (0.9–1.8 kg). The remaining 4–9 lb (1.8–4.1 kg) is extravascular fluid and fat reserves.

Water metabolism   Increased water retention is a basic alteration of pregnancy. Several interrelated factors cause this phenomenon. The increased level of steroid sex hormones affects sodium and fluid retention. The lowered serum protein also influences the fluid balance, as do the increased intracapillary pressure and permeability. The extra water is due to the products of conception—the fetus, placenta, and amniotic fluid—and the mother's increased blood volume, interstitial fluids, and enlarged organs.

Endocrine System

Thyroid   The thyroid gland often enlarges slightly during pregnancy. Its capacity to bind thyroxine is greater, resulting in an increase in serum protein-bound iodine (PBI). These changes are due to higher blood levels of estrogen.

The basal metabolic rate increases by 25% in late pregnancy. However, within a few weeks after delivery, all thyroid function returns to normal limits.

Pituitary   Pregnancy is made possible by the hypothalamic stimulation of the anterior pituitary gland, which in turn produces the hormones FSH, which stimulates ova growth, and LH, which brings about ovulation. Stimulation of the pituitary also prolongs the ovary's corpus luteal phase, which maintains the endometrium for development of the pregnancy. Prolactin, another anterior pituitary hormone, is responsible for initial lactation.

The posterior portion of the pituitary secretes oxytocin. Oxytocin promotes uterine contractility and stimulates ejection of milk from the breasts (the *let-down reflex*).

Adrenals   The adrenal cortex enlarges during pregnancy in response to high estrogen levels. Circulating cortisol, which regulates carbohydrate and protein metabolism, increases. Cortisol blood levels return to normal 1–6 weeks postpartum.

Pancreas   The pregnant woman has increased insulin needs, and the islets of Lang-

erhans, which secrete insulin, are stressed. Thus a latent deficiency state may become apparent, and the woman may show signs of gestational diabetes.

Placental hormones

Human chorionic gonadotrophin (hCG)   The trophoblast secretes hCG in early pregnancy. hCG stimulates progesterone and estrogen production by the corpus luteum to maintain the pregnancy until the placenta is developed sufficiently to assume that function.

Human placental lactogen (hPL)   Also called human chorionic somatomammotropin, hPL is produced by the syncytiotrophoblast. hPL is an antagonist of insulin; it increases the amount of circulating free fatty acids for maternal metabolic needs and decreases maternal metabolism of glucose.

Estrogen   Estrogen, secreted originally by the corpus luteum, is produced primarily by the placenta as early as the seventh week of pregnancy. Estrogen stimulates uterine development to provide a suitable environment for the fetus. It also helps to develop the ductal system of the breasts in preparation for lactation.

Progesterone   Progesterone, also produced initially by the corpus luteum and then by the placenta, plays the greatest role in maintaining pregnancy. It maintains the endometrium and inhibits spontaneous uterine contractility, thus preventing early spontaneous abortion due to uterine activity. Progesterone also helps develop the acini and lobules of the breasts in preparation for lactation.

Psychologic Responses of the Expectant Family to Pregnancy

Pregnancy as a Crisis

Whether pregnancy terminates in elective or spontaneous abortion, or in a term infant, it is a turning point in a couple's life. Pregnancy is a *maturational crisis* because it is a common event in the normal growth and development of a family—an event that requires intrapersonal and interpersonal changes and reorganization. Because pregnancy is a crisis, stress and anxiety are common responses to the many adjustments the couple must make.

The expectant couple may be unaware of the physical, emotional, and cognitive changes of pregnancy and may anticipate no problems from such a normal event. Thus, they may be confused and distressed by feelings and behaviors that are essentially normal.

Parenthood brings significant role changes for the couple. Career goals and mobility may be affected, and the couple's relationship takes on new meanings to themselves and within their families and community. Routines and family dynamics are altered with each pregnancy, and require readjustment and realignment.

The couple must make decisions about financial matters—whether the woman will work during her pregnancy, and whether she will return to work after her child is born. They may also need to decide about the division of domestic tasks. Any differences of opinion must be discussed openly and resolved so that the family can meet the needs of its members.

The couple must face the anxieties of labor and delivery and must also deal with fears that the baby may be ill or disfigured. Classes in prepared childbirth can help the couple overcome concerns that are based on misinformation or lack of information.

Even if the pregnant woman has no stable partner or plans to place the infant for adoption, she must deal with the role changes, fears, and adjustments of pregnancy. She is no longer a separate individual; she must consider the needs of another being who depends on her totally, at least during pregnancy.

Duvall (1977) views the period of pregnancy and childbirth as part of the first major phase in the family life cycle—*the expanding family*. This phase lasts from the beginning of the marriage until the children leave home. The second major phase, the *contracting family*, extends from the launching of the children to the death of one of the spouses. These two phases are further divided into stages.

During the expanding family phase the couple plans for the child's arrival, continues to participate in joint and separate activities, and assumes distinct roles—often the man as breadwinner and the woman as homemaker. Each member of the family must adjust to the experience of pregnancy and its implications. This can be a period of support or conflict for the couple, depending on the amount of adjustment each is willing to make to maintain the family's equilibrium. Both partners' possible reactions to the pregnancy are given in Table 5-3.

The Mother

Initially, even if the pregnancy is planned, there is an element of surprise. Many women commonly experience feelings of ambivalence during early pregnancy. This may be related to a feeling that the timing is somehow wrong, the need to modify existing relationships or career plans, fears about assuming a new role, unresolved emotional conflicts with one's own mother, and fears about pregnancy, labor, and delivery. These feelings may be more pronounced if the pregnancy is unplanned or unwanted.

First trimester　During the first trimester, feelings of disbelief and ambivalence are paramount. The woman's baby does not seem real to her, and she focuses on herself and her pregnancy (Colman and Colman, 1971). She may experience early symptoms of pregnancy, such as breast tenderness or morning sickness, which are unsettling and at times unpleasant.

During the first trimester, the expectant mother begins to exhibit some characteristic behavioral changes. She becomes increasingly introspective and passive. She is also emotionally labile, with characteristic mood swings from joy to despair and tears. She may also fantasize about a miscarriage and feel guilt because of these fantasies.

Second trimester　During the second trimester, quickening occurs. This perception of fetal movement helps the woman to think of her baby as a separate person, and she generally becomes excited about the pregnancy even if she was not earlier.

The woman becomes increasingly introspective as she evaluates her life, her plans, and her child's future. This introspection helps the woman prepare for her new mothering role. Emotional lability, which may be unsettling to her partner, persists. In some instances, he may react by withdrawing. This is especially distressing to the woman because she needs increased love and affection. Once the couple understands

Table 5-3
Parental Reactions to Pregnancy

First trimester		Second trimester Continued	
Mother's reactions	**Father's reactions**	**Mother's reactions**	**Father's reactions**
Informs father secretly or openly	Differ according to age, parity, desire for child, economic stability	Remains regressive and introspective; all problems with authority figures projected onto partner; may become angry as if lack of interest is sign of weakness in him	If he can cope, will give her extra attention she needs; if he cannot cope, will develop a new time-consuming interest outside of home
Feels ambivalent toward pregnancy; anxious about labor and responsibility of child	Acceptance of pregnant woman's attitude or complete rejection and lack of communication		
Is aware of physical changes; daydreams of possible miscarriage	Is aware of his own sexual feelings; may develop more or less sexual arousal	Continues to deal with feelings as a mother and looks for furniture as something concrete	May develop a creative feeling and a "closeness to nature"
Develops special feelings for, renewed interest in mother, with formation of own mother identity	Accepts, rejects, or resents mother-in-law		
	May develop new hobby outside of family as sign of stress	May have other extreme of anxiety and wait until ninth month to look for furniture and clothes for baby	May become involved in pregnancy and buy or make furniture

Second trimester		Third trimester	
Mother's reactions	**Father's reactions**	**Mother's reactions**	**Father's reactions**
Feels movement and is aware of fetus and incorporates it into herself	Feels for movement of baby, listens to heartbeat, or remains aloof, with no physical contact	Experiences more anxiety and tension, with physical awkwardness	Adapts to alternative methods of sexual contact
		Feels much discomfort and insomnia from physical condition	Becomes concerned over financial responsibility
Dreams that partner will be killed, telephones him often for reassurance	May have fears and fantasies about himself being pregnant; may become uneasy with this feminine aspect in himself	Prepares for delivery, assembles layette, picks out names	May show new sense of tenderness and concern; treats partner like doll
Experiences more distinct physical changes; sexual desires may increase or decrease	May react negatively if partner is too demanding; may become jealous of physician and of his/her importance to partner and her pregnancy	Dreams often about misplacing baby or not being able to deliver it; fears birth of deformed baby	Daydreams about child as if older and not newborn; dreams of losing partner
		Feels ecstasy and excitement; has spurt of energy during last month	Renewed sexual attraction to partner
			Feels he is ultimately responsible for whatever happens

that these behaviors are characteristic of pregnancy, it is easier for the couple to deal with them effectively, although they will be sources of stress to some extent throughout pregnancy.

As pregnancy becomes more noticeable, the woman's body image changes. She may feel great pride, she may feel embarrassed or even concerned. Generally, women feel best during the second trimester, which is a relatively tranquil time.

Third trimester   In the third trimester, the woman feels both pride about her pregnancy and anxiety about labor and delivery. Physical discomforts increase, and the woman is eager for the pregnancy to end. She experiences increased fatigue, her body movements are more awkward, and her interest in sexual activity may decrease. Toward the end of this period, there is often a surge of energy as the woman prepares a "nest" for the infant. Many women report bursts of energy during which they vigorously clean and organize their homes.

Psychologic tasks of the mother   During her pregnancy, a woman undertakes several psychologic tasks to establish a foundation for a healthy, mutually gratifying relationship with her infant.

- *Acceptance of pregnancy*. She must resolve any ambivalence about the pregnancy and accept the infant as part of herself so that bonds of attachment can be established.

- *Acceptance of termination of pregnancy*. Toward the end of pregnancy, the woman prepares herself psychologically for physical separation from the fetus. Quickening has helped her form bonds of attachment, but it also helps her perceive the fetus as a separate individual. The discomforts of late pregnancy and her desire for pregnancy to end also help the new mother relinquish her fetus.

- *Acceptance of the mother role*. Most women begin to think of themselves as mothers during their first pregnancy. The self-concept is reinforced by actual experience as a mother and continues to grow throughout subsequent childbearing and childrearing.

- *Resolution of fears about childbirth*. During pregnancy, fears and fantasies about childbirth arise. Some women suppress their fears and make no preparations for labor. Others attempt to master their fears by taking classes in childbirth preparation, reading, and the like.

- *Attachment*. The attachment of a woman to her child and her binding commitment to nurture the child begin during pregnancy. This response may be influenced by how positively or negatively she views the pregnancy.

The Father

For the expectant father, pregnancy is a psychologically stressful time because he, too, must adjust to a new child. Initially, expectant fathers may feel pride in their virility, which pregnancy confirms, but may also have many of the same ambivalent feelings expectant mothers have. The extent of ambivalence depends on many factors, including his relationship with his partner, previous experience with pregnancy, and his age and economic stability. Another important factor is whether the pregnancy was planned.

Recent evidence suggests that anxiety in the father-to-be during pregnancy is lessened if both parents agree on the paternal role the man is to assume. For example, if both see his role as that of breadwinner, the man's stress is low. If the man views his role as that of breadwinner, however, and the woman expects him to be involved actively in child care, his stress increases (Fishbein, 1984).

First trimester   After the initial excitement attending the announcement of the pregnancy, an expectant father may begin to feel left out. He may be confused by his partner's mood changes. He may resent the attention she receives and her need to modify their relationship as she experiences fatigue and possibly a decreased interest in sex. In addition, he is concerned about what kind of father he will be.

Some expectant fathers experience **mitleiden** and develop symptoms similar to those of the pregnant woman: weight gain, nausea, and various aches and pains. The exact significance of this phenomenon is unknown.

Second trimester   The father's role in the pregnancy is still vague in the second trimester, but his involvement may increase by watching and feeling fetal movement and by listening to the fetal heartbeat during a visit to the nurse or physician.

Like expectant mothers, expectant fathers need to confront and resolve some of their conflicts about the fathering they received. A father needs to sort out which behaviors of his own father he wants to imitate and which he does not.

As the woman's appearance begins to change, her partner may have several reactions. Her changed appearance may decrease his sexual interest, or it may have the opposite effect. Because of the variety of emotions both partners may feel, continued communication and acceptance are important.

Third trimester   If the couple's relationship has grown through effective communication of their concerns and feelings, the third trimester is a special and rewarding time. They may attend childbirth classes and make concrete preparations for the arrival of the baby. If the father has developed a detached attitude about the pregnancy prior to this time, it is unlikely he will become a willing participant, even though his role becomes more obvious.

Concerns and fears may recur. The father may worry about hurting the unborn baby during intercourse or become concerned about labor and delivery. Also, he may wonder what kind of parents he and his partner will be or may worry about financial stability.

Siblings

Bringing a new baby home usually marks the beginning of sibling rivalry. The siblings view the baby as a threat to the security of their relationships with their parents. Parents who recognize this potential problem early in pregnancy and begin constructive actions can help minimize the problem of sibling rivalry.

Preparation of the young sibling begins several weeks prior to the anticipated birth. Because they do not have a clear concept of time, young children should not be told too early about the pregnancy. The mother may let the child feel the baby moving in her uterus, explaining that the uterus is "a special place where babies grow." The child can help the parents put the baby clothes in drawers or prepare the nursery.

If the child is ready, toilet training is most effective several months before or after the baby's arrival. It is not unusual for the older, toilet-trained child to regress to wetting or soiling due to the attention the newborn gets for such behavior. The older, weaned child may want to nurse or drink from the bottle again after the baby comes. If the new mother anticipates these behaviors, they will be less frustrating during her early postpartum days.

Pregnant women may find it helpful to bring their children to a prenatal visit to the nurse or physician. The children may become involved in the prenatal care and are also given an opportunity to listen to the fetal heartbeat. These activities help make the baby more real to them (Figure 5-5).

If siblings are school-age children, pregnancy should be viewed as a family affair. Teaching should be appropriate to the child's level of understanding and may be supplemented with appropriate books. Taking part in family dis-

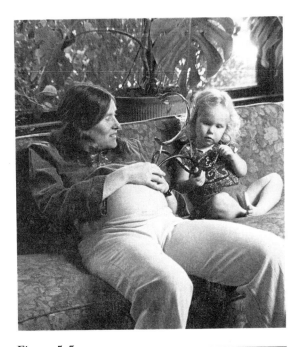

Figure 5-5
Children respond positively when they hear the heartbeat of their sibling-to-be.

cussions, attending sibling preparation classes, feeling fetal movement, and listening to the fetal heartbeat help the school-age child take part in the experience of pregnancy and not feel like an outsider.

The older child or adolescent may appear to have sophisticated knowledge but in reality may have many misconceptions. Thus, opportunities should be provided for discussion and participation.

Even after the birth, siblings need to feel that they are taking part. Permitting siblings to visit their mother and the new baby at the hospital helps this process. After the baby comes home, siblings can share in "showing off" the new baby.

Sibling preparation is essential, but other factors are equally important. These include how much parental attention the new arrival receives, how much attention the older child receives after the baby comes home, and how well the parents handle regressive or aggressive behavior.

For further information about sibling preparation, see Chapter 9.

Grandparents

The first relatives told about a pregnancy are usually the grandparents. Often, the expectant grandparents become increasingly supportive of the couple, even if conflicts previously existed. But it can be difficult for even sensitive grandparents to know how deeply to become involved in the childrearing process.

Younger grandparents leading active lives may not demonstrate as much interest as the young couple would like. In other cases, expectant grandparents may give advice and gifts unsparingly. For grandparents, conflict may be related to the expectant couple's need to feel in control of their own lives, or it may stem from events signalling changing roles in their own lives (for example, retirement, financial concerns, menopause, death of a friend). Some parents of expectant couples may already be grandparents with a developed style of grandparenting. This fact influences their response to the pregnancy.

Because childbearing and childrearing practices have changed, family cohesiveness is promoted by frank discussion among young couples and interested grandparents about the changes and the reasons for them. Effective communication among new parents and grandparents is important. Clarifying the role of the helping grandparent ensures a comfortable situation for all.

Cultural Values and Reproductive Behavior _____

Generalization about cultural characteristics or values is difficult because not every individual in a culture may display these characteristics. For example, a third generation Chinese-American family might have very different values and beliefs because of their exposure to the American culture. For this reason, the nurse needs to supplement a general knowledge of cultural values and practices with a complete assessment of the individual's values and practices.

Knowledge about cultural values helps the nurse understand and predict reactions and behaviors related to pregnancy. Understanding how a culture views male-female roles, family

life-styles, and children may explain reactions of joy or shame. Knowing health values and beliefs is also important in understanding reactions and behaviors. If a culture views pregnancy as a sickness, certain behaviors can be expected. If pregnancy is viewed as a natural occurrence, other behaviors may be expected.

Blacks usually consider pregnancy as a state of wellness. Mexican Americans view pregnancy as a natural and desirable condition (Kay, 1978). Most American Indian tribes consider pregnancy a normal process (Farris, 1978). For the Oriental woman, pregnancy is a normal and natural process, but it is also a time of anticipation and anxiety (Char, 1981).

In all these cultures, children are desired. In fact, children can improve the social standing of the traditional Chinese family. A woman who gives birth, especially to a son, achieves higher status. In Mexican-American society, having children proves the male's virility and is a sign of manliness or *machismo*, a desired trait among Mexican-American men.

Health Beliefs

Although many cultures view pregnancy as a natural occurrence, it may also be seen as a time of increased vulnerability. Individuals belonging to groups who believe in evil spirits may take certain protective precautions. For example, pregnant Vietnamese women are warned to avoid funerals, places of worship, and streets at noon and five o'clock in the afternoon since spirits are present at these places and times (Stringfellow, 1978). In the Mexican-American culture, the concept of *mal aire*, or bad air, is sometimes related to evil spirits (Baca, 1969). It is thought that air, especially night air, may enter the body and cause harm.

Most of the taboos stemming from the belief in evil spirits are grounded in fear of injuring the unborn child. Taboos also arise from the belief that a pregnant woman has evil powers (Brown, 1976). For this reason, women are sometimes prohibited from taking part in certain activities.

The hot-cold classification exists in Latin American, the Near Eastern, Far Eastern, and Asian cultures. The meanings of this classification vary among cultures. For example, Mexicans often view the body as unusually warm in pregnancy, and thus pregnant women avoid cold foods (Currier, 1978). Malays view pregnancy as a hot state, while the Vietnamese consider it a cold state (Manderson, 1981).

The concepts of hot and cold are not as important in American Indian or Black American cultures. There are some similarities in all these groups because they all emphasize achieving a natural balance. Black Americans believe that health is harmony with nature and a balance between good and evil, while American Indians have traditionally seen health as harmony with nature (Henderson and Primeaux, 1981).

Health Practices

Health care practices during pregnancy are influenced by numerous factors, including the following:

- The prevalence of traditional home remedies and folk beliefs
- The importance of local or native healers
- Socioeconomic status
- The influence of professional health care workers

An awareness of alternative health practices is crucial for health professionals, since these practices affect health outcomes. Local healers are important in several cultures. In the Mexican-American culture, the healer is called a *curandero*. In some American Indian tribes, the medicine man may fulfull the role of healer. Herbalists are often used by Orientals. Blacks sometimes consult faith healers, root doctors, and spiritualists.

The importance of assessing health care practices becomes evident when one looks at current maternal and infant mortality rates. One study found that hemorrhage, infection, and preeclampsia-eclampsia (PIH) are leading causes of maternal death, and the rates of these among nonwhites is more than four times greater than among whites (Schaffner et al., 1977). Another study found that perinatal mortality in the United States for whites is 34 deaths in 1000 births; for Blacks, 51 in 1000; for Puerto Ricans, 41 in 1000; and for Orientals, 23 in 1000. Disorders causing these deaths included premature rupture of the membranes, placental growth retardation, amniotic fluid infections,

and major congenital malformations (Naeye, 1979).

Many of these conditions can be prevented with prenatal care. Health care professionals must make the effort to overcome cultural barriers so that proper prenatal care can be provided. This may be accomplished by working with healers respected in other cultures, eliminating communication difficulties, and reducing economic barriers. These measures will lead to trust and use of the professional health care system. Certainly, sensitivity to cultural differences will result in greater understanding between health professionals and clients of all cultures.

Couvade

The term **couvade** refers to the observance of certain rituals and taboos by the male to signify the transition to fatherhood. This affirms his psychosocial and biophysical relationship to the woman and child. Some taboos restrict his actions. For example, in some cultures or primitive groups he may be forbidden to eat certain foods, kill certain animals, or carry certain weapons prior to and immediately after the birth.

A father who observes couvade plays an active and vital role during labor. In one culture, the father writhes, cries out in agony, and is attended by others to draw the attention of evil spirits while his partner delivers quietly alone or with one attendant, safe from the harmful spirits.

Summary

Although each pregnancy is unique, certain changes are common to all normal pregnancies. Deviations from normal may indicate pathology. The nurse must be able to detect these abnormalities during prenatal care so that appropriate interventions can be instituted. A basic understanding of the physical and psychologic changes of pregnancy, along with knowledge of significant cultural influences, form a foundation on which the nurse can base effective assessment of (Chapter 6) and intervention in (Chapters 7, 8, and 10) the health problems of the expectant woman.

References _____

Baca JE: Some health beliefs of the Spanish speaking. *Am J Nurse* 1969; 69:2172.

Brown MS: A cross-cultural look at pregnancy, labor, and delivery. *J Obstet Gynecol Neonatal Nurs* September/October 1976; 5:35.

Char EI: The Chinese American. In: *Culture and Childrearing.* Clark AL (editor). Philadelphia: Davis, 1981.

Colman A, Colman L: *Pregnancy: The Psychological Experience.* New York: Herder and Herder, 1971.

Currier RL: The hot-cold syndrome and symbolic balance. In: *Hispanic Culture and Health Care.* Martinez RA (editor). St. Louis: Mosby, 1978.

Danforth DN (editor): *Obstetrics and Gynecology,* 4th ed. Philadelphia: Harper & Row, 1982.

Duvall EM: *Marriage and Family Development,* 5th ed. Philadelphia: JB Lippincott, 1977.

Farris L: The American Indian. In: *Culture Childbearing Health Professionals.* Clark AL (editor). Philadelphia: Davis, 1978.

Fishbein EG: Expectant father's stress—due to mother's expectations? *J Obstet Gynecol Neonatal Nurs* September/October 1984; 13:325.

Henderson G, Primeaux M: The importance of folk medicine. In: *Transcultural Health Care.* Henderson G, Primeaux M (editors): Menlo Park, Calif.: Addison-Wesley, 1981.

Kay MA: The Mexican American. In: *Culture Childbearing Health Professionals.* Clark AL (editor). Philadelphia: Davis, 1978.

Manderson L: Roasting, smoking, and dieting in response to birth: Malay confinement in cross-cultural perspective. *Soc Sci Med* 1981; 15B:509.

Naeye R: Causes of fetal and neonatal mortality by race in a selected U.S. population. *Am J Public Health* 1979; 69:857.

Pritchard JA, MacDonald P, Gant NF: *Williams' Obstetrics,* 17th ed. New York: Appleton-Century-Crofts, 1985.

Schaffner W et al: Maternal mortality in Michigan: An epidemiologic analysis, 1950–1971. *Am J Public Health* 1977; 67:821.

Stringfellow L: The Vietnamese. In: *Culture Childbearing Health Professionals.* Clark AL (editor). Philadelphia: Davis, 1978.

Additional Readings _____

Anderson R, Lewis SZ, Giachello AL et al: Access to medical care among the Hispanic population of Southwestern United States. *J Health Soc Behav* 1981; 22:78.

Bullough VL, Bullough B: *Health Care of the Other Americans.* New York: Appleton-Century-Crofts, 1982.

Charles D, Larson B: How pregnancy alters infection defenses. *Contemp Ob/Gyn* June 1984; 23:96.

Ebrahim GJ: Cross-cultural aspects of pregnancy and breast feeding. *Proc Nutrition Soc* 1980; 39:13.

Griffith S: Childbearing and the concept of culture. *J Obstet Gynecol Neonatal Nurs* May/June 1982; 11:181.

Hershey DW, Vieira L: Problems of pregnancy at high altitude. *Contemp Ob/Gyn* February 1984; 23:47.

Marrs RP, Mischell DR: Placental trophic hormones. *Clin Obstet Gynecol* 1980; 23:721.

Mercer RT, Hackley KC, Bostrom AG: Relationship of psychosocial and perinatal variables to perception of childbirth. *Nurs Res* July/August 1983; 32:202.

Tilden VP: The relation of life stress and social support to emotional disequilibrium during pregnancy. *Research Nurs Health* December 1983; 6:167.

Tyson JE: Changing role of placental lactogen and prolactin in human gestation. *Clin Obstet Gynecol* 1980; 23:737.

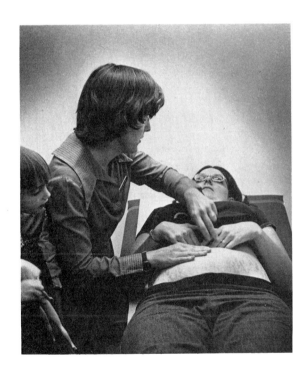

6

Antepartal Nursing Assessment

Chapter Contents

Objectives

- Identify the essential components of a prenatal history.

- Explain the common obstetric terminology used in the history of a maternity client.

- Identify factors related to the father's health that should be recorded on the prenatal record.

- Describe the normal physiologic changes one would expect to find when performing a physical assessment of a pregnant woman.

- Explain how a woman's attitude toward childbearing can affect the course of her pregnancy.

Key Terms ▰▰▰▰▰▰▰▰

abortion

antepartum

diagonal conjugate

gestation

gravida

intrapartum

multigravida

multipara

Nägele's rule

nullipara

obstetric conjugate

para

postpartum

postterm labor

preterm or prema-
   ture labor

primigravida

primipara

risk factors

stillbirth

The course of a pregnancy depends on many factors, including the prepregnancy health of the woman, presence of disease states, emotional status, and past health care. Ideally, health care during pregnancy will be a continuation of established and adequate medical care.

If maternal health is to be maintained, a thorough history and physical examination are essential to identify problem areas. The history and physical examination may be done by a nurse, a physician, or both.

Client History _____

Definition of Terms

The following terms are used in the obstetric history of maternity clients:

Gestation: Time elapsed (measured in weeks) since the first day of the LMP.

Abortion: Delivery that occurs prior to the end of 20 weeks' gestation.

Preterm or premature labor: Labor that occurs after 20 weeks but before the completion of 37 weeks of gestation (pregnancy).

Postterm labor: Labor that occurs after 42 weeks of gestation.

Antepartum: Time between conception and the onset of labor; usually used to describe the period during which a woman is pregnant.

Intrapartum: Time from the onset of true labor until the delivery of the infant and placenta.

Postpartum: Time from delivery until the woman's body returns to an essentially prepregnant condition.

Gravida: Any pregnancy, regardless of duration, including present pregnancy.

Primigravida: A woman who is pregnant for the first time.

Multigravida: A woman who is in her second or any subsequent pregnancy.

Para: Delivery after 20 weeks of gestation (pregnancy) regardless of whether the infant is born alive or dead.

Nullipara: A woman who has not had a delivery at more than 20 weeks' gestation.

Primipara: A woman who has had one delivery at more than 20 weeks' gestation, regardless of whether the infant is born alive or dead.

Multipara: A woman who has had two or more deliveries at more than 20 weeks' gestation.

Stillbirth: An infant born dead after 20 weeks of gestation.

The terms *gravida* and *para* are used in relation to pregnancies, not to the number of fetuses.

The following examples illustrate how these terms are applied in clinical situations:

1. Jean Smith has one child born at 38 weeks and is pregnant for the second time. At her initial prenatal visit, the nurse indicates her obstetric history as "gravida II para I ab 0." Jean Smith's present pregnancy terminates at 16 weeks' gestation. She is now "gravida II para I ab I."

2. Mrs. Alexander is pregnant for the fourth time. She has twins born at 35 weeks at home. One pregnancy ended at 10 weeks' gestation, and she delivered another infant stillborn at term. At her prenatal assessment the nurse records her obstetric history as "gravida IV para II ab I." Note that twins are considered as one pregnancy and delivery.

Because of the confusion that may result from this system when a multiple pregnancy occurs, a more detailed approach is used in some settings. Using the detailed system, *gravida* keeps the same meaning, while *para* changes to mean the number of infants born rather than the number of deliveries. A useful acronym for remembering the system is TPAL.

First digit, T—number of *term* infants born; that is, the number of infants born after 37 weeks' gestation or more.

Second digit, P—number of *preterm* infants born; that is, the number of infants born before 37 weeks' gestation.

Third digit, A—number of pregnancies ending in either spontaneous or therapeutic *abortion*.

Fourth digit, L—number of currently *living* children.

Using this approach, the nurse would have described Jean Smith (see the first example above) initially as "gravida 2 para 1001." Following her abortion she would be "gravida 2 para 1011." Mrs. Alexander would be described as "gravida 4 para 1212."

Client Profile

The history is essentially a screening tool that identifies factors that may negatively affect the course of a pregnancy. The following information should be obtained for each maternity client at the first prenatal assessment:

1. Current pregnancy
   a. First day of LMP
   b. Presence of cramping, bleeding, or spotting since LMP
   c. Woman's attitude toward pregnancy (is this pregnancy planned? Wanted?)
   d. Results of pregnancy tests, if completed
2. Past pregnancies
   a. Number of pregnancies
   b. Number of abortions, spontaneous or induced
   c. Number of living children
   d. History of previous pregnancies—length of pregnancy, complications (antepartal, intrapartal, postpartal), length of labor
   e. Perinatal status of previous children—birth weights, general development, complications, feeding patterns
   f. Blood type and Rh factor (if negative—medication after delivery for immunization)
   g. Prenatal education classes

3. Gynecologic history
   a. Previous infections—vaginal, cervical, sexually transmitted
   b. Previous surgery
   c. Age at menarche
   d. Regularity, frequency, and duration of menstrual flow
   e. History of dysmenorrhea
   f. Contraceptive history (if birth control pills were used, did pregnancy occur immediately following cessation of pills? If not, how long after?)
4. Current medical history
   a. Weight
   b. Blood type and Rh factor, if known
   c. Any medications presently being taken (including nonprescription medications) or taken since the onset of pregnancy
   d. Alcohol and tobacco intake
   e. Illicit drug use and/or abuse
   f. Drug allergies
   g. Potential teratogenic insults to this pregnancy (such as viral infections, medications, x-ray examinations, surgery)
   h. Presence of disease conditions (such as diabetes, hypertension, cardiovascular disease, renal problems)
   i. Record of immunizations (especially rubella)
   j. Presence of any abnormal symptoms
5. Past medical history
   a. Childhood diseases
   b. Past treatment for any disease condition
   c. Surgical procedures
   d. Presence of bleeding disorders or tendencies (has she received blood transfusions?)
6. Family medical history
   a. Presence of diabetes, cardiovascular disease, hypertension, hematologic disorders, preeclampsia-eclampsia (PIH)
   b. Occurrence of multiple births
   c. History of congenital diseases or deformities
   d. Occurrence of cesarean deliveries
7. Partner's history
   a. Presence of genetic conditions or diseases
   b. Age
   c. Significant health problems
   d. Previous or present alcohol intake, drug use
   e. Blood type and Rh factor

8. Personal information
   a. Age
   b. Educational level
   c. Previous or present use of drugs, alcohol, and cigarettes
   d. Cultural patterns that could influence pregnancy (such as dietary practices or self-medication)
   e. Acceptance of pregnancy
   f. Race or ethnic group (to identify need for prenatal genetic screening or counseling)
   g. Religion (for example, Jehovah's Witnesses—refusal of blood transfusions)
   h. Stability of living conditions
   i. Economic level
   j. Housing
   k. Any history of emotional or physical deprivation (herself or children)
   l. History of emotional problems
   m. Support systems
   n. Overuse or underuse of health care system

Obtaining Data

A questionnaire is used in many instances to obtain information. The woman should complete the questionnaire in a quiet place with a minimum of distractions.

The nurse can obtain further information in a direct interview, which allows the pregnant woman to expand or clarify her responses to questions, and gives the nurse and client the opportunity to begin developing a good relationship.

The expectant father should be encouraged to attend the prenatal examinations. He is often able to contribute information to the history and may use the opportunity to ask questions or express concerns.

Prenatal High-Risk Screening

Risk factors are any findings that suggest the pregnancy may have a negative outcome, either for the woman or her unborn child. Screening for high-risk factors is an important part of the prenatal assessment.

Many risk factors can be identified during the initial prenatal assessment; others may be detected during subsequent prenatal visits. It is important to identify high-risk pregnancies early so that appropriate interventions can be started immediately. Not all high-risk factors threaten the pregnancy equally; thus many agencies use a risk scoring sheet to determine the degree of risk. Information must be updated throughout pregnancy as necessary. It is always possible that a pregnancy may begin as low risk and change to high risk because of complications.

Table 6-1 identifies the major risk factors currently recognized. The table also identifies maternal and fetal/neonatal implications if the risk is present in the pregnancy.

Initial Physical Assessment

After a complete history is obtained, the woman is prepared for a physical examination. The physical examination begins with assessment of vital signs, then the woman's body is examined. The pelvic examination is performed last.

Before the examination, the woman should provide a clean urine specimen. When the bladder is empty, the woman is more comfortable during the pelvic examination, and the examiner can palpate the pelvic organs more easily. After emptying her bladder, she is asked to disrobe and is given a sheet or some other protective covering.

The extent of the initial physical assessment varies greatly according to examiner preference and agency policy. The accompanying Initial Prenatal Physical Assessment Guide identifies those areas commonly assessed during an initial prenatal examination (it is not a complete physical examination). The assessment guide is divided into three columns: area to be assessed and the normal findings, alterations and possible causes for them, and nursing responses to the data collected. The nurse should be aware that certain organs and systems are assessed concurrently with other systems. More information on pelvic assessment and determination of delivery date follows the assessment guide.

Table 6-1
Prenatal High-Risk Factors

Factor	Maternal implication	Fetal/neonatal implication
Social-personal		
Low income level	Poor antenatal care Poor nutrition ↑risk of preeclampsia	Low birth weight Intrauterine growth retardation (IUGR)
Poor diet	Inadequate nutrition ↑risk anemia ↑risk preeclampsia	Fetal malnutrition Prematurity
Living at high altitude	↑hemoglobin	Prematurity IUGR
Multiparity > 3	↑risk antepartum/postpartum hemorrhage	Anemia Fetal death
Weight < 100 lb	Poor nutrition Cephalopelvic dysproportion Prolonged labor	IUGR Hypoxia associated with difficult labor and delivery
Weight > 200 lb	↑risk hypertension ↑risk cephalopelvic dysproportion	↓fetal nutrition
Age < 16	Poor nutrition Poor antenatal care ↑risk preeclampsia ↑risk cephalopelvic dysproportion	Low birth weight ↑fetal wastage
Age > 35	↑risk preeclampsia ↑risk cesarean delivery	↑risk congenital anomalies ↑chromosomal aberrations
Smoking — one pack/day or more	↑risk hypertension ↑risk cancer	↓placental perfusion →↓O_2 and nutrients available Low birth weight IUGR Preterm birth
Use of addicting drugs	↑risk poor nutrition ↑risk of infection with IV drugs	↑risk congenital anomalies ↑risk low birth weight Neonatal withdrawal Lower serum bilirubin
Excessive alcohol consumption	↑risk poor nutrition Possible hepatic effects with long-term consumption	↑risk fetal alcohol syndrome
Preexisting medical disorders		
Diabetes mellitus	↑risk preeclampsia, hypertension Episodes of hypoglycemia and hyperglycemia ↑risk cesarean delivery	Low birth weight Macrosomia Neonatal hypoglycemia ↑risk congenital anomalies ↑risk respiratory distress syndrome
Cardiac disease	Cardiac decompensation Further strain on mother's body ↑maternal death rate	↑risk fetal wastage ↑perinatal mortality
Anemia:* hemoglobin < 9 g/dL (white) < 29% hematocrit (white) < 8.2 g/dL hemoglobin (black) < 26% hematocrit (black)	Iron deficiency anemia Low energy level Decreased oxygen carrying capacity	Fetal death Prematurity Low birth weight
Hypertension	↑vasospasm ↑risk central nervous system (CNS) irritability →convulsions ↑risk cerebral vascular accident (CVA) ↑risk renal damage	↓placental perfusion →low birth weight Preterm birth

Continued

Table 6-1
Prenatal High-Risk Factors (continued)

Factor	Maternal implication	Fetal/neonatal implication

Thyroid disorder
    hypothyroidism
	↑ infertility
	↓ Basal metabolic rate (BMR)
	    goiter, myxedema
		↑ spontaneous abortion
		↑ risk congenital goiter
		Mental retardation → cretinism
		↑ incidence congenital anomalies

hyperthyroidism	↑ risk postpartum hemorrhage ↑ risk preeclampsia Danger of thyroid storm	↑ incidence preterm birth ↑ tendency to thyrotoxicosis
Renal disease (moderate to severe)	↑ risk renal failure	↑ risk IUGR ↑ risk preterm delivery
Obstetric considerations *Previous pregnancy* Stillborn	↑ emotional/psychologic distress	↑ risk IUGR ↑ risk preterm delivery
Habitual abortion	↑ emotional/psychologic distress ↑ possibility diagnostic work-up	↑ risk abortion
Cesarean delivery	↑ probability repeat cesarean delivery	↑ risk preterm birth ↑ risk respiratory distress
Rh or blood group sensitization	↑ financial expenditure for testing	Hydrops fetalis Icterus gravis Neonatal anemia Kernicterus Hypoglycemia
Current pregnancy Rubella (first trimester)		Congenital heart disease Cataracts Nerve deafness Bone lesions Prolonged virus shedding
Rubella (second trimester)		Hepatitis Thrombocytopenia
Cytomegalovirus		IUGR Encephalopathy
Herpesvirus type 2	Severe discomfort	Neonatal herpesvirus type 2 Neurologic abnormalities
Syphilis	↑ incidence abortion	↑ fetal wastage Congenital syphilis
Abruptio placentae and placenta previa	↑ risk hemorrhage Bed rest Extended hospitalization	Fetal/neonatal anemia Intrauterine hemorrhage ↑ fetal wastage
Preeclampsia/eclampsia	See hypertension	↓ placental perfusion → low birth weight
Multiple gestation	↑ risk postpartum hemorrhage	↑ risk preterm birth ↑ risk fetal demise

Elevated hematocrit*
    > 41% (White)
    > 38% (Black)
	Increased viscosity of blood	Fetal death rate 5 times normal rate

*Data from Garn, S. M., et al. April 1981. Maternal hematologic levels and pregnancy outcomes. *Sem Perinatol* 5:155.

Assess/Normal findings	Alterations and possible causes*	Nursing responses to data†
VITAL SIGNS Blood pressure (BP): 90–140/60–90	High BP (essential hypertension; renal disease; pregestational hypertension; apprehension or anxiety associated with pregnancy diagnosis, exam, or other crises)	BP > 150/90 requires immediate consideration; establish client's BP; refer to physician if necessary. Assess patient's knowledge about high BP; counsel on self-care and medical management
Pulse: 60–90 beats/min. Rate may increase 10 beats/min during pregnancy	Increased pulse rate (excitement or anxiety, cardiac disorders)	Count for one full minute; note irregularities
Respiration: 16–24 breaths/min (or pulse rate divided by four). Pregnancy may induce a degree of hyperventilation; thoracic breathing predominant	Marked tachypnea or abnormal patterns	Assess for respiratory disease
Temperature: 36.2–37.6C (98–99.6F)	Elevated temperature (infection)	Assess for infection process or disease state if temperature is elevated; refer to physician
WEIGHT Depends on body build	Weight < 100 lb or > 200 lb; rapid, sudden weight gain (preeclampsia-eclampsia [PIH])	Evaluate need for nutritional counseling; obtain information on eating habits, cooking practices, foods regularly eaten, income limitations, need for food supplements, pica and other abnormal food habits Note initial weight to establish baseline for weight gain throughout pregnancy
SKIN Color: Consistent with racial background; pink nail beds	Pallor (anemia); bronze, yellow (hepatic disease, other causes of jaundice)	The following tests should be performed: complete blood count (CBC), bilirubin level, urinalysis, and blood urea nitrogen (BUN)
	Bluish, reddish, mottled; dusky appearance or pallor of palms and nail beds in dark-skinned women (anemia)	If abnormal, refer to physician
Condition: Absence of edema (slight edema of lower extremities is normal during pregnancy)	Edema (preeclampsia); rashes, dermatitis (allergic response)	Counsel on relief measures for slight edema Initiate preeclampsia assessment; refer to physician
Lesions: Absence of lesions	Ulceration (varicose veins, decreased circulation)	Further assess circulatory status; refer to physician if lesion severe
Spider nevi common in pregnancy	Petechiae, multiple bruises, ecchymosis (hemorrhagic disorders)	Evaluate for bleeding or clotting disorder
Moles	Change in size or color (carcinoma)	Refer to physician
Pigmentation: Pigmentation changes of pregnancy include linea nigra, striae gravidarum, chloasma, spider nevi		Assure patient that these are normal manifestations of pregnancy and explain the physiologic basis for the changes
Café-au-lait spots	Six or more (Albright's syndrome or neurofibromatosis)	Consult with physician

*Possible causes of alterations are in parentheses.
†This column provides guidelines for further assessment and initial nursing intervention.

INITIAL PRENATAL PHYSICAL ASSESSMENT GUIDE (continued)

Assess/Normal findings	Alterations and possible causes*	Nursing responses to data†
NOSE Character of mucosa: Redder than oral mucosa; in pregnancy nasal mucosa is edematous in response to increased estrogen, resulting in nasal stuffiness and nosebleeds	Olfactory loss (first cranial nerve deficit)	Counsel client about possible relief measures for nasal stuffiness and epistaxis; refer to physician for olfactory loss
MOUTH May note hypertrophy of gingival tissue because of estrogen	Edema, inflammation (infection); pale in color (anemia)	Assess hematocrit for anemia; counsel regarding dental hygiene habits Refer to physician or dentist if necessary
NECK Nodes: Small, mobile, nontender nodes	Tender, hard, fixed or prominent nodes (infection, carcinoma)	Examine for local infection; refer to physician
Thyroid: Small, smooth lateral lobes palpable on either side of trachea; slight hyperplasia by third month of pregnancy	Enlargement or nodule tenderness (hyperthyroidism)	Listen over thyroid for bruits, which may indicate hyperthyroidism Question woman about dietary habits (iodine intake) Ascertain history of thyroid problems; refer to physician
BREASTS Supple; symmetrical in size and contour; darker pigmentation of nipple and areola; may have supernumerary nipples, usually 5–6 cm below normal nipple line	"Pigskin" or orange-peel appearance, nipple retractions, swelling, hardness (carcinoma); redness, heat, tenderness, cracked or fissured nipple (infection)	Encourage monthly breast checks; instruct client how to examine own breasts Refer to physician
Axillary nodes unpalpable or pellet-sized	Tenderness, enlargement, hard node (carcinoma); may be visible bump (infection)	Refer to physician if evidence of inflammation
Pregnancy changes: 1. Size increase noted primarily in first 20 weeks 2. Become nodular 3. Tingling sensation may be felt during first and third trimester; woman may report feeling of heaviness 4. Pigmentation of nipples and areolas darkens 5. Superficial veins dilate and become more prominent 6. Striae seen in multiparas 7. Tubercles of Montgomery enlarge 8. Colostrum may be present after twelfth week 9. Secondary areola appears at 20 weeks, characterized by series of washed-out spots surrounding primary areola 10. Breasts less firm, old striae may be present in multiparas		Discuss normalcy of changes and their meaning with the client Teach and/or institute appropriate relief measures Encourage use of supportive brassiere

*Possible causes of alterations are in parentheses.
†This column provides guidelines for further assessment and initial nursing intervention.

INITIAL PRENATAL PHYSICAL ASSESSMENT GUIDE (continued)

Assess/Normal findings	Alterations and possible causes*	Nursing responses to data†
HEART Normal rate, rhythm, and heart sounds Pregnancy changes: 1. Palpitations may occur due to sympathetic nervous system disturbance 2. Short systolic murmurs that ↑ in held expiration are normal due to increased volume	Enlargement, thrills, thrusts, gross irregularity or skipped beats, gallop rhythm or extra sounds (cardiac disease)	Complete an initial assessment Explain normalcy of pregnancy-induced changes Refer to physician if indicated
ABDOMEN Normal appearance, skin texture, and hair distribution; liver nonpalpable; abdomen nontender Pregnancy changes: 1. Purple striae may be present (or silver striae on a multipara) 2. Diastasis of the rectus muscles late in pregnancy	Muscle guarding (anxiety, acute tenderness); tenderness, mass (ectopic pregnancy, inflammation, carcinoma)	Assure client of normalcy of diastasis Provide initial information about appropriate postpartum exercises Evaluate client anxiety level. Refer to physician if indicated
3. Size: Flat or rotund abdomen; progressive enlargement of uterus due to pregnancy 10–12 weeks: Fundus slightly above symphysis pubis 16 weeks: Fundus halfway between symphysis and umbilicus 20–22 weeks: Fundus at umbilicus 28 weeks: Fundus three fingerbreadths above umbilicus 36 weeks: Fundus just below ensiform cartilage	Size of uterus inconsistent with length of gestation (intrauterine growth retardation [IUGR] multiple pregnancy, fetal demise, hydatidiform mole)	Reassess menstrual history regarding pregnancy dating Evaluate increase in size using McDonald's method Use ultrasound to establish diagnosis
4. Fetal heartbeats: 120–160 beats/min may be heard with Doppler at 10–12 weeks' gestation; may be heard with fetoscope at 17–20 weeks	Failure to hear fetal heartbeat after 17–20 weeks (fetal demise, hydatidiform mole)	Refer to physician Administer pregnancy tests Use ultrasound to establish diagnosis
5. Fetal movement not felt prior to 20 weeks' gestation by examiner	Failure to feel fetal movements after 20 weeks' gestation (fetal demise, hydatidiform mole)	Refer to physician for evaluation of fetal status
6. Ballottement: During fourth to fifth month, fetus rises and then rebounds to original position when uterus is tapped sharply	No ballottement (oligohydramnios)	Refer to physician for evaluation of fetal status
EXTREMITIES Skin warm, pulses palpable, full range of motion; may be some edema of hands and ankles in late pregnancy; varicose veins may become more pronounced	Unpalpable or diminished pulses (arterial insufficiency); marked edema (preeclampsia)	Evaluate for other symptoms of heart disease; initiate follow-up if client mentions that her rings feel tight Discuss prevention and self-treatment measures for varicose veins; refer to physician if indicated

*Possible causes of alterations are in parentheses.
†This column provides guidelines for further assessment and initial nursing intervention.

INITIAL PRENATAL PHYSICAL ASSESSMENT GUIDE (continued)

Assess/Normal findings	Alterations and possible causes*	Nursing responses to data†
SPINE Normal spinal curves: Concave cervical, convex thoracic, concave lumbar	Abnormal spinal curves: flatness, kyphosis, lordosis	Refer to physician for assessment of cephalopelvic disproportion (CPD)
In pregnancy, dorsal and lumbar spinal curve may be accentuated	Backache	May have implications for administration of spinal anesthetics; see p. 139 for relief measures
Shoulders and iliac crests should be even	Uneven shoulders and iliac crests (scoliosis)	Refer very young clients to a physician; discuss back-stretching exercises with older clients
REFLEXES Normal and symmetrical	Hyperactivity, clonus (preeclampsia)	Evaluate for other symptoms of preeclampsia
PELVIC AREA External female genitals: Normally formed with female hair distribution; in multiparas, labia majora loose and pigmented; urinary and vaginal orifices visible and appropriately located	Lesions, hematomas, varicosities, inflammation of Bartholin's glands; clitoral hypertrophy (masculinization)	Explain pelvic examination procedure (Procedure 6-1) Encourage woman to minimize her discomfort by relaxing her hips Provide privacy (Figure 6-1)
Vagina: Pink or dark pink; vaginal discharge odorless, non-irritating; in multiparas, vaginal folds smooth and flattened; may have episiotomy scar	Abnormal discharge associated with vaginal infections	Obtain vaginal smear Provide understandable verbal and written instructions about treatment for client and partner, if indicated
Cervix: Pink color; os closed except in multiparas, in whom os admits fingertip	Eversion, reddish erosion, Nabothian or retention cysts, cervical polyp; granular area that bleeds (carcinoma of cervix)	Provide client with a hand mirror and identify genital structures for her; encourage her to view her cervix if she wishes Refer to physician if indicated
	Presence of string or plastic tip from cervix (intrauterine device [IUD] in uterus)	Advise client of potential serious risks of leaving an IUD in place during pregnancy; refer to physician for removal
Pregnancy changes: 1–4 weeks' gestation: Enlargement in anteroposterior diameter 4–6 weeks' gestation: Softening of cervix (Goodell's sign), softening of isthmus of uterus (Hegar's sign); cervix takes on bluish coloring (Chadwick's sign) 8–12 weeks' gestation: Vagina and cervix appear bluish-violet in color (Chadwick's sign)	Absence of Goodell's sign (inflammatory conditions, carcinoma)	Refer to physician
Uterus: Pear-shaped, mobile, smooth surface	Fixed (pelvic inflammatory disease—PID); nodular surface (fibromas)	Refer to physician
Ovaries: Small, walnut-shaped, nontender	Pain on movement of cervix (PID); enlarged or nodular ovaries (cyst, tumor, tubal pregnancy, corpus luteum of pregnancy)	Evaluate adnexal areas; refer to physician

*Possible causes of alterations are in parentheses.
†This column provides guidelines for further assessment and initial nursing intervention.

INITIAL PRENATAL PHYSICAL ASSESSMENT GUIDE (continued)

Assess/Normal findings	Alterations and possible causes*	Nursing responses to data†
PELVIC MEASUREMENTS Internal measurements: 1. Diagonal conjugate 12.5 cm (Figure 6-4,A)	Measurement below normal	Vaginal delivery may not be possible if deviations are present Consider possibility of cesarean delivery Determine CPD by radiological examination and ultrasound
2. Obstetric conjugate estimated by subtracting 1.5–2 cm from diagonal conjugate	Disproportion of pubic arch	
3. Inclination of sacrum	Abnormal curvature of sacrum	
4. Motility of coccyx; external intertuberosity diameter > 8 cm	Fixed or malposition of coccyx	
ANUS AND RECTUM No lumps, rashes, excoriation, tenderness; cervix may be felt through rectal wall	Hemorrhoids, rectal prolapse; nodular lesion (carcinoma)	Counsel about appropriate prevention and relief measures; refer to physician for further evaluation
LABORATORY EVALUATION Hemoglobin: 12–16 g/dL; women residing in high altitudes may have higher levels of hemoglobin	< 12 g/dL (anemia)	Hemoglobin < 12 g/dL requires iron supplementation and nutritional counseling
ABO and Rh typing: Normal distribution of blood types	Rh negative	If Rh negative, check for presence of anti-Rh antibodies Check partner's blood type; if partner is Rh positive, discuss with client the need for antibody titers during pregnancy, management during the intrapartal period, and possible candidacy for RhoGAM
Complete blood count (CBC) Hematocrit: 38%–47%; physiologic anemia may occur Red blood cells (RBC): 4.2–5.4 million/μL	Marked anemia or blood dyscrasias	Perform CBC and Schilling differential cell count
White blood cells (WBC): 4500–11,000/μL	Presence of infection; may be elevated in pregnancy and with labor	Evaluate for other signs of infection
Differential Neutrophils 40%–60% Bands up to 5% Eosinophils 1%–3% Basophils up to 1% Lymphocytes 20%–40% Monocytes 4%–8%		
Syphilis tests—serologic test for syphilis (STS), complement fixation test, Venereal Disease Research Laboratory (VDRL) test—Nonreactive	Positive reaction STS—tests may have 25%–45% incidence of biologic false positive results; false results may occur in individuals who have acute viral or bacterial infections, hypersensitivity reactions, recent vaccination, collagen disease, malaria, or tuberculosis	Positive results may be confirmed with the fluorescent treponemal antibody absorption (FTA-ABS) tests; all tests for syphilis give positive results in the secondary stage of the disease; antibiotic tests may cause negative test results
Gonorrhea culture: Negative	Positive	Refer for treatment

*Possible causes of alterations are in parentheses.
†This column provides guidelines for further assessment and initial nursing intervention.

INITIAL PRENATAL PHYSICAL ASSESSMENT GUIDE (continued)

Assess/Normal findings	Alterations and possible causes*	Nursing responses to data†
Urinalysis (u/a): Normal color, specific gravity; pH 4.6–8.0	Abnormal color (porphyria, hemoglobinuria, bilirubinemia); alkaline urine (metabolic alkalemia, *Proteus* infection, old specimen)	Repeat u/a; refer to physician
Negative for protein, red blood cells, white blood cells, casts	Positive findings (contaminated specimen, kidney disease)	Repeat u/a; refer to physician
Glucose: Negative (small degree of glycosuria may occur in pregnancy)	Glycosuria (low renal threshold for glucose, diabetes mellitus)	Assess blood glucose; test urine for ketones
Rubella titer: hemagglutination-inhibition test (HAI) > 1:10 indicates woman is immune	HAI titer < 1:10	Immunization will be given on postpartum or within 6 weeks after delivery. Instruct client whose titers are < 1:10 to avoid children who have rubella
Antibody screen: Negative	Positive	If results are positive, further testing should be done to identify specific antibodies; in addition, antibody titers may be done during pregnancy
Sickle cell screen for Black clients: Negative	Positive; test results would include a description of cells	Refer to physician
Papanicolaou (Pap) test: Negative	Test results that show atypical cells	Refer to physician. Discuss the meaning of the various classes with the client and importance of follow-up

*Possible causes of alterations are in parentheses.
†This column provides guidelines for further assessment and initial nursing intervention.

Determination of Delivery Date

Nägele's Rule

The delivery date, or estimated date of confinement (EDC), can be determined in a number of different ways. The most common method is **Nägele's rule**. To use this method, take the first day of the LMP, subtract 3 months, and add 7 days. For example:

First day of LMP	November 21
Subtract 3 months	− 3 months
Add 7 days	August 21
EDC	+ 7 days
	August 28

If a woman with a history of menses every 28 days remembers her LMP and was not taking oral contraceptives prior to becoming pregnant, Nägele's rule may be a fairly accurate determiner of her delivery date. However, if her cycle is irregular or 35–40 days long, the time of ovulation may be delayed by several days. If she has been using oral contraceptives, ovulation may be delayed several weeks following her last menses. Ovulation usually occurs 14 days before the onset of the next menses, not 14 days after the previous menses.

Uterine Size

Physical examination When a woman is examined in the first 10–12 weeks of her pregnancy and her uterine size is compatible with her menstrual history, uterine size may be the single most important clinical method for dating her pregnancy. In many cases, however, women do not seek obstetric attention until well into their second trimester, when it becomes much more difficult to evaluate specific uterine size. In the obese woman, it is most difficult to determine uterine size early in a pregnancy.

PROCEDURE 6-1
Assisting with Pelvic Examination

Objective	Nursing action	Rationale
Prepare client	Explain procedure.	Explanation of procedure decreases anxiety.
	Instruct client to empty her bladder and to remove clothing below waist. She may be encouraged to keep her shoes on and may be given a disposable drape to hold in front of herself.	Comfort is promoted during internal examination. She may feel more comfortable with shoes on rather than supporting her weight with bare heels against cold stirrups.
	Position client in lithotomy position with thighs flexed and adducted. Place her feet in stirrups. Buttocks should extend slightly beyond end of examining table (Figure 6-1).	
	Drape client with a sheet, leaving flap so perineum can be exposed.	
Ensure smooth accomplishment of procedure	Prepare and arrange following equipment so that they are easily accessible:	Examination is facilitated.
	1. Various-sized vaginal specula, warmed prior to insertion.	Warmed speculum assists in lubrication and facilitates initial insertion when culture and smears are to be taken; many standard lubricants cannot be utilized.
	2. Glove.	
	3. Lubricant.	
	4. Pelvimeter.	
	5. Materials for Pap smear and gonorrhea culture.	
	6. Good light source.	
Provide support to client as physician or nurse practitioner carries out examination	Explain each part of examination as it is performed: inspection of external genitals, vagina, and cervix; bimanual examination of internal organs.	Relaxation is promoted.
	Instruct client to relax and breathe slowly.	
	Advise client when speculum is to be inserted and ask her to bear down.	When speculum is inserted, woman may feel intravaginal pressure. Bearing down helps open vaginal orifice and relax perineal muscles.
	Lubricate examiner's finger well prior to bimanual examination.	
Provide client comfort at end of examination	Assist client to sitting position.	Supine position may create postural hypotension.
	Provide tissues to wipe lubricant from perineum.	When she sits, vaginal secretions along with lubricant may be discharged.
	Provide privacy for client to dress.	Comfort and sense of privacy is promoted.

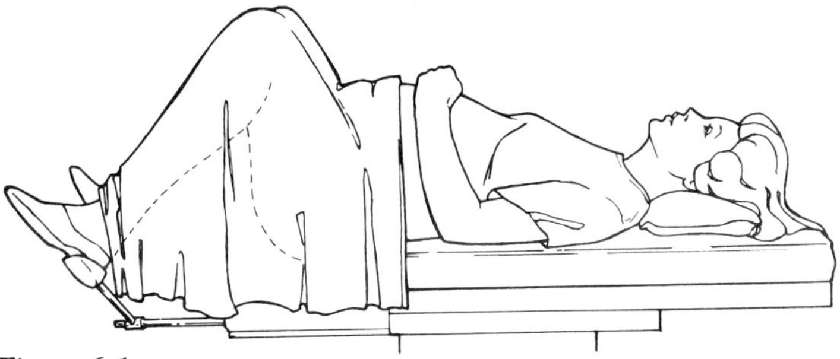

Figure 6-1
Woman in lithotomy position and draped for a pelvic examination.

Fundal height   Fundal height may be used as an indicator of uterine size, although this method of dating the pregnancy is at best accurate only within about 4 weeks and cannot be used late in pregnancy. A centimeter tape measure is used to measure the distance abdominally from the top of the symphysis pubis to the top of the uterine fundus (McDonald's method) (Figure 6-2). Fundal height usually correlates with gestational age until the third trimester, when fetal weights vary considerably. Thus, at 26 weeks' gestation, fundal height is probably about 26 cm. At 20 weeks' gestation, the fundus is about 20 cm and at the level of the umbilicus in an average female.

McDonald's rule may also be used to measure fundal height in the second and third trimesters. Calculation is done as follows:

Height of fundus (in centimeters) × 2/7 = Duration of pregnancy in lunar months
  Example: 28 cm × 2/7 = 8 lunar months
Height of fundus (in centimeters) × 8/7 = Duration of pregnancy in weeks
  Example: 28 cm × 8/7 = 32 weeks

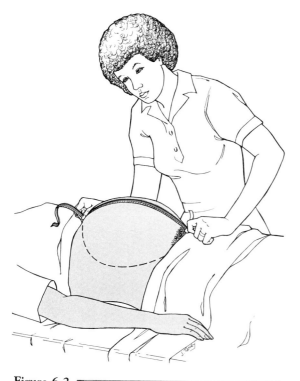

Figure 6-2 ▰▰▰▰▰
Use of McDonald's method to measure fundal height.

If the woman is very tall or very short, fundal height will differ.

Measurements of fundal height from month to month and week to week may signal intrauterine growth retardation (IUGR) if there is a lag in progression. A sudden increase in fundal height may indicate twins or hydramnios.

Fetal Development

Quickening   Fetal movements felt by the mother may indicate that the fetus is nearing 20 weeks' gestation. However, quickening may be experienced between 16 and 22 weeks' gestation, so this method is not completely accurate.

Fetal heartbeat   The fetal heartbeat can be detected with a fetoscope as early as week 16 and almost always by 19 or 20 weeks of gestation. Fetal heartbeat may be detected with the ultrasonic Doppler device (Figure 6-3) as early as 8 weeks, but it is first heard, on average, at 10–12 weeks' gestation.

Ultrasound findings   In the first trimester, ultrasound scanning can detect a gestational sac as early as 5–6 weeks after the LMP, fetal heart activity by 9–10 weeks, and fetal breathing movement by 11 weeks of pregnancy. C-R measurements can be used to assess fetal age until the fetal head can be visualized clearly. Biparietal diameter (BPD) can then be used. The BPD can be measured at approximately 12–13 weeks. This diameter is a more accurate determiner of

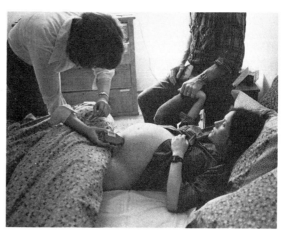

Figure 6-3 ▰▰▰▰▰
Listening to fetal heartbeat with Doppler device.

age early in pregnancy, when less biologic variation occurs.

Assessment of Pelvic Adequacy

The pelvis is usually assessed during the prenatal course. Some agencies assess the pelvis as part of the initial physical assessment. Others wait until later in the pregnancy, when hormonal effects are greatest and it is possible to make some determination of fetal size.

The method of measurement is depicted in Figures 6-4 and 6-5. The parts of the pelvis that are evaluated and their typical measurements include the following:

1. Pelvic inlet (Figure 6-4)
   a. **Diagonal conjugate**, 12.5 cm
   b. **Obstetric conjugate**, 11 cm (this measurement is approximately 1.5 cm smaller than the diagonal conjugate)
2. Pelvic cavity (midpelvis)
   a. Plane of greatest dimensions or midplane, 12.75 cm
   b. Plane of least dimension, 11.5–12.0 cm
3. Pelvic outlet (Figure 6-5)
   a. Anteroposterior diameter, 9.5–11.5 cm
   b. Transverse diameter, 8 cm

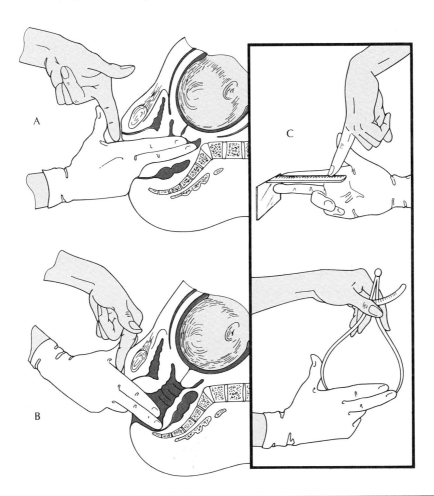

Figure 6-4

Manual measurement of pelvic inlet and outlet. **A**, Estimation of diagonal conjugate, which extends from lower border of symphysis pubis to sacral promontory. **B**, Estimation of anteroposterior diameter of the outlet, which extends from the lower border of the symphysis pubis to the tip of the coccyx. **C**, Manual estimation of anteroposterior measurements may be checked using a wall-mounted measure or hand-held device.

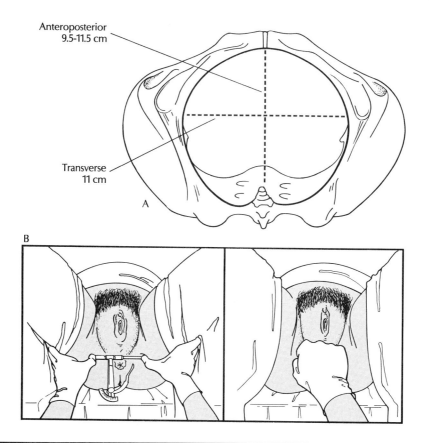

Figure 6-5

A, Diameters of the pelvic outlet. **B**, Measurement of the transverse diameter of the outlet. Left, use of Thom's pelvimeter; right, use of closed fist for measuring.

Initial Psychologic Assessment

At the initial visit, the woman (and her partner, if he is present) evaluates the health team that she has chosen. The establishment of the nurse-client relationship helps the woman to evaluate the health team. A good nurse-client relationship is conducive to interviewing, support, and education.

Many clients are excited and anxious on the initial visit. Because of this, the initial psychologic assessment is general. The goal is to set the foundation for a trusting nurse-client relationship. See the Initial Psychologic Assessment Guide.

INITIAL PSYCHOLOGIC ASSESSMENT GUIDE

Assess/Normal findings	Alterations and possible causes*	Nursing responses to data†
PSYCHOLOGIC STATUS		
Excitement and/or apprehension; ambivalence	Marked anxiety (fear of pregnancy diagnosis, fear of medical facility)	Establish lines of communication; active listening is useful Establish trusting relationship; encourage woman to take active part in her care
	Apathy; display of anger with pregnancy diagnosis	Establish communication and begin counseling; use active listening techniques

INITIAL PSYCHOLOGIC ASSESSMENT GUIDE (continued)

Assess/Normal findings	Alterations and possible causes*	Nursing responses to data†
EDUCATIONAL NEEDS May have questions about pregnancy or may need time to adjust to reality of pregnancy		Establish educational, supporting environment that can be expanded throughout pregnancy
SUPPORT SYSTEMS Can identify at least two or three individuals with whom woman is emotionally intimate (partner, parent, sibling, friend, etc.)	Isolated (no telephone, unlisted number); cannot name a neighbor or friend whom she can call upon in an emergency; does not perceive parents as part of her support system	Institute support system through community groups Develop trusting relationship with health care professionals
ECONOMIC STATUS Source of income is stable and sufficient to meet basic needs of daily living and health care needs	Limited prenatal care; poor physical health; limited use of health care system; unstable economic status	Discuss available resources for health maintenance and delivery. Institute appropriate referral for meeting expanding family's needs—food stamps, etc.
STABILITY OF LIVING CONDITIONS Adequate, stable housing for expanding family's needs	Crowded living conditions; questionable supportive environment for newborn	Refer to appropriate community agency. Work with family on self-help ways to improve situation

*Possible causes of alterations are in parentheses.
†This column provides guidelines for further assessment and initial nursing interventions.

Subsequent Physical Assessment

The recommended frequency of prenatal visits is as follows:

- Monthly for the first 32 weeks of gestation.
- Every 2 weeks to week 36.
- After week 36, every week until delivery.

The accompanying Subsequent Physical Assessment Guide provides a systematic approach to the regular physical examinations that the pregnant woman should undergo for optimal prenatal care.

SUBSEQUENT PHYSICAL ASSESSMENT GUIDE

Assess/Normal findings	Alterations and possible causes*	Nursing responses to data†
VITAL SIGNS Pulse: 60–90 beats/min Rate may increase 10 beats/min during pregnancy	Increased pulse rate (anxiety, cardiac disorders)	Note irregularities; evaluate anxiety and stress
Respiration: 16–24 breaths/min	Marked tachypnea or abnormal patterns (respiratory disease)	Refer to physician
Blood Pressure: 90–140/60–90 (falls in second trimester)	> 140/90 (preeclampsia)	Assess for edema, proteinuria, hyperreflexia. Refer to physician; schedule appointments more frequently

*Possible causes of alterations are in parentheses.
†This column provides guidelines for further assessment and initial nursing interventions.

SUBSEQUENT PHYSICAL ASSESSMENT GUIDE (continued)

Assess/Normal findings	Alterations and possible causes*	Nursing responses to data†
WEIGHT GAIN First trimester: 2–4 lb Second trimester: 11 lb Third trimester: 11 lb	Excessive weight gain (excessive caloric intake, edema, preeclampsia)	Discuss appropriate weight gain; provide nutritional counseling; assess for presence of edema
EDEMA Small amount of dependent edema, especially in last weeks of pregnancy	Edema in hands, face, legs, feet (preeclampsia)	Identify any correlation between edema and activities, blood pressure or proteinuria; refer to physician if indicated
UTERINE SIZE See Initial Physical Assessment Guide for normal changes during pregnancy	Unusually rapid growth (multiple gestation, hydatidiform mole, hydramnios, miscalculation of EDC)	Evaluate fetal status Determine height of fundus using McDonald's rule; use diagnostic ultrasound
FETAL HEART BEAT 120–160 beats/min Funic souffle	Absence of fetal heartbeat after 20 weeks of gestation (maternal obesity, fetal demise)	Evaluate fetal status
LABORATORY EVALUATION Hemoglobin: 12–16 g/dL; pseudoanemia of pregnancy	< 12 g/dL (anemia)	Provide nutritional counseling; hemoglobin may be repeated at 7 months' gestation
Antibody screen: negative	Positive	Refer for further testing to identify specific antibodies Titers may be indicated
Urinalysis: See Initial Physical Assessment Guide for normal findings	See Initial Physical Assessment Guide for deviations	Repeat urinalysis at 7 months' gestation
Protein: Negative	Proteinuria (contamination by vaginal discharge, urinary tract infection, preeclampsia)	Obtain dipstick urine sample at each visit; refer to physician if deviations are present
Glucose: Negative	Persistent glycosuria (diabetes mellitus)	Refer to physician
DANGER SIGNS OF PREGNANCY Client should know the danger signs of pregnancy and be instructed to report them immediately (see Essential Facts to Remember— Danger Signs in Pregnancy)	Lack of information	Provide appropriate teaching

*Possible causes of alterations are in parentheses.
†This column provides guidelines for further assessment and initial nursing interventions.

Subsequent Psychologic Assessment ——————

Periodic prenatal examinations offer the nurse an opportunity to assess the maternity client's psychologic needs and emotional status. If the woman's partner attends the prenatal visits, his needs and concerns can also be identified.

ESSENTIAL FACTS TO REMEMBER

Danger Signs in Pregnancy

The woman should report the following danger signs in pregnancy immediately:

Danger sign	Possible cause
1. Sudden gush of fluid from vagina	Premature rupture of membranes
2. Vaginal bleeding	Abruptio placentae, placenta previa Lesions of cervix or vagina "Bloody show"
3. Abdominal pain	Premature labor, abruptio placentae
4. Temperature above 38.3C (101F) and chills	Infection
5. Dizziness, blurring of vision, double vision, spots before eyes	Hypertension, preeclampsia
6. Persistent vomiting	Hyperemesis gravidarum
7. Severe headache	Hypertension, preeclampsia
8. Edema of hands, face, legs, and feet	Preeclampsia
9. Muscular irritability, convulsions	Preeclampsia, eclampsia
10. Epigastric pain	Preeclampsia-ischemia in major abdominal vessels
11. Oliguria	Renal impairment, decreased fluid intake
12. Dysuria	Urinary tract infection
13. Absence of fetal movement	Maternal medication, obesity, fetal death

A friendly, trusting environment facilitates the interchange between the nurse and client. If the nurse provides time and demonstrates genuine interest, the client will feel more at ease bringing up questions that she may believe are silly or concerns that she has been afraid to verbalize.

During the prenatal period, it is essential to begin assessing the ability of the woman (and her partner, if possible) to assume their responsibilities as parents successfully. Table 6-2 identifies areas for assessment and provides some sample questions the nurse might use to obtain necessary information. If the woman's responses are primarily negative, interventions can be planned for the prenatal and postpartal periods.

As the pregnancy progresses, the woman may exhibit psychologic problems, such as the following:

- Increasing anxiety
- Inability to establish communication
- Inappropriate responses or actions
- Denial of pregnancy
- Inability to cope with stress
- Failure to acknowledge quickening
- Failure to plan and prepare for the baby (for example, living arrangements, clothing, feeding methods)

If the client appears to have these or other critical psychologic problems, the nurse should refer her to the appropriate professionals.

The Subsequent Psychologic Assessment Guide on pp. 130–131 provides a model for the psychologic evaluation of both the pregnant woman and the expectant father.

Role of the Nurse

As pregnancy is increasingly viewed as a normal physiologic process and not a disease condition, the nurse is assuming a more important role in prenatal clinics and obstetricians' offices. It is often the nurse who develops the initial rapport with the client and with whom the client identifies. This contact between the nurse and the client simplifies the nurse's task of providing prenatal counseling and education. A nurse who is also a certified nurse-midwife may be the primary caregiver during an uncomplicated pregnancy. A nurse who is a nurse prac-

Text continued on p. 131.

Table 6-2
Prenatal Assessment of Parenting Guide*

Areas assessed	Sample questions

I. Perception of complexities of mothering
   A. Baby is desired for itself.
   Positive:
     1. Feels positive about pregnancy.
   Negative:
     1. Wants baby to meet own needs such as someone to love her, someone to get her out of unhappy home.
	1. Did you plan on getting pregnant?
	2. How do you feel about being pregnant?
	3. Why do you want this baby?

B. Expresses concern about impact of mothering role on other roles (wife, career, school).
   Positive:
     1. Realistic expectations of how baby will affect job, career, school, and personal goals.
     2. Interested in learning about child care.
   Negative:
     1. Feels pregnancy and baby will make no emotional, physical, or social demands on self.
     2. No insight that mothering role will affect other roles or life-style.
   C. Gives up routine habits because "not good for baby"; e.g., quits smoking, adjusts time schedule, etc.†
   Positive:
     1. Gives up routines not good for baby — quits smoking, adjusts eating habits, etc.
	1. What do you think it will be like to take care of baby?
	2. How do you think your life will be different after you have your baby?
	3. How do you feel this baby will affect your job, career, school, and personal goals?
	4. How will the baby affect your relationship with boyfriend or husband?
	5. Have you done any reading, babysitting, or made any things for a baby?

II. Attachment
   A. Strong feelings regarding sex of baby.
     Why?
   Positive:
     1. Verbalizes positive thoughts about the baby.
   Negative:
     1. Baby will be like negative aspects of self and partner.
   B. Interested in data regarding fetus; e.g., growth and development, heart tones, etc.
   Positive:
     1. As above.
   Negative
     1. Shows no interest in fetal growth and development, quickening, and fetal heart tones.
     2. Negative feelings about fetus expressed by rejection of counseling regarding nutrition, rest, hygiene.
	1. Why do you prefer a certain sex? (Is reason inappropriate for a baby?)
	2. Note comments client makes about baby not being normal and why client feels this way.

C. Fantasies about baby.
   Positive:
     1. Follows cultural norms regarding preparation.
     2. Time of attachment behaviors appropriate to her history of pregnancy loss.
   Negative:
     1. Bonding is conditional depending on sex, age of baby, and/or labor and delivery experience.
	1. What did you think or feel when you first felt baby move?
	2. Have you started preparing for the baby?
	3. What do you think your baby will look like — what age do you see your baby at?
	4. How would you like your new baby to look?

*Modified and used with permission of the Minneapolis Health Dept., Minneapolis, MN.
†When "Negative" is not listed in a section, the reader may assume that negative is the absence of positive responses.

Table 6-2
Prenatal Assessment of Parenting Guide (continued)

Areas assessed	Sample questions
2. Patient only considers own needs when making plans for baby. 3. Exhibits no attachment behaviors after critical period of previous pregnancy. 4. Failure to follow cultural norms regarding preparation.	

III. Acceptance of child by significant others
 A. Acknowledges acceptance by significant other of the new responsibility inherent in child.
 Positive:
  1. Acknowledges unconditional acceptance of pregnancy and baby by significant others.
  2. Partner accepts new responsibility inherent with child.
  3. Timely sharing of experience of pregnancy with significant others.
 Negative:
  1. Significant others not supportively involved with pregnancy.
  2. Conditional acceptance of pregnancy depending on sex, race, age of baby.
  3. Decision making does not take in needs of fetus; e.g., spends food money on new car.
  4. Take no/little responsibility for needs of pregnancy, woman/fetus.
	1. How does your partner feel about pregnancy?
	2. How do your parents feel?
	3. What do your friends think?
	4. Does your partner have preference regarding sex of baby and why?
	5. How does partner feel about being a father?
	6. What do you think he'll be like as a father?
	7. What do you think he'll do to help you with child care?
	8. Have you and partner talked about how the baby might change your lives?
	9. Who have you told about pregnancy?

B. Concrete demonstration of acceptance of pregnancy/baby by significant others; e.g., baby shower, significant other involved in prenatal education.†
 Positive:
  1. Baby shower.
  2. Significant other attends prenatal class with client.
	1. Note if partner attends clinic with client (degree of interest); e.g., listens to heart tones, etc. Significant other plans to be with client in labor and delivery.
	2. Is partner contributing financially?

IV. Ensures physical well-being
 A. Concerns about having normal pregnancy, labor and delivery, and baby.
 Positive:
  1. Client preparing for labor and delivery, attends prenatal classes, interested in labor and delivery.
  2. Client aware of danger signs of pregnancy.
  3. Seeks and utilizes appropriate health care: e.g., time of initial visit, keeps appointments, follows through on recommendations.
 Negative:
  1. Denial of signs and symptoms that might suggest complications of pregnancy.
  2. Verbalizes extreme fear of labor and delivery — refuses to talk about labor and delivery.
  3. Fails appointments, failure to follow instructions, refuses to attend prenatal classes.
 B. Family/client decisions reflect concern for health of mother and baby; e.g., use of finances, time.†
 Positive:
  1. As above.
	1. What have you heard about labor and delivery?
	2. Note data about client's reaction to prenatal class.

SUBSEQUENT PSYCHOLOGIC ASSESSMENT GUIDE

Assess/Normal findings	Alterations and possible causes*	Nursing responses to data†
EXPECTANT MOTHER		
Psychologic Status		
First trimester: Incorporates idea of pregnancy, may feel ambivalent, especially if she must give up desired role; usually looks for signs of verification of pregnancy, such as increase in abdominal size, fetal movement, etc.	Increasing stress and anxiety; inability to establish communication; inability to accept pregnancy; inappropriate responses; denial of pregnancy; inability to cope	Encourage woman to take an active part in her care Establish lines of communication Establish a trusting relationship Counsel as necessary. Refer to appropriate professional as needed
Second trimester: Baby becomes more real to woman as abdominal size increases and she feels movement; she becomes more introspective.		
Third trimester: Begins to think of baby as separate being; may feel restless and may feel that time of labor will never come; remains self-centered and concentrates on preparing place for baby		
Educational Needs		
Self-care measures and knowledge about following: breast care, hygiene, rest, exercise, nutrition, relief measures for common discomforts of pregnancy	Inadequate information	Teach and/or institute appropriate relief measures (see Chapter 7)
Sexual activity: Client knows how pregnancy affects sexual activity	Lack of information about effects of pregnancy and/or alternate positions during sexual intercourse	Provide counseling
Preparation for Parenting		
Appropriate preparation; see Table 6-2, Prenatal Assessment of Parenting	See Table 6-2, Prenatal Assessment of Parenting	Counsel. If lack of preparation is due to inadequacy of information, provide appropriate information. Social service referral may be indicated for alterations.
Preparation for Childbirth		
Client aware of following:		
1. Prepared childbirth techniques		If couple chooses particular technique, refer to classes (Chapter 9 description of childbirth preparation techniques)
2. Normal processes and changes during childbirth		Encourage prenatal class attendance; educate woman during visits as current physical status makes appropriate Provide reading list for more specific information
3. Problems that may occur as a result of drug, tobacco, and alcohol use	Continued abuse of tobacco, drugs, and alcohol; denial of possible effect on self and baby	Review danger signs that were presented on initial visit
Woman has met other physician and/or nurse-midwife who may be attending her delivery in the absence of primary caregiver	Introduction of new individual at delivery may increase stress and anxiety for patient and partner	Introduce woman to all members of group practice

*Possible causes of alterations are in parentheses.
†This column provides guidelines for further assessment and initial nursing interventions.

SUBSEQUENT PSYCHOLOGIC ASSESSMENT GUIDE (continued)

Assess/Normal findings	Alterations and possible causes*	Nursing responses to data†
Impending Labor Client knows signs of impending labor: 1. Uterine contractions that increase in frequency, duration, intensity 2. Bloody show 3. Expulsion of mucous plug 4. Rupture of membranes	Lack of information	Provide appropriate teaching, stressing importance of seeking appropriate medical assistance
EXPECTANT FATHER **Psychologic Status** First trimester: May express excitement over confirmation of pregnancy and of his virility; concerns move toward providing for financial needs; energetic; may identify with some discomforts of pregnancy and may even exhibit symptoms	Increasing stress and anxiety; inability to establish communication; inability to accept pregnancy diagnosis; withdrawal of support; abandonment of the mother	Encourage expectant father to come to prenatal visits Establish lines of communication Establish trusting relationship
Second trimester: May feel more confident and be less concerned with financial matters; may have concerns about wife's changing size and shape, her increasing introspection		Counsel. Let expectant father know that it is normal for him to experience these feelings
Third trimester: May have feelings of rivalry with fetus, especially during sexual activity; may make changes in his physical appearance and exhibit more interest in himself; may become more energetic; fantasizes about child but usually imagines older child; fears of mutilation and death of woman and child arise		Include expectant father in pregnancy activities as he desires; provide education, information, and support Increasing number of expectant fathers are demonstrating desire to be involved in many or all aspects of prenatal care, education, and preparation

*Possible causes of alterations are in parentheses.
†This column provides guidelines for further assessment and initial nursing interventions.

titioner may be sharing this role with a physician. An office nurse may complement the physician's role by performing additional assessments while focusing on the counseling and psychologic aspects of pregnancy.

With each antepartal visit, an environment of comfort and open communication should be established. The nurse should convey an attitude of concern for the client and an availability to listen to and discuss the woman's concerns and desires. This rapport can be initiated as the nurse evaluates the vital signs and weight of the client. A supportive atmosphere, coupled with the guidelines found in the physical and psychologic assessments, help the nurse to identify needed areas of education and counseling.

Summary

Assessment of psychologic, social, cultural, and physical data forms the framework of specific medical and nursing interventions throughout a woman's pregnancy. The nurse must have a thorough understanding of the normal physical changes that occur during pregnancy so that deviations can be recognized and treated in an appropriate manner.

References

Garn SM et al: Maternal hematologic levels and pregnancy outcomes. *Semin Perinatol* April 1981; 5:155.

Additional Readings —————————

Becker CH: Comprehensive assessment of the healthy gravida. *J Obstet Gynecol Neonatal Nurs* November/December 1982; 11(6):375.

Bennett EC: The first trimester. *J Obstet Gynecol Neonatal Nurs* March/April 1984; 13 (Suppl 2):935.

Donaldson PJ et al: The impact of prenatal care on birth weight: Evidence from an international data set. *Med Care* February 1984; 22(2):177.

Grimes L et al: Phenomenological risk-screening for childbirth: Successful prospective differentiation of risk for medically low-risk mothers. *J Nurse Midwifery* September/October 1983; 28(5):27.

Malnory ME: A prenatal assessment tool for mothers and fathers. *J Nurse Midwifery* November/December 1982; 27(6):26.

Shepard TH: Teratogens: An update. *Hosp Pract* January 1984; 19(1):191.

7

The Expectant Family: Needs and Care

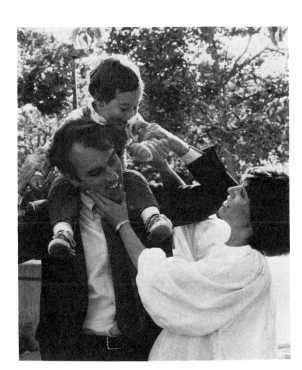

Objectives

- Identify nursing interventions that might be effective in helping a family adjust to pregnancy.

- Identify common discomforts that occur during pregnancy, their possible causes, and appropriate measures to alleviate the discomforts.

- Identify some of the concerns that the expectant couple may have concerning sexual activity.

- Discuss the basic information that the nurse should provide to the expectant family to allow them to carry out appropriate self-care.

- Determine differences between nursing management for adolescent childbirth and adult childbirth.

Key Terms

fetal alcohol
   syndrome (FAS)
Kegel's exercises

lightening
ptyalism
teratogens

The many physical changes that occur during pregnancy may cause a number of annoying and possibly painful conditions. This chapter focuses on antepartal nursing management of the common discomforts and concerns arising during pregnancy. Most of the common discomforts of pregnancy can be relieved by self-care measures. The primary nursing intervention in these cases is client education. Occasionally, however, other nursing actions are required, depending on the severity of the problem or the ability of the woman to assume responsibility for her own care.

A discussion of antepartal needs and care that does not consider the pregnant adolescent would be incomplete. Adolescent needs are considered in depth in this chapter and then highlighted throughout the remainder of the book.

Antepartal Nursing Management

Assessment: Establishing the Data Base

As described in Chapter 6, during the initial contact with the expectant mother or couple,

the nurse obtains a complete client profile that includes information about the following:

- The family's environment, life-style, habits, and relationships
- Sources and adequacy of income
- Race and/or culture
- Client's temperament and usual way of coping with stressful situations
- An average day in the life of the family
- Impact of the pregnancy on self, family, and significant others
- Personal habits relevant to pregnancy (patterns of diet, sleep, and sexual activity; exercise; hobbies; and use of alcohol, tobacco, caffeine, and other drugs
- Health history
- Family history to determine expected support of family members

The data base is completed after a description of body functioning, a complete physical examination, laboratory tests, and a psychologic evaluation (Chapter 6) are made.

During subsequent visits, the nurse may ask the woman what *mother* means to her, what she thinks an average day with the baby will be like, and what she expects from the father. The nurse can ask the father similar questions about his expectations of himself and his partner as parents.

Many nonparents are not prepared for the sleep and feeding patterns of newborns. They have not considered their feelings about the inevitable crying of the newborn and what they will do when the baby cries. Many couples are surprised to discover the sometimes extreme discrepancy between one partner's view of parenthood and the expectations of the other. Guided discussion of these topics allows parents-to-be to attack problems, to arrive at compromises, and to appreciate each other's uniqueness.

From the health assessment, the nurse develops an initial plan for interventions during the couple's preparation for childbearing and childrearing. The plan anticipates the need for information, guidance, and physical care. Interventions are timed to coincide with the woman's (couple's) readiness and needs.

Interventions

Any crisis makes the involved parties more vulnerable but also more accepting of intervention. The nurse is often in a good position to intervene therapeutically. Two primary functions of the nurse caring for the expectant family are (a) to support the family unit and (b) to provide prenatal education. If these functions are performed well, family members may gain greater problem-solving ability, self-esteem, self-confidence, and greater ability to participate in health care. In addition, parents who feel good about themselves have a solid foundation on which to build meaningful relationships with their children.

Support of family unit   The problems and concerns of the pregnant woman, the relief of her discomforts, and the maintenance of her physical health receive much attention. However, her well-being also depends on the well-being of those she is closest to. Thus, the nurse must help meet the needs of the woman's family to maintain the integrity of the family unit.

Father   Anticipatory guidance of the expectant father is a necessary part of any plan of care. He may need information about the anatomic, physiologic, and emotional changes that occur during pregnancy and postpartum, the couple's sexuality and sexual response, and the reactions that he may experience. He may wish to express his feelings about breast- versus bottle-feeding, the sex of the child, and other topics. If it is culturally and personally acceptable to him, the nurse refers the couple to expectant parents' classes for further information and support from other couples.

The nurse assesses the father's intended degree of participation during labor and delivery and his knowledge of what to expect. If the couple prefers that his participation be minimal or restricted, the nurse supports their decision. With this type of consideration and collaboration, the father is less apt to develop feelings of alienation, helplessness, and guilt during the intrapartal period. Thus the relationship between the couple may be strengthened and his self-esteem raised. He is then better able to provide physical and emotional support to his partner during labor and delivery.

Siblings   The nurse incorporates in the plan for prenatal care a discussion about the negative feelings that older children may have. Parents may be distressed to see an older child become aggressive toward the newborn. Parents who are unprepared for the older child's feelings of anger, jealousy, and rejection may respond inappropriately in their confusion and surprise. The nurse emphasizes that open communication between parents and children (or acting out feelings with a doll if the child is too young to verbalize) helps children to master their feelings and may prevent them from hurting the baby when they are unsupervised. Children may feel less neglected and more secure if they know that their parents are willing to help with their anger and aggressiveness.

Parents may be encouraged to bring their children to antepartal visits. For siblings, seeing what is involved and listening to the fetal heartbeat may make the pregnancy more real. Many agencies also provide sibling classes geared to different ages and levels of understanding.

Prenatal education   Throughout the prenatal period, the nurse provides informal and formal education to the childbearing family. This education is designed to help the family carry out self-care when appropriate and to report changes that may indicate a possible health problem. The nurse also provides anticipatory guidance to help the family plan for changes that will occur following childbirth. Issues that could be possible sources of postpartal stress should be discussed by the expectant couple. Some issues to be resolved beforehand may include the sharing of infant and household chores, help in the first few days, options for babysitting to allow the mother and couple some free time, the mother's return to work after the baby's birth, and sibling rivalry. Couples resolve these issues in different ways; however, postpartal adjustment is easier for a couple that agrees on the issues beforehand than for a couple that does not confront and resolve these issues.

Cultural considerations in pregnancy   As discussed in Chapter 6, specific actions during pregnancy are often determined by cultural beliefs. Some beliefs, which are passed down from generation to generation, may be called "old wives' tales." At one time, these beliefs certainly had some meaning, but with the passing of time the meanings have often been lost. Other beliefs have definite meanings that are retained. Tables 7-1 and 7-2 present activities prescribed and proscribed by certain cultures. The tables are not meant to be all-inclusive; they offer a few examples of cultural activities impor-

tant during the prenatal period.

In working with clients of another culture, the health professional is as open as possible to other beliefs. If certain activities are not harmful, there is no need to impose one's beliefs and practices upon a person of another culture. If the activities are harmful, the nurse can consult or work with someone within the culture or

Table 7-1
Activities or Rituals During Pregnancy

Culture	Activity	Cultural meaning or belief	Nursing intervention
Mexican-American	Certain clothing is worn (muneco-cord worn beneath the breasts and knotted over the umbilicus, Brown, 1976)	Ensures a safe delivery	If practice does not cause any danger, do not interfere with it
	Use of spearmint or sassafras tea or Benedictine (Brown, 1976)	Eases morning sickness	Assess use of herbs and determine safety of their use
	Use of cathartics during the last month of pregnancy (Brown, 1976)	Ensures a good delivery of a healthy boy	Assess use of cathartics Provide teaching about dangers of the practice and explore other culturally acceptable means of resolving constipation (high fiber foods)
Black American	Use of self-medication for many discomforts of pregnancy is common (Epsom salts, castor oil for constipation; herbs for -nausea and vomiting; vinegar and baking soda for heartburn) (Carrington, 1978)	Improves health and builds resistance	Assess use of self-medication; discourage those practices that may present problems
American Indian (selected examples)	*Navajo* Meets with the medicine man 2 months prior to delivery (Farris, 1976) Exercise is important during pregnancy; woman is also taught to concentrate on good thoughts and to be joyful (Farris, 1976)	Prayers are said to ensure safe delivery and healthy baby "Body movement is said to produce efficiency and promote joy" (Sevcovic, 1979, p. 39)	Encourage the use of support systems
	Muckeshoot Indians Keep busy and walk a lot (Horn, 1982)	The baby will be born earlier, and the labor and delivery will be easier	
	Tonawanda Seneca Eat sparingly and exercise freely (Evaneshko, 1982)	Delivery will be easier	Assess nutritional patterns and provide teaching if needed
Vietnamese	Consume ginseng tea Woman is expected to carry on conversations with and counsel fetus (Hollingsworth et al., 1980)	Gives strength	Assess use and be certain it is not taken to the exclusion of necessary nutrients

Table 7-2
Proscribed Activities

Culture	Activity	Rationale
Mexican-American	Pregnant woman should not look at the full moon (Brown, 1976)	It will cripple or deform the unborn child
	She should not hang laundry or reach high	This will cause knots in the umbilical cord
	Baby showers should not be planned until delivery time (Kay, 1978)	Earlier would invite bad luck or the "evil eye"
	The woman should not allow herself to quarrel or express anger (Kay, 1978)	Consequences are spontaneous abortion, premature labor, or knots in the cord
Black American	Avoid any emotional fright (Carrington, 1978)	Baby will have a birthmark
	Avoid reaching up	The umbilical cord may wrap around the baby's neck
American Indian (selected examples)	*Navajo*	
	Rug weaving is forbidden; carrying and lifting also avoided (Sevcovic, 1979)	Puts unnatural strain on the body
	Avoid funerals or looking at dead animals (Sevcovic, 1979)	Exposes the baby to the realm of the dead and may cause later illness to the baby
	Laguna Pueblo	
	Do not sew with a bone or a needle (Farris, 1978)	This will have an unkind effect on the baby
Vietnamese	Do not attend weddings or funerals (Hollingsworth et al., 1980)	Bad luck for the newlyweds; the baby may cry

someone aware of cultural beliefs and values to help modify a client's behavior.

Common Discomforts of Pregnancy

The common discomforts of pregnancy are a result of physical and anatomic changes and are fairly specific to each of the three trimesters. Health professionals often refer to these discomforts as minor, but they are not minor to the pregnant woman. They can make her quite uncomfortable and, if they are unexpected, anxious.

Pregnancy aggravates some preexisting problems, such as hemorrhoids and varicose veins. For women who do not have these preexisting conditions, the second trimester may be a relatively comfortable time. The discomforts caused by the enlarging uterus do not affect women until the last trimester or even until the last month.

Table 7-3 identifies the common discomforts of pregnancy, their possible causes, and the *self-care* measures that might relieve the discomfort.

First Trimester

Nausea and vomiting   Nausea and vomiting are early symptoms in pregnancy. Some degree of nausea occurs in the majority of pregnant women. These symptoms appear sometime after the first missed menstrual period and usually cease by the fourth missed menstrual period. Some women develop an aversion only to specific foods, many experience nausea upon arising in the morning, and others experience nausea throughout the day. Vomiting does not occur in the majority of these women.

Nausea and vomiting in early pregnancy are believed to be caused by elevated hCG levels and changes in carbohydrate metabolism, but fatigue and emotional factors may also play a part.

A physician may order antiemetics for women suffering extreme nausea and vomiting in the first trimester. However, antiemetics should be avoided if possible during this time

Table 7-3
Common Disorders of Pregnancy

Discomfort	Influencing factors	Interventions
First trimester		
Nausea and vomiting	Increased levels of hCG Changes in carbohydrate metabolism Emotional factors Fatigue	Avoid odors or causative factors Dry crackers or toast before arising in morning Small but frequent meals Avoid greasy or highly seasoned foods Dry meals with fluids between meals Carbonated beverages
Urinary frequency	Pressure of uterus on bladder in both first and third trimester	Important to void when urge is felt Increase fluid intake during the day Decrease fluid intake *only* in the evening to decrease nocturia
Breast tenderness	Increased levels of estrogen and progesterone	Well-fitting supportive bra
Increased vaginal discharge	Hyperplasia of vaginal mucosa and increased production of mucus by the endocervical glands due to the increase in estrogen levels	Cleanliness, daily bathing Avoid douching, nylon underpants and panty hose; cotton underpants are more absorbent; powder can be used to maintain dryness if not allowed to cake
Nasal stuffiness and epistaxis	Elevated estrogen levels	May be unresponsive but cool air vaporizers may help; avoid use of nasal sprays and decongestants
Ptyalism	Specific causative factors unknown	Astringent mouthwashes, chewing gum, or sucking hard candy
Second and third trimester		
Heartburn (pyrosis)	Increased production of progesterone; decreasing gastrointestinal motility and increasing relaxation of cardiac sphincter; displacement of stomach by enlarging uterus; thus regurgitation of acidic gastric contents into esophagus	Small and more frequent meals Low sodium antacids Avoid overeating, fatty and fried foods, lying down after eating, and sodium bicarbonate
Ankle edema	Prolonged standing or sitting Increased levels of sodium due to hormonal influences Circulatory congestion of lower extremities Increased capillary permeability Varicose veins	Frequent dorsiflexion of feet when prolonged sitting or standing occurs Elevate legs when sitting or resting Avoid tight garters or restrictive bands around the legs
Varicose veins	Venous congestion in the lower veins which increases with pregnancy Hereditary factors (weakening of walls of veins, faulty valves) Increased age and weight gain	Frequent elevation of legs Supportive hose Avoid crossing legs at the knees, standing for long periods, garters, and hosiery with constricting bands
Hemorrhoids	Constipation (see following discussion) Increased pressure from gravid uterus on hemorrhoidal veins.	Avoid constipation Ice packs, topical ointments, anesthetic agents, warm soaks, or sitz baths; gentle reinsertion into rectum as necessary
Constipation	Increased levels of progesterone cause general bowel sluggishness Pressure of enlarging uterus on intestine Iron supplements Diet, lack of exercise, and decreased fluids	Increase fluid intake, fiber in the diet, exercise Develop regular bowel habits Stool softeners as recommended by physician

Table 7-3
Common Disorders of Pregnancy (continued)

Discomfort	Influencing factors	Interventions
Backache	Increased curvature of the lumbosacral vertebras as the uterus enlarges Increased levels of hormones cause softening of cartilage in body joints Fatigue Poor body mechanics	Proper body mechanics Use of the pelvic tilt exercise Comfortable working heights Avoid wearing high-heeled shoes Avoid lifting heavy loads Avoid fatigue
Leg cramps	Imbalance of calcium/phosphorus ratio Increased pressure of uterus on nerves Fatigue Poor circulation to lower extremities Pointing the toes	Dorsiflexion of feet in order to stretch affected muscle Evaluation of diet Heat to affected muscles
Faintness	Postural hypotension Sudden change of position causing venous pooling in dependent veins Standing for long periods in warm area Anemia	Arise slowly from resting position Avoid prolonged standing in warm or stuffy environments Evaluation of hematocrit/hemoglobin
Dyspnea	Decreased vital capacity from pressure of enlarging uterus on the diaphragm	Proper posture when sitting and standing At night sleep propped up with pillows for relief if problem occurs

because of possible harmful effects on embryo development.

Urinary frequency and urgency   Two common discomforts of pregnancy are urinary frequency and urgency. They occur early in pregnancy and again during the last trimester due to pressure of the enlarging uterus on the bladder. If no other symptoms of urinary tract infection exist, these are considered normal. The woman should be encouraged to maintain an adequate fluid intake—at least 2000 mL/day. If symptoms of urinary tract infection develop, she should contact her caregiver.

Breast tenderness   Sensitivity of the breasts occurs early and continues throughout the pregnancy. Increased levels of estrogen and progesterone contribute to soreness and tingling of the breasts and increased sensitivity of the nipples.

Increased vaginal discharge   Increased whitish vaginal discharge (leukorrhea) is common in pregnancy. It occurs as a result of hyperplasia of the vaginal mucosa and increased mucus production by the endocervical glands.

Nasal stuffiness and epistaxis   Once pregnancy is well established, elevated estrogen levels may produce edema of the nasal mucosa. This results in nasal stuffiness, nasal discharge, and obstruction. Epistaxis (nosebleeds) may also result. Cool air vaporizers may help, but the problem is often unresponsive to treatment. Women experiencing these problems find it difficult to sleep and may resort to nasal sprays and decongestants. Such interventions can increase nasal stuffiness and create other discomforts. In addition, the use of any medications in pregnancy should be avoided unless approved by the woman's caregiver.

Ptyalism   Ptyalism is a rare discomfort of pregnancy in which excessive, often bitter saliva is produced. The cause is unknown, and effective treatments are limited.

Second and Third Trimesters

It is more difficult to classify discomforts as specifically occurring in the second or third trimesters, since many problems are due to individual variations in women. The symptoms discussed in this section usually do not appear until the third trimester in primigravidas but occur earlier with each succeeding pregnancy.

Heartburn (pyrosis) Heartburn is the regurgitation of acidic gastric contents into the esophagus. It creates a burning sensation in the esophagus and radiates upward, sometimes leaving a bad taste in the mouth. Heartburn appears to be primarily a result of the displacement of the stomach by the enlarging uterus. The increased production of progesterone in pregnancy, decreases in gastrointestinal motility, and relaxation of the cardiac (esophageal) sphincter also contribute to heartburn.

The caregiver may recommend an antacid, such as aluminum hydroxide (Amphojel) or a combination of aluminum hydroxide and magnesium hydroxide (Maalox). Common household remedies containing sodium bicarbonate (baking soda) should never be used for heartburn during pregnancy because they may lead to electrolyte imbalance.

Ankle edema Most women experience ankle edema in the last part of their pregnancy because of the increasing difficulty of venous return from the lower extremities. Prolonged standing or sitting and warm weather increase the edema. It is also associated with varicose veins.

Varicose veins Varicose veins are a result of weakening of the walls of veins or faulty functioning of the valves. Poor circulation in the lower extremities predisposes to varicose veins in the legs and thighs, as does prolonged standing or sitting. Pressure of the gravid uterus on the pelvic veins prevents good venous return and may therefore aggravate existing problems or contribute to obvious changes in the veins of the legs.

Treatment of varicose veins by the injection method or by surgery is not recommended during pregnancy. The woman should be aware that treatment may be needed after pregnancy because the problem will be aggravated by a succeeding pregnancy.

Although they are less common, varicosities in the vulva and perineum may also develop. They produce aching and a sense of heaviness in these areas. The woman may relieve uterine pressure on the pelvic veins by resting on her side.

Hemorrhoids Hemorrhoids are varicosities of the veins in the lower rectum and the anus. During pregnancy, the gravid uterus presses on the veins and interferes with venous circulation. In addition, the straining that accompanies constipation frequently is a contributing cause of hemorrhoids.

Some women may not be bothered by hemorrhoids until the second stage of labor, when the hemorrhoids appear as they push. These usually become asymptomatic during the early postpartal period.

Symptoms of hemorrhoids include itching, swelling, pain, and bleeding. Women who had hemorrhoids prior to pregnancy will probably experience difficulties with them during pregnancy.

The woman can find relief by gently reinserting the hemorrhoid. The woman lies on her side or in the knee-chest position. She places some lubricant on her finger and presses against the hemorrhoids, pushing them inside. She holds them in place for 1–2 minutes and then gently withdraws her finger. The anal sphincter should then hold them inside the rectum. The woman will find it especially helpful if she can then maintain a side-lying (Sims') position for a time, so this method is best done before bed or prior to a daily rest period.

Constipation Conditions that predispose the pregnant woman to constipation include general bowel sluggishness caused by increased progesterone and steroid metabolism; displacement of the intestines, which increases with the growth of the fetus; and the oral iron supplements some women need.

In severe or preexisting cases of constipation, the physician may prescribe stool softeners, mild laxatives, or suppositories.

Backache Many pregnant women experience backache, due primarily to exaggeration of the lumbosacral curve that occurs as the uterus enlarges and becomes heavier.

The use of good posture and proper body mechanics throughout pregnancy are important in preventing backache. The woman should avoid bending over to pick up objects but should bend from the knees instead (Figure 7-1). She should place her feet 12–18 in apart to maintain body balance. If the woman uses work surfaces that require her to bend, the

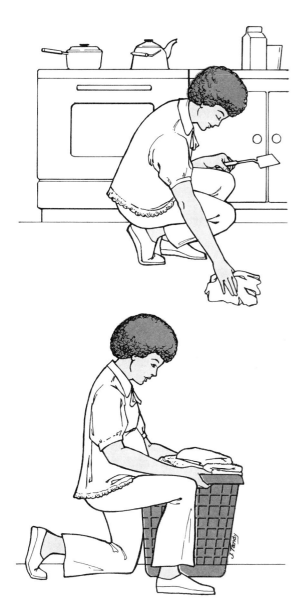

Figure 7-1
Proper body mechanics must be used by the pregnant woman when picking up objects from floor level or when lifting objects.

nurse should advise the woman to adjust the height of the surfaces.

Leg cramps   Leg cramps are painful muscle spasms in the gastrocnemius muscles. They occur most frequently at night after the woman has gone to bed but may occur at other times. Extension of the foot can often cause leg cramps; the nurse should warn the pregnant woman not to extend the foot during childbirth preparation exercises or during rest periods.

Leg cramps are most common in women who consume large quantities of dairy products. They may be caused by an imbalance of the calcium/phosphorus ratio of the body.

Leg cramps are more common in the third trimester because of increased weight of the uterus on the nerves supplying the lower extremities. Fatigue and poor circulation in the lower extremities contribute to this problem.

Immediate relief of the muscle spasm is achieved by stretching the muscle (Figure 7-2). The woman may also stand and put her foot flat on the floor. Massage and warm packs can alleviate the discomfort of leg cramps.

The physician may recommend that the woman drink no more than a pint of milk daily and take calcium carbonate. When planning a treatment regimen, caregivers must be careful not to exclude milk from the woman's diet totally because it is an excellent source of other essential nutrients.

Faintness   Many pregnant women feel faint, especially in warm, crowded areas. Faintness is caused by changes in the blood volume and postural hypotension due to pooling of blood in the dependent veins. Sudden change of position or standing for prolonged periods

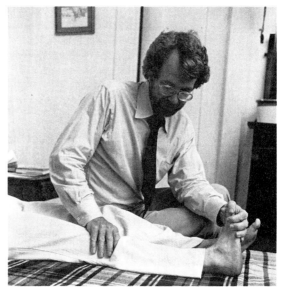

Figure 7-2
The expectant father can help relieve the woman's painful leg cramps by dorsiflexing her foot while holding her knee flat.

can cause the pregnant woman to feel faint or to faint.

If a woman begins to feel faint from prolonged standing or from being in a warm, crowded room, she should sit down and lower her head between her legs. If this procedure does not help, the woman should be assisted to an area where she can lie down and get fresh air. When arising from a resting position, she should move slowly.

Shortness of breath   Shortness of breath occurs as the uterus rises into the abdomen and causes pressure on the diaphragm. This problem worsens in the last trimester as the enlarged uterus presses directly on the diaphragm, decreasing vital capacity. In the last few weeks of pregnancy in the primigravida, the fetus and uterus move down in the pelvis, and the woman experiences considerable relief. This feeling is called **lightening**. Because the multigravida does not usually experience lightening until labor, she feels short of breath throughout her pregnancy.

Nursing Responsibilities

As described in this chapter, there is a fairly predictable pattern of concerns specific to the different trimesters of pregnancy. The nurse caring for the pregnant woman continually assesses and anticipates the presence of discomforts. The nurse knows the appropriate interventions and evaluates the effectiveness of the relief measures used. If these methods are not effective, the nurse must determine why they are not helpful. Are they ineffective because the source of discomfort was incorrectly assessed or because the woman did not receive sufficient instruction? After the situation is reevaluated, nursing interventions can be changed as necessary to meet the woman's comfort and safety needs.

Education for Self-Care

Breast Care

Whether the pregnant woman plans to bottle- or breast-feed her infant, proper support of the breasts is important to promote comfort, retain breast shape, and prevent back strain, particularly if the breasts become large and pendulous. The sensitivity of the breasts in pregnancy is also relieved by good support.

A well-fitting, supportive brassiere has the following qualities:

- The straps are wide and do not stretch (elastic straps soon lose their tautness with the weight of the breasts and frequent washing).
- The cup holds all breast tissue comfortably.
- The brassiere has tucks or other devices that allow it to expand, thus accommodating the enlarging chest circumference.
- The brassiere supports the nipple line approximately midway between the elbow and shoulder. At the same time, the brassiere is not pulled up in the back by the weight of the breasts.

Cleanliness of the breasts is important, especially as the woman begins producing colostrum. Colostrum that crusts on the nipples should be removed with warm water. The woman planning to breast-feed should not use soap on her nipples because of its drying effect. Toughening the nipples, which prevents soreness when the baby begins to nurse, is recommended as a preparation for breast-feeding. After a daily bath, the woman should use a rough towel to dry the nipples but should not rub to the point of soreness or irritation. Rolling the nipple—grasping it between thumb and forefinger and gently rolling it for a short time each day—also prepares the nipple for breast-feeding. A woman with a history of preterm labor is advised not to do this because nipple stimulation triggers the release of oxytocin. (See Chapter 18 for a discussion of oxytocin.)

Nipple-rolling is more difficult for women with flat or inverted nipples but still a useful preparation for breast-feeding. Breast shields designed to correct inverted nipples can be worn during pregnancy. The shields appear to be the only measure that really helps women with inverted nipples. For further discussion of inverted nipples, see Chapter 24.

Oral stimulation of the nipple by the woman's partner during sex play is also an excellent technique for toughening the nipple in preparation for breast-feeding. The couple who enjoys this stimulation should be encouraged to continue it throughout the pregnancy.

Clothing

Clothing in pregnancy can be an important factor in how the woman feels about herself and her appearance. Clothes affect her general comfort and should be loose and nonconstricting. Maternity clothes can be expensive, however, and are worn for a relatively short time. Women who can afford the maternity clothes they want, and women who know how to sew, can dress stylishly. For women in lower socioeconomic levels, the expense may be a problem. Possible solutions include buying used clothing and exchanging maternity clothes with friends or relatives.

Maternity girdles are not necessary for most pregnant women, but women who are accustomed to wearing girdles may wish to continue wearing them during pregnancy. These women should be made aware that the girdle is for support, not for constriction of the abdomen. Women who have large, pendulous abdomens benefit considerably from a well-fitting, supportive girdle but should avoid girdles with tight leg bands.

High-heeled shoes aggravate back discomfort by increasing the curvature of the lower back. They should not be worn if the woman experiences backache or problems with balance. Shoes should fit properly and feel comfortable.

Bathing

Daily bathing is important because perspiration and mucoid vaginal discharge increase during pregnancy. The woman may take showers or tub baths, but tub baths are contraindicated when the membranes are ruptured because of the possibility of introducing infection.

Caution is needed because balance becomes a problem in pregnancy. Rubber mats in the tub and hand grips are important safety devices. Extremely warm bath water causes vasodilatation; after a hot bath, the woman may feel faint when she attempts to get out of the tub. Because of this possibility, she may need help getting out of the tub, especially during the last trimester.

Employment

Most women continue working outside the home throughout pregnancy. Some women work because they need the money or because their work is personally satisfying and important to them. Others work to overcome boredom.

Fetotoxic hazards in the environment, overfatigue, excessive physical strain, and medical or obstetric complications are the major deterrents to employment during pregnancy. Employment involving balance may be terminated during the last half of pregnancy to protect the mother.

Fetotoxic hazards are always a concern to the expectant couple. The pregnant woman (or the woman contemplating pregnancy) who works in industry should contact her company physician or nurse about possible hazards in the work environment.

Travel

Pregnant women often have many questions about the effects of travel on themselves and their unborn children. If there are no medical or obstetric complications, travel is not restricted.

Travel by automobile can be especially fatiguing, aggravating many of the discomforts of pregnancy. The pregnant woman needs frequent opportunities to get out of the car and walk. A good pattern for the woman to follow is to stop every 2 hours and walk around for approximately 10 minutes. Seat belts should be worn low, under the abdomen, and should not fit tightly. Although seat belts can cause internal damage during a collision, without them the woman could be fatally injured.

As pregnancy progresses, long-distance trips are best taken by plane or train. The availability of medical care at the destination is an important factor for the near-term woman who travels.

Activity and Rest

Normal participation in exercise can continue throughout an uncomplicated pregnancy. The woman should check with her physician or nurse-midwife about taking part in strenuous sports, such as skiing, diving, and horseback riding. In general, however, the skilled sportswoman is no longer discouraged from participating in these activities if her pregnancy is uncomplicated. Pregnancy, however, is not the appropriate time to learn strenuous sports. Swimming and bicycling are safe, non–weight-bearing exercises for the pregnant woman. They eliminate the bouncing associated with other exercise and are well tolerated physically (Ketter and Shelton, 1984).

Exercise helps prevent constipation, condition the body, and maintain a healthy mental state. However, an important rule to follow, especially during pregnancy, is not to overdo.

Adequate rest in pregnancy is important for both physical and emotional health. Women need more sleep throughout pregnancy, particularly in the first and last trimesters, when they tire easily. Without adequate rest, pregnant women have less resilience.

Finding time to rest during the day may be difficult for women who work or have small children. The nurse can help the expectant mother examine her daily schedule to develop a realistic plan for short periods of rest and relaxation.

Sleeping becomes more difficult during the last trimester because of the enlarged abdomen, increased frequency of urination, and greater activity of the fetus. Finding a comfortable position becomes difficult for the pregnant woman.

Figure 7-3 shows a position most pregnant women find comfortable. Progressive relaxation techniques similar to those taught in prepared childbirth classes can help prepare the woman for sleep.

Exercises

In pregnancy, exercises help strengthen muscle tone in preparation for delivery and promote more rapid restoration of muscle tone after delivery. Certain physical changes of pregnancy can be reduced considerably by faithfully practicing prescribed body conditioning exercises early in the prenatal period, as well as during the puerperium. A great variety of body conditioning exercises are taught, but only a few are discussed here.

The pelvic tilt, or pelvic rocking, helps prevent or reduce back strain and strengthens abdominal muscle tone. To do the pelvic tilt, the pregnant woman lies on her back and puts her feet flat on the floor. This bent position of the knees helps prevent strain and discomfort (Figure 7-4). She decreases the curvature in her back by pressing her spine toward the floor. With her back pressed to the floor, the woman tightens her buttocks and abdominal muscles as she tucks in her buttocks. The pelvic tilt can also be performed on hands and knees, while sitting in a chair, or while standing with the back against a wall. The body alignment that results

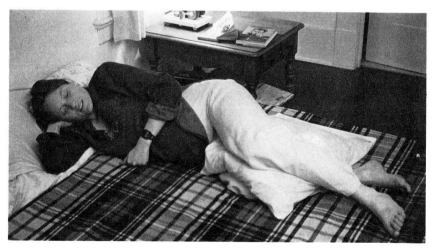

Figure 7-3
Position for relaxation and rest as pregnancy progresses.

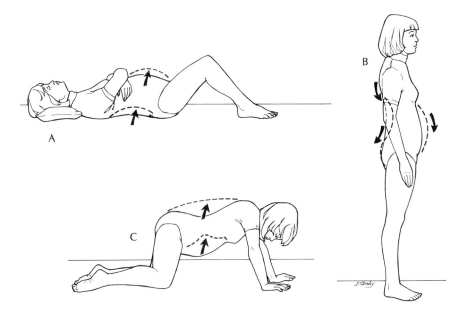

Figure 7-4

Pelvic tilt exercise relieves exaggerated lumbosacral curvature of pregnancy. This exercise may be done in three ways: **A**, lying supine; **B**, standing; **C**, on hands and knees.

when the pelvic tilt is correctly done should be maintained as much as possible throughout the day.

Abdominal exercises   A basic exercise to increase abdominal muscle tone is tightening abdominal muscles in synchronization with respirations. It can be done in any position, but it is best learned while the woman lies supine. With knees flexed and feet flat on the floor, the woman expands her abdomen and slowly takes a deep breath. As she slowly exhales, she gradually pulls in her abdominal muscles until they are fully contracted. She relaxes for a few seconds, and then repeats the exercise.

Partial sit-ups strengthen abdominal muscle tone and are done according to individual comfort levels. When doing a partial sit-up, the woman lies on the floor as described above. It is imperative that this exercise be done with the knees flexed and the feet flat on the floor to avoid undue strain on the lower back. She stretches her arms toward her knees as she slowly pulls her head and shoulders off the floor to a comfortable level (if she has poor abdominal muscle tone, she may not be able to pull up very far). She then slowly returns to the starting position, takes a deep breath, and repeats

the exercise. To strengthen the oblique abdominal muscles, she repeats the process, but stretches the left arm to the side of her right knee, returns to the floor, takes a deep breath, and then reaches with the right arm to the left knee.

These exercises can be done approximately five times in a sequence, and the sequence can be repeated at other times during the day as desired. It is important to do the exercises slowly to prevent muscle strain and overtiring.

Perineal exercises   Perineal muscle tightening, also referred to as **Kegel's exercises**, strengthens the pubococcygeus muscle and increases its elasticity (Figure 7-5). The woman can feel the specific muscle group to be exercised by stopping urination mid-stream. Doing Kegel's exercises while urinating, however, is discouraged because this practice has been associated with urinary stasis and urinary tract infection. Childbirth educators sometimes use the following technique to teach Kegel's exercises. They tell the woman to think of her perineal muscles as an elevator. When she relaxes, the elevator is on the first floor. To do the exercises, she contracts, bringing the elevator to the second, third, and fourth floors. She keeps the

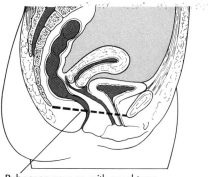

Pubococcygeus m. with good tone

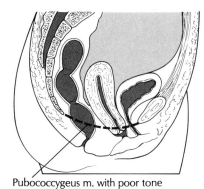

Pubococcygeus m. with poor tone

Figure 7-5 ▬▬▬▬

Kegel's exercises. The woman learns to tighten the pubococcygeus muscle, which improves support to the pelvic organs.

elevator on the fourth floor for a few seconds, and then gradually relaxes the area (Fenlon et al., 1979). If the exercise is properly done, the woman does not contract the muscles of the buttocks and thighs.

Kegel's exercises can be done at almost any time. Some women use ordinary events—for instance, stopping at a red light—as a cue to remember to do the exercise. Others do Kegel's exercises while waiting in a check-out line, talking on the telephone, or watching television.

Inner thigh exercises The pregnant woman should assume a cross-legged sitting position whenever possible. The *tailor sit* stretches the muscles of the inner thighs in preparation for labor and delivery.

Sexual Activity

As a result of the physiologic, anatomic, and emotional changes of pregnancy, the couple usually has many questions and concerns about sexual activity during pregnancy. Often, these questions are about possible injury to the baby or the woman during intercourse and about changes in the desire each partner feels for the other.

In the past, couples were frequently warned to avoid sexual intercourse during the last 6–8 weeks of pregnancy to prevent complications such as infection or premature rupture of the membranes. However, these fears seem to be unfounded. In a healthy pregnancy, there is no valid reason to limit sexual activity (Alouf and Barglow, 1981; Lion, 1982). Intercourse is contraindicated only when bleeding is present, membranes are ruptured, or other complications that might lead to premature delivery exist.

The expectant mother may experience changes in sexual desire and response. Often, these are related to the various discomforts that occur throughout pregnancy. For instance, during the first trimester, fatigue or nausea and vomiting may decrease desire, while breast tenderness may make the woman less responsive to fondling of her breasts. During the second trimester, many of the discomforts have lessened, and, with the vascular congestion of the pelvis, the woman may experience greater sexual satisfaction than she experienced prior to pregnancy.

During the third trimester, interest in coitus may again decrease as the woman becomes more uncomfortable and fatigued. In addition, shortness of breath, painful pelvic ligaments, urinary frequency, and decreased mobility may lessen sexual desire and activity (Swanson, 1980). If they are not already being used, coital positions other than male superior, such as side-by-side, female superior, and rear-entry, should be considered.

Sexual activity does not have to include intercourse. Many of the nurturing and sexual needs of the pregnant woman can be satisfied by cuddling, kissing, and being held. The warm, sensual feelings that accompany these activities can be an end in themselves. Her partner, however, may need to masturbate more frequently than before. The sexual desires of men are also affected by many factors in pregnancy. These include the previous relationship with the partner, acceptance of the pregnancy, attitudes toward the partner's change of appearance, and concern about hurting the expectant mother or baby.

The expectant couple should be aware of their changing sexual desires, the normality of these changes, and the importance of communicating these changes to each other so that they can make nurturing adaptations. The nurse has an important role in helping the expectant couple adapt. It is essential that nurses feel comfortable about their own sexuality and be well informed about the subject. When nurses counsel expectant couples, an accepting and nonjudgmental attitude is important. The couple must feel free to express concerns about sexual activity, and the nurse must be able to respond and give anticipatory guidance in a comfortable manner.

Occasionally, a woman initiates discussion about her sexual concerns, especially if she has good rapport with the nurse. More often, the nurse must broach the subject.

A statement such as "Many couples experience changes in sexual desire during pregnancy" can initiate the discussion. This generalization can be followed by an exploration of the couple's personal experience. The question "What kind of changes have you experienced?" stimulates discussion more effectively than "Have you experienced any changes?"

The presence of both partners during sexual counseling is most effective in fostering communication between them.

Dental Care

Proper dental hygiene is important during pregnancy. However, problems such as gum hypertrophy and tenderness, nausea and vomiting, and even heartburn may discourage a woman from taking care of her teeth. The nurse can encourage the pregnant woman who experiences these problems to use a softer toothbrush or even a soft cloth wrapped over her finger. Gentle flossing should also be continued.

Immunizations

All women of childbearing age should be aware of the risks of receiving certain immunizations if pregnancy is possible. Immunizations with attenuated live viruses should not be given in pregnancy because of the teratogenic effect of the live viruses on the developing embryo. Vaccinations using killed viruses can be used.

Teratogenic Substances

Substances that adversely affect the normal growth and development of the fetus are called **teratogens**. Many of these effects are readily apparent at birth, but others may not be identified for years. A well-known example is the development of cervical cancer in adolescent females whose mothers took diethylstilbestrol (DES) during pregnancy.

Many suspected teratogenic substances exist. The harmful effects of others, such as some pesticides and exposure to x-rays in the first trimester of pregnancy, have been documented. During pregnancy, women need to have a realistic attitude about environmental hazards. Those factors that are suspected as hazards to the general population should obviously be avoided if possible.

Much research is being conducted on the teratogenic effects of medications, alcohol, and smoking. This information is discussed in the following sections.

Medications   The use of medications during pregnancy, including both prescription and over-the-counter drugs, is of great concern. Even when a woman is highly motivated to avoid taking any medications, she may ingest potentially teratogenic medications before her pregnancy is diagnosed, especially if she has an irregular menstrual cycle.

The greatest potential for gross abnormalities in the fetus occurs during the first trimester of pregnancy, when initial organ development is taking place. Many factors influence this, including medication dosage and timing of ingestion as correlated with specific organ development. Individual metabolic and circulatory factors in the mother, placenta, and fetus are also important, as are other factors about the substance. Table 7-4 identifies the possible effects of selected drugs on the fetus and neonate.

Although the first trimester is the critical period for teratogenesis, some medications are known to have teratogenic effect when taken in the second and third trimesters. Two examples of prescription drugs include tetracycline and sulfonamides. Tetracycline taken in late pregnancy is commonly associated with staining of teeth in children and has been shown to retard limb growth in premature infants. Sulfonamides

Table 7-4
Possible Effects of Selected Drugs on the Fetus and Neonate*

Maternal drug	Effects on fetus and neonate
Risk outweighs benefits if the following drugs are given in the first trimester:	
Thalidomide	Limb, auricle, eye, and visceral malformations
Tolbutamide (Orinase)	Increase of anomalies
Streptomycin	Eighth nerve damage; multiple skeletal anomalies
Tetracycline	Inhibition of bone growth, syndactyly, discoloration of teeth
Iodide	Congenital goiter; hypothyroidism; mental retardation
Methotrexate	Multiple anomalies
Diethylstilbestrol	Clear-cell adenocarcinoma of the vagina and cervix; genital tract anomalies
Warfarin (Coumarin)	Skeletal and facial anomalies; mental retardation
Risk vs. benefits uncertain in the first trimester:	
Gentamicin	Eighth cranial nerve damage
Kanamycin	Eighth cranial nerve damage
Lithium	Goiter; eye anomalies; cleft palate
Barbiturates	Increase of anomalies
Quinine	Increase of anomalies
Septra or Bactrim	Cleft palate
Cytotoxic Drugs	Increase of anomalies
Benefit outweighs risk in the first trimester:	
Clomiphene (Clomid)	Increase of anomalies; neural tube defects; Down syndrome
Glucocorticoids	Cleft palate; cardiac defects
General anesthesia	Increase of anomalies
Tricyclic antidepressants	CNS and limb malformations
Sulfonamides	Cleft palate; facial and skeletal defects
Antacids	Increase of anomalies
Salicylates	Central nervous system, visceral, and skeletal malformations
Acetominophen	None
Heparin	None
Terbutaline	None
Phenothiazines	None
Insulin	Skeletal malformations
Penicillins	None
Chloramphenicol	None
Isoniazide (INH)	Increase of anomalies

*Adapted from Howard, F.M., Hill, J.M. 1979. *Obstet Gynecol Surv* 34:643. Modified and used with permission from Danforth, D.N. 1982. *Obstetrics and gynecology*. 4th ed. Philadelphia: Harper & Row, pp. 496–497.

in the last few weeks of pregnancy are known to compete with bilirubin attachment of protein-binding sites, resulting in the occurrence of jaundice in the newborn and occasional kernicterus (Hayes, 1981). Thus, use of tetracycline and sulfonamides should be avoided in pregnancy.

Many pregnant women need medication for therapeutic purposes, such as the treatment of infections, allergies, or other pathologic processes. In these situations, the problem can be extremely complex. Known teratogenic agents are not prescribed and usually can be replaced by medications considered safe. Unfortunately, reliable data about how many medications affect a fetus are lacking.

Caution is the watchword for nurses caring for pregnant women who have been taking medications. It is essential that the pregnant woman check with her physician about medications that she was taking when pregnancy occurred and about any nonprescription drugs that she is contemplating using. A good rule to follow is that the advantage of using a particular medication must outweigh the risks. Any medication with possible teratogenic effects must be avoided.

Smoking   Many studies in the last several years have shown that infants of mothers who smoke have a lower birth weight than infants of mothers who do not smoke. In addition, many studies have found that intrauterine growth retardation (IUGR) increases with the number of cigarettes smoked; IUGR was minimal or avoided when women stopped smoking early in the pregnancy (Naeye, 1981).

The exact reason for this IUGR is not known. Many authorities believe that the passage of carbon monoxide through the placenta produces intrauterine hypoxia (Longo, 1977). Others suggest that the vasoconstrictive effect of nicotine influences the fetus directly or indirectly by decreasing placental perfusion (Haworth et al., 1980).

Hundreds of chemical compounds are found in tobacco smoke. It may be some time before the mechanisms actually causing IUGR are known. Studies demonstrate, however, that any decrease in smoking during pregnancy improves the fetal outcome. Pregnancy may be a difficult time for a woman to stop smoking, but the nurse should encourage her to reduce the number of cigarettes she smokes daily. The need to protect her unborn baby can increase her motivation.

Alcohol   Alcohol was first recognized as a teratogenic substance during pregnancy in 1968 (Lemoine et al., 1968). Newborns with a specific combination of characteristics were identified as having **fetal alcohol syndrome (FAS)**. Most of the research demonstrates that heavy alcohol consumption increases the risk of FAS, but the effect of moderate consumption of alcohol is still not clear. The general conclusion currently is that the risk of teratogenic effects increases proportionately with the consumption of alcohol (Hanson et al., 1978). Pregnant women who have an occasional drink should not be unduly alarmed about the effect it will have on the fetus.

In most cases, once a woman becomes aware of her pregnancy, she decreases her consumption of alcohol. However, the alcohol consumed immediately after conception and before pregnancy is diagnosed remains a cause for concern.

Assessment of alcohol intake should be a chief part of every woman's medical history; any questions should be asked in a direct and nonjudgmental manner. All women should be counseled about the role of alcohol in pregnancy. If heavy consumption is involved, these women should be referred immediately to an alcoholic treatment program. Counselors in these programs should be made aware of a woman's pregnancy before drug therapy is suggested, since certain drugs may be harmful to the developing fetus. For example, the drug disulfiram (Antabuse), often used in conjunction with alcohol treatment, is suspected as a teratogenic agent.

CASE STUDY

Pamela Paulson is a 24-year-old gravida 2 para 0, whose first pregnancy ended in spontaneous abortion a year ago. Pam is a secretary for a construction firm and plans to continue working as long as possible. Her husband, Steve, is an electrician and has a fairly stable year-round income. Pam initially was seen in the clinic when she was 9 weeks pregnant. Her first contact was Marie Carlson, an RN. Marie checked Pam's vital signs, weight, and urine specimen; drew blood for laboratory tests; and completed the health history. She then asked Pam if she had any questions or concerns. Pam revealed that her pregnancy had been planned, and both she and Steve were eager to have a baby. However, she was constantly afraid that she would do something that might result in another miscarriage. Marie reassured her that it was not unusual for a woman to have one miscarriage. She then asked Pam if there was anything in her life-style or environment that might be a risk factor. Pam stated she was an avid swimmer and generally stopped at the YWCA on her way home from work to swim. However, she had given that up once she suspected she was pregnant for fear of causing another miscarriage. Marie reassured her that as long as she was not having any bleeding or other problems that might interfere, swimming was a wonderful exercise that she certainly could continue. She was advised to monitor her level of fatigue to avoid overdoing it. Marie and Pam discussed Pam's life-style further, and Marie was able to reassure her that it was a healthy one. The remainder of the visit went well. Pam's physician reported that her physical exam was normal and her pelvis appeared large enough for successful vaginal delivery. She was started on a vitamin and iron supplement; the warning signs of potential problems in pregnancy were reviewed; and she left with literature to read about all other aspects of pregnancy.

The early months of Pam's pregnancy went smoothly. She did not suffer from nausea, and the urinary frequency she experienced eased in her fourth month. She continued prenatal visits every 4 weeks. As Pam began wearing maternity clothes, her fear of miscarriage abated.

Pam felt the first flutterings of fetal movement at 19 weeks, and the fetal heart tones (FHT) were auscultated a week later. Pam persuaded Steve to accompany her on a prenatal visit, and he obviously enjoyed hearing the FHT with the Doppler.

In her seventh month, Pam began to develop varicose veins in her legs and had problems with hemorrhoids. Marie and Pam discussed Pam's schedule and habits, identifying some changes Pam might make to ease her discomfort. Pam began wearing maternity support hose to work and walking around her office every hour. During her breaks and at lunch, Pam laid on her side in the staff lounge with her feet elevated. She continued her evening swims. A review of Pam's diet showed it had sufficient fiber, fresh fruit, and vegetables. She also drank several glasses of water every day. Nevertheless, constipation was still a problem. Marie reported these findings to the physician, and a mild stool softener was prescribed. Pam continued to follow this regimen, and her symptoms eased.

At 37 weeks, Pam began experiencing urinary frequency again, and physical assessment showed that lightening had occurred. Pam reported to Marie that the nursery was ready and that her suitcase was packed. She and Steve had taken the childbirth preparation classes offered at the clinic, and Pam felt well prepared.

Pam and Marie spent some time talking about what being a parent meant, and Marie gave Pam some interesting articles on adjusting to a new baby. Marie also spoke with Pam about some of the sexual changes she might experience. At the end of the conversation, Pam said, "You know, Marie, I'm so glad you brought this

up. I wondered what sex would be like afterward but felt a little embarrassed about asking."

One day before her EDC, Pam went into labor and, following a 12-hour labor, successfully delivered a 7 lb 2 oz son—Ryan Erik Paulson.

Preparing the Adolescent for Childbirth and Childrearing

Pregnancy is a crisis situation no matter what the age of the individual involved. However, many factors make it more complicated for the adolescent. Physically, her development is incomplete. Psychologically, she has not yet completed the developmental tasks of adolescence, and her available support systems may be limited. In addition, her education is unfinished and plans for its completion may be jeopardized.

The teenage pregnancy rate has continued to increase during the last decade, with at least one in 10 young women becoming pregnant each year (Guttmacher, 1981). Although contraceptive use has increased among adolescents, it has not kept pace with the increasing incidence of sexual activity.

Many factors contribute to the increase of adolescent pregnancy. Menarche is occurring at an earlier age, as is the age of first sexual intercourse. Marriage is being delayed until later years, and cohabitation is far more accepted than in the past.

Some pregnant adolescents are continuing school, usually with their classmates, thus increasing their visibility in the community. Twenty years ago, pregnant adolescents were expelled from school and generally not seen for 9 months. Fewer young women are choosing to "legitimize" their newborns by marriage, and more of them are choosing to keep their newborns rather than relinquishing them for adoption.

Even though the incidence of adolescent pregnancy has increased, the birth rate is declining, partially because of the availability of legal abortion services. Nevertheless, adolescents are becoming pregnant in greater numbers, and the consequences of this must be addressed by the health care profession.

Psychosocial Effects of Adolescence

The adolescent years are often turbulent because of the effort required to deal with physical changes, changing relationships, and the increasing need for independence. Developmental tasks of the adolescent have been described by many writers. Mercer (1979) identified six of these tasks as follows:

- Acceptance and achievement of comfort with body image
- Determination and internalization of sexual identity and role
- Development of a personal value system
- Preparation for productive citizenship
- Achievement of independence from parents
- Development of an adult identity

These tasks may be overwhelming for many adolescents; the guidance, nurturing, and support offered by the family and community play a large part in determining successful achievement. Rebellion is one way for adolescents to accomplish developmental tasks, enhancing their ability to make the transition to adult social roles.

The young adolescent (under 14 years) still sees authority in parents; the middle adolescent (14–16 years) relies on the peer group for authority and decision making. Middle adolescence is the critical time for challenging: experimenting with drugs, alcohol, and sex are avenues for rebellion. Older adolescents (17 years and older) are more at ease with their individuality and decision making.

Cognitive development is another crucial change of adolescence. Young people move from the concrete and egocentric thinking of childhood to abstract conceptualization (Piaget, 1972). The ability of the young adolescent to see herself in the future or forsee the consequences of her behavior is minimal. She perceives her focus of control as external; that is, that her destiny is controlled by others, especially parents and other authority figures. As she matures, she

learns to solve problems, to conceptualize, and to make decisions, she gradually will see herself as having control. She will then be able to see the consequences of her behavior.

The Pregnant Adolescent

Many possible explanations for adolescent pregnancy have been suggested. The oedipal conflicts of adolescence may serve as motivation—the adolescent girl uses pregnancy to maintain dependence on her own mother. Deficits in ego functioning also have been suggested as a cause for acting out sexually. The adolescent may have little sense of self-worth and some hopelessness regarding the future. Other psychologic rationales include unstable family relationships; needing someone to love; competition with her mother; punishment of her father and/or mother; emancipation from an undesirable home situation; and seeking attention. Pregnancy may be a young woman's form of delinquency.

Another school of thought suggests that pregnancy is a result of unmotivated accidents. She has sex infrequently, often without planning it, and therefore does not consider contraception. She may have guilt feelings surrounding sex and may not be able to admit she is sexually active. She is incapable of understanding how pregnancy will affect her future. Rationale may include such comments as, "I don't have intercourse often enough," or "It was the safe time of the month." Many adolescent girls have no idea of when they ovulate and how they conceive.

Physiologic risks   Adolescents over 15 years of age who receive early, thorough prenatal care are at no greater risk during pregnancy than women over 20 years. The young adolescent (under 14 years of age) remains at high risk for premature births, low-birth-weight (LBW) infants, cephalopelvic disproportion (CPD), pregnancy-induced hypertension (PIH) and its sequelae, and iron deficiency anemia (Carey et al., 1981). In this age group, prenatal care is the critical factor that most influences pregnancy outcome.

Teenagers between 15 and 19 years old have the second highest incidence of sexually transmitted diseases in the United States. The impact of herpesvirus, syphilis, and gonorrhea during a pregnancy increases the dangers greatly. In addition, the incidence of chlamydial infection increases (Osofsky, 1985). Other problems seen in adolescents are cigarette smoking and alcohol and drug abuse. By the time pregnancy is confirmed in young women, the fetus already may be damaged by these substances.

Psychologic risks   The major psychologic risk to the pregnant adolescent is the interruption in completing her developmental tasks. Add to this the tasks of pregnancy, and the young woman has an overwhelming amount of psychologic work to do, the completion of which will affect her own and her newborn's future.

Table 7-5 lists adolescent developmental tasks (as identified by Mercer), the impact on the pregnant adolescent, and nursing implications. Tasks of pregnancy are listed in Table 7-6.

Through the nursing process, the nurse should assist the client in completing these tasks during prenatal visits. An interdisciplinary approach, with a social worker, nutritional counselor, and school counselor, will benefit the client.

Sociologic risks   The adolescent pregnancy not only affects the adolescent but society as well. The syndrome of failure (Waters, 1969) describes the sequence of events that the adolescent is at risk for, the brunt of which society must carry. This syndrome includes:

- Failure to fulfill the functions of adolescence
- Failure to remain in school
- Failure to limit family size
- Failure to establish stable families
- Failure to be self-supporting
- Failure to have healthy infants

Table 7-5
Developmental Tasks of Adolescence and Their Implications During Pregnancy

Developmental tasks of adolescence (Mercer, 1979)	Impact on pregnant adolescent	Nursing implications
Acceptance and comfort with body image	Must learn to deal with changing body: enlarging breasts and abdomen, striae, chloasma, weight gain; she may not have yet incorporated the changes of puberty	Assist the client in determining what the changes of puberty meant to her; how she feels about the changes of pregnancy Help her think of ways in which she can feel good about herself
	May be reticent about wearing maternity clothes	Assess at what point in the pregnancy she begins to wear maternity clothes; ask why if she is not wearing them at the appropriate time
	May try fad diets or eat junk food, due to peer pressure and the slender image society has of women; does not want to get fat	Nutrition counseling will be in order for every adolescent Emphasize that pregnant women do not diet, she can lose the weight later; give exercises for pregnant women
	Must learn to cope with looking different from her peers	Elicit feelings about how she is coping with this; support from friends, family
Determination and internalization of sexual role and identity	May not be able to perceive of herself as a sexual being (pregnancy confers overt sexuality)	Elicit feelings about sexuality
	Must learn to incorporate the concept of becoming a mother	What does motherhood mean to the client?
	Must cope with possible changes in relationships with friends, boyfriend, and family	How does she see relationships changing? How is she dealing with this?
	May see her role as solely procreator, other opportunities for development of other female roles may be temporarily abandoned	What other roles does she see for herself now? In 5 years?

Table 7-5
Developmental Tasks of Adolescence and Their Implications During Pregnancy (continued)

Developmental tasks of adolescence (Mercer, 1979)	Impact on pregnant adolescent	Nursing implications
Development of a personal value system	Must cope with and adjust to the fact that she became pregnant; is this in conflict with her self ideal of chastity? Adjust to premature motherhood and the inherent responsibilities	Discuss her feelings of conflict, if any: Is she living up to her expectations and how can she do so? Explore the value the client places on becoming a mother and having children How does she see her relationship with her newborn, now and 5 years from now?
	Incorporate problem-solving skills and decision-making skills	Explore values regarding career, school, marriage Reality test: "Tell me how you see a typical day with a 2-month-old infant?"
Preparation for productive citizenship	Adjust to interruption of school May see school as unnecessary, or postpone indefinitely	Explore provisions for school while pregnant: when can she return? Refer to Social Service; discuss importance of education regarding her career and future
	Incorporate career goals with parenting; she may not consider working important	Discuss future economic consolidation Assist problem solving in this area
Achievement of independence from parents	Cope with realities of pregnancy, and dependence on family (or someone) for financial help	Elicit what changes she perceives and how she feels about them Discuss the reality of her situation (reality testing is constructive) How can she adjust? How can she plan independence? Living at home may be out of the question; she may end up on welfare Check her home and family situation often during the pregnancy
	Adjust to need for financial assistance until she can earn her own living	What role will the father of the child play? If she does not live at home, who will support her?
Development of an adult identity	Learn to accept the responsibilities of adulthood and parenthood Learn to accept the responsibilities for her actions Learn to plan for her future	Encourage prenatal classes, parenting classes Discuss prenatal care and the effects on her pregnancy Explore options through all of the above

The frustration of being forced into adult roles before completing adolescent developmental tasks causes a negative series of events that affects the adolescent's entire life.

Many adolescents who become pregnant drop out of school and never complete their education. Lack of education reduces the quality of jobs available to these individuals. Programs for pregnant adolescents and adolescent mothers may help decrease this problem.

Although adolescent women are more immediately affected by a pregnancy, adolescent husbands also are adversely affected in that they tend to pursue less prestigious careers, earn less income, and have less job satisfaction than men who marry at an older age.

Failure to limit family size is another element of the syndrome. The younger the adolescent at her first pregnancy, the more likely she is to become pregnant again while still an adolescent. These young women frequently fail to establish a stable family. Their family structure tends to be single parent and matriarchal, often the same family structure in which the adolescent was raised. If such women do marry, their divorce rate is the highest of any age group

Table 7-6

Tasks of Pregnancy and the Adolescent

Task	Impact on adolescent	Nursing implications
Acceptance of pregnancy	May deny until well into pregnancy, thus having no alternative but to carry pregnancy	Counsel or refer for counseling regarding whether she will keep or relinquish her newborn Discuss importance of early prenatal care
	May have difficulty bonding with fetus, which may carry over to unresponsiveness to newborn	Elicit feelings about pregnancy (see Table 7-5, developmental task I)
Acceptance of termination of pregnancy	Toward end of pregnancy may focus on "wanting it to be over"; may have trouble individuating fetus	Elicit why she has these feelings Assist with coping mechanisms Discuss preferred sex, names, showers, and readiness for newborn's arrival
Acceptance of mother role	May not perceive of newborn as being her own, especially if client's mother will be caring for the newborn; may think of newborn as a doll or sister	Discuss plans for newborn, include client's mother as indicated Elicit client's perception of motherhood (see Table 7-5, developmental task II) Discuss dreams, role playing, fantasies that she experiences Does she know any new mothers? Encourage prenatal classes
Resolution of fears about childbirth	May focus on labor and delivery as mutilating to her body	Encourage attendance at prenatal classes, childbirth education Offer literature or references
	May not see childbirth education as necessary for coping and learning	Elicit expectations, knowledge, and fears about childbirth Discuss analgesia, labor process; offer tour of facilities
	May have fantasies, dreams or nightmares about childbirth	Reinforce that fantasies or dreams are normal Encourage support person to attend classes with client
Bonding	May feel ambivalent about pregnancy and motherhood	Assess all parameters of feelings about pregnancy in other developmental tasks and tasks of pregnancy (Table 7-5) Refer for counseling if there is any sign of maladjustment to pregnancy

in the United States. Certainly situations of poverty aggravate this problem.

Failure to be self-supporting logically follows lack of education and lost career goals. Many adolescents with children end up on welfare.

Finally, adolescents are at risk for having unhealthy babies because of potential complications and lack of prenatal care.

The Adolescent Father

The unwed adolescent father historically has been met with less than supportive services. His stresses, concerns, and needs have been ignored by society.

Adolescent fathers are usually within 3 to 4 years of age of the adolescent mother. The mother and father are generally from similar socioeconomic backgrounds and have similar education. Many are involved in meaningful relationships. Frequently, the fathers are involved in the decision making regarding abortion or adoption. Many fathers are very involved in the pregnancy and in the childrearing.

Psychologic and sociologic risks to the adolescent father are in many ways similar to the adolescent mother's risks. Card and Wise (1978) found that adolescent fathers achieve less formal education than older fathers, and they enter the labor force earlier with less education. They also found that adolescent fathers marry at a younger age and have larger families than older fathers. The divorce rate of adolescent fathers is two to four times greater than that of couples who postpone childbearing and marriage.

Psychologically the adolescent father's developmental tasks will be interrupted. Because he is not yet mature, his level of cognitive development and decision-making skills will influence whether he remains supportive or flees the situation. Certainly, he will be more vulnerable to emotional stressors than will an adult man.

The stresses of pregnancy on the adolescent male come from many sources. He faces negative reactions from people in his environment, including his own family and the family of the young woman. Feelings of anger, shame, and disappointment will be aimed at him. Although both young people were involved in the act of intercourse, the young man is usually considered the guilty party. He will feel isolated and alone, and if the young woman's parents refuse to allow him to see her, his sole emotional support may be gone.

Another source of stress arises from changes in his life. His educational and career goals may be threatened as he anticipates marriage or quitting school to support the young woman and his forthcoming child. His relationship with his peers may be altered as well.

A third stressor will be his concerns regarding the health of the young woman and the fetus. He may be protective, yet may not understand the physical and psychologic changes of pregnancy.

The adolescent father faces a serious situation, which may be overwhelming for him. The unresolved stress may lead to a severe crisis, manifested by abnormal adaptive behavior, marked depression, somatic symptoms, sexually deviant behavior, or even acute psychosis.

The implications for the health care team are important. Even if the couple has severed their relationship, the father should be sought to assess how he is coping and to offer him counseling. He may not understand why he needs to come to the clinic and the nurse must let him know that the staff would like to help him, too.

If the couple is still together, the father should be told that his participation is important, that he is an excellent support person for the young woman, and that he is welcome to attend clinic and classes. Many clinics interview the couple routinely on the first prenatal visit.

The young man will need education regarding pregnancy, childbirth, childcare, and parenting. Some clinics have couples attend classes together; others offer "father" classes. In becoming parents, men need to learn rates of growth and development so they understand their newborn's potential and do not become frustrated and dissatisfied with the child's behavior.

As part of his counseling, the nurse should assess the young man's stressors, his support systems, his plans for involvement in the pregnancy and childrearing, his future plans, and his health care needs. He should be referred to social services for an opportunity to be counseled regarding his educational and vocational future. When the father is involved in the pregnancy, the young mother feels less deserted, more confident in her decision making, and better able to discuss her future.

Parents' Reactions to Adolescent Pregnancy

Telling her parents that she is pregnant often is very difficult for the adolescent, and she may avoid it until her pregnancy is obvious. Her mother is usually the first to find out, often attempting to prevent the young woman's father from discovering his daughter's pregnancy.

Parents' initial reactions to the news are usually shock, anger, shame, guilt, and sorrow. The angry mother may accompany her daughter to the clinic. The nurse should assess the disharmony that is occurring and explain the process of adaptation that follows.

The mother frequently feels guilty about her daughter's pregnancy and feels that she has been an inadequate parent. She may also be angry over having to help her daughter deal with a crisis just as her children are growing up and she is experiencing a new sense of freedom. The idea of being a grandmother may also be upsetting. Once these reactions are faced, normalcy returns to the mother–daughter relationship. The mother may become involved in decision making and in dealing with the father-to-be and his family. Family communication is important in the adolescent's decision making. The adolescent's decisions regarding abortion, relinquishing her newborn for adoption, or keeping the infant are influenced greatly by her family's reactions.

As the pregnancy progresses the mother begins to take on the grandmother role. She may buy presents for the newborn and plan for the future. She may participate in prenatal care and classes and can be an excellent support for her daughter. She should be encouraged to participate if the mother–daughter relationship is positive. The mother should be updated on maternity care to clarify any misconceptions she might have. During labor and delivery, the mother will be a key figure for her daughter. She can offer reassurance and instill confidence in the adolescent.

The last stages of a mother's acceptance occur after her daughter's child is born. As the mother attempts to integrate her role of grandmother, an initial blurring of roles occurs. The grandmother now sees her daughter as a mother, and the daughter begins to identify herself as a mother. Role confusion may develop and sometimes continues for years—the grandmother may essentially do all the mothering and caretaking activities for the newborn, while the daughter remains only a daughter and becomes a sibling of her newborn. Until the daughter is able to internalize her role as mother, the grandmother will be unable to completely identify as a grandmother.

This new role development is clouded by the adolescent's struggle to complete her tasks of adolescence. The wise mother will gently encourage a balance between helping her daughter to be a parent and allowing her to complete the tasks of adolescence. As her daughter becomes more confident in the role of parent, the grandmother can gradually encourage more independence for the daughter.

Nursing Management of the Pregnant Adolescent

Early and thorough prenatal care is the main factor in reducing morbidity and mortality for the adolescent and her newborn. The nurse must understand the special needs of the adolescent to successfully meet this challenge. The major objectives in the prenatal care of the pregnant adolescent are to:

- Assure quality health care to eliminate complications of pregnancy
- Develop a trusting relationship with the client
- Assist the client in increasing her self-esteem
- Help the adolescent develop her decision-making and problem-solving skills so that she may proceed with her developmental tasks and begin to assume responsibility for her life as well as her newborn's life

Assessment: establishing the data base Within any one age group, the maturity level varies from one individual to another. Adolescent life-styles and support systems also vary greatly. It is essential that the interdisciplinary health team have information regarding the expectant adolescents' feelings and perceptions about themselves, their sexuality, and the coming baby; their knowledge of, attitude toward, and anticipated ability to physically care for and financially support the infant; and their maturational level and needs.

The nurse must establish a data base to plan her interventions for the adolescent mother-to-be. This includes information about family and personal history, medical history, menstrual history, and obstetric history as described in Chapter 6.

Nursing Responsibilities   The nurse in a prenatal clinic must be alert to the special problems of adolescents. The young woman's first visit to the clinic or office may be fraught with anxiety. Not only will she be nervous because of her situation, but this may be her first exposure to the health care system since childhood. Making this experience as positive as possible will encourage her to return for follow-up care and ensure a favorable attitude toward the importance of health care for both her and her newborn.

Developing a trusting relationship with the pregnant adolescent is essential. Honesty and respect for the young woman and a caring attitude promote self-esteem. As a role model, the nurse's attitudes about self-care and responsibility affect the adolescent's maturation process.

An overview of what the client will experience over the prenatal course, including thorough explanations and rationale for each procedure as it occurs, will help the client's understanding and give her a feeling of control. Actively involving the young woman in her care will give her a sense of participation and responsibility in her own health care (Figure 7-6).

Since this first office or clinic visit may include the young woman's first pelvic examination, a thorough explanation of the procedure is essential to lessen the inevitable anxiety provoked by this situation. Gentle and thoughtful examination technique will help put the client at ease. A mirror is useful in allowing the client to see her cervix, educating her about her anatomy, and giving her an active role in the examination. Clinical pelvimetry is an important tool in predicting CPD, but it may be postponed until the next visit if the client is extremely nervous and uncomfortable during the first pelvic exam.

Baseline weight and blood pressure measurements are valuable in assessing weight gain and predisposition to PIH. The client may be encouraged to take part in her care by measuring and recording her weight. The nurse may use this time as an opportunity for assisting the young woman in problem solving: "Have I gained too much or too little weight?" "What influence does my diet have on my weight?" "How can I change my eating habits?"

Another way to introduce the subject of nutrition is during measurement of baseline and subsequent hemoglobin and hematocrit values. Since the adolescent is at risk for anemia, she will need education regarding the importance of iron in her diet. A nutritional consultation is indicated for all adolescents. Group classes are helpful because peer pressure is strong among this age group.

Adolescents may fear laboratory tests, which can evoke early childhood memories of being "stuck" with needles or hurt. Explanations help relieve anxiety and coordination of services will avoid multiple venous punctures.

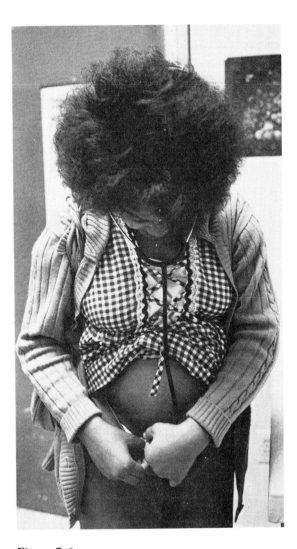

Figure 7-6

The nurse provides this young mother with an opportunity to listen to her baby's heartbeat. (Photo by Suzanne Arms.)

As mentioned earlier, adolescents have an increased incidence of sexually transmitted diseases. The initial prenatal examination should include a gonoccocal culture and wet prep for *Candida*, *Trichomonas*, and *Gardnerella*. Tests for syphilis should also be done. Education about sexually transmitted disease is important, as is careful observation of herpetic lesions or other symptoms throughout the client's pregnancy.

Substance abuse should be discussed with adolescents. It is important to review the risks associated with the use of cigarettes, caffeine, drugs, and alcohol with the young woman. She should be aware of the effects of these substances on her development as well as the development of the fetus.

Ongoing prenatal care should include the same assessments that the older client receives. Special attention is paid to evaluating fetal growth by measurement of fundal height, fetal heart tones, quickening, and fetal movement. If there is a discrepancy of 2 cm either way in size–date evaluation, an ultrasound is warranted to establish fetal age and for diagnosis and early treatment of IUGR.

PIH is the most common medical complication of pregnant adolescents. The average diastolic blood pressure of a normal young woman, aged 14–20 years, is usually between 50 and 66 mm Hg. thus, the criteria of a blood pressure reading of 140/90 mm Hg cannot be used in determining PIH in adolescents. Instead, gradual increases from the prepregnant diastolic readings, as well as any excessive weight gain must be carefully assessed. This is one reason why early prenatal care is vital to management of the adolescent.

Adolescents tend to be egocentric and may not regard as important the fact that their health and habits affect the fetus. It is often useful to emphasize the effects of these practices on the client herself. The young woman will also need help in problem solving and in visualizing the future so she can plan effectively. It is essential for the nurse to understand that the adolescent must meet the developmental tasks of pregnancy in addition to the developmental tasks of adolescence. Table 7-6 identifies the tasks of pregnancy and their impact on the adolescent.

The nurse assesses the family situation during the first prenatal visit. The nurse determines what level of involvement the adolescent desires from each of her family members. A sensitive approach to the daughter-mother relationship helps motivate their communication. If the mother and daughter agree, the mother should participate in the client's care. Encouraging the mother to become part of the maternity team, grandmother crisis support groups, and counseling helps the mother adapt to her role and support her daughter.

The nurse should also help the mother assess her daughter's needs and help her meet them. Some adolescents become more dependent during pregnancy, and some become more independent. The mother can ease and encourage her daughter's self-growth by understanding how to respond to and support the adolescent.

Prenatal Education for the Adolescent

Ideally prenatal education programs should include the clinic and the school system. The clinic can benefit the adolescent by offering workshops on prenatal education, parenting skills, and childbirth classes. Schools are taking a larger role by supplementing academic classes with special classes in these areas.

The clinic can offer rap sessions, pamphlets, or films in the waiting room. Giving the clients something to do while they wait for their appointments may encourage them to return and also may help them learn. Decorating the clinic with attractive educational posters and creating an informal atmosphere establishes an environment where adolescents feel free to interact with professionals.

Areas that might be included in prenatal classes are anatomy and physiology, sex education, exercises for pregnancy and postpartum, contraception, labor and delivery, and growth and development of the fetus. Adolescents may want to participate in the teaching of these classes and should be encouraged to do so. Peer support and friendships can blossom among these young women, helping them all to mature (Figure 7-7).

Many adolescents cite the school as a preferred agency for education during pregnancy and early parenting. School systems are currently attempting to meet this need in a variety of ways. The most effective method appears to be mainstreaming the pregnant adolescent in academic classes with her peers and adding classes appropriate to her needs during pregnancy and early parenting. This is an ideal way to keep the adolescent in school while helping her to learn the skills she needs to cope with childbearing and childrearing. She also receives vocational guidance, which is most beneficial to her future.

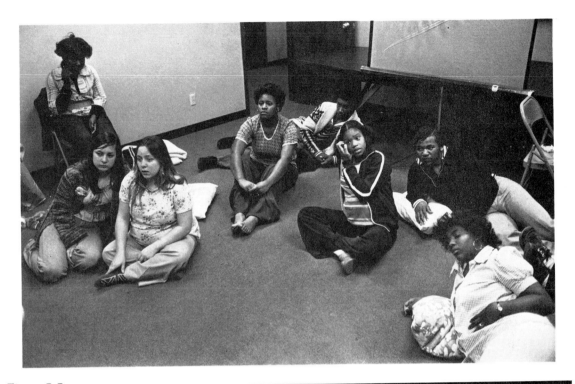

Figure 7-7
Prenatal classes may be designed especially for adolescents. (Photo by Suzanne Arms.)

Summary

The nurse needs comprehensive knowledge of the physiologic and psychologic aspects of pregnancy to counsel the pregnant woman and her family about hygiene, relief measures for the discomforts of pregnancy, and general health care practices. This teaching allows the woman to practice appropriate self-care measures and assume a great measure of responsibility for her own well-being. The nurse's chief responsibilities during the antepartal period are summarized in the Essential Facts to Remember box.

The pregnant adolescent requires special attention from the nurse. The young woman is at physical, psychologic, and sociologic risk because of her incomplete development. The expectant adolescent couple must be prepared to assume the role of mother and father while they are still dependent on their own parents. If the expectant family is properly prepared for childbirth, this experience can be one of growth and development for all members. The nurse has a crucial role in ensuring that the family receives the opportunity to make the event a positive experience.

 ESSENTIAL FACTS TO REMEMBER

Key Antepartal Nursing Interventions

Antepartal nursing interventions focus on:

- Explaining the normal changes of pregnancy to the childbearing family

- Specifying those signs or symptoms that indicate a problem may be developing

- Providing appropriate information about self-care measures the pregnant woman may employ to relieve the common discomforts of pregnancy

- Answering questions about the common concerns that arise during pregnancy

- Referring the woman for additional or more specialized assistance when necessary

Resource Groups ⎯⎯⎯⎯⎯⎯

International Childbirth Education Association (ICEA) (P.O. Box 20048, Minneapolis, Minn. 55420).

Maternity Center Association (48 East 93rd Street, New York, NY 10028).

References ⎯⎯⎯⎯⎯⎯

Alouf FE, Barglow P: Sexual counseling for the pregnant and postpartum patient. In: *Gynecology and Obstetrics*, vol. 2, Sciarra JJ et al (editors). Hagerstown, Md.: Harper & Row, 1981.

Brown MS: A cross-cultural look at pregnancy, labor, and delivery. *J Obstet Gynecol Nurs* September/October 1976; 5:35

Card JJ, Wise LL: Teenage mothers and teenage fathers: The impact of early childbearing on the parent's personal and professional lives. *Fam Plan Perspect* July/August 1978; 10:199.

Carey WB et al: Adolescent age and obstetric risk. *Seminars Perinatol* January 1981; 5:9.

Carrington BW: The Afro American. In: *Culture Childbearing Health Professionals.* Clark AL (editor). Philadelphia: Davis, 1978.

Evaneshko V: Tonawanda Seneca childbearing culture. In: *Anthropology of Human Birth.* Kay MA (editor). Philadelphia: Davis, 1982.

Farris LS: Approaches to caring for the American Indian maternity patient. *MCN* March/April 1976; 1:81.

Fenlon A, McPherson E, Dorchak L: *Getting Ready for Childbirth.* Englewood Cliffs, N.J.: Prentice-Hall, 1979.

The Alan Guttmacher Institute. *Teen pregnancy: The problem that hasn't gone away.* New York, 1981.

Hanson JW, Streissgrith AP, Smith DW: The effects of moderate alcohol consumption during pregnancy on fetal growth and morphogenesis. *J Pediatr* 1978; 92:457.

Haworth JC et al: Fetal growth retardation in cigarette smoking mothers is not due to decreased maternal food intake. *Am J Obstet Gynecol* July 1980; 137:719.

Hayes D: Teratogenesis: A review of the basic principles with a discussion of selected agents. 3. *Drug Intell Clin Pharm* September 1981; 15:639.

Hollingsworth AO, Brown LP, Brooten DA: The refugees and childbearing: What to expect. *RN* November 1980; 43:45.

Horn BM Northwest coast Indians: The Muckleshoot. In: *Anthropology of Human Birth.* Kay MA (editor). Philadelphia: Davis, 1982.

Kay MA: The Mexican American. In: *Culture Childbearing Health Professionals.* Clark AL (editor). Philadelphia, Davis, 1978.

Ketter DE, Shelton BJ: Pregnant and physically fit, too. *MCN* March/April 1984; 9:120.

Lemoine P et al: Children of alcoholic parents, observed anomalies (127 cases). *Quest Med* 1968; 21:476.

Lion EM (editor): *Human Sexuality in Nursing Process.* New York: Wiley, 1982.

Longo D: The biological effect of carbon monoxide on the pregnant woman, fetus and newborn infant. *Am J Obstet Gynecol* 1977; 129:69.

Mercer R: *Perspectives on Adolescent Health Care.* New York: Lippincott, 1979.

Naeye RL: Influence of maternal cigarette smoking during pregnancy on fetal and childhood growth. *Obstet Gynecol* January 1981; 57(1):18.

Osofsky HJ: Mitigating the adverse effects of early parenthood. *Contemp Ob/Gyn* January 1985; 25:57.

Piaget J: Intellectual evolution of adolescence to adulthood. *Human Development* 1972; 15:1.

Sevcovic: Traditions of pregnancy which influence maternity care of the Navajo people. In: *Transcultural Nursing.* Leininger M (editor). New York: Masson Publishing, 1979.

Swanson J: The marital sexual relationship during pregnancy. *J Obstet Gynecol Neonatal Nurs* 1980; 9:267.

Waters JL: Pregnancy in young adolescents: A syndrome of failure. *South Med J* June 1969; 62:655.

Additional Readings ⎯⎯⎯⎯⎯⎯

Alley NM: Morning sickness: The client's perspective. *J Obstet Gynecol Neonatal Nurs* May/June 1984; 13:185.

Ashley MJ: Alcohol use during pregnancy: A challenge for the 80's. *Can Med Assoc J* 1981; 125(2):141.

Baldwin W: Adolescent pregnancy and childbearing: An overview. *Semin Perinatol* January 1981; 5:1.

Becerea RM et al: Pregnancy and motherhood among Mexican-American adolescents. *Health Soc Work* Spring 1984; 9(2):106.

Blum RW, Goldhagen J: Teenage pregnancy in perspective. *Clin Pediatr* May 1981; 20:335.

Horan M: Discomfort and pain during pregnancy. *MCN* July/August 1984; 9(4):267.

Luke B, Hawkins MM, Petrie RH: Influence of smoking, weight gain and pregravid weight for height on intrauterine growth. *Am J Clin Nutr* 1981; 34(7):1410.

Olson ML: Fitting grandparents into new families. *MCN* 1981; 6:419.

Porter LS: Parenting enhancement among high-risk adolescents: Testing a holistic patient-centered nursing practice model. *Nurs Clin North Am* March 1984; 19(1):89.

Speroff L: Exercise during pregnancy. *Contemp Ob/ Gyn* June 1984; 23:25.

Wiles LS: The effect of prenatal breastfeeding education on breastfeeding success and maternal perception of the infant. *J Obstet Gynecol Neonatal Nurs* 1984; 13(4):253.

Zacharis J: A rational approach to drug use in pregnancy. *J Obstet Gynecol Neonatal Nurs* May/June 1983; 12:183.

Zellman GL: Public school programs for adolescent pregnancy and parenthood. *Fam Plan Perspect* January/February 1982; 14:15.

8
Maternal Nutrition

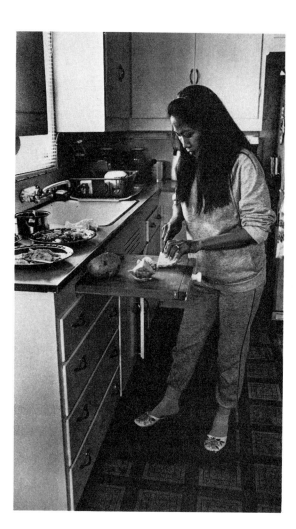

Chapter Contents

Maternal Weight Gain

Nutritional Requirements
Calories
Protein
Fat
Carbohydrates
Minerals
Vitamins

Vegetarianism

Factors Influencing Nutrition
Lactose Intolerance
Pica
Food Myths
Cultural, Ethnic, and Religious Influences
Psychosocial Factors

The Pregnant Adolescent

Nursing Responsibilities

Objectives

- Identify the role of specific nutrients in the diet of the pregnant woman.

- Compare nutritional needs during pregnancy and lactation with normal requirements.

- Discuss the specific dietary needs of pregnant women of various ethnic backgrounds.

- Describe basic factors a nurse should consider when offering nutritional counseling to a pregnant adolescent.

Key Terms

calorie	pica
folic acid	recommended
lacto-ovovegetarian	dietary allowances
lactose intolerance	(RDA)
lactovegetarian	vegan

A woman's nutritional status prior to and during pregnancy can influence her health and that of her unborn child significantly. In most prenatal clinics and offices, nurses offer nutritional counseling directly or work closely with the nutritionist in providing necessary nutritional assessment and teaching.

This chapter focuses on the special nutritional needs of a normal pregnant woman. A special section considers the nutritional needs of the pregnant adolescent.

Good prenatal nutrition is the result of proper eating for a lifetime, not just during pregnancy. Many factors influence the ability of a woman to achieve good prenatal nutrition:

• *General nutritional status prior to pregnancy*. Nutritional deficits present at the time of conception and continuing into the early prenatal period may influence the outcome of the pregnancy.

• *Maternal age*. An expectant adolescent must meet her own growth needs in addition to the nutritional needs of pregnancy. This may be especially difficult because teenagers often have nutritional deficiencies.

• *Maternal parity*. The mother's nutritional needs and the outcome of the pregnancy are influenced by the number of pregnancies she has had and the interval between them.

A mother's nutritional status does affect her fetus. Factors influencing fetal well-being are interrelated, but research suggests that nutrient deficiency can produce measurable effects on cell and organ growth.

Growth occurs in three overlapping stages: (a) growth by increase in cell number, (b) growth by increases in cell number and cell size, and (c) growth by increase in cell size alone. It is now thought that nutritional problems that interfere with cell division may have permanent consequences. If the nutritional insult occurs when cells are mainly enlarging, the changes are reversible when normal nutrition occurs.

Growth of fetal and maternal tissues requires increased quantities of essential dietary components. Table 8-1 compares the **recommended dietary allowances (RDA)** for nonpregnant females with those for pregnant and lactating teenage and adult women.

Table 8-1
Recommended Dietary Allowances for Women 15–40 Years of Age*

Nutrient	(15–18 years)	Nonpregnant (19–22 years)	(23–40 years)	Pregnant	Lactating
Energy, calories	2100	2100	2000	+300	+500
Protein (g)	46	44	44	+30	+20
Vitamin A (μg RE)	800	800	800	+200	+400
Vitamin D (μg)	10	7.5	5	+5	+5
Vitamin E (IU)	8	8	8	+2	+3
Ascorbic acid (mg)	60	60	60	+20	+40
Folacin (μg)	400	400	400	+400	+100
Niacin (mg)	14	14	13	+2	+5
Riboflavin (mg)	1.3	1.3	1.2	+0.3	+0.5
Thiamine (mg)	1.1	1.1	1.0	+0.4	+0.5
Vitamin B_6 (mg)	2.0	2.0	2.0	+0.6	+0.5
Vitamin B_{12} (μg)	3.0	3.0	3.0	+1.0	+1.0
Calcium (mg)	1200	800	800	+400	+400
Phosphorus (mg)	1200	800	800	+400	+400
Iodine (μg)	150	150	150	+25	+50
Iron (mg)	18	18	18	†	†
Magnesium (mg)	300	300	300	+150	+150
Zinc (mg)	15	15	15	+5	+10

*From *Recommended dietary allowances*. 9th ed. 1980. Washington D.C.: Committee on Dietary Allowances Food and Nutrition Board, National Academy of Sciences, National Research Council.
†This iron requirement cannot be met by ordinary diets. Therefore, the use of 30–60 mg supplemental iron is recommended.

Most of the recommended nutrients can be obtained by eating a well-balanced diet each day. The basic food groups and recommended amounts during pregnancy and lactation are presented in Table 8-2.

Table 8-2
Daily Food Plan for Pregnancy and Lactation*

Food group	Nutrients provided	Food source	Recommended daily amount during pregnancy	Recommended daily amount during lactation
Dairy products	Protein; riboflavin; vitamins A, D, and others; calcium; phosphorus; zinc; magnesium	Milk — whole, 2%, skim, dry, buttermilk Cheeses — hard, semisoft, cottage Yogurt — plain, low-fat Soybean milk — canned, dry	3-4 eight-ounce cups; used plain or with flavoring, in shakes, soups, puddings, custards, cocoa Calcium in 1 c milk equivalent to 1½ c cottage cheese, 1½ oz hard or semisoft cheese, 1 c yogurt, 1½ c ice cream (high in fat and sugar)	4-5 eight-ounce cups; equivalent amount of cheeses, yogurts, etc.
Meat group	Protein; iron; thiamine, niacin, and other vitamins; minerals	Beef, pork, veal, lamb, poultry, animal organ meats, fish, eggs; legumes; nuts, seeds, peanut butter, grains in proper vegetarian combination (vitamin B_{12} supplement needed)	2 servings (1 serving = 3-4 oz) Combination in amounts necessary for same nutrient equivalent (varies greatly)	2½ servings
Grain products, whole grain or enriched	B vitamins; iron; whole grain also has zinc, magnesium, and other trace elements; provides fiber	Breads and bread products such as cornbread, muffins, waffles, hot cakes, biscuits, dumplings; cereals; pastas; rice	4-5 servings daily: 1 serving = 1 slice bread, ¾ c or 1 oz dry cereal, ½ c rice or pasta	5 servings
Fruits and fruit juices	Vitamins A and C; minerals; raw fruits for roughage	Citrus fruits and juices, melons, berries, all other fruits and juices	3-4 servings (1 serving for vitamin C): 1 serving = 1 medium fruit, ½-1 c fruit, 4 oz orange or grapefruit juice	Same as for pregnancy
Vegetables and vegetable juices	Vitamins A and C; minerals; provides roughage	Leafy green vegetables; deep yellow or orange vegetables such as carrots, sweet potatoes, squash, tomatoes; green vegetables such as peas, green beans, broccoli; other vegetables such as beets, cabbage, potatoes, corn, lima beans	3-4 servings (1 or 2 servings should be raw; 1 serving of dark green or deep yellow vegetable for vitamin A): 1 serving = ½-1 c vegetable, 2 tomatoes, 1 medium potato	Same as for pregnancy, except 1-2 servings of foods that provide vitamin A

Table 8-2
Daily Food Plan for Pregnancy and Lactation* (continued)

Food group	Nutrients provided	Food source	Recommended daily amount during pregnancy	Recommended daily amount during lactation
Fats	Vitamins A and D; linoleic acid	Butter, cream cheese, fortified table spreads; cream, whipped cream, whipped toppings; avocado, mayonnaise, oil, nuts	As desired in moderation (high in calories): 1 serving = 1 tbsp butter or enriched margarine	Same as for pregnancy
Sugar and sweets		Sugar, brown sugar, honey, molasses	Occasionally, if desired, but not recommended	Same as for pregnancy
Desserts		Nutritious desserts such as puddings, custards, fruit whips, and crisps; other rich, sweet desserts and pastries	Occasionally, if desired (high in calories)	Same as for pregnancy
Beverages		Coffee, decaffeinated beverages, tea, bouillon, carbonated drinks	As desired, in moderation	Same as for pregnancy
Miscellaneous		Iodized salt, herbs, spices, condiments	As desired	Same as for pregnancy

*The pregnant woman should eat regularly, three meals a day, with nutritious snacks of fruits, cheese, milk, or other foods between meals if desired. (More frequent but smaller meals are also recommended.)
One should diet only under the guidance of one's primary health care provider.
Four to six glasses (8 oz) of water and a total of eight to ten cups (8 oz) total fluid should be consumed daily. Water is an essential nutrient.
An occasional alcoholic drink is permissible, but the expectant woman should avoid frequent or heavy drinking.

Maternal Weight Gain

Maternal weight gain and infant birth weight are related. A weight gain of 11–13.6 kg (25–30 lb) is generally recommended. The optimal weight gain depends on the woman's height, bone structure, and the prepregnant nutritional state. The ideal pattern of weight gain during pregnancy consists of a gain of 1–2 kg (2–4.4 lb) during the first trimester, followed by an average gain of 0.4 kg (slightly less than a pound) per week during the last two trimesters. The pattern of gain is important. Sharp increases may indicate excessive fluid retention and should be evaluated.

There are special concerns for weight gain in the obese woman. Pregnancy is not a time for dieting, and severe weight restriction during pregnancy can result in maternal ketosis, a threat to fetal well-being. Although obesity is a complex problem, pregnancy is a practical time for the obese woman to evaluate the quality of her diet.

Women who are 10% or more below their recommended weight prior to conception also have special nutritional concerns in pregnancy. These women tend to have a higher incidence of low-birth weight (LBW) infants than women who are at normal weight and gain the same amount of weight during their pregnancy (Edwards et al., 1978). Inadequate weight gain in pregnancy for both underweight and normal weight women, however, increases the risk of delivering LBW babies for both groups.

Individualizing optimal weight gain from conception has gained favor. Naeye (1979) demonstrated that optimal weight gain needs to be based on the woman's body build (classified as overweight, underweight, or normal weight for height), rather than on an average weight gain for all women. He found that for the best outcome of pregnancy, the optimum weight gain for grossly overweight women was 16 lb and for underweight women, 30 lb.

Nutritional Requirements _____

Calories

The term **calorie** (cal) designates that amount of heat required to raise the temperature of 1 g of water 1C. The *kilocalorie* (kcal) is equivalent to 1000 cal and is the unit used to express the energy value of food.

An extra daily caloric allowance of about 300 cal above the individual requirement, or a total of 2300–2400 calories per day, throughout pregnancy is considered adequate for most women. This allowance does not take into consideration such factors as physical activity.

Protein

Protein supplies the amino acids (nitrogen) required for the growth and maintenance of tissue and other physiologic functions. Protein also contributes to the body's overall energy metabolism.

The body uses the increased protein that is retained, beginning in early pregnancy, for hyperplasia and hypertrophy of maternal tissues, such as the uterus and breasts, and to meet fetal needs. The fetus makes its greatest demands during the last half of pregnancy, when fetal growth is greatest.

The protein requirement for the pregnant woman is at least 74–76g/day, a 30 g increase. Approximately half this requirement can be met with milk. A quart of whole milk supplies 32 g of protein, whereas the same quantity of skim or 2% low-fat milk yields 40 g.

Milk can be incorporated into the diet in a variety of dishes, including soups, puddings, custards, sauces, and yogurt. Beverages such as hot chocolate and milk-and-fruit drinks can also be included, but they are high in calories. Various kinds of hard and soft cheeses and cottage cheese are excellent protein sources, although cream cheese is categorized as a fat source only.

Women who have allergies to milk (lactose intolerance) or who practice vegetarianism may find dried or canned soybase milk acceptable. It can be used in cooked dishes or as a beverage. Tofu, or soybean curd, can replace cottage cheese. Those who are allergic to cow's milk can sometimes tolerate goat's milk and cheese. Frequently, cooked milk is readily tolerated.

Some women make a high-protein drink from a mixture of ingredients. They prepare a quart of this drink in the morning to drink between meals throughout the day as an easy way to increase protein intake. Ingredients may vary but generally include 3 cups of milk (cow, goat, or soy), ½ cup nonfat milk powder (cow or soy), 2 tbsp wheat germ, 2 tbsp brewer's yeast or protein powders, fruit, and vanilla (eggs are optional). These ingredients are mixed together and stored in a covered container in the refrigerator.

Meat, poultry, fish, eggs, and legumes are also good sources of protein. Small amounts of complete animal protein can be combined with partially complete plant protein for an excellent, easily utilized supply of protein. Several examples of complementary proteins are eggs and toast, tuna and rice, cereal and milk, spaghetti with meat sauce, macaroni and cheese, and peanut butter and bread. Except in unusual medical situations, dietary protein should be obtained through natural foods, and the use of protein supplements should be avoided (Johnstone, 1984).

Fat

Fats are valuable sources of energy for the body. Fats are more completely absorbed during pregnancy, resulting in a marked increase in serum lipids, lipoproteins, and cholesterol and decreased elimination of fat through the bowel. Fat deposits in the fetus increase from about 2% at midpregnancy to almost 12% at term.

Carbohydrates

Carbohydrates provide protective substances, bulk, and energy. Carbohydrates contribute to the total caloric intake required. If the total caloric intake is not adequate, the body uses protein for energy. Protein then becomes unavailable for growth needs. In addition, protein breakdown leads to ketosis. Ketosis can be a problem, especially in diabetic women, due to glycosuria, reduced alkaline reserves, and lipidemia.

The carbohydrate and caloric needs of the pregnant woman increase, especially during the last two trimesters. Carbohydrate intake promotes weight gain and growth of the fetus, placenta, and other maternal tissues. Milk, fruits, vegetables, and whole-grain cereals and breads all contain carbohydrates and other important nutrients.

Minerals

The absorption of minerals improves during pregnancy, and mineral allowances are increased to allow for the growth of new tissue.

Calcium and phosphorus   Calcium and phosphorus are involved in energy and cell production and in acid-base buffering. Calcium is absorbed and used more efficiently during pregnancy, so the woman may store more than needed. Some calcium and phosphorus are required early in pregnancy, but most of the fetus's bone calcification occurs during the last 2–3 months. Teeth begin to form at about the eighth week of gestation and are formed by birth. The 6-year molars begin to calcify just before birth.

Thus calcium is a particularly important structural element. If the pregnant woman's reserves of calcium are low, she should increase her calcium intake early in pregnancy. The minimum daily requirement of calcium for the pregnant adult woman is 1200 mg.

The pregnant woman gets all the calcium and phosphorus she needs from an adequate diet that includes 3–4 cups of milk or an equivalent alternate. Frequently, the dietary intake of phosphorus exceeds the calcium intake. An excess of phosphorus can be avoided by limiting milk to 1 pint and meat to one serving daily and by ensuring that the intake of magnesium, which is necessary for the proper utilization of calcium, is adequate. Sources of calcium are listed in nutrition textbooks. Phosphorus is supplied by calcium- and protein-rich foods, especially milk, eggs, and meat.

Iodine   Inorganic iodine is excreted in the urine during pregnancy. Enlargement of the thyroid gland may occur if iodine is not replaced by adequate dietary intake or additional supplement.

The iodine allowance of 175 μg/day can be met by using iodized salt. When sodium is restricted, the physician may prescribe an iodine supplement.

Sodium   The sodium ion is essential for proper metabolism. Sodium intake in the form of salt is never entirely curtailed during pregnancy, even when hypertension or PIH is present. Food may be seasoned to taste during cooking. Salty foods such as potato chips, ham, sausages, and sodium-based seasonings can be eliminated to avoid excessive intake.

Zinc   Zinc was recognized as a nutrient factor affecting growth in 1974. The RDA in pregnancy is 20 mg. Sources include milk, liver, shellfish, and wheat bran.

Magnesium   Magnesium is essential for cellular metabolism and structural growth. The RDA for pregnancy is 450 mg. Sources include milk, whole grains, beet greens, nuts, legumes, and tea.

Iron   Anemia in pregnancy is mainly caused by low iron stores, although it may also be caused by inadequate intake of other nutrients, such as vitamins B_6 and B_{12}, folic acid, ascorbic acid, copper, and zinc. Anemia is generally defined as a decrease in the oxygen-carrying capacity of the blood. Anemia leads to a significant reduction in hemoglobin in the volume of packed red cells per decaliter of blood (hematocrit), or in the number of erythrocytes.

The normal hematocrit in the nonpregnant woman is 38%–47%. In the pregnant woman, the level may drop as low as 34%, even when nutrition is adequate. This condition is called the *physiologic anemia of pregnancy*. It is a result of increased plasma volume, which dilutes the blood and causes a drop in hematocrit level between 24 and 32 weeks' gestation.

Fetal demands for iron further contribute to symptoms of anemia in the pregnant woman. The fetal liver stores iron, especially during the third trimester. The infant needs this stored iron during the first 4 months of life to compensate for the normally inadequate levels of iron in breast milk and non–iron-fortified formulas.

To prevent anemia, the woman must balance iron requirements and intake. This is a problem for nonpregnant women and a greater one for pregnant ones. A supplement of simple iron salt, such as ferrous gluconate, ferrous fumarate, or ferrous sulfate (30–60 mg daily) should be taken during the second and third trimesters of pregnancy when fetal demand is the greatest. Supplements are not usually given during the first trimester because the increased demand is still minimal, and iron may increase the woman's nausea.

Vitamins

Vitamins are organic substances necessary for life and growth. They are found in small amounts in specific foods and generally cannot be synthesized by the body.

Vitamins are grouped according to solubility. Those vitamins that dissolve in fat are A, D, E, and K; those soluble in water include vitamin C and the B complex. An adequate intake of all vitamins is essential during pregnancy; however, several are required in larger amounts to fulfill specific needs.

Fat-soluble vitamins   The fat-soluble vitamins A, D, E, and K are stored in the liver and thus are available should the dietary intake become inadequate. The major complication related to these vitamins is not deficiency but toxicity due to overdose. Unlike water-soluble vitamins, excess amounts of A, D, E, and K are not excreted in the urine. Symptoms of vitamin toxicity include nausea, gastrointestinal upset, dryness and cracking of the skin, and loss of hair.

Vitamin A is involved in the growth of epithelial cells, which line the entire gastrointestinal tract and compose the skin. Vitamin A plays a role in the metabolism of carbohydrates and fats. In the absence of A, the body cannot synthesize glycogen, and the body's ability to handle cholesterol is also affected. The protective layer of tissue surrounding nerve fibers does not form properly if vitamin A is lacking.

Probably the best-known function of vitamin A is its effect on vision in dim light. A person's ability to see in the dark depends on the eye's supply of retinol, a form of vitamin A. In this manner, vitamin A prevents night blindness. Vitamin A is associated with the formation and development of healthy eyes in the fetus.

If maternal stores of vitamin A are adequate, the overall effects of pregnancy on the woman's vitamin A requirements are not remarkable. The blood serum level of vitamin A decreases slightly in early pregnancy, rises in late pregnancy, and falls before the onset of labor.

Excessive intake of preformed vitamin A is toxic to both children and adults. There are indications that excessive intake of vitamin A in the fetus can cause eye, ear, and bone malformation, cleft palate, possible renal anomalies, and central nervous system damage (Luke, 1985).

Rich plant sources of vitamin A include deep green and yellow vegetables; animal sources include liver, liver oil, kidney, egg yolk, cream, butter, and fortified margarine.

Vitamin D is best known for its role in the absorption and utilization of calcium and phosphorus in skeletal development. To supply the needs of the developing fetus, the woman should increase vitamin D intake by 5 μg/day.

A deficiency of vitamin D results in rickets, a condition caused by improper calcification of the bones. It is treated with relatively large doses of vitamin D under a physician's direction.

Main food sources of vitamin D include fortified milk, margarine, butter, liver, and egg yolks. Drinking a quart of milk daily provides the vitamin D needed during pregnancy.

Excessive intake of vitamin D is not usually a result of eating but of taking high-potency vitamin preparations. Overdoses during pregnancy can cause hypercalcemia or high blood calcium levels due to withdrawal of calcium from the skeletal tissue. In the fetus, cardiac defects, especially aortic stenosis, may occur (Luke, 1985). Continued overdose can also cause hypercalcemia and eventually death, especially in young children. Symptoms of toxicity are excessive thirst, loss of appetite, vomiting, weight loss, irritability, and high blood calcium levels.

The major function of *vitamin E*, or tocopherol, is as an antioxidant. Vitamin E takes on oxygen, thus preventing another substance from undergoing chemical change. For example, vitamin E helps spare vitamin A by preventing its oxidation in the intestinal tract and in the tissues. It decreases the oxidation of polyunsaturated fats, thus helping to retain the flexibility and health of the cell membrane. In protecting the cell membrane, vitamin E affects the health of all cells in the body. Its role during pregnancy is not known.

Vitamin E is also involved in certain enzymatic and metabolic reactions. It is an essential nutrient for the synthesis of nucleic acids required in the formation of red blood cells in the bone marrow. Vitamin E is beneficial in treating certain types of muscular pain and intermittent claudication, in surface healing of wounds and burns, and in protecting lung tissue from the damaging effects of smog. These functions may help explain the abundant claims and cures attributed to vitamin E, many of which have not been scientifically proved.

The newborn's need for vitamin E has been widely recognized. Human milk provides adequate vitamin E, whereas cow's milk is lower in E content. Deficiency symptoms of vitamin E are related to long-term inability to absorb fats. In humans, malabsorption problems exist in cases of cystic fibrosis, liver cirrhosis, postgastrectomy, obstructive jaundice, pancreatic problems, and sprue.

The recommended intake of vitamin E increases from 8 IU for nonpregnant females to 10 IU for pregnant women. The vitamin E requirement varies with the polyunsaturated fat content of the diet. Vitamin E is widely distributed in foodstuffs, especially vegetable fats and oils, whole grains, greens, and eggs.

Some pregnant women use vitamin E oil on the abdominal skin to make it supple and possibly prevent permanent stretch marks. It is questionable whether taking high doses internally will accomplish this goal or satisfy any other claims related to vitamin E's role in reproduction or virility.

Vitamin K, or menadione as used synthetically in medicine, is an essential factor for the synthesis of prothrombin; its function is thus related to normal blood clotting. Synthesis occurs in the intestinal tract by the *Escherichia coli* bacteria normally inhabiting the large intestine. These organisms generally provide adequate vitamin K. Newborn infants, having a sterile intestinal tract and receiving sterile feeding, lack vitamin K. Thus newborns often receive a dose of menadione as a protective measure.

Intake of vitamin K is usually adequate in a well-balanced prenatal diet; an increased requirement has not been identified. Secondary problems may arise if an illness is present that results in malabsorption of fats or if antibiotics are used for an extended period, which would inhibit vitamin K synthesis.

Water-soluble vitamins   Water-soluble vitamins are excreted in the urine. Only small amounts are stored, so there is little protection from dietary inadequacies. Thus, adequate amounts must be ingested daily. During pregnancy, the concentration of water-soluble vita-

mins in the maternal serum falls, whereas high concentrations are found in the fetus.

The requirement for *vitamin C* (ascorbic acid), increases in pregnancy. The major function of vitamin C is to aid the formation and development of connective tissue and the vascular system. Ascorbic acid is essential to the formation of collagen. Collagen is like a cement that binds cells together, just as mortar holds bricks together. If the collagen begins to disintegrate due to a lack of ascorbic acid, cell functioning is disturbed and cell structure breaks down, resulting in muscular weakness, capillary hemorrhage, and eventual death. These are symptoms of scurvy, the disease caused by vitamin C deficiency. Infants fed mainly cow's milk become deficient in vitamin C, and they constitute the main population group that develops these symptoms (Food and Nutrition Board, 1980). Surprisingly newborns of women who have taken megadoses of vitamin C may experience a rebound form of scurvy (Bean, 1978).

Maternal plasma levels of vitamin C progressively decline throughout pregnancy, with values at term being about half those at mid-pregnancy. It appears that ascorbic acid concentrates in the placenta; thus levels in the fetus are 50% or more above maternal levels.

A nutritious diet should meet the pregnant woman's needs for vitamin C without additional supplementation. Common food sources of vitamin C include citrus fruit, tomatoes, cantaloupe, strawberries, potatoes, broccoli, and other leafy greens. Ascorbic acid is readily destroyed by oxidation. Therefore, foods containing vitamin C must be stored and cooked properly.

The *B vitamins* include thiamine (B_1), riboflavin (B_2), niacin, folic acid, pantothenic acid, vitamin B_6, and vitamin B_{12}. These vitamins serve as vital coenzyme factors in many reactions, such as cell respiration, glucose oxidation, and energy metabolism. The quantities needed, therefore, invariably increase as caloric intake increases to meet the metabolic and growth needs of the pregnant woman.

The *thiamine* requirement increases from the prepregnant level of 1.1 mg/day to 1.5 mg/day. Sources include pork, liver, milk, potatoes, enriched breads, and cereals.

Riboflavin deficiency is manifested by cheilosis and other skin lesions. During pregnancy, women may excrete less riboflavin and still require more, because of increased energy and protein needs. An additional 0.3 mg/day is recommended. Sources include milk, liver, eggs, enriched breads, and cereals.

An increase of 2 mg daily in *niacin* intake is recommended during pregnancy and 5 mg during lactation, although no information on the niacin requirements of pregnant and nursing women is available. Sources of niacin include meat, fish, poultry, liver, whole grains, enriched breads, cereals, and peanuts.

Folic acid is directly related to the outcome of pregnancy and to maternal and fetal health. Folate deficiency has been associated with abortion, fetal malformation, abruptio placentae, and other late bleeding conditions. Severe maternal folate deficiency may have other unrecognized effects on the fetus and newborn. Hemorrhagic anemia in the newborn is attributed to this deficiency.

Megaloblastic anemia due to folate deficiency is rarely found in the United States, but those caring for pregnant women must be aware that it does occur. Folate deficiency can also be present in the absence of overt anemia. Because of the risks associated with deficiency during pregnancy, folic acid supplementation often begins with the onset of pregnancy or even before.

Normal serum folic acid levels in pregnancy range from 3–15 mg/mL; less than 3 mg/mL constitutes acute deficiency. If no other complications are present, this deficiency can be easily remedied with folic acid therapy. For pregnant women, an intake of 400 μg (0.4 mg) daily is usually effective. After the baby is born, a routine nutritious diet generally provides adequate folic acid to alleviate the woman's symptoms; however, it is wise to give additional folate therapy to build up stores and promote rapid hematologic changes. Iron supplementation is also recommended, since iron is an essential factor in hemoglobin formation. The latest revision of the RDA recommends 800 μg (0.8 mg) for all dietary sources during pregnancy. Pure sources of folic acid are effective in less than a fourth of this amount.

Folic acid and iron are the only nutritional supplements generally recommended during pregnancy. The increased need for other vitamins and minerals can be met with an adequate diet.

The best food sources of folates are green leafy vegetables, kidney, liver, food yeasts, and peanuts. As indicated by the list of food sources in Table 8-3, many foods contain small amounts of folic acid. In a well-planned diet, folate intake should be adequate. Cow's milk contains a small amount of folic acid, but goat's milk contains none. Therefore, infants and children who are given goat's milk must receive a folate supplement to prevent a deficiency. Adults can generally receive adequate folate from other food sources.

Folic acid content of foods can be altered by preparation methods. Since folic acid is a water-soluble nutrient, care must be taken in cooking. Loss of the vitamin from vegetables and meats can be considerable when they are cooked in large amounts of water.

No allowance has been set for *pantothenic acid* in pregnancy. Some studies suggest that it is advisable to supplement the diet with 5–10 mg of pantothenic acid daily. Sources include liver, egg yolk, yeast, and whole-grain cereals and breads.

Vitamin B$_6$ (pyridoxine) has long been associated biochemically with pregnancy. The RDA for vitamin B$_6$ during pregnancy is 2.6 mg, an increase of 0.6 mg over the allowance for nonpregnant women. Since pyridoxine is associated with amino acid metabolism, a higher-than-average protein intake requires increased pyridoxine intake. Generally, the slightly increased need can be supplied by dietary sources, which include wheat germ, yeast, fish, liver, pork, potatoes, and lentils.

Vitamin B$_{12}$, or cobalamin, is the cobalt-containing vitamin found only in animal sources. Rarely is B$_{12}$ deficiency found in women of reproductive age. Vegetarians can develop a deficiency, however, so it is essential that their dietary intake be supplemented with this vitamin. Occasionally vitamin B$_{12}$ levels decrease during pregnancy but increase again after delivery. The RDA during pregnancy is 4 μg/day.

A deficiency may be due to inability to absorb vitamin B$_{12}$. Pernicious anemia results; infertility is a complication of this type of anemia.

Table 8-3
Folic Acid Content of Selected Foods*

Food	Amount	Folic acid (μg)	Food	Amount	Folic acid (μg)
Yeast, torula	1 tbsp	240.0	Chocolate	1 oz	28.1
Beef liver, cooked	2 oz	167.6	Corn, fresh	3½ oz	28.0
Yeast, brewer's	1 tbsp	161.8	Snap beans, green fresh	3½ oz	27.5
Cowpeas, cooked	½ c	140.5	Peas, green, fresh	3½ oz	25.0
Pork liver, cooked	2 oz	126.0	Shredded wheat cereal	1 biscuit	16.5
Asparagus, fresh	3½ oz	109.0	Figs, fresh	3 small	16.0
Wheat germ	1 oz	91.5	Sweet potatoes, fresh	½ medium	12.0
Spinach	3½ oz	75.0	Walnut halves, raw	8–15	11.5
Soybeans, cooked	½ c	71.7	Oysters, canned	3½ oz	11.3
Wheat bran	1 oz	58.5	Pork (ham)	3½ oz	10.6
Kidney beans, cooked	½ c	57.6	Banana, fresh	1 medium	9.7
Broccoli, fresh	⅔ c	53.5	Cantaloupe, diced, fresh	⅔ c	9.0
Brussels sprouts, fresh	3½ oz	49.0	Cottage cheese	1 oz	8.8
Whole-wheat flour	1 c	45.6	White flour	1 c	8.8
Garbanzos, cooked	½ c	40.0	Peanut butter	1 tbsp	8.5
Wheat bran cereal	1 c	35.0	Blueberries, fresh	⅔ c	8.0
Beans, lima, fresh	3½ oz	34.0	Turkey	3½ oz	7.5
Asparagus, green, fresh	3½ oz	32.4	Celery, diced, fresh	1 c	7.0

*Modified from Hardinga, M. G., and Crooks, H. N. Lesser known vitamins in food. ©The American Dietetic Association. Reprinted by permission from *J. Am. Diet. Assoc.* 38:240, 1961.

Vegetarianism

Vegetarianism is the dietary choice of many persons. Some are vegetarians for religious reasons (Seventh-Day Adventists); others believe that this practice leads to a healthier body and mind.

There are several types of vegetarians. **Lacto-ovovegetarians** include milk, dairy products, and eggs in their diet. Occasionally fish, poultry, and liver are allowed. **Lactovegetarians** include dairy products but no eggs in their diets. **Vegans** are "pure" vegetarians; these individuals will not eat any food from animal sources.

Whether the family is currently practicing vegetarianism or is considering it as an alternative, it is vital that the expectant woman eat the proper combination of foods to obtain adequate nutrients. An adequate pure vegetarian diet contains protein from unrefined grains (brown rice and whole wheat), legumes (beans, split peas, lentils), nuts in large quantities, and a variety of cooked and fresh vegetables and fruits. Complete protein may be obtained by eating any of the following food combinations at the same meal: legumes and whole-grain cereals, nuts and whole-grain cereals, or nuts and legumes. Seeds may be used in the vegetarian diet if the quantity is large enough. Because proteins are less concentrated in plant tissue than in animal tissue, vegetarians must eat larger quantities of food to meet body needs.

Sample vegetarian menus that meet the requirements of good prenatal nutrition are given in Table 8-4.

Table 8-4
Suggested Menus for Adequate Prenatal Vegetarian Diets

Meal pattern	Mixed diet	Lacto-ovovegetarian	Lacto-vegetarian	Seventh-Day Adventist	Vegan
BREAKFAST					
Fruit	¾ c orange juice	Same as mixed diet	Same	Same	Same
Grains	½ c granola, 1 slice whole wheat toast				1 c granola, 1 slice whole grain toast
Meat group	1 scrambled egg with cheese		1 oz cheese melted over toast (no egg)		
Fat	1 tsp butter		Same		1 tsp sesame butter
Milk	½ c milk				1 c soy milk
MIDMORNING					
Milk	1 c hot chocolate				1 c protein drink*
LUNCH					
Meat group/ vegetable	1 c lentil chowder† (made with ground beef)	1 c lentil chowder† (no ground beef)	1 c lentil chowder† (no ground beef)	1c lentil chowder† (made with vegeburger)‡	1½ c lentil chowder† (1 tbsp torula yeast, wheat germ added)
Grains	1 corn muffin	Same	Same	Same	2 corn muffins§
Fat	1 tsp butter, honey				2 tsp margarine, honey
Fruit/dessert	½ peach, ½ c cottage cheese salad				½ peach, ½ c tofu salad
Tea	1 c tea			Decaffeinated or herbal tea	Same as Seventh-Day Adventist
MIDAFTERNOON					
Milk	¾ c vanilla pudding			Same	1 c pudding (soy milk)
Fruit	¼ c sliced banana				½ banana
Grain	1 graham cracker				1 graham cracker with peanut butter
DINNER					
Meat group/ vegetable	¾ c meat sauce (onion, celery, carrot, tomato, mushroom in sauce), parmesan cheese	¾ c tomato sauce (same vegetables as in mixed diet), ¼ c cheese	Same as lacto-ovovegetarian	Same (add vegeburger‡ to tomato sauce)	Same (use tofu instead of cheese)

*Protein drink recipe is given on p. 166. Use soy milk instead of cow's or goat's milk. Do not use eggs.
†Lentil chowder is made from lentils, celery, carrots, potatoes, onion, and tomatoes.
‡Vegeburger is made from meat analogs.
§Wheat germ and soy flour are added to corn muffin mixture.

Table 8-4
Suggested Menus for Adequate Prenatal Vegetarian Diets (continued)

Meal pattern	Mixed diet	Lacto-ovovegetarian	Lacto-vegetarian	Seventh-Day Adventist	Vegan
Grains	¾ c spaghetti, bread	1 c whole-wheat spaghetti, 1 slice French bread	↓	↓	↓
Vegetable	Mixed vegetable salad	Mixed vegetable salad with ¼ c sprouts, ½ egg, ½ oz cheese, ¼ c kidney beans added	(No egg in salad)		(Add tofu; no egg in salad)
Fat	Oil-vinegar dressing, ½ tsp butter	Same as mixed diet	Same		1 tsp margarine
Fruit	Fresh pear or baked pear half			↓	Same as mixed diet
Tea	1 c tea			Decaffeinated or herbal tea	Same as 7th-Day Adventist
BEDTIME Milk	1 c milk			Same	
Meat group/ vegetable	2 tsp peanut butter on celery or on wheat crackers				1 c protein drink*
Grain		↓	↓	↓	Corn muffins§

Register and Sonnenberg (1973) recommend that families changing from a nonvegetarian to a lacto-ovovegetarian diet follow these principles:

1. Decrease all empty-calorie foods as much as possible.

2. Increase the intake of foods from the basic food groups to provide sufficient calories.

3. Eat more legumes, nuts, and possibly meat analogs (food products derived from soy and wheat) to replace meat.

4. Increase the intake of whole-grain products that supply protein, B vitamins, and iron to the diet.

5. Increase the intake of dairy products, using nonfat and low-fat milk, cottage cheese, cheeses, and other foods, to provide additional protein and vitamin B_{12}.

For those changing from a lacto-ovovegetarian diet to a pure vegetarian diet, Register and Sonnenberg (1973) have additional recommendations:

1. Maintain an adequate calorie intake so that the body will not burn protein for caloric needs.

2. Increase the intake of foods that contain nutrients such as calcium and riboflavin, which most people get from foods in the milk group. Alternate sources of these nutrients include fortified soybean milk preparations; leafy green vegetables; legumes, especially soybeans; nuts, particularly almonds; and dried fruits.

3. Supplement the diet with vitamin B_{12}, since there is no practical plant source.

Factors Influencing Nutrition

Besides having knowledge of nutritional needs and food sources, the nurse needs to be aware of other factors that affect a client's nutrition. What is the age, life-style, and culture of the pregnant woman? What food beliefs and habits does she have? What a person eats is determined by availability, economics, and symbolism. These factors and others influence the expectant mother's acceptance of the nurse's intervention.

Lactose Intolerance

Some individuals have difficulty digesting milk and milk products. This condition, known as **lactose intolerance**, results from an inadequate amount of the enzyme lactase, which breaks down the milk sugar lactose into smaller digestible substances.

Lactose intolerance is found in the majority of Blacks, Mexican Americans, American Indians, Ashkenazic Jews, and Orientals (Rosenberg, 1977). Symptoms include abdominal distention, discomfort, nausea, vomiting, loose stools, and cramps.

In counseling pregnant women who might be intolerant of milk and milk products, the nurse should be aware that even one glass of milk can produce symptoms (Bayless et al., 1975). Milk in cooked form, such as in custards, or mixed with Ovaltine, is sometimes tolerated. Green leafy vegetables are a nondairy source of calcium (Campbell and Chang, 1973). In some instances, the enzyme lactase may be taken to alleviate this problem.

Pica

Pica is the eating of substances that are not ordinarily considered edible or to have nutritive value. Most women who practice pica in pregnancy eat such substances only during that time. Women usually explain this practice by saying it relieves various discomforts of pregnancy or that it ensures a beautiful baby (Curda, 1977).

Pica is most commonly practiced in poverty-stricken areas, where diets tend to be inadequate, but may also be found in other socioeconomic levels. The substances most commonly ingested in this country are dirt, clay, starch, and freezer frost. Iron-deficiency anemia is the most common concern in pica. Studies indicate that ingestion of laundry starch contributes to iron deficiency because it interferes with iron absorption. Other problems with pica

have been reported, including severe hypokalemia and intestinal obstruction (Curda, 1977). The ingestion of starch may be associated with excessive weight gain.

Nurses should be aware of pica and its implications for the woman and fetus. Assessment for the practice of pica is an important part of a nutritional history. Nurses may detect this practice as they help determine appropriate and effective relief measures for discomforts the woman is experiencing. Reeducation of the expectant woman is important in helping her to decrease or eliminate this practice.

Food Myths

The relationship of food to pregnancy is reflected in some common beliefs or sayings. Nurses frequently hear that the pregnant woman must eat for two or that the fetus takes from the mother all the nutrients it needs. The practice of pica, for example, has roots in myth. Common beliefs regarding pica include (a) that laundry starch will make the newborn lighter in color, and (b) that the baby will "slide out" more easily during delivery (Curda, 1977).

Cultural, Ethnic, and Religious Influences

Cultural, ethnic, and occasionally religious background determines one's experiences with food and influences food preferences and habits. People of different nationalities are accustomed to eating different foods because of the kinds of foodstuffs available in their countries of origin. The way food is prepared varies, depending on the customs and traditions of the ethnic and cultural group. In addition, the laws of certain religions sanction particular foods, prohibit others, and direct the preparation and serving of meals.

In each culture, certain foods have symbolic significance. Generally, these symbolic foods are related to major life experiences such as birth, death, or developmental milestones. (General food practices of different cultural and ethnic groups are presented in Table 8-5. Sample daily menus for differing cultural groups that meet minimal nutritional requirements during pregnancy are presented in Table 8-6.)

For example, Navajo Indian women believe that eating raisins will cause brown spots on the

Table 8-5
Food Practices of Various Ethnic and Religious Groups

Cultural group	Staple foods	Prohibitions or foods not used	Food preparation
Jewish Orthodox	Meat: Forequarter of cattle, sheep, goat, deer Poultry: chicken, pheasant, turkey, goose, duck Dairy products	No blood may be eaten in any form Combining milk and meat at meal not allowed; milk and cheese may be eaten before meal, but must not be eaten for 6 hours after meal containing meat No shellfish or eels	Animal slaughter must follow certain rules, including minimal pain to animal and maximal blood drainage Two sets of dishes are used: one for meat, one for milk meals
	Fish with fins and scales No restrictions on cereals, fruits, or vegetables		
Mexican American	Main vegetables: corn (source of calcium) and chili peppers (source of vitamin C); pinto beans or calice beans; potatoes Coffee and eggs Grain products: corn is basic grain; tortillas from enriched flour made daily	Milk rarely used	Chief cooking fat is lard Usually beans are served with every meal
Chinese	Rice is staple grain and used at most meals Traditional beverage is green tea Most meats are used, but in limited amounts Fruits are usually eaten fresh	Milk and cheese rarely used Meat considered difficult to chew, so may be eliminated from child's diet	Foods are kept short time and are cooked quickly at high temperature so that natural flavors are enhanced and texture and color are maintained Chief cooking fat is lard or peanut oil
Japanese	Seafood (raw fish) eaten frequently Most meats; large variety of vegetables and fresh fruits Rice is staple grain, but corn and oats also used	Milk and cheese rarely used	Chief cooking fat is soybean oil

mother or baby. Many Black Americans believe that craving one food excessively can cause the baby to be "marked"; some say the shape of the birthmark echoes the shape of the food the mother craved during pregnancy. This belief is also held by some Mexican-American women. Also, some Mexican Americans believe drinking milk makes their babies too big, thereby creating difficult deliveries.

The traditional Chinese classify food as either hot or cold, and these classifications are related to the balance of forces for good health. Since childbirth is considered a cold condition, it must be treated with hot foods, such as chicken, squash, and broccoli. Vietnamese women believe that eating "unclean foods," such as beef, dog, and snake, during pregnancy will cause the baby to be born an imbecile. Cabbage is also avoided because it is believed to produce flatulence that might bring on false labor (Clark, 1978).

Psychosocial Factors

Sharing food has long been a symbol of friendliness, warmth, and social acceptance in many cultures. Food is also symbolic of motherliness; that is, taking care of the family and feeding them well is a part of the traditional mothering role. The mother influences her chil-

Table 8-6
Sample Menus for Adequate Prenatal Diet for Various Cultural Groups*

Caucasian	Mexican-American	Southern U.S.	Oriental	Jewish	Italian
BREAKFAST					
Peaches	Peaches	Peaches	Peaches	Peaches	Peaches
Oatmeal/milk	Oatmeal/milk	Oatmeal/milk	Steamed rice/	Oatmeal/milk	Oatmeal/milk
Toast with peanut	Corn tortilla	Cornbread with	milk (soy)	Bagel with	Bread with
butter	Refried beans	molasses	Rice cracker	unsalted butter	butter
Milk	Milk	Milk	Tea	Milk	Cheese
					Coffee/milk
MIDMORNING					
Fruit/juice	Fruit/juice	Fruit	Fruit	Fruit	Fruit/juice
LUNCH					
Cheese omelet	1 fried egg	1 fried egg	Miso soup	Cheese omelet	Cheese omelet
and vegetables	Refried beans	Black-eyed peas	Chinese omelet	Brown rice	Zucchini, green
Whole grain	with cheese	and salt pork	(with bean	Lettuce and	salad
muffin with butter	Corn tortilla	Cornbread with	sprouts, pepper,	tomato salad	Grapes/cheese
Lettuce and tomato	Fresh tomato	molasses	green onion,	Honey cookie	Milk
salad	and chillies	Turnip greens	mushroom) and	Milk	
Raw apple	Banana	Ice cream	fried rice		
Milk	Milk		Spinach		
			Tea		
MIDAFTERNOON					
Fruit	Fruit	Fruit	Fruit	Fruit	Fruit
Cottage cheese	Cottage cheese		Tofu		Cheese
DINNER					
Roast beef	Refried beans	Beef stew with	Beef strips with	Beef stew with	Spaghetti and
and gravy	with cheese	vegetables	pan-fried	vegetables	meatballs with
Whole grain	Fried macaroni	(carrots, greens)	vegetables	Barley pilaf	tomato sauce
roll with butter	Tortilla	Dumplings	Brown rice,	Cooked cabbage	Italian bread
Parsley, carrots,	Carrots, steamed	Steamed potato,	steamed	Unsalted butter	with butter
cabbage slaw	tomato, chillies	cabbage slaw	Milk custard	Coffeecake	Sauteed
Banana cream pie	Corn pudding	Corn pudding		Fruit/juice	eggplant,
Tea	milk				cabbage, salad
					Fruit
					Coffee/milk
BEDTIME					
Milk	Milk	Milk	Ice cream	Ice cream	Ice cream
Wheat crackers	Tortilla with	Corn pudding			
1 oz cheese	beans				
	Cheese				

*Modified from American Dietetic Association. *Cultural food patterns in the U.S.A.*

dren's likes and dislikes by what she prepares and by her attitude about foods. Certain foods are assigned positive or negative values, as reflected in the statements "Milk helps you grow" and "Coffee stunts your growth."

Socioeconomic factors Socioeconomic level may be a determinant of nutritional status.

Poverty-level families are unable to afford the same foods that higher-income families can. Thus, pregnant women with low incomes frequently are at risk for poor nutrition.

Education Knowledge about the basic components of a balanced diet is essential. Often educational level is related to economic status, but even people on very limited incomes can prepare well-balanced meals if their knowledge of nutrition is adequate.

Psychologic factors   Emotions affect nutritional well-being directly. For example, anorexia nervosa, a psychologic disorder that occurs primarily in adolescent girls, is due chiefly to self-inflicted starvation, resulting in malnutrition and ultimately death if not treated. Loss of appetite is also a common symptom of serious depression.

The expectant woman's attitudes and feelings about her pregnancy influence her nutritional status. The woman who is depressed or who does not wish to be pregnant may manifest these feelings by loss of appetite or by improper food practices, such as overindulgence in sweets or alcohol.

The Pregnant Adolescent ──────

Healthy adolescents often have irregular eating patterns. Many skip breakfast, and most tend to be frequent snackers. Teens rarely follow the traditional three-meal-a-day pattern; their day-to-day intake often varies drastically; and they eat food combinations that may seem bizarre to adults. Despite this, adolescents usually achieve a better nutritional balance than most adults would expect.

Inadequate iron intake is the main concern about the adolescent diet, although for some teens inadequate calcium intake is also a problem. Estimates suggest that 20% of the adolescent population is at risk of iron-deficiency anemia (Mellendick, 1983.) Because iron demands increase during pregnancy, iron-deficiency anemia may become a problem for the pregnant adolescent. Consequently, iron supplements are definitely indicated, and for those teens with an aversion to milk, calcium supplementation may also be indicated.

In assessing the diet of the pregnant adolescent, the nurse should consider the eating pattern over time, not simply a single day's intake. This pattern is critical because of the irregularity of most adolescent eating patterns. Once the pattern is identified, counseling can be directed toward correcting deficiencies.

The pregnant teenager will soon become a parent, and her understanding of nutrition will influence not only her well-being but also that of her child. However, teens tend to live in the present, and counseling that stresses long-term changes may be less effective than more concrete approaches. In many cases, group classes are effective, especially those with other teens. In a group atmosphere, adolescents often work together to plan adequate meals including foods that are special favorites.

Nursing Responsibilities ──────

Each person's view of nutrition and its relationship to pregnancy depends on previous teaching and dietary habits. A member of the health care team takes a complete diet history and assesses nutritional status to help each woman plan a suitable diet. During the data-gathering, the nurse has an opportunity to discuss important aspects of nutrition in the context of the family's needs and life-style.

The nurse can use a nutritional questionnaire such as the one shown in Figure 8-1 to gather and record important facts. This information serves as the data base on which the nurse bases an intervention plan to fit the woman's individual needs. The sample questionnaire has been filled in to demonstrate this process.

The nurse begins to assess nutritional status as the questionnaire is completed. From these assessments, the nurse can develop a nursing diagnosis and plan an approach to correct any nutritional deficiencies or improve the overall quality of the diet. To be truly effective, this plan must be made in cooperation with the pregnant woman. Once a plan has been developed, the nurse and client may wish to identify ways of evaluating its effectiveness. Evaluation may involve keeping a food journal, writing out weekly menus, and the like. If anemia is a special problem, periodic hematocrit assessments are also indicated. The Essential Facts to Remember box on p. 179 summarizes the basic information the nurse should stress when providing prenatal nutrition counseling.

Women with serious nutritional deficiencies are referred to a nutritionist. The nurse can then work closely with the nutritionist and the client to improve the pregnant woman's health by modification of her diet.

NUTRITIONAL QUESTIONNAIRE

Name Susan Longmont   Date 1-16-84

Age 20

Ethnic group white middle class

Religion Protestant

Gravida 1   Para 0   EDC 8-7-84

Age of youngest child? NA

Birth weights of previous children? NA

Usual nonpregnant weight 115   Present weight 125

Weight gain during last pregnancy? NA

Vitamin supplements? none

Current medications? aspirin for headache

Do you smoke? yes   How much per day? 1-1½ packs

Eating patterns:

1. How many meals per day? 2   when 12:30 pm 6:30 pm

2. How many snacks per day? 3   when 10:30 am 4:00 pm 10:00 pm

3. What other foods are important to your usual diet? chocolate and candy bars

4. Amount per day 4 bars/week

5. Do you have any different food preferences now? no

6. Do you eat nonfoods such as:

	Amount
laundry starch	no NA
ice	yes 10 cubes/day
other (name)	no NA

7. What foods do you dislike or do not eat? spinach and dried beans

8. For added information complete a typical daily intake (24 hour recall is suggested).

Do you have special problems in food preparation such as:

1. Physical disability   yes ____ no ✓ Explain ____
2. Cooking appliances   yes ____ no ✓ Explain ____
3. Refrigeration of food   yes ____ no ✓ Explain ____

Who does the meal planning? I do. ____ shopping? We both do.
cooking? I do most of the time but my husband likes to help.

Are there transportation problems? We have only one car but we go in the evening.

Financial situation: My husband is working and going to school.
I am not working.   Foodstamps yes   w/c no

Do you have any previous nutritional problems? No. I have never paid much attention
to food before, but now I have a lot of questions.

Are there any problems with this pregnancy? Nausea Yes, in the morning.

Constipation No   Other NA

Assessment by the nurse following the completion of the questionnaire.

Basic estimated nutrient and caloric value of typical daily intake.

Please circle one of the following:

Protein intake was   low   (adequate)   high
Caloric intake was   low   adequate   high
Calcium intake was   (low)   adequate   high
Iron intake was   (low)   adequate   high
Vitamin C intake was   low   (adequate)   high

Figure 8-1

Sample nutritional questionnaire used in nursing management of a pregnant client.

✸ ESSENTIAL FACTS TO REMEMBER

Prenatal Nutrition

- The pregnant woman should eat regularly, three meals a day, and snack on fruits, cheese, milk, or other nutritious foods between meals if desired.
- More frequent but smaller meals are also recommended.
- The woman should diet *only* under the guidance of her primary health care provider.
- Water is an essential nutrient. The woman should drink four to six (8-ounce) glasses of water and a total of eight to ten glasses of fluid daily.
- If the diet is adequate, folic acid and iron are the only supplements generally recommended during pregnancy.
- To avoid possible deficiencies, many caregivers also recommend a daily vitamin supplement.
- Taking (megadoses) of vitamins during pregnancy is unnecessary and potentially dangerous.

Summary

The importance of adequate nutrition in maternal and fetal well-being cannot be overstressed. Nutritional assessment and counseling should be an integral part of prenatal care. The nurse must understand the importance of essential nutrients and be able to offer suggestions, incorporating cultural and individual client preferences, for meeting nutritional needs.

References

Bayless TM et al: Lactose and milk intolerance: Clinical implications. *N Engl J Med* 1975; 292:1156.

Bean WB: Some aspects of pharmacologic use and abuse of water-soluble vitamins. In *Nutrition and Drug Interrelations* Hathock JN, Coon J (editors). New York: Academic Press, 1978.

Campbell T, Chang B: Health care of the Chinese in America. *Nurs Outlook* April 1973; 21:245.

Clark AL (editor): *Culture Childbearing Health Professionals*. Philadelphia: Davis, 1978.

Curda LR: What about pica? *J Nurse-Midwifery* Spring 1977; 23:8.

Edwards LE et al: Pregnancy in the massively obese: Course, outcome and obesity prognosis of the infant. *Am J Obstet Gynecol* 1978; 131:479.

Food and Nutrition Board: *Recommended Dietary Allowances*. Washington, DC: National Academy of Sciences, National Research Council, 1980.

Johnstone FD: Nutrition intervention and pregnancy: What are clinicians' choices? *Contemp Ob/Gyn* January 1984; 23:211.

Luke B: Megavitamins and pregnancy: A dangerous combination. *MCN* January/February 1985; 10:18.

Mellendick GJ: Nutritional issues in adolescence. In: *Adolescent Medicine* Hofmann AD (editor). Menlo Park, Calif.: Addison-Wesley, 1983.

Naeye RL: Weight gain and the outcome of pregnancy. *Am J Obstet Gynecol* September 1979; 135:3.

Register UD, Sonnenberg LM: The vegetarian diet. *J Am Diet Assoc* 1973; 62:253.

Rosenberg FH: Lactose intolerance. *Am J Nurs* May 1977; 77:823.

Additional Readings

Bull N et al: Food habits of 15–25 year olds: Dietary patterns and nutrient intakes of young women. Part 1. *Health Visit* March 1984; 57(3):84.

Corbett MA et al: Nutritional interventions in pregnancy. *J Nurse Midwifery* July/August 1983; 28(4):23.

Deskins BB, Laska MF: The community health nurse's nutrition guidelines: A trimester approach for expectant mothers. *MCN* May/June 1982; 7:202.

Henley EC et al: Symposium on maternal and newborn nursing. Nutrition across the woman's life cycle: Special emphasis on pregnancy. *Nurs Clin North Am* March 1982; 17:99.

Leonard LG: Twin pregnancy: Maternal-fetal nutrition. *J Obstet Gynecol Neonatal Nurs* May/June 1982; 11:139.

Metzler S et al: Teaching prenatal nutrition in an outpatient clinic: A change project. *Issues Health Care Women* September/December 1981; 3 (5/6):341.

Perkins J: Evaluating a nutrition education program for pregnant teenagers: Cognitive vs. behavioral outcomes. *J Sch Health* September 1983; 53(7):420.

Suter CB et al: Maternal and infant nutrition recommendations: A review. *J Am Diet Assoc* May 1984; 84(5):572.

Udall JN: Nutrition in pregnancy: Dietary adjustments that benefit mother and fetus. *Consultant* July 1983; 23(7):170.

9
Preparation for Childbirth

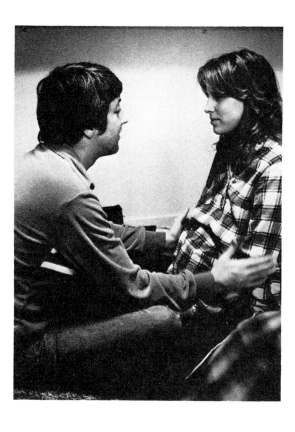

Chapter Contents

Classes for Family Members during Pregnancy
Prenatal Education
Prepared Sibling Programs
Classes for Grandparents

Education of the Family Having Cesarean Birth
Preparation for Cesarean Birth
Preparation for Repeat Cesarean Birth

Selected Methods of Childbirth Preparation
Read Method
Psychoprophylactic (Lamaze) Method
Bradley Method
Hypnosis
Other Methods

Objectives

- Identify the various issues related to pregnancy, labor, and delivery that require decision making by the parents.

- Discuss the basic goals of childbirth education.

- Describe the types of antepartal education programs available to expectant couples and their families.

- Discuss ways of making group teaching effective for maternity clients.

- Compare methods of childbirth preparation.

Key Terms

antepartal education
abdominal effleurage
Bradley method

hypnoreflexogenous
  method
Lamaze method
Read method

Today, expectant couples are seeking a more active role in their childbearing experience. A participatory childbirth experience requires that the couple participate in all the decisions about the birth, including the timing of the pregnancy and the method and setting of childbirth.

A couple's preparation for childbirth begins with their own birth into a family. Their knowledge and feelings about parenthood are influenced by the experiences they encountered as they grew up. The information the couple has may or may not be accurate; their experiences with parenting or children may have been pleasant or frightening.

As parent advocates and supporters, nurses need to provide information that reflects respect for the dignity and the rights of the couple and promotes the safety of mother and fetus. The health care information given should focus on:

1. The right of the couple to know the mother's health status

2. The parent's options
3. Their participation in decision-making
4. Responsibilities for self-care
5. Treatments and their reason
6. Maintenance of family support systems
7. Consideration and respect of each individual's needs

Prospective parents have a right to be an integral part of the decision-making process. For instance, the couple must make decisions about who will provide health care, where the child will be born, who will attend the birth, and whether to attend prepregnancy or prenatal classes. The woman must also make decisions about whether to allow analgesia, perineal preparation, an enema, or the use of stirrups; what position to use during labor and delivery; and whether to breast-feed her child. She needs to discuss these issues with her partner, and the couple should be given information about the

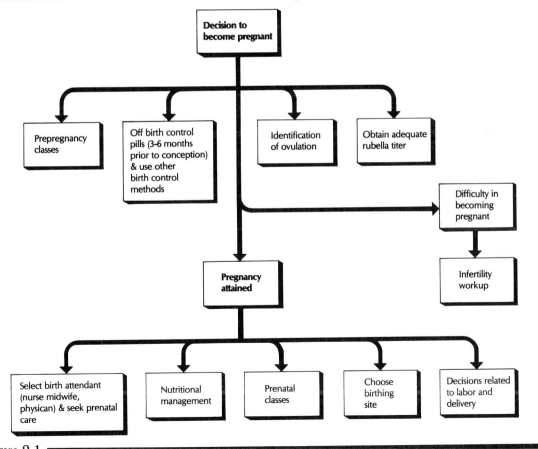

Figure 9-1
Pregnancy decision tree.

risks and benefits of each option. Their decisions should then be discussed with the health care provider. See Figure 9-1 and Table 9-1.

Each couple should have access to individualized health care and prenatal care information. This individualized health care helps the couple to recognize their feelings and fears, reassures them that such feelings are normal, dispels myths and misconceptions, and prepares them for the coming event.

Classes for Family Members during Pregnancy

Prenatal Education

Antepartal educational programs vary in their goals, content, leadership techniques, and method of teaching. The content of a class is generally dictated by its goals. For example, the

Table 9-1
Consumer Decisions During Pregnancy and Labor and Delivery*

Issue	Benefits	Risks
Breast-feeding	No additional expense Contains maternal antibodies Decreases incidence of infant otitis media, vomiting, and diarrhea Easier to digest than formula Immediately after delivery, promotes uterine contractions and decreases incidence of postpartum hemorrhage	Transmission of pollutants to newborn Can facilitate reinfection of neonate with *Candida albicans* Irregular ovulation and menses can cause false sense of security and nonuse of contraceptives. Increased nutritional requirement in mother Not advised in insulin-dependent diabetic women
Perineal prep	May decrease risk of infection Facilitates episiotomy repair	Nicks can be portal for bacteria Discomfort as hair grows back
Enema	May facilitate labor Increases space for infant in pelvis Increases strength of contractions Prevents contamination of sterile field	Increases discomfort and anxiety Coach is asked to leave, disrupting childbirth techniques
Ambulation during labor	Comfort for laboring woman May assist in labor progression by: a. Stimulating contractions b. Allowing gravity to help descent of fetus c. Giving sense of independence and control	Cord prolapse with ruptured membranes unless engagement has occurred Delivery of infant in undesirable situations Feelings of dependence and helplessness
Electronic fetal monitoring	Helps evaluate fetal well-being Helps diagnose fetal distress Useful in diagnostic testing Helps evaluate labor progress	Supine postural hypotension Intrauterine perforation (with internal monitoring) Infection (with internal monitoring) Decreases personal interaction with mother because of attention paid to the machine Mother is unable to ambulate or change her position freely
Oxytocin	Decreases incidence of cesarean birth with augmentation of labor Restimulates labor in cases of slowing contractions resulting from epidural blocks or uterine atony	Hyperstimulation contractions interfere with oxygenation of fetus Uterine rupture Early placental separation

*Compiled from Burst, H. October, 1983. The influence of consumers on the birthing movement. *Topics Clin Nurs* 5:42.
Hotchner, T. 1979. *Pregnancy and childbirth: a complete guide for a new life.* New York: Avon Books.

Table 9-1
Consumer Decisions During Pregnancy and Labor and Delivery* (continued)

Issue	Benefits	Risks
Analgesia	Maternal relaxation facilitates labor	All drugs reach the fetus in varying degrees and with varying effects
Delivery position (lithotomy) (see Chapter 6 for further discussion of positions)	Ease of visualization of perineum by birth attendant Facilitates elective operative intervention, if necessary	Increases need for episiotomy May decrease normal intensity of contractions
Stirrups	Assist in positioning for pushing (can be used in side-lying position) Comfortable for some women Convenient for the person delivering the baby	Supine postural hypotension Uncomfortable for some women Leg cramping and/or palsy Increased chance of tearing the perineum Thrombophlebitis Prolonged 2nd stage due to ineffective positioning for pushing
Episiotomy	Decreases irregular tearing of perineum May decrease stretch and loss of sexual pleasure after pregnancy	Painful healing May spasm during sexual intercourse due to poor repair Permanent scarring with certain episiotomies Infection

goal of some classes is to prepare the couple for childbirth, and therefore they do not address the discomforts of pregnancy and the care of the newborn. Other classes may focus only on pregnancy, not labor and delivery. Special classes are also available for couples who know that the woman will be having a cesarean delivery. Nurses should be aware of the couple's goals before directing them to specific classes.

One-to-one teaching Teaching on an individual basis occurs when the client needs it. Anticipatory guidance is also a positive part of teaching and is useful for discussing such topics as care of the breasts in pregnancy, sexual activity, and preparation for labor and delivery.

Nurses' teaching skills improve as they broaden their base of knowledge and become more aware of the needs of expectant families. A continuous evaluation of the effectiveness of one's teaching is essential in developing these skills.

Group teaching Group discussion is a useful teaching method. In group teaching, the nurse assesses the needs of the group instead of the needs of an individual. Skill in dealing with groups thus becomes essential. Skill in

teaching groups can be developed in several ways, and nurses have access to some excellent books on how to be an effective group leader. The following guidelines identify some basic principles of effective group teaching: Groups of couples should contain no more than 20 individuals, groups of mothers only should be smaller. The environment must be informal and friendly. The members must attend consistently, and other activities should be encouraged to increase group cohesiveness.

Helping the group to set an agenda at the initial session is one way of assessing members' needs. The individuals in the group must first become comfortable with each other so that they feel free to share concerns, questions, and information.

Nursing intervention during group discussion takes many forms and frequently overlaps with assessment and evaluation as specific interests and concerns are clarified. The nurse may need to draw other members into the discussion or to clarify information. However, most prenatal classes are not purely discussion groups but include films, tours of maternity wards, demonstrations, and lengthy explanations. In classes concerned with selected methods of childbirth preparation, many group members may have read extensively on the subject and can contribute considerably to the discussion. Other members may know nothing about it and thus require more explanations and demonstrations by the nurse. In situations where group members know little about the method, a more structured approach to discussion and exercises may be useful.

Evaluation of the effectiveness of the teaching-learning process is continuous and difficult. Checking each individual's performance after demonstration of an exercise is the most concrete way to evaluate learning. Evaluating members' changes in attitude or misconceptions is more difficult. A general evaluation of the series may be conducted in the last class, or the nurse can give group members evaluation forms to return by mail.

Prepared Sibling Programs

Many hospitals now have children's visiting hours on maternity wards. Children who are able to visit their mothers during labor and delivery and the postpartal recovery period may experience less separation anxiety. In addition, some hospitals and community groups sponsor classes to prepare children for their visits and to make them more comfortable in the hospital setting. Another purpose of many of these classes is to help the parents prepare their children for the new baby.

Usually, there is only one class, and the youngest child accepted is no less than 3 years old. Children younger than 3 years generally have little interest in pregnancy or birth, but older preschool children are interested in babies and where they come from. Involvement in the pregnancy, preparations for the birth, and seeing the birth itself may help reduce unspoken fears and misconceptions of some children.

Parents bring their children to the hospital, but parents are not included in the class unless a child will not participate without them. On the one hand, most instructors find it difficult to focus on the children when accompanying parents are asking their own questions. On the other hand, instructors of the classes want the children to feel positive about the hospital environment and do not force a child to attend without a parent.

The classes usually involve a tour of the maternity ward where the children will visit their mothers. Children usually show interest in such items as television sets, electric beds, and telephones the mothers will use to call them. The youngsters can climb on footstools at the nursery window to see the new babies. Most tours involve a visit to a birthing room, but not to delivery rooms. After the tour, the children have an opportunity to see and hear more about what happens to the parents and newborn in the hospital, how babies are born, and what babies are like. This teaching usually involves a combination of books, audiovisual materials, models, parental discussion, formal classes, and play experiences. They also have the opportunity to discuss their feelings about having a new baby in the family (MacLaughlin and Johnston, 1984). Discussion sessions may be divided into two age groups, if the ages of the children attending vary greatly.

Within the limits of their cognitive development, children should be exposed to certain essential points. These include the anatomy and physiology of pregnancy, labor, and birth and some information about fetal development. It is important to tell them what they are likely to see or hear during the birth process. For example, they may be told:

- Labor is hard, intense work, and mother will need to concentrate during her contractions. Between the contractions she may be able to talk and answer questions.

- The work of labor may be accompanied by sounds, such as groaning and panting, that the child has not heard before.

- Labor is uncomfortable and sometimes painful, but women's bodies are made in a special way to do this work without coming apart.

- Birth is generally very "wet": this is to be expected and is OK.

Teaching children about the placenta and its delivery is also necessary, and information concerning the episiotomy and its repair is included when appropriate (Parma, 1979). Children as young as 3 years can be given basic information tailored to meet their understanding. Some practitioners recommend that children under 4 years old should be discouraged from attending the birth because they are less likely to question what they do not understand and are more dependent on their mothers for emotional support (Leonard et al., 1979).

It is highly recommended that the child be accompanied by a support person or coach whose sole responsibility is tending to the needs of the child. The support person should be well known to the child, warm, sensitive, flexible, knowledgeable about the birth process, and comfortable with sexuality and birth. He or she must be prepared to interpret what is happening as the child requires and to intervene when necessary (Daniels, 1983).

After the class, parents usually receive additional resources that tell how to prepare children for a baby in the family. Some programs award certificates to the children who attended, offer refreshments to the children and their parents, and give gift packets with articles similar to those new mothers receive (lotion, diapers for the new baby).

An increasing number of hospitals allow siblings to attend the birth in birthing room settings. These hospitals usually require the siblings to attend special classes to prepare them for this experience. In addition, a sibling-support person whom the child trusts must accompany the child so that he or she can be present without distracting the mother. A grandparent often fills this role.

Classes that prepare children for attendance at birth vary. It is important that the children be at least familiar with what to expect during the labor and delivery: how the parents will act, especially the sounds and faces the mother may make; what they will see, including the messiness, blood, and equipment; and how the baby will look and act at birth. In addition, parents are encouraged to involve the child early in the pregnancy, including taking the child on a prenatal visit to see the birth attendant and listen to the fetal heart beat. Most advocates feel the child also needs to be comfortable with seeing the mother without clothes prior to seeing her during labor and delivery.

Classes for Grandparents

For many years, hospital regulations have prevented grandparents of the newborn from having much contact until mother and baby arrive home. Those regulations are changing considerably. Health professionals are beginning to recognize the important role grandparents play in the arrival of a newborn and the potential influence they have on the childbearing family. Hospital visiting hours are more open and extended, and some communities are establishing classes for grandparents. The major purpose of these classes is twofold: to increase grandparents' awareness of the changes that have occurred in approaches to childbearing and childcare and to increase grandparents' awareness of their feelings and the potential areas of conflict.

Education of the Family Having Cesarean Birth

Preparation for Cesarean Birth

Cesarean birth is an alternative method of delivery. Since one out of every five or six deliveries is a cesarean, preparation for this possibility should be an integral part of every childbirth education curriculum. The instructor should treat cesarean birth as a normal event and present factual information that will allow a couple to make choices and participate in their birth experience. The instructor can emphasize the similarities between cesarean and vaginal births to minimize undertones of "normal" versus "abnormal" delivery (Affonso, 1981). This will diminish feelings of anger, loss, and grief.

All couples should be encouraged to discuss with their physician or nurse-midwife what the approach would be in the event of a cesarean. They can also discuss their needs and desires. Their preferences may include the following:

- Participating in the choice of anesthetic
- Father (or significant other) being present during the procedures and/or delivery

Preparation for Repeat Cesarean Birth

When a couple is anticipating a repeat cesarean birth, they have time to analyze and synthesize the information and to prepare for some of the specifics. Many hospitals or local groups (such as C-Sec, Inc.) provide preparation classes for cesarean birth. Couples who have had previous negative experiences need an opportunity to describe what they felt contributed to their feelings. They should be encouraged to identify what they would like to change and to list interventions that would make the experience more positive. Those who have had positive experiences need reassurance that their needs and desires will be met in the same manner. In addition, an opportunity should be given to discuss any fears or anxieties.

A specific concern of the client facing a repeat cesarean is anticipation of the pain. She needs reassurance that subsequent cesareans are often less painful than the first. If her first cesarean was preceded by a long or strenuous labor, she will not experience the same fatigue. Giving this information will help her cope more effectively with stressful stimuli, including pain. The nurse can remind the client that she has already had experience with how to prevent, cope with, and alleviate painful stimuli.

Selected Methods of Childbirth Preparation

Various methods of childbirth preparation are taught in North America. Some antepartal classes are more specifically oriented to preparation for labor and delivery, have a name indicating a theory of pain reduction in childbirth, and teach specific exercises to reduce pain. The three most common methods of this type are the Read (natural childbirth), the Lamaze (psychoprophylactic), and the Bradley (partner-coached childbirth) methods. Hypnosis is also discussed here because it is sometimes used to help the expectant mother reduce or even eliminate pain in labor and delivery.

Each of these methods is designed to provide the woman with self-help measures so that her pregnancy and delivery are healthy and happy events in which she participates.

Expectant parents are taught that childbirth exercises and preparation for childbirth do not exclude the use of analgesics but that they often reduce the amount necessary. Some women will not require medication. Unfortunately, some groups teach that painless childbirth is the desired goal, causing those women who experience discomfort and accept pain medication to feel as failures. This feeling can be extremely destructive to the woman's self-concept at a time when she needs positive reinforcement in her abilities to achieve and perform competently. Fortunately, current thinking recognizes that individuals vary in their responses to stress, that the character of individual labors differs, and that pain medication used judiciously may enhance the woman's ability to use relaxation techniques.

The programs in prepared childbirth have some similarities. All have an educational component to help eliminate fear (Peterson, 1983). The classes vary in the amount of coverage of various subjects related to the maternity cycle, but they all teach relaxation techniques and all prepare the participants for what to expect during labor and delivery. Except for hypnosis, these methods also feature exercises to condition muscles and breathing patterns used in labor. The greatest differences among the methods lie in the theories of why they work and in the relaxation techniques and breathing patterns they teach.

The advantages of these methods of childbirth preparation are several. The most important is that the baby may be healthier because of the reduced need for analgesics and anesthetics. Another advantage is the satisfaction of the couples for whom childbirth becomes a shared and profound emotional experience. In addition, proponents of each method claim that it shortens the labor process, a claim that has been clinically validated.

All maternity nurses must know how these methods differ so that they can support each couple in their chosen method. It is important to assess the couple's emotional resources and their expectations so that the nurse can help them achieve their goals more effectively.

Read Method

Dr. Grantly Dick-Read (1959) was an English physician and a pioneer in the childbirth preparation movement. After observing many women in labor and assisting them in delivery, he developed a theory of preparation for childbirth. In 1933, his first book, entitled *Natural Childbirth*, was published. It created a considerable furor among physicians in his country.

Dick-Read called his method *natural childbirth* because he felt the process of labor and delivery was originally a natural process. He believed that pain experienced during this time was mental in origin, stating that "theoretically nature made no provision for parturition to be painful." Most women experience pain because of the culturally induced fear that they associate with childbirth. Thus his preparation method centers on eliminating the fear-tension-pain syndrome: If the fear of childbirth is removed, tension will be reduced and pain will be minimized.

Dick-Read believed that education was the key in overcoming fear of childbirth. The mother learns the physiology of pregnancy, labor, and delivery and ways to help herself during the various phases of labor. Achievement of relaxation is also important since tension can interfere with cervical dilatation. Dick-Read advocated exercises to condition muscles that would be used in childbirth and exercises to help the woman control respiration during contractions. His program of physical preparation has been further developed.

Classes teaching the Read method follow a basic pattern. Part of the class is devoted to lecture, discussion, and the like and the other part to demonstration and practice of exercises.

The woman is taught to use passive relaxation methods, such as progressive contraction and relaxation of muscle groups from her head to her toes, that promote sleep. She is encouraged to use this technique in labor to help her sleep or nap between contractions. If she is not able to sleep, at least she can relax her muscles.

The pattern of respiration used in labor is basically abdominal. The woman concentrates on forcing the abdominal muscles to rise. When she begins the class, she probably takes several breaths per minute, but she is gradually taught to take one breath per minute, with a 30-second inhalation and 30-second exhalation. This pattern of breathing lifts the abdominal muscles as the uterus rises forward with a contraction. Proponents of this method suggest the pressure of the abdominal muscles on the contracting uterus increases pain. The woman is encouraged to practice her breathing in various positions and while involved in various activities.

She begins the breathing technique with the first contraction in labor. *Slow* abdominal breathing is used during the first stage of labor and is helpful in avoiding painful spasms of the abdominal muscles. Rapid chest breathing is learned for use toward the end of labor if abdominal breathing becomes difficult at that time. Laboring women utilizing the Read method should not be interrupted in the middle of a contraction while doing their breathing.

An effective "pushing" position is also taught, but pushing is not done until the second stage of labor, when it is needed. Exercises condition the appropriate muscles. Panting is also taught to prevent pushing when it is not necessary.

Dick-Read emphasized the importance of a supportive environment throughout labor and delivery. He believed that a major source of discomfort for a woman during labor was the suggestion of pain, which "emanates from doctors, nurses, and relatives who believe in pain" (Dick-Read, 1959).

Dick-Read believed husbands should be educated because of their influence on their wives but that husbands should not be with their wives during labor if they were not helpful to them. He emphasized that analgesia and anesthesia were available for women using his method of natural childbirth but implied throughout his book that a woman is either improperly prepared or remiss in her duty as a mother if she requests them.

Psychoprophylactic (Lamaze) Method

The terms *psychoprophylactic* and **Lamaze** are used interchangeably. *Psychoprophylactic* means "mind prevention," and Dr. Fernand Lamaze, a French obstetrician, was the first person to introduce this method of childbirth preparation to the Western world. Psychoprophylaxis actually originated in Russia and is based on Pavlov's research with conditioned reflexes. Pavlov found that the cortical centers of the brain can respond to only one set of signals at a time and that they accept only the strongest signal; the weaker signals are inhibited. Pavlov's research also demonstrated that verbal representation of a stimulus can create a response. When the real stimulus is substituted, the conditioned response continues to be produced. This theory was successfully applied to preparation for childbirth by Russian physicians.

Lamaze first became familiar with the psychoprophylaxis method when attending a conference in Russia. He introduced the method in France in 1951, adding innovations of his own. It was popularized soon after in this country through Marjorie Karmel's book *Thank You, Dr. Lamaze* (1965). The method was called "painless childbirth" and thus received much resistance from the medical profession in this country because many believed that pain in childbirth is inevitable. Also, with the development of many analgesics and anesthetics, it did not seem necessary to condition women for childbirth.

Proponents of the method gradually organized and in 1960 formed a nonprofit group called the American Society for Prophylaxis in Obstetrics (ASPO). Two of the founders were Marjorie Karmel and Elizabeth Bing, a physical therapist who had also written about childbirth preparation using this method (Bing, 1967). This organization helped establish many programs throughout the country and has become one of the most popular methods of childbirth education.

The two components of Lamaze classes are education and training.

Class content originally was confined to exercises, relaxation, breathing techniques, and the normal labor and delivery experience.

Childbirth educators have added information on prenatal nutrition, infant feeding, cesarean birth, and other variations from usual labor as well as discussions concerning sexuality, early parenting, and coping skills for the postpartum period.

Instructors teaching the method in this country have modified many of the original exercises, but the basic theory of conditioned reflex remains the same. Women are taught to substitute favorable conditioned responses for unfavorable ones. Rather than restlessness and loss of control in labor, the woman learns to respond to contractions with conditioned relaxation of the uninvolved muscles and a learned respiratory pattern. Exercises taught in these classes include proper body mechanics and body conditioning, breathing techniques for labor, and relaxation.

A specific type of cutaneous stimulation used prior to the transitional phase of labor is known as **abdominal effleurage** (Figure 9-2). This light abdominal stroking is used in the Lamaze method of childbirth preparation. It effectively relieves mild to moderate pain, but not intense pain. Deep pressure over the sacrum is more effective for relieving back pain. In addition to the measures just described, the nurse can promote relaxation by encouraging and supporting the client's controlled breathing.

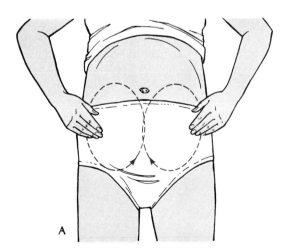
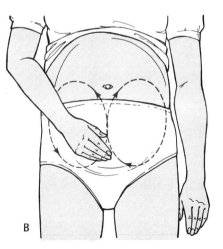

Figure 9-2

Effleurage is light stroking of the abdomen with the fingertips. **A,** Starting at the symphysis, the woman lightly moves her fingertips up and around in a circular pattern. **B,** An alternate approach involves the use of one hand in a figure-eight pattern. This technique is used primarily during labor.

Some of the body conditioning exercises, such as the pelvic tilt, pelvic rock, and Kegel's exercises, are similar to those taught in other childbirth preparation classes. Other exercises strengthen the abdominal muscles for the expulsive phase of labor. The method of relaxing uninvolved muscle groups (neuromuscular control) is unique to Lamaze. This pattern of active relaxation is in contrast to the Read method of passive relaxation. The woman is taught to become familiar with the sensation of contracting and relaxing the voluntary muscle groups throughout her body. She then learns to contract a specific muscle group and relax the rest of her body. This process of isolating the action of one group of voluntary muscles from the rest of the body is called *neuromuscular disassociation* and is basic to the psychoprophylaxis method of prepared childbirth. This exercise conditions the woman to relax uninvolved muscles while the uterus contracts.

The breathing patterns used in the Lamaze method are also different from those of other methods. Some educators feel that Lamaze's chest breathing is easier to use and more comfortable throughout labor than Read's abdominal breathing. Chest breathing patterns vary according to the phase of labor, with breathing becoming progressively more shallow (see Table 9-2). A major modification of the original breathing pattern has been to use moderately shallow breathing rather than rapid panting. Shallow, effortless breathing, moderate in pace and high in the chest, is now taught in combination with the slower chest breathing. This shallow breathing is used as labor intensifies,

when slow chest breathing is no longer effective by itself. Using this combined pattern, the woman begins her contraction with slow chest breathing, switches to shallow chest breathing for the peak of the contraction, and returns to slow chest breathing as the contraction declines. The shallow breathing itself has several variations, and an acceleration-deceleration pattern or a pant-blow pattern may be used as transition nears (Figure 9-3). In the second stage of labor, the woman may assume any comfortable physiologic position (a 35° semisitting, squatting, or sidelying position), take several deep breaths, then hold her breath, bulge abdominal muscles, relax the perineum, and push out through the vagina. This pushing effort is repeated throughout the contraction, timed and coached by the partner.

Proponents of this method believe that the variety of chest breathing patterns helps keep the pressure of the diaphragm off the contracting uterus. The patterns of breathing taught in different classes vary. The woman is taught to use one pattern until it is no longer effective rather than in conjunction with the phases of labor.

Another major modification in the Lamaze method involves the goals of expectant couples. Lamaze and his supporters implied that, if the childbirth experience was to be successful (painless with no anesthetic), specific criteria must be adhered to. Couples using this method are now encouraged to set their own goals for success. Lamaze childbirth education in this country supplies them with the tools to accomplish these goals. The couple is encouraged to

Table 9-2
Lamaze Method: Breathing Patterns

First level (slow chest). The first breathing level is a slow and even chest breathing. The breath is taken in through the nose and exhaled through the nose or mouth. The rate should be approximately 6 to 9 breaths per minute. *Second level (accelerated-decelerated)*. The second breathing pattern is useful when the contractions become more intense. It is more shallow and rapid and can be accelerated at the acme of the contraction and slowed as the contraction intensity decreases. The breath is taken in through the nose and exhaled through the mouth.	*Third level (pant-blow)*. The third breathing level is useful in the transition phase. The client takes more rapid and shallow breaths throughout the contraction, inhaling and exhaling through the mouth. After taking a cleansing breath, the woman holds the mouth in a semismiling position and exhales making a sound like "hee." After three of these "hee" breaths, she purses her lips slightly as she exhales the next breath, making a "hoo" sound. This pattern (hee-hee-hee-hoo) continues through the contraction and ends with a cleansing breath. "Hee-hoo" breathing is shallow and rhythmic. If the mouth gets too dry, the tongue can be placed against the roof of the mouth (Fenlon et al., 1979).

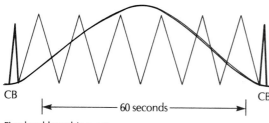

First level breathing pattern

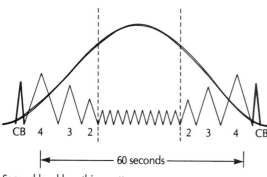

Second level breathing pattern

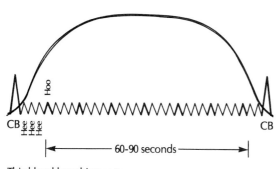

Third level breathing pattern

Figure 9-3

Lamaze breathing patterns. Each diagram represents a different breathing pattern. The curved line represents the uterine contraction. The peaked lines represent breaths that are taken during the contraction. Each breathing pattern begins and ends with a cleansing breath (CB). (From Fenlon, A., Oakes, E., and Dorchak, L. 1979. *Getting ready for childbirth*. Englewood Cliffs, N.J.: Prentice-Hall, Inc.)

discuss their goals with the obstetrician and maternity nursing personnel in labor and delivery. The nursing staff who knows the couple's goals and resources is able to offer effective support.

In France, *monitrices* are specially trained to assist the woman in labor and delivery. In North America, the partner is the specially trained individual. In the United States, the Lamaze method no longer means childbirth without anesthetics or pain. The couple's training, however, helps the woman to reduce pain and even to eliminate the need for anesthetics. More important, the woman is prepared to be an active participant and to be in control of her experience.

Bradley Method

The **Bradley method**, frequently referred to as partner- or husband-coached natural childbirth, is basically Read's method with the active participation of the partner or support person. The support person plays a vital role in coaching the woman throughout pregnancy in preparation for labor and delivery.

In his writings and talks, Bradley compares his method of natural childbirth to the instincts of animals. After observing that animals do not suffer pain during the birthing process, he suggests that women can adopt animal birthing behaviors to alleviate pain. Bradley lists environmental characteristics that birthing animals seek and their natural birthing behaviors. These, he feels, are necessary to achieve natural childbirth: darkness, quiet, physical comfort, physical relaxation, controlled breathing, and the appearance of sleep (Bradley, 1981). The exercises used to accomplish relaxation and slow controlled breathing are basically those used in the Read method. Hartman (1975) gives more explicit instructions on how to do these exercises.

Bradley's goal is to help women achieve an unmedicated pregnancy, labor, and delivery. Proponents of his method have established the American Academy of Husband-Coached Childbirth for certifying teachers in his method. The teachers are usually individuals who have used the method successfully.

Hypnosis

The use of hypnosis in childbirth is not as common as the other methods of preparation just discussed. It does not include active exercising and is not always taught in a group situation. However, hypnosis is similar to the other methods in that it reduces fear of childbirth by preparing the woman for what to expect, promotes relaxation, and reduces or eliminates pain.

The basic technique of hypnosis used in obstetrics is known as the **hypnoreflexogenous method** first described in the Western hemisphere by Roig-Garcia (1961). The method is a combination of hypnosis and conditioned reflexes. Proponents believe that if a woman's response to labor has been verbally conditioned through posthypnotic suggestion, only rarely does the woman need enter a hypnotic state during labor.

During the sessions, hypnosis is used to modify the woman's existing perceptions of labor and delivery, eliminating fear and anxiety and allowing her to perceive contractions as painless sensations. In addition, a low excitability level of the cortex accompanies hypnosis and posthypnotic suggestion. Proponents of this method feel that they are preparing the woman for a normal physiologic process, not a surgical procedure. Although specific techniques of producing anesthesia and analgesia are not taught, they are believed to be by-products of the method (Werner et al., 1982). Roig-Garcia (1961) describes the woman prepared hypnotically as managing the labor and delivery process "in a state of vigilance and wakefulness without the presence of a pain component."

Practitioners of the hypnoreflexogenous method prepare their clients for the recovery period as well as for labor and delivery. Posthypnotic suggestions to aid elimination, breastfeeding, and other postpartum activities are incorporated into the training sessions.

Hypnotists in obstetrics sometimes modify the hypnoreflexogenous method and include the concept of "glove anesthesia." When the client achieves a medium or complete trance, the hypnotist suggests that she is losing sensation in her hand from the wrist to her fingertips. The hypnotist describes the tingling and the eventual numbness of her hand. When the subject is able to achieve the numbness in her hand, she can transfer this anesthesia to other parts of her body by suggestion and touch. Throughout these suggestions, the woman's experience in labor and delivery is described in a positive manner, and the hypnotist attempts to prepare her for her experience step by step to eliminate any element of surprise. By the last session, the client may achieve autohypnosis (Tinterow, 1972). The woman uses posthypnotic suggestions automatically in labor, achieving numbness from the abdominal area to the knees rapidly, inside and out. During labor, the woman is never unconscious and can carry out such activities as voiding. She should be disturbed as seldom as possible and spoken to softly; discomfort should never be suggested.

The sessions just described are time-consuming because they are often done on a one-to-one basis. The obstetrician is frequently the hypnotist and begins preparing the woman around the fifth or sixth month of pregnancy. Six to eight sessions may be incorporated as part of the woman's prenatal visits.

The hypnoreflexogenous method without the additional introduction of "glove anesthesia" seems to be the most common method of hypnosis now used in childbirth, probably because it can be taught in group sessions in less time.

Much controversy has surrounded the use of hypnosis, perhaps because the mechanism of hypnosis is only vaguely understood. Hypnotic trance also seems to connote mysticism and lack of control. Proponents of hypnosis, however, say that the subject does not adopt suggestions that she ordinarily would reject. There is no physical danger to the woman and baby, especially with the reduction or elimination of medications in labor and delivery.

The greatest disadvantage of hypnosis to the couple is that the man is usually not involved. In addition, some are concerned about the risk of producing psychosis in a woman who has an emotional disorder. Others feel that this would be impossible (Tinterow, 1972).

Other Methods

The *Wright method* is based on psychoprophylaxis but uses less active breathing than the Lamaze method. The breathing levels become more complex as labor progresses.

The *Kitzinger method* is not based on psychoprophylaxis principles. It uses sensory memory to help the woman understand and work with her body in preparation for birth. It incorporates the Stanislavsky method of acting as a way to teach relaxation. This method uses chest breathing in conjunction with abdominal release.

Summary

Pregnancy is an extremely stressful period for the expectant family. Knowledge about childbirth and childrearing do much to strengthen the family's ability to cope with fears.

Nurses are often responsible for providing prenatal education to expectant families. Information about labor and delivery is supplied to the childbearing couple.

The expectant couple can also learn various methods of childbirth preparation that use relaxation and breathing techniques to reduce discomfort.

If the expectant family is properly prepared for childbirth, this experience can help all family members grow. The nurse has an important role in giving the family the opportunity to have this positive experience.

Resource Groups

American Society for Prophylaxis in Obstetrics (ASPO) (1411 K St., N.W. Washington DC 20005).
Cesarean Association for Research, Education, Support, and Satisfaction in Birthing (CARESS) (Burbank, Calif., 91510).
Cesarean Birth Council (San Jose, Calif., 95101).
Cesarean/Support, Education, and Concern (C/Sec., Inc.) (Dedham, Mass. 02026).
International Childbirth Education Association (P.O. Box 20048, Milwaukee, WI 55420).

References

Affonso DD: *Impact of Cesarean Childbirth*. Philadelphia: Davis, 1981.
Bing E: *Six Practical Lessons for an Easier Childbirth*. New York: Bantam Books, 1967.
Bradley RA: *Husband-Coached Childbirth*, 3rd ed. New York: Harper & Row, 1981.
Burst H: The influence of consumers on the birthing movement. *Topics Clin Nurs* October 1983; 5:42.
Daniels MB: The birth experience for the sibling: description and evaluation of a program. *J Nurse-Midwifery* September/October 1983; 28(5):15.
Dick-Read G: *Childbirth Without Fear*, 2nd ed. New York: Harper & Row, 1959.
Fenlon A, McPherson E, Dorchak L: *Getting Ready for Childbirth*. Englewood Cliffs, N.J.: Prentice-Hall, 1979.
Hartman R: *Exercises for True Natural Childbirth*. New York: Harper & Row, 1975.
Hotchner T: *Pregnancy and Childbirth: A Complete Guide for a New Life*. New York: Avon Books, 1979.
Karmel M: *Thank You, Dr. Lamaze*. New York: Doubleday, 1965.
Leonard CH et al: Preliminary observations on the behavior of children present at the birth of a sibling. *Pediatrics* 1979; 64:950.
MacLaughlin SM, Johnston KB: The preparation of young children for the birth of a sibling. *J Nurse-Midwifery* November/December 1984; 29(6):371.
Parma S: A family-centered event? Preparing the child for sharing in the experience of childbirth. *J Nurse-Midwifery* 1979; 24:6.
Peterson G: Addressing complications of childbirth in the prenatal setting. *J Nurse-Midwifery* March/April 1983; 28(2):25.
Roig-Garcia S: The hypnoreflexogenous method: a new procedure in obstetrical psychoanalgesia. *Am J Clin Hypnosis* July 1961; 4:1.
Tinterow MM: Techniques of hypnosis. In: *Obstetric Analgesia and Anesthetics*, Bonica JJ (editor). Philadelphia: Davis, 1972.
Werner ME et al: An argument for the revival of hypnosis in obstetrics. *Am J Clin Hypnosis* January 1982; 24:149.

Additional Readings

Lamb GS, Lipkin M Jr.: Somatic symptoms of expectant fathers. *MCN* 1982; 7:110.
May KA: Active involvement of expectant fathers in pregnancy: Some further considerations. *J Obstet Gynecol Neonatal Nurs* March/April 1978; 7:7.
Olson ML: Fitting grandparents into new families. *MCN* 1981; 6:419.
Richards MPM: The trouble with "choice" in childbirth. *Birth* Winter 1982; 9:253.

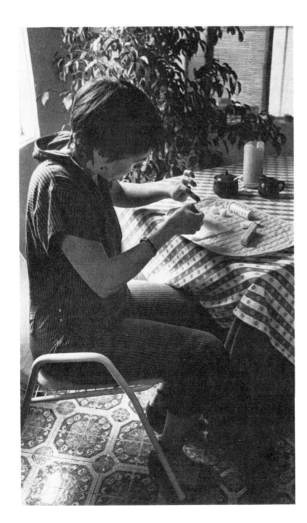

10

Complications of Pregnancy

Chapter Contents

Objectives

- Discuss the effects of selected preexisting medical conditions on pregnancy.

- Compare the bleeding problems associated with pregnancy.

- Describe the development and course of hypertensive disorders associated with pregnancy.

- Explain the cause and prevention of Rh hemolytic disease of the newborn.

- Describe effects of surgical procedures on pregnancy, and how pregnancy may complicate diagnosis.

- Discuss some common infections that may be contracted during pregnancy or may coexist with pregnancy.

- Discuss possible teratogenic effects of infections and drugs.

- Discuss drug use and abuse during pregnancy.

Key Terms

abortion	preeclampsia
eclampsia	pregnancy-induced
erythroblastosis	hypertension
fetalis	(PIH)
hydrops fetalis	RhoGAM
macrosomia	TORCH

Pregnancy puts stress on the healthy female biologically, physiologically, and psychologically. In the presence of certain factors, pregnancy can become a life-threatening event. Thus, prenatal care is aimed toward specific identification, assessment, and management of the high-risk client.

In this chapter, the discussion focuses on pregestational medical disorders and specific disorders that are unique to the pregnant woman. The possible effects of these disorders on the outcome of pregnancy are examined. In addition, surgical procedures, accidents and trauma, and infectious processes that may influence maternal and fetal well-being are described.

Pregestational Medical Disorders

Cardiac Disease

Heart disease is estimated to occur in 1%–2% of pregnant women (Danforth, 1982). Rheumatic heart disease formerly accounted for the great majority of cases, but recently congenital heart disease has become the leading cause of heart disease associated with pregnancy (Pritchard, MacDonald, and Gant, 1985). Other less common causes of heart disease in pregnancy are syphilis; arteriosclerosis; coronary occlusion; and renal, pulmonary, and thyroid disorders.

The majority of expectant women with heart disease are able to complete a pregnancy successfully. Although heart disease is the major nonobstetric cause of maternal death, the incidence of death is less than 1% (Leman et al., 1981).

For women with congenital heart disease, the implications of pregnancy depend on the specific defect. If the heart defect has been surgically repaired and no evidence of organic heart disease remains, pregnancy may be undertaken with confidence. In such cases, antibiotic prophylaxis is recommended to prevent subacute bacterial endocarditis at the time of delivery (Noller, 1981a). Women with congenital heart disease who experience cyanosis should be counseled to avoid pregnancy because the risk to mother and fetus is high.

Classification   Depending on the severity of cardiac disease, an individual's physical activities may be limited because of discomfort and risk. The Criteria Committee of the New York Heart Association, Inc. (1955) classifies cardiac disease in terms of functional capacity as follows:

- Class I. No limitation of physical activity. Ordinary physical activity causes no discomfort; patients do not have anginal pain.

- Class II. Slight limitation of physical activity. Ordinary physical activity causes fatigue, dyspnea, palpitation, or anginal pain.

- Class III. Moderate to marked limitation of physical activity. During less than ordinary physical activity, patients experience excessive fatigue, dyspnea, palpitation, or anginal pain.

- Class IV. Unable to carry on any physical activity without experiencing discomfort. Even at rest, they experience symptoms of cardiac insufficiency or anginal pain.

Clients in classes I and II usually experience a normal pregnancy and have few complications, whereas those in classes III and IV are at risk for more severe complications.

Clinical Manifestations Pregnancy results in increased cardiac output, heart rate, and blood volume. The normal heart is able to adapt to these changes without undue difficulty. These changes, however, may strain the cardiac reserve of the woman with heart disease. Initially, her heart compensates by ventricular dilatation, ventricular hypertrophy, and tachycardia. When these mechanisms maintain adequate blood flow to the tissues in the presence of pathologic changes, the heart is in a state of compensation. When these mechanisms fail and the heart is no longer able to cope with the demands placed on it, decompensation occurs. At this point, symptoms develop when the woman increases her activity because her cardiac reserve is reduced. In addition to manifesting a decreased tolerance of activity, the pregnant woman with impending cardiac decompensation exhibits other clinical symptoms, including:

- Cough (frequent, with or without hemoptysis)
- Dyspnea (progressive, upon exertion)
- Edema (progressive, generalized, including extremities, face, eyelids)
- Heart murmurs (heard on auscultation)
- Palpitations
- Rales (auscultated in lung bases)

These progressive symptoms are indicative of congestive heart failure, the heart's signal of its decreased ability to meet the demands of pregnancy. It should be noted that this cycle is *progressive*, because some of these same behaviors are seen to a minor degree in a pregnancy without cardiac involvement.

Careful monitoring of these women during the prenatal period is essential. If such symptoms appear, prompt medical actions are required to correct the cardiac status. Until cardiac function is improved, delivery should not be attempted, since even the slightest stimulus might lead to cardiac failure.

Fetal-neonatal implications If maternal decompensation occurs, the risk of fetal mortality increases. In addition, the fetus may gain less weight than usual, and the possibility of premature labor increases. The respiratory and metabolic acidosis suffered by the fetus in utero as a result of inadequate oxygenation leads to cellular damage and predisposes the fetus to intrauterine fetal distress when labor begins.

The neonate who has suffered hypoxia in utero and during birth is at increased risk during the neonatal period, particularly if born prematurely. Favorable prognosis for the newborn of the cardiac client is based on maintenance of normal respiratory and metabolic functioning.

Interventions Nursing management is directed toward maintaining a balance between cardiac reserve and cardiac workload. This involves varying tasks in the antepartal, intrapartal, and postpartal periods.

Antepartal interventions The pregnant woman with cardiac disease has specific physiologic and psychologic needs. The priority assigned to these needs varies with the severity of the cardiac disease.

A diet that is high in iron, protein, and essential nutrients but low in sodium and calories best meets the nutrition needs of the client with cardiac disease. To help preserve her cardiac reserves, the woman may need to restrict her activities. In addition, 8–10 hours of sleep, with frequent daily rest periods, is essential. Because upper respiratory infections may tax the heart and lead to decompensation, the woman must avoid contact with sources of infection.

The woman may also require specific drug therapy to maintain her health. Congestive heart failure, if it develops, may be treated with thiazide diuretics and furosemide (Lasix). Cardiac failure and arrythmias are treated with digitalis glycosides and antiarrythmic drugs. Coagulation problems are treated with the anticoagulant heparin. Penicillin prophylaxis, if not contraindicated by allergy, is encouraged.

The pregnancy of a woman with cardiac disease is monitored closely. One or two prenatal visits per week for assessment of cardiac status are encouraged, especially between weeks 28–30, when the blood volume is greatest.

Intrapartal interventions During labor and delivery, the woman and fetus undergo tremendous stress (see Chapter 13). This stress could be fatal to the fetus of a woman with cardiac disease because it may be receiving a decreased oxygen and blood supply. The intrapartal management of such a patient, therefore, is aimed at reducing the amount of physical exertion and accompanying fatigue. The goal of nursing actions is to minimize the duration of the second stage of labor by encouraging and supporting relaxation.

Maternal vital signs, fetal heart rate, and the progress of labor are closely monitored, and any signs of possible decompensation are assessed. To ensure cardiac emptying and proper oxygenation, the nurse encourages the laboring woman to assume either a semi-Fowler's or side-lying position with her head and shoulders elevated. Oxygen by mask, diuretics to decrease fluid retention, sedatives and analgesics, and digitalis may also be used as indicated by the woman's status.

The nurse should remain with the patient to support and encourage her. The nurse keeps the patient and her family informed of labor progress and management plans, collaborating with them to fulfill their wishes for the birth experience as much as possible. The nurse needs to maintain an atmosphere of calm to lessen anxiety of the woman and her family.

The safest method of delivery is by low forceps and the use of a regional or local anesthetic to maintain controlled vaginal delivery. The stress of pushing is reduced, and the risk of trauma to the newborn is decreased. Cesarean delivery should be performed only if fetal or obstetric indications are present and not on the basis of heart disease alone.

Postpartal interventions   The postpartal period is a most significant time for the patient with cardiac disease. As extravascular fluid returns to the blood stream for excretion, cardiac output and blood volume increase. This physiologic adaptation places great strain on the heart and may lead to decompensation, especially in the first 48 hours postpartum.

So that the health team can detect any possible problems, the patient remains in the hospital for approximately 1 week to rest and recover. She stays in the semi-Fowler's or side-lying positions, with her head and shoulders elevated, and begins a gradual, progressive activity program. Appropriate diet and stool softeners facilitate bowel movement without undue strain.

For the first few days, as determined by the mother's cardiac status, the nurse will provide care for the newborn. This is best done at the mother's bedside to increase her contact with her newborn and to provide teaching opportunities. If the mother's cardiac condition is class I or class II, she may breast-feed her baby in bed. The nurse can assist her to a comfortable side-lying position with her head moderately elevated or to a semi-Fowler's position. The nurse should position the newborn at the breast and be available to burp the baby and reposition it at the other breast.

The advisability of breast-feeding for the class III or class IV cardiac patient must be evaluated carefully. In many cases, because of the excessive fatigue factor and because the mother may be taking several medications that pass into the breast milk, breast-feeding may not be advisable. The caregiver should give the woman accurate, understandable information about the associated risk so that she can make an informed decision.

In addition to providing the normal postpartum discharge teaching, the nurse should plan an activity schedule with the woman and her family. Visiting nurse referrals may also be necessary, depending on the woman's status.

Diabetes Mellitus

Diabetes mellitus, an endocrine disorder of carbohydrate metabolism, disrupts approximately 1 in 300 pregnancies (Moore et al., 1981). It results from inadequate production or utilization of insulin. Insulin, produced by the cells of the islets of Langerhans in the pancreas, enables glucose to move from the blood into muscle and adipose tissue cells. Without adequate insulin, glucose does not enter the cells and they become energy depleted. Blood glucose levels remain high (hyperglycemia), and the cells then break down their stores of fats and protein for energy. Protein breakdown results in a negative nitrogen balance; fat metabolism causes ketosis.

These are the four cardinal signs and symptoms of diabetes mellitus:

• Polyuria (frequent urination) results because water is not reabsorbed by the renal tubules due to the osmotic activity of glucose.

• Polydipsia (excessive thirst) is caused by dehydration from polyuria.

- Weight loss (seen in insulin-dependent diabetes, also called type I diabetes) is due to the use of fat and muscle tissue for energy.
- Polyphagia (excessive hunger) is caused by tissue loss and a state of starvation, which results from the inability of the cells to utilize the blood glucose.

Classification   States of altered carbohydrate metabolism have been classified in several ways. Table 10-1 shows the current accepted classification, a result of the 1979 report of a special committee of the National Institutes of Health (National Diabetes Data Group, 1979). This classification contains three main categories: diabetes mellitus (DM), impaired glucose tolerance (IGT), and gestational diabetes mellitus (GDM).

GDM is diabetes mellitus that has its onset or is first diagnosed during pregnancy. Except for showing an impaired tolerance to glucose, the woman may remain asymptomatic or may have a mild form of the disease. Diagnosis of GDM is very important, however, because even mild diabetes causes increased risk for perinatal morbidity and mortality.

Table 10-2 shows White's classification of diabetes in pregnancy. This classification is still used in many agencies.

Influence of pregnancy on diabetes   In the healthy, nondiabetic woman, pregnancy produces significant changes in her metabolism. She produces increased levels of insulin, which are counterbalanced by the placenta's increased production of the hormone human placental

Table 10-1 ▰▰▰▰▰▰▰▰▰▰▰▰
Classification of Diabetes Mellitus (DM) and Other Categories of Glucose Intolerance*

1. Diabetes mellitus
   a. Type I, insulin-dependent (IDDM)
   b. Type II, noninsulin-dependent (NIDDM)
      (1) Nonobese NIDDM
      (2) Obese NIDDM
   c. Secondary diabetes
2. Impaired glucose tolerance (IGT)
3. Gestational diabetes (GDM)

*From National Diabetes Data Group of National Institutes of Health, 1979.

Table 10-2 ▰▰▰▰▰▰▰▰▰▰▰▰
Classification of Diabetes in Pregnancy*

Class	Criterion
A	Chemical diabetes
B	Maturity onset (age over 20 years), duration under 10 years, no vascular lesions
C_1	Age 10 to 19 years at onset
C_2	10 to 19 years' duration
D_1	Under 10 years at onset
D_2	Over 20 years' duration
D_3	Benign retinopathy
D_4	Calcified vessels of legs
D_5	Hypertension
E	No longer sought
F	Nephropathy
G	Many failures
H	Cardiopathy
R	Proliferating retinopathy
T	Renal transplant (added by Tagatz and colleagues of the University of Minnesota)

*From White, P. 1978. Classification of obstetric diabetes. *Am. J. Obstet. Gynecol.* 130:228.

lactogen (hPL), which diminishes the effectiveness of maternal insulin. The hPL levels rise tenfold over the last 20 weeks of pregnancy, with the highest levels in the third trimester. In addition, the elevated levels of estrogen and progesterone may help block insulin action (Burrow and Ferris, 1982).

Pregnancy can affect diabetes in the following ways:

1. Diabetic control
   a. Change in insulin requirements
      (1) Frequently, the need for insulin decreases during the first trimester. Levels of hPL, an insulin antagonist, are low, and the woman and developing fetus use more glycogen and glucose.
      (2) Insulin requirements begin to rise in the second trimester and may double or quadruple by the end of pregnancy as a result of placental maturation and hPL production.
      (3) Increased energy needs during labor may require increased insulin to balance intravenous glucose.

(4) Usually an abrupt decrease in insulin requirement occurs after the passage of the placenta and the resulting loss of hPL in maternal circulation.
b. Decreased renal threshold
c. Dietary fluctuations due to nausea, vomiting, and cravings
d. Increased risk of ketoacidosis, insulin shock, and coma
2. Possible accelerations of vascular disease
a. Hypertension: increase in blood pressure of greater than 30 mm Hg systolic and 15 mm Hg diastolic
b. Nephropathy: renal impairment
c. Retinopathy

Influence of diabetes mellitus on pregnancy outcome   The course of the pregnancy in a woman with diabetes mellitus is characterized by an increased incidence of maternal, fetal, and neonatal complications. The longer the woman has been diabetic, the higher the risk to the health of the fetus and the woman, especially if control of the diabetes has been poor in the years preceding pregnancy. However, perinatal mortality is now less than 5% for mothers and infants who receive high-quality prenatal care (Spellacy, 1984).

Maternal implications   Hydramnios, or an increase in the volume of amniotic fluid, occurs in 6%–25% of pregnant diabetics (Burrow and Ferris, 1982). The exact mechanism causing the increase is unknown, although osmotic pressure, hypersecretion of amniotic fluid, and diuresis due to fetal hyperglycemia are suspected. Premature rupture of membranes and onset of labor may be a problem, but only occasionally.

Hypertensive disorders of pregnancy occur in about 12%–13% of diabetics. These conditions may be due to vascular changes resulting from the diabetes (Burrow and Ferris, 1982).

Hyperglycemia can lead to a state of ketoacidosis as a result of the increase in ketone bodies (which are mildly acidic) in the blood released in metabolism of fatty acids. Ketosis develops slowly but can eventually lead to coma in the woman. The risk of fetal death is increased to 50% or higher if ketoacidosis is not promptly treated (Burrow and Ferris, 1982) because the fetal enzyme systems cease functioning in an acidotic environment.

Since infants of diabetic women are often large (see the following discussion), dystocia may occur as a result of cephalopelvic disproportion (CPD).

Anemia may develop as a result of vascular involvement and of nausea and vomiting caused by hormonal changes. Infections of the genital tract, particularly monilial vaginitis, may develop because of glycosuria. The client should not be allowed to go past term because of the increased incidence of intrauterine fetal death. Because of the excessive size of the fetus, induction of labor is often not successful; then cesarean delivery is performed.

Fetal-neonatal implications   The incidence of stillbirths increases markedly with gestations carried beyond 36 weeks. In some instances, these intrauterine deaths can be attributed to poor diabetic control and acidosis. Careful control of the pregnant woman's diabetes significantly reduces the incidence of mortality and morbidity in the neonate, especially morbidity associated with hypoglycemia (Guthrie and Guthrie, 1982). However, even in the well-controlled diabetic, the fetus is in jeopardy. At present, congenital anomalies are the leading cause of fetal-neonatal mortality in diabetic pregnancy. These defects frequently involve the nervous system, heart, and skeletal system.

Characteristically, infants of type I diabetic mothers (or classes A, B, and C) are large for gestational age (LGA) as a result of the high maternal levels of blood glucose, from which the fetus derives its glucose. These elevated levels continually stimulate the fetal islets of Langerhans to produce insulin. This hyperinsulin state causes the fetus to utilize the available glucose. This leads to excessive growth (known as **macrosomia**) and fat deposits.

Infants of mothers with more advanced diabetes, by contrast, may demonstrate IUGR, which occurs because vascular changes in the diabetic woman decrease the efficiency of placental perfusion and the infant is not as well sustained in utero. (See the discussion in Chapter 22).

Tests for diabetes mellitus   The pregnant woman's urine should be tested for glucose at every prenatal visit. Further testing for diabetes should be done if she has one or more of the following:

- Glycosuria
- The cardinal symptoms of diabetes
- Obesity
- Family history of diabetes
- An obstetric history that includes a neonate weighing 4000 g or more at birth, hydramnios, unexplained stillbirth, neonatal death, or congenital anomalies.

Urine tests   Tes-Tape, Diastix, and Clinitest tablets may be used to test urine. Because the renal threshold is lower during pregnancy, glucose may spill into the urine when blood glucose levels are 130 mg/dL. Thus glycosuria is not considered diagnostic of diabetes but does indicate the need for further testing.

Blood tests

1. A *fasting plasma glucose test (FPG)*, commonly called a *fasting blood sugar test (FBS)*, is done to determine the amount of glucose that remains in the blood after a period of fasting. Two elevations are indicative of diabetes mellitus.
2. *Two-hour postprandial (after meal) testing* is a more sensitive test than FPG but is not considered totally diagnostic of diabetes.
3. *Oral glucose tolerance test (OGTT)* is the most sensitive (with IGTT, discussed next) method for detecting diabetes mellitus or impaired glucose tolerance. OGTT measures response to a specific amount of glucose.
4. *Intravenous glucose tolerance test (IGTT)* is the preferred test in pregnancy, since glucose absorption from the intestinal tract may vary and alter findings of OGTT.

Antepartal nursing care   The major goals of nursing care are (a) to maintain a physiologic equilibrium of insulin production and glucose utilization during pregnancy and (b) to deliver an optimally healthy mother and neonate. To achieve these goals, the health care team must give good prenatal care top priority (see Nursing Care Plan—Diabetes Mellitus, pp. 201–204).

Antepartal nursing care is based on careful assessment and knowledge of the woman's condition and of the plan of care developed by the health team.

Assessment of disease process and client information   Thorough physical examination is necessary at the first visit to detect any complications or sign of infection. Assessment will also yield information about the woman's coping abilities and her ability to follow a recommended regimen of care. Follow-up visits are usually scheduled twice a month during the first two trimesters and weekly during the last trimester.

Instruction and support   A woman with gestational diabetes may require more teaching and support than a woman whose diabetes is well established. She may feel angry and overwhelmed and need time for adjustment. The nurse must recognize this reaction and allow time for adjustment. Teaching should be individualized and should include the woman's partner or support person. Teaching sessions should be well planned and tailored to the couple's needs. Repetition and review are often necessary; and visual aids, demonstrations, and written material are useful.

The nurse also helps the couple learn to administer insulin. The basic responsibility is the woman's, but the support person should be able to help in an emergency. The woman and her support person should also know the signs of hypoglycemia and hyperglycemia and know what actions to take if these occur.

Dietary control is essential. It is best managed by a dietitian who can work with the woman to plan meals that match her culture and life-style. Smoking is contraindicated for both pregnancy and diabetes and should be discouraged. Travel is not contraindicated for the pregnant diabetic. She may carry insulin and glucagon with her in a small travel kit. Diabetic meals can be arranged with the airlines if necessary. The woman should wear a bracelet or necklace identifying her as a diabetic, and she should check with her physician for any prescriptions or instructions before leaving.

Many communities have diabetes support groups or education classes, which can be most helpful to clients with newly diagnosed diabetes. Learning that others have faced a similar situation and hearing how they managed can help the person trying to cope with a chronic disease.

Chances for a cesarean birth are increased if the pregnant woman is diabetic. This possibility should be anticipated, and enrollment in cesarean birth preparation classes may be suggested. Many hospitals offer classes, and information is available through organizations such as the Resource Groups listed at the end of Chapter 9 (p. 192). The couple may prefer simply to discuss cesarean birth with the nurse and their obstetrician and read some books on the topic.

Dietary regulation   Recommended daily food intake should be 30–35 kcal/kg, 150–200 g of carbohydrates, 125 g of protein, and 60–80 g of fat. The carbohydrates ingested should be primarily complex starches rather than concentrated sweets (Burrow and Ferris, 1982). The goal is to increase caloric intake with sufficient insulin to force glucose into the cells. Meals and snacks must be distributed to coincide with peaks in insulin activity. This is especially important when multiple doses of insulin are used. A regimen of three meals and three to four snacks per day, equally spaced, is best.

Urinary and blood glucose determinations   Ideally, the blood glucose should be maintained at 60–90 mg/dL after fasting and less than 120 mg/dL 2 hours after meals (Skyler et al., 1981). Fractional urine testing is done four times a day as needed. However, when circumstances permit, home blood glucose monitoring is the most desirable approach.

Recently, a method of determining long-term diabetic control, measuring hemoglobin A_{1c} (Hb A_{1c}) levels, has gained widespread clinical use. When plasma glucose levels are increased, hemoglobin A_o is converted to Hb A_{1c}. This reaction is nonenzymatic and essentially irreversible. Because it is a relatively slow process, the Hb A_{1c} levels give a picture of the average serum glucose concentrations during the preceding 60 days. Lower levels occur with better control. (Jovanovic and Peterson, 1982). Fetal outcome is enhanced when good control is maintained.

Establishment of insulin requirements   It has generally been held that women with gestational diabetes (White's class A) could be managed with dietary control alone. Evidence is increasing, however, that insulin therapy begun early and continued through pregnancy improves fetal outcome (Guthrie and Guthrie, 1982). For these women, a low-dosage mixture of regular- and intermediate-acting (NPH or Lente) insulin given twice a day seems the best management. Oral hypoglycemics are contraindicated in pregnancy because of possible teratogenic effects.

Women with type I diabetes (White's classes B through F) are most often controlled with multiple insulin injections (Guthrie and Guthrie, 1982). Various combinations of regular- and intermediate-acting insulin are used. With multiple-injection therapy, tighter control can be achieved and more flexibility allowed in the timing and amount of foods than with single-injection therapy. Insulin dosage may be determined by finger-stick home blood-glucose monitoring. Hospitalization may be needed to achieve control and establish insulin requirements, as mentioned earlier.

Some physicians now insert long-acting insulin pumps into the pregnant woman with diabetes. These pumps continuously infuse insulin subcutaneously, allowing the woman to approximate normal functioning.

Evaluation of fetoplacental functioning   Fetal assessment throughout the prenatal course is essential. The following techniques are usually used:

- Monitoring serum estriol levels
- Monitoring insulin requirements (If the woman does not need increased insulin dosages after the first trimester or has a sudden drop in requirement, the caregiver should suspect placental malfunction.)
- Assessing fetal growth with ultrasonography
- Measuring fundal height
- Administering nonstress and contraction stress tests, begun at 30–32 weeks' gestation and performed at least once a week.

Assessment of fetal maturity   Fetal lung maturity may be confirmed by obtaining a sample of amniotic fluid by amniocentesis and then determining the lecithin/sphingomyelin (L/S) ratio (see p. 240). Caution must be used in evaluating L/S ratio results, since they may be falsely elevated in the diabetic woman.

An L/S ratio as high as 3:1 may be needed to indicate fetal lung maturity in the pregnant diabetic, compared with a ratio of 2:1 in the nondiabetic. Because of this, some agencies also use PG determinations to assess fetal lung maturity. (See Chapter 11.)

Text continued on p. 205.

NURSING CARE PLAN
Diabetes Mellitus in Prenatal, Intrapartal, and Postpartal Periods

CLIENT ASSESSMENT

Nursing History

1. Complete assessment: client and family
2. Identification of client's predisposition to diabetes
   a. Recurrent preeclampsia-eclampsia
   b. Previous LGA infants ($\geq$ 4000 g)
   c. Hydramnios
   d. Unexplained fetal death
   e. Obesity
   f. Family history of diabetes

Physical Examination

1. Length of gestation
2. Complaints of thirst and hunger
3. Recurrent monilial vaginitis
4. Frequent urination beyond first trimester and prior to third trimester
5. Fundal height greater than expected for gestation
6. Obesity

Laboratory Evaluation

1. Fasting plasma glucose (FPG)
2. 2-hour postprandial GTT
3. 3-hour IGTT or OGTT
4. Urine test for glucose
5. 24-hour urinary estriol

Nursing Priorities

1. Observe for signs of hypoglycemia, hyperglycemia, preeclampsia
2. Test blood or urine as necessary for glucose
3. Regulate diet and insulin as needed
4. Assess client and family needs for referral
5. Assess client's knowledge of diabetes
6. During labor, monitor labor and maternal and fetal status

Client/Family Education Focus

1. Discuss importance of strict dietary control, maintenance of appropriate blood glucose levels, adequate insulin coverage, and regular prenatal care for successful pregnancy outcome
2. Review signs and symptoms of hypoglycemia and hyperglycemia and the actions the client or her family should take if they appear
3. Provide appropriate literature about diabetes in pregnancy and refer the client/family to available resource and support groups

Note for diagnosis: 2 hr pp of 140 mg/dL or above is indicative of diabetes mellitus, and a level of 110–140 mg/dL is suggestive of subclinical diabetes. May be confirmed with IGTT.

Problem	Nursing interventions and actions	Rationale
Dietary regulation	Maintain strict diet: 1. 30–35 kcal/kg 2. 150–200 g carbohydrate 3. 125 g protein 4. 60–80 g fat 5. Sodium intake may be restricted	Maintain ideal weight in first trimester and average gain in last two trimesters (no more than 3–3.5 lb/month)
Insulin needs	Assess insulin needs: 1. Check lab results of FPG and 2-hour postprandial 2. Test urine four times daily using Tes-Tape, Clinitest tablets, or Diastix 3. Teach client use of home blood glucose monitoring device. Determine amount of insulin based on sliding scale. 4. Administer regular insulin or NPH or Lente insulin, or combination, as ordered	Sufficient insulin must be present to enable proper carbohydrate metabolism to take place; pregnancy requires a marked increase in circulating insulin to maintain normal blood glucose Fasting glucose level tends to be lower than nonpregnant value Effectiveness of insulin may be reduced by presence of hPL Insulin requirements fluctuate widely during pregnancy because of factors mentioned in text; in addition, conversion of blood glucose into lactose during lactation may cause marked changes in glucose tolerance and/or hypoglycemia
Hypoglycemia	1. Teach client early signs of hypoglycemia and treatment 2. Observe for signs of hypoglycemia such as shakiness; hunger; sweaty, cold, clammy skin; pallor; headache; double vision; shallow respirations; disorientation; convulsion; coma	Self-care at home is a preventive measure so hypoglycemia will not become serious Correction of hypoglycemia and maintenance of controlled state provide optimal fetal health

NURSING CARE PLAN (continued)
Diabetes Mellitus in Prenatal, Intrapartal, and Postpartal Periods

Problem	Nursing interventions and actions	Rationale
	3. Treat within minutes of onset	Rapid treatment of hypoglycemia is essential to prevent brain damage because the brain requires glucose to function (skeletal and heart muscles can derive energy from ketones and free fatty acids)
	a. Obtain immediate blood samples for testing	Provides baseline information on glucose levels
	b. If client is alert give half a glass of orange juice or other liquid containing sugar; notify physician	Liquids are absorbed from the GI tract faster than solids; 10 g of glucose, which will reverse most hypoglycemic reactions, is the amount found in one-half glass orange juice, 2 tsp sugar or 1 or 2 hard candies
	c. If client is not alert enough to swallow give 1 mg glucagon subcutaneously or intramuscularly; notify physician	Glucagon triggers the conversion of glycogen stored in the liver to glucose
	d. If client is in labor with intravenous lines in place, 10–20 mL of 50% dextrose may be given IV	
	Standing order should be available; notify physician	
Hyperglycemia	1. Teach client early signs of hyperglycemia and treatment	Client can recognize signs and administer self-treatment Client can also report any symptoms that may occur
	2. Observe for signs of hyperglycemia such as polyuria, polydipsia, dry mouth, increased appetite, fatigue, nausea, hot flushed skin, rapid deep breathing, abdominal cramps, acetone breath, headache, drowsiness, depressed reflexes, oliguria or anuria, stupor, coma	Administer insulin to restore body's normal metabolism of carbohydrate, protein, and fat
	3. Administer treatment; notify physician	
	a. Obtain frequent measurement of blood and urine glucose; measure urine acetone	Need to establish a baseline and to determine additional insulin dosage and prevent overtreatment; urine acetone indicates development of ketoacidosis
	b. Administer prescribed amount regular insulin subcutaneously or intravenously, or combination of routes	Regular insulin used because it acts immediately and is of short duration
	c. Replace fluids IV, orally, or both	Fluids are depleted in the process of ketoacidosis; hypotension can result from decreased blood volume due to dehydration
	d. Measure intake and output	Polyuria is an early sign of hyperglycemia; oliguria develops with hypotension and decreased bloodflow to kidneys
	e. Observe for symptoms of circulatory collapse; monitor BP and pulse	Circulatory collapse can result from hypotension
Preeclampsia (PIH)	Observe and report any signs of preeclampsia	Preeclampsia is more prevalent in the pregnant woman with diabetes
Vaginitis	Observe for symptoms of burning, itching, and leukorrhea; obtain vaginal smear; treat with prescription based on the causative organism and gestation	Vaginitis is more common in the woman with diabetes; treatment is specific to the organism

NURSING CARE PLAN (continued)
Diabetes Mellitus in Prenatal, Intrapartal, and Postpartal Periods

Problem	Nursing interventions and actions	Rationale
Urinary tract infections (UTI)	Observe for symptoms of frequency, urgency, and burning on urination; low back pain with kidney involvement Obtain urine specimen for culture and sensitivity Administer prescribed antibiotics Encourage fluids; measure intake and output	Incidence of UTI is increased in diabetes, possibly because the existence of glycosuria provides rich medium for bacterial growth Antibiotic prescribed is specific to causative organism Increased fluid intake promotes urinary removal of organisms
Inadequate rest	Instruct client to rest frequently during day in lateral position	Lateral position increases uteroplacental circulation and diminishes myometrial tone
Fear and lack of knowledge	Support and encourage client and partner: 1. Explain procedures 2. Allow them to ask questions 3. Assess their level of knowledge of childbirth and utilize this to teach about what is happening 4. Involve partner as much as possible 5. Utilize breathing and relaxation techniques to minimize amount of medication needed, especially if gestation is 36 or 37 weeks, to decrease fetal narcosis. 6. Administer analgesics as needed in labor	When less afraid, the client will be more effective as a member of the antepartal-intrapartal health team Fetal narcosis should be avoided
Compromise of fetoplacental status	Periodic assessments: 1. Level of plasma and/or urine estriol 2. Creatinine clearance 3. Regular assessment of fetal size 4. Ultrasonographs 5. L/S ratio, or phosphatidylglycerol or phosphatidylinositol levels 6. NST or contraction stress test (CST)	Continued slow rise of estriol indicates adequate functioning of maternal system, placental function, and fetal status because estriol and creatinine require interplay of all three systems Assess fetal growth Evaluate fetal size 2:1 ratio usually indicates fetal lung maturity sufficient to sustain infant in extrauterine environment. In one-third of insulin-dependent women, L/S ratio fails to show a terminal rise; others show early excessive rise.
Size of fetus	Assessments: 1. Ultrasonographs 2. Measuring fundal height	Increased circulating glucose leads to increased deposition of fatty tissue of fetus Indicates uterine size, not necessarily size of fetus
Frequent hospitalization	Orient patient to surroundings and routines: 1. Provide support 2. Promote rest	Admit prenatally to assess diabetic status Admit if there are signs of incipient preeclampsia or infection Admit for most of third trimester if patient has microvascular disease so that rest can be maintained and patient can be closely supervised
Hydramnios	Assess size of uterus Assess signs of distress from hydramnios: 1. Respiratory distress 2. Stasis of fluid in legs Slow removal of amniotic fluid by transabdominal amniotomy may be done	Diabetic clients are more prone to hydramnios, and it may develop rapidly Remove fluid slowly to prevent abruptio placentae and amniotic fluid embolus

NURSING CARE PLAN (continued)
Diabetes Mellitus in Prenatal, Intrapartal, and Postpartal Periods

Problem	Nursing interventions and actions	Rationale
Labor	Admit to unit: 1. Perform routine admission 2. Assess size of fetus and capacity of pelvis: ultrasonograph, x-ray pelvimetry 3. Administer IV fluids to maintain hydration and glucose to avoid depleting glycogen stores	Induction of labor at about 37 weeks, once fetal lung maturity is ascertained, may be recommended to ensure safe fetal outcome Macrosomia is often associated with diabetes
	4. Assess insulin needs by frequent blood glucose monitoring 5. Check urine acetone every hour 6. Continuously monitor fetal status 7. Alleviate induction concerns (see Nursing Care Plan on induction, Chapter 18)	Increased exertion during labor alters insulin needs Ketonuria indicates increased need for insulin
Postpartum		
Insulin needs	Assess insulin needs by blood glucose; client may not require insulin for first 24 hours after delivery	Removal of hPL from circulation permits more efficient utilization of insulin
Parent-infant bonding	Provide parents with frequent opportunities for contact with their newborn especially if in special care nursery Encourage rooming-in if newborn's condition permits Support breast-feeding if it is mother's chosen feeding method	Increased fears for the newborn's health may impede bonding
Postpartum hemorrhage	Frequently assess for vaginal bleeding and fundal firmness; massage to stimulate contraction if boggy; monitor BP and pulse	Higher incidence of postpartal hemorrhage in women with diabetes due to overdistended uterus if LGA infant or hydramnios present

NURSING CARE EVALUATION
Client's diabetes will be controlled
Client will consume needed calories and nutrients
Client will have sufficient insulin to maintain control
Fetoplacental status will be monitored to avoid complications
Client education will be enhanced and client questions will be answered

NURSING DIAGNOSIS*	SUPPORTING DATA	NURSING ORDERS
Knowledge deficit related to diet	Expressed concerns or questions about diet and changes needed with pregnancy Episodes of hypoglycemia or hyperglycemia	Increase client's dietary knowledge base 1. Assess current intake 2. Arrange for counseling with dietitian 3. If hospitalized, have client choose own menus with assistance of dietitian
Alteration in nutrition related to impaired carbohydrate metabolism	Episodes of hyperglycemia or hypoglycemia Abnormal weight gain pattern during pregnancy	Help client stabilize diabetic condition 1. Assess for signs of hypoglycemia or hyperglycemia 2. Assess client's knowledge of signs and symptoms and treatment actions to be taken if hypoglycemia or hyperglycemia develop

*These are examples of nursing diagnoses that may be appropriate for a person with this condition. It is not an inclusive list and must be individualized for each woman.

Nursing care during labor In the last 8–10 weeks of pregnancy the woman and fetus are monitored closely, usually on an ambulatory-care basis. If the fetal or maternal condition warrants it, the woman may be hospitalized the last few weeks for more careful observation. The woman whose blood glucose level remains within acceptable limits, whose estriol levels are rising, and whose fetus has a reactive nonstress test is doing well and can probably continue to term and deliver spontaneously. If intrauterine conditions threaten fetal survival, labor may be induced by oxytocin if the cervix is ready, or cesarean delivery may be needed.

During labor, the blood glucose level is monitored closely, and intravenous fluids and nutrients are provided. Regular insulin is generally added to the intravenous infusion of glucose and regulated with an infusion pump. The intravenous insulin is discontinued with the third stage of labor.

Vital signs are monitored closely throughout labor and the woman is encouraged to lie on her side to promote placental perfusion.

The fetus is also observed closely during labor. Continuous electronic fetal monitoring provides the best information about the fetus and fetal response to maternal contractions.

The diabetic woman and her support person, like any woman in labor and her partner, need physical comfort, support, reassurance, information about progress, and explanation of all procedures. The nurse should collaborate with the couple to plan care that meets their realistic expectations for the childbirth experience.

Postpartal nursing care After birth, the mother requires much less insulin because the levels of hPL, progesterone, and estrogen fall after placental separation. Their anti-insulin effect ceases, resulting in decreased blood glucose levels. The diabetic mother may require no insulin for the first 24 hours or only one-fourth to one-half of her previous dose. It is then necessary to reestablish insulin needs based on blood sugar testing. Diet and exercise levels must also be redetermined.

Diabetes control and the establishment of parent-child relationships are the priorities of this period. If her newborn must be cared for in a special care nursery, the mother needs support and information about the neonate's con-dition. Every effort must be made to provide as much contact as possible between the parents and their newborn.

Contraceptive options should also be explored. Oral contraceptives increase the risk of vascular complications and should be used only on a short-term basis by diabetic women with no vascular involvement. Intrauterine devices are associated with a slight increase in the incidence of pelvic infection. They should be used only by women with well-controlled diabetes (Spellacy, 1984).

Mechanical devices offer the lowest health risk to the diabetic woman. A diaphragm that is well fitted and used with spermicidal cream or jelly is very reliable. Reliability is almost 100% if the man also uses a condom.

If the couple is certain that they want no more children, vasectomy may be the method of choice. Tubal ligation carries slightly more risk for the diabetic woman than the nondiabetic woman.

Other Medical Conditions and Pregnancy

Table 10-3 describes some other medical conditions that may occur in women of childbearing age. The table briefly identifies the maternal and fetal-neonatal implications of each disease.

Medical Disorders Associated with Pregnancy

Disruptive conditons that arise during the gestational period are the result of many high-risk factors, such as age, blood type, socioeconomic status, parity, psychologic well-being, and predisposing chronic illnesses. Prenatal nursing care is directed toward screening clients for these complications and toward supportive therapies that will promote good maternal and fetal outcomes.

Hyperemesis Gravidarum

Hyperemesis gravidarum is pernicious vomiting during pregnancy. It may be mild at first, but true hyperemesis progresses to a point at which the woman not only vomits everything she swallows but retches between meals.

Table 10-3
Selected Medical Conditions and Pregnancy

Condition	Brief description	Maternal implications	Fetal-neonatal implications
Hyperthyroidism (Thyrotoxicosis)	Condition characterized by overactivity of the thyroid gland resulting in increased metabolic rate, increased protein-bound iodine values and increased ^{131}I intake. Symptoms include muscle wasting, elevated pulse, enlarged thyroid, sweating, and exophthalmos. Treatment is pharmacologic or surgical.	Increased incidence of premature delivery, postpartum hemorrhage, and preeclampsia. Major complication is thyroid storm characterized by elevated temperature, tachycardia, severe dehydration, sweating, possible heart failure, and erratic mental function.	Extremely rare in newborns. Overtreatment of mother with hyperthyroid drugs may result in fetal hypothyroidism, fetal goiter, and mental deficiencies. Breast-feeding is contraindicated for women taking antithyroid medication because it is excreted in the milk.
Hypothyroidism	Condition characterized by inadequate thyroid secretions. In extreme form it is often accompanied by amenorrhea and anovulation. Symptoms include decreased metabolic rate, fatigue, cold intolerance, myxedema, dry skin, headache, constipation, and possibly goiter. Treatment includes replacement thyroid therapy and serial assessment of fetal status.	Increased incidence of infertility or, if pregnancy occurs, increased incidence of abortion. Weekly nonstress test (NST) after 35 weeks gestation.	Newborn has a slightly increased risk of being born with congenital goiter or true cretinism. If newborn has hypothyroidism, there is an increased risk of hyperbilirubinemia. To detect hypothyroidism, newborns are now routinely screened in many states for serum thyroxine levels.
Iron deficiency anemia	Condition caused by inadequate iron intake resulting in hemoglobin levels below 11 gm/dL. To prevent this, most women are advised to take supplemental iron during pregnancy.	Pregnant woman with this anemia tires easily, is more susceptible to infection, has increased chance of postpartal hemorrhage, and cannot tolerate even minimal blood loss during delivery.	Abortion and prematurity rates are increased, and the neonate may be SGA. Fetus may be hypoxic during labor due to impaired uteroplacental oxygenation (Danforth, 1982).
Sickle cell anemia	Recessive autosomal disease present in about 0.7% of the Blacks in the US. The sickle cell trait is carried by 8% of American Blacks (Danforth, 1982). The disease is characterized by sickling of the RBCs in the presence of decreased oxygenation. Condition may be marked by crisis with profound anemia, jaundice, high temperature, and infarction.	Pregnancy may aggravate anemia and bring on more crises. Increased risk of developing preeclampsia exists. There is also increased risk of urinary tract infection, pneumonia, congestive heart failure, and pulmonary infarction. The goal of treatment is to reduce the anemia and maintain good health. Oxygen supplementation should be used continuously during labor. Additional blood should be available if transfusion is necessary following delivery.	Abortion, fetal death, and prematurity lead to a perinatal death rate of about 50% (Danforth, 1982). IUGR is also a characteristic finding in neonates of women with sickle cell anemia.

The exact cause of hyperemesis is probably related to trophoblastic activity and gonadotrophin production. Psychologic factors may stimulate or exaggerate the condition.

In severe cases, dehydration may lead to fluid-electrolyte imbalances, alkalosis, hypovolemia, hypotension, tachycardia, increased hematocrit and BUN, and decreased urine output.

Severe potassium loss may disrupt cardiac functioning. Starvation may also cause severe protein and vitamin deficiencies. Fetal or embryonic death may result, and the woman may suffer irreversible metabolic changes or death.

Treatment involves intravenous administration of fluid containing glucose, vitamins (B-complex, C, A, and D), and electrolytes. Intake and output are measured, and oral hygiene is given. In 48 hours, the woman's condition usually improves sufficiently to begin controlled oral feedings.

Nursing care should be supportive and directed at maintaining a relaxed, quiet environment. Because emotional factors may play a role in this condition, psychotherapy is often recommended. With proper treatment, prognosis is favorable.

Bleeding Disorders

During the first and second trimesters of pregnancy, the major cause of bleeding is abortion. **Abortion** is the termination of a pregnancy prior to the viability of the fetus. Abortions are either *spontaneous*, occurring naturally, or *induced*, occurring as a result of artificial or mechanical interruption. *Miscarriage* is a lay term applied to spontaneous abortion.

Other complications that can cause bleeding in the first half of pregnancy are ectopic pregnancy (1 in every 200 pregnancies) and hydatidiform mole (1 in every 2000 pregnancies). In the second half of pregnancy, particularly in the third trimester, placenta previa (1 in every 200 pregnancies) and abruptio placentae (1 in every 50 to 270 pregnancies) may cause bleeding (Bernstine, 1981).

General principles of nursing intervention   All bleeding during pregnancy should be carefully evaluated. Therefore, antepartal teaching about bleeding as a warning sign should be emphasized. It is often the nurse's responsibility to make the initial assessment of bleeding. In general, the following nursing measures should be implemented for pregnant women being treated for bleeding disorders:

- Frequent monitoring of blood pressure and pulse is imperative.

- Observe the woman for behaviors indicative of shock, such as pallor, clammy skin, perspiration, dyspnea, or restlessness.

- Count pads to assess amount of bleeding over a given time period; any tissue or clots expelled should be saved.

- If pregnancy is of 20 weeks' gestation or beyond, assess fetal heart tones.

- Prepare for intravenous therapy.

- Prepare equipment for physical examination.

- Have oxygen therapy available.

- Collect and organize all data, including antepartal history, onset of bleeding episode, laboratory studies (hemoglobin, hematocrit, and hormonal assays).

- Assess coping mechanisms of woman in crisis. Give emotional support to enhance her coping abilities by staying with her, clearly explaining procedures, and by communicating her status to the family. Most important, prepare the woman for possible fetal loss. Assess her expressions of anger, denial, silence, depression, or self-blame.

Spontaneous abortion   Many pregnancies end in the first trimester because of spontaneous abortion. Often the woman assumes she is having a heavy menstrual period when in reality she is having an early abortion. Statistics are inaccurate, but estimates suggest that 15%–20% of all pregnancies end in spontaneous abortion (Borg and Lasker, 1981).

Etiology   The most common causes of spontaneous abortion are related to abnormal development of the embryo or fetus. This abnormal development may be due to:

- Genetic defects

- Teratogenic drugs

- Abnormalities of the woman's reproductive tract, such as double uterus, incompetent cervix, or uterine fibroids

- Maternal infections

- Endocrine imbalances, especially a reduction in progesterone and estrogen in early pregnancy

- Maternal malnutrition or maternal thyroid disorders

- Chronic maternal disease, such as hypertensive vascular disease, ABO incompatability, or chronic nephritis

Classification   Spontaneous abortions are subdivided into the following categories so that they can be differentiated clinically:

1. *Threatened abortion.* The fetus is jeopardized by unexplained bleeding, cramping, and backache. Bleeding may persist for days. The cervix is closed. It may be followed by partial or complete expulsion of the products of pregnancy (Figure 10-1).

2. *Imminent abortion.* Bleeding and cramping increase. The internal cervical os dilates. Membranes may rupture. The term *inevitable abortion* applies.

3. *Complete abortion.* All the products of conception are expelled.

4. *Incomplete abortion.* Part of the products of conception are retained, most often the placenta. The internal cervical os is dilated slightly.

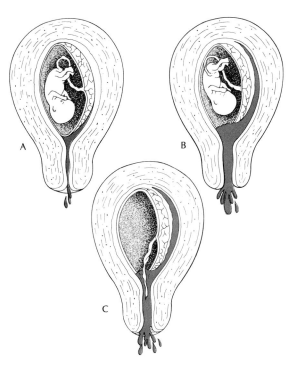

Figure 10-1 ▬▬▬▬▬▬▬
Types of spontaneous abortion. **A**, Threatened abortion. **B**, Imminent abortion. **C**, Incomplete abortion.

5. *Missed abortion.* The fetus dies in utero but is not expelled. Uterine growth ceases, breast changes regress, and the woman may report a brownish vaginal discharge. The cervix is closed. Diagnosis is made based on history, pelvic examination, a negative pregnancy test, and may be confirmed by ultrasound if necessary. If the fetus is retained beyond 6 weeks, the breakdown of fetal tissues results in the release of thromboplastin and disseminated intravascular coagulation (DIC) may develop.

6. *Habitual abortion.* Abortion occurs consecutively in three or more pregnancies.

Diagnosis   A primary consideration in the differential diagnosis of a bleeding condition is to determine whether vaginal bleeding is related to spontaneous abortion or other factors. One of the more reliable criteria is the presence of pelvic cramping and backache. These symptoms are usually absent in bleeding caused by polyps, ruptured cervical blood vessels, or cervical erosion. Results of pregnancy tests are not particularly helpful because hCG levels may remain elevated for as long as 2 weeks after fetal death.

Interventions   The therapy prescribed for the pregnant woman with bleeding includes restriction of activities, bed rest, abstinence from coitus, and perhaps sedation. If bleeding persists and abortion is imminent or incomplete, the woman is hospitalized. Fluid may be replaced by intravenous therapy or blood transfusions, and the remaining products of conception are removed by dilatation and curettage (D&C) or suction evacuation. If the woman is Rh-negative and not sensitized, Rh_o (D) immune globulin (**RhoGAM**) is given within 72 hours.

In missed abortions, the products of conception are eventually expelled spontaneously. If this does not occur within 4–6 weeks, the woman is hospitalized and a D&C is performed.

Chances for carrying the next pregnancy to term after one spontaneous abortion are as good as they are for the general population. Chances of successful pregnancy decrease with each succeeding abortion, however. If the cause of the abortion can be determined, specific therapy can often be implemented to correct it.

Providing emotional support is an important task for nurses caring for women who have aborted. Feelings of shock or disbelief are normal at first. Couples who approached the pregnancy with feelings of joy and a sense of expectancy now feel grief, sadness, and possibly anger. Those who were perhaps less than joyful or even negative about their pregnancy may feel guilt and blame. The woman may harbor negative feelings about herself or even believe that the abortion may be a punishment for some wrongdoing.

The nurse can offer invaluable psychologic support to the woman and her family by encouraging them to talk about their feelings, by allowing them the privacy to grieve, and by sympathetically listening to their concerns about this pregnancy and future ones. Feelings of guilt or blame may be decreased by informing the woman and her family about the causes of spontaneous abortion. The nurse can also refer them to other health care professionals for additional help as necessary.

Ectopic pregnancy   *Ectopic pregnancy* is an implantation of the blastocyst in a site other than the endometrial lining of the uterus. It may result from many causes, including tubal damage caused by pelvic inflammatory disease (PID), previous pelvic or tubal surgery, hormonal factors that may interfere with forward motion of the egg in the fallopian tube, tubal atony or spasms, and blighted ovum.

The most common type is a tubal pregnancy, in which implantation occurs in a fallopian tube. Other less common types of ectopic pregnancy are shown in Figure 10-2. Incidence of ectopic pregnancy in the United States ranges from 1 in 80 to 1 in 200 live births (Danforth, 1982).

Initially, the normal symptoms of pregnancy may be present, specifically amenorrhea, breast tenderness, and nausea. hCG is present in the blood and urine. As time passes the woman may experience spotting or irregular bleeding, lower abdominal pain, and faintness. As the pregnancy progresses, the chorionic villi grow into the wall of the tube or site of implantation, and a blood supply is established. Thus, bleeding occurs when the tube ruptures, causing the characteristic symptoms of sharp pain, syncope, and referred shoulder pain as the abdomen fills with blood.

Characteristically, physical examination reveals pain in the area over the tube and ovary (*adnexa*), and often an adnexal mass is palpable. Bleeding tends to be slow and chronic, and the abdomen gradually becomes rigid and tender. With extensive bleeding into the abdominal cavity, vaginal examination causes extreme pain.

Laboratory tests may reveal low hemoglobin and hematocrit levels and rising leukocyte levels. The hCG titers are lower than in intrauterine pregnancy.

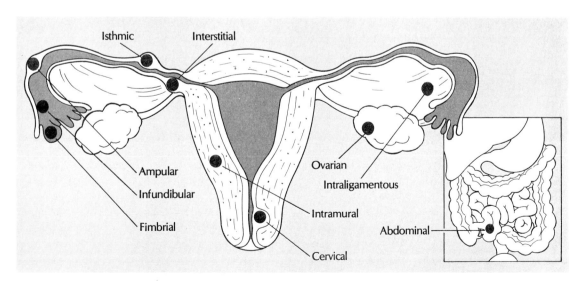

Figure 10-2

Implantation sites in ectopic pregnancy. Implantation also may occur within the abdominal cavity.

The following procedures help to establish the diagnosis:

- A careful assessment of menstrual history, particularly the LMP
- Careful pelvic exam to identify any abnormal pelvic masses
- Ultrasound to identify a gestational sac in an unruptured tubal pregnancy, or confirm an intrauterine pregnancy and rule out an ectopic one
- Laparoscopy to reveal an extrauterine pregnancy and perhaps prevent the rupture of a tube
- Culdocentesis to reveal clotted blood, possibly including an aborted fetus
- Laparotomy to confirm the diagnosis and allow opportunity for immediate treatment

Interventions Once the diagnosis of ectopic pregnancy has been made, surgery is performed. The affected tube and sometimes the ovary are removed surgically. If massive infection is found, a complete removal of uterus, tubes, and ovaries may be necessary. However, every effort is made to leave a normal tube, ovary, and uterus so that childbearing may be a future possibility. If childbearing is a consideration and the woman's other tube has been damaged, salpingostomy (incision into the tube to remove the fetus) may be done. The risk of a subsequent tubal pregnancy is 10%–20% (Danforth, 1982).

The woman and her family will need emotional support during this difficult time. Their feelings and responses to this crisis will probably be similar to those that occur in cases of spontaneous abortion. As a result, similar nursing actions are required for these individuals (see p. 209).

Hydatidiform mole Hydatidiform mole (molar pregnancy) is a relatively rare condition in which the trophoblastic epithelium proliferates and numerous clear, avascular vesicles derived from the chorionic villi are formed. These vesicles are filled with fluid and form grapelike clusters. Usually no embryo is present. The cause is unknown.

Initially, the clinical picture is similar to that of pregnancy. However, by the end of the first trimester, classic symptoms appear. Bright red or brownish vaginal bleeding (called *prune juice*) occurs, and, because of the rapid proliferation of the trophoblastic cells, uterine size may be greater than appropriate for gestational age. Because serum hCG levels are higher than those in a normal pregnancy, severe nausea and vomiting are present. Some women (approximately 7%) will also show signs of hyperthyroidism (Berkowitz and Goldstein, 1984). Symptoms of PIH prior to 24 weeks' gestation strongly suggest a molar pregnancy. No fetal heart tones are heard, and no fetal movement is palpated. Sonography reveals no fetal skeleton and often shows a characteristic pattern.

Interventions Although the mole may be aborted spontaneously, it is generally removed surgically by curettage. Women who have one molar pregnancy are at risk for developing recurring moles or choriocarcinoma, a rare but highly malignant form of cancer.

The patient treated for hydatidiform mole should receive follow-up therapy for a year. Pregnancy is avoided during that time because the elevated hCG levels associated with pregnancy would cause confusion as to whether choriocarcinoma had developed.

Continued high or rising hCG titers are abnormal. If this occurs, dilatation and curettage are performed, and tissue is examined. If malignant cells are found, chemotherapy for choriocarcinoma is started, using either methotrexate or dactinomycin. If therapy is ineffective, the choriocarcinoma has a tendency to metastasize rapidly.

If, after a year of monitoring, the hCG serum titers are within normal limits, a couple may be assured that subsequent normal pregnancy can be anticipated with low probability of recurrent hydatidiform mole.

Placenta previa In placenta previa, the placenta is improperly implanted in the lower uterine segment, perhaps on a portion of the lower segment or over the internal os. As the lower uterine segment contracts and the cervix dilates in the later weeks of pregnancy, the placental villi are torn from the uterine wall. Thus the uterine sinuses are exposed at the placental site. The classic symptom is painless vaginal bleeding usually occurring after 20 weeks' gestation. See Chapter 17 for an in-depth discussion of placenta previa.

Abruptio placentae   Abruptio placentae is the premature separation of the placenta from the uterine wall. It occurs prior to delivery and usually during labor. See Chapter 17 for an in-depth description of abruptio placentae.

Incompetent Cervix

Cervical incompetence is characterized by repeated second trimester abortion. It may be caused by previous cervical trauma associated with D&C, conization, or cervical lacerations with previous deliveries (Pritchard, MacDonald, and Gant, 1985).

The woman usually has a history of repeated, relatively painless and bloodless second trimester abortions. Serial pelvic exams early in the second trimester reveal progressive effacement and dilatation of the cervix and bulging of the membranes through the cervical os.

Interventions   Incompetent cervix is managed surgically with a Shirodkar-Barter operation or a modification of it by McDonald. The surgery reinforces the weakened cervix by encircling it at the level of the internal os with a purse-string suture (cerclage). The surgery is performed between 14 and 18 weeks of gestation.

Once the suture is in place, a cesarean delivery may be planned (to prevent repeating the procedure in subsequent pregnancies), or the suture may be released at term and vaginal delivery permitted. Success rate for carrying the pregnancy to term is approximately 80%.

Hypertensive Disorders in Pregnancy

Pregnancy-Induced Hypertension (Preeclampsia and Eclampsia)

Pregnancy-induced hypertension or PIH is a broad term for a specific hypertensive disorder that includes **preeclampsia** and **eclampsia** as conditions (Willis, 1982). PIH is characterized by the development of three cardinal signs: *hypertension*, *edema*, and *proteinuria*. PIH is seen most often in the last 10 weeks of gestation, during labor, or in the first 12–48 hours after delivery.

The only cure for preeclampsia is termination of the pregnancy. Severe preeclampsia can progress to eclampsia. Eclampsia is manifested by development of convulsions and coma in a woman with preeclampsia. If prompt and intensive antepartal care is given to pregnant women, eclampsia may be prevented.

PIH occurs in 5%–7% of all pregnancies. For teenagers, young primigravidas, and women of low income the risk of developing PIH is 10%–30% (Gant and Worley, 1980). For women with chronic hypertension, the chances are 25%–35%. The cause of PIH is unknown. Known predisposing factors include diabetes mellitus, hypertension, renal disease, malnutrition (especially low protein diet), obesity, hydatidiform mole, multiple pregnancy, hydramnios, previous diagnosis of PIH, and a familial tendency to PIH.

Pathophysiology   Vasospasm with arteriolar vasoconstriction is a major finding in PIH and results in increased peripheral vascular resistance. This may be due to an increased sensitivity of the vascular system to vasopressors such as angiotensin II.

Clinical manifestations   *Mild preeclampsia*   Women with mild preeclampsia may exhibit an almost asymptomatic pregnancy. Little or no peripheral edema may be present following bed rest. The blood pressure is elevated to 140/90 or more, or increases 30 mm Hg systolic and 15 mm Hg diastolic. Thus, a young woman who normally has a blood pressure of 90/60 would be hypertensive at 120/76. Therefore, a baseline blood pressure obtained early in the pregnancy is essential. Urine testing may show a +1 or +2 albumin, although proteinuria is the last of the three cardinal signs to appear.

Severe preeclampsia   Severe preeclampsia may develop suddenly. Edema becomes generalized and readily apparent in face, hands, sacral area, lower extremities, and the abdominal wall. Edema is also characterized by an excessive weight gain of more than 0.9 kg (2 lb) over a couple of days to a week. Blood pressure is 160/100 or higher, a dipstick albumin measurement is +3 to +4, and the 24-hour urine protein is greater than 5 g. Hematocrit, serum creatinine, and uric acid levels are elevated.

Other characteristic symptoms are frontal headaches, blurred vision, scotomata, nausea, vomiting, irritability, hyperreflexia, cerebral disturbances, oliguria (less than 400 mL of urine in 24 hours), pulmonary edema or cyanosis, and finally, epigastric pain. The epigastric pain is often the sign of impending convulsion and is thought to be caused by increased vascular engorgement of the liver.

Eclampsia.   Eclampsia is characterized by a grand mal seizure. An elevated temperature may accompany the seizure. The seizure usually has a tonic phase, then a clonic phase. As the convulsive movements gradually cease, the woman often slips into a coma that may last for an hour or more. In other cases, the coma may be quite brief and, if the woman is not treated, convulsions may recur in a few minutes. Some women experience only one convulsion. Others may have several. Unless they occur quite frequently, the woman often regains consciousness between convulsions.

Fetal-neonatal implications   Infants of women with hypertension during pregnancy tend to be small for gestational age (SGA). The cause is related specifically to maternal vasospasm and hypovolemia, which result in fetal hypoxia and malnutrition. In addition, the neonate may be premature because of the necessity for early delivery. Perinatal mortality associated with preeclampsia is approximately 10%, and that associated with eclampsia is 24% (Zuspan, 1984).

At the time of delivery, the neonate may be oversedated because of medications administered to the woman. The neonate may also have hypermagnesemia due to treatment of the woman with large doses of magnesium sulfate.

Fetal assessment   Tests to evaluate fetal status are done more frequently as a pregnant woman's PIH progresses and are essential to achieving a safe outcome for the fetus. The following tests are used:

• Fetal movement

• Nonstress test

• Ultrasonography for serial determination of growth

• Contraction stress test

• Estriol and creatinine determinations

• Amniocentesis to determine fetal lung maturity

These tests are described in detail in Chapter 11.

Interventions—mild preeclampsia

Blood pressure   The client's baseline blood pressure and weeks of gestation must be determined early in prenatal care. Blood pressure is assessed at each antepartal visit. If the blood pressure rises or even if the slight decrease in blood pressure expected between 8–28 weeks does not occur, the client should be followed more closely.

Diet   Women with mild preeclampsia or women at risk for PIH are advised to follow a high-protein diet to replace proteins lost in the urine. Salt intake should be moderate (2.5–6.0 g/day); thus, the woman should avoid salty food and extra salting at the table. Fluid intake of 6–8 glasses of water a day is recommended.

Lateral recumbent position   Bed rest in the left lateral recumbent position is often beneficial to women with PIH. This position permits increased blood flow to the kidneys and results in increased renal plasma flow, glomerular filtration rate (GFR), and placental perfusion. Bed rest need not be complete but should increase if the condition worsens.

Support and teaching   The woman with a high-risk pregnancy is often concerned about losing her baby and about the costs of prolonged hospitalization and increased testing. Sexual activities may be another concern: She and her partner may fear intercourse will harm the baby. Finally, the woman's partner may become resentful or feel neglected, and the woman may also feel depressed or resentful (Weil, 1981).

The nurse should identify and discuss each area of concern with the couple. It is necessary to explain to them the reasons for bed rest. A woman with mild preeclampsia may feel very well and be unable to see the need for resting even a few hours each day. The nurse can refer the couple to community resources such as homemaking services, a support group for the partner, or a hot line to answer questions as they arise. In addition, the woman needs to know which symptoms are significant and should be reported at once. Usually, the woman with mild preeclampsia is seen every 2 weeks, but she may need to come in earlier if symptoms indicate the condition is worsening. She must understand her diet plan, which must match her culture, finances, and life-style.

Interventions—severe preeclampsia If the preeclampsia progresses to the severe stage, hospitalization is essential. The goal of care is to prevent convulsions by decreasing blood pressure and establishing adequate renal function, and to continue pregnancy until the fetus is mature. If the pregnancy is 36 weeks' gestation or more and fetal lung maturity is confirmed, labor is induced. If labor is unsuccessful, cesarean delivery is necessary. When the pregnancy is less than 36 weeks' gestation or when L/S ratio indicates immaturity, interventions are aimed at alleviating maternal symptoms to allow the fetus to mature.

Assessment Pulse, respiration, and blood pressure should be monitored every 2–4 hours or more frequently if necessary because of medication being administered or changes in patient status. The fetal heart rate is determined at the same time or continuously monitored electronically if the situation warrants. Temperature is determined regularly.

All urinary output should be measured. If an indwelling catheter is in place, hourly urine output can be assessed and should be at least 30 mL/hr. Urine protein and specific gravity are also assessed hourly.

The patient should be weighed at the same time daily and carefully assessed for evidence of edema. Since pulmonary edema may also develop, the patient is observed for coughing, and the lungs are auscultated for rales.

Deep tendon reflexes (DTRs) are assessed for evidence of hyperreflexia. Clonus should also be assessed by vigorously dorsiflexing the foot while the knee is held in a fixed position. Normally no clonus is present. If it is present, it is measured as 1–4 beats and is recorded as such.

The patient should be questioned about any headache, visual changes, or epigastric pain. Her alertness and mood are also noted. Because placental separation is another potential complication, the patient should be assessed frequently for vaginal bleeding and uterine rigidity. Daily blood tests and a daily fundoscopic examination are also indicated.

The patient's emotional responses are also carefully assessed so that support and teaching can be planned accordingly.

Therapy Complete bed rest is essential. The woman should be encouraged to maintain the left lateral recumbent position as much as possible. Stimuli should be reduced and visitors limited to reduce the possibility of convulsion. A high-protein, moderate-sodium diet is given if tolerated. Fluid therapy may be oral or supplemented with intravenous fluids. Often an intravenous line is maintained for the administration of medication.

Magnesium sulfate ($MgSO_4$) is the medication of choice for preventing convulsions (see Drug Guide on p. 214). With severe hypertension (diastolic pressure above 110 mm Hg), the drug of choice is the vasodilator hydralazine hydrochloride (Apresoline) (Gant and Worley, 1980).

The development of severe preeclampsia is a cause for concern to the patient and her family. Increased stress can elevate the blood pressure. Thus, decreasing anxiety and providing an atmosphere of confidence and calm is a major nursing goal. The nurse can provide accurate information, give the woman and her partner opportunities to voice their fears, and keep them informed of fetal status. The nurse can also seek other sources of information or aid for the family as needed.

Interventions—eclampsia A convulsion is a frightening event for any family member who may be present, and the woman will not be able to recall it when she becomes conscious. Therefore, offering explanations to family members, and later to the woman herself, is essential.

Assessment During the convulsion, the woman must be protected from injury. When it subsides, fetal heart tones and maternal vital signs are monitored closely. The patient is also assessed for evidence of pulmonary edema, cerebral edema, signs of placental separation, and the onset of labor.

Therapy Magnesium sulfate is administered intravenously. When the patient's condition is stabilized, delivery of the fetus should be

DRUG GUIDE
Magnesium Sulfate (MgSO$_4$)

OVERVIEW OF OBSTETRIC ACTION

MgSO$_4$ acts as a CNS depressant by decreasing the quantity of acetylcholine released by motor nerve impulses and thereby blocking neuromuscular transmission. This action reduces the possibility of convulsion; this is why MgSO$_4$ is used in the treatment of preeclampsia. Because magnesium sulfate secondarily relaxes smooth muscle it may decrease the blood pressure, although it is not considered an antihypertensive, and may also decrease the frequency and intensity of uterine contractions.

ROUTE, DOSAGE, FREQUENCY

MgSO$_4$ may be given intramuscularly (IM) or intravenously (IV).

IV: The intravenous route allows for immediate onset of action and avoids the discomfort associated with IM administration. It must be given by an infusion pump for accurate dosage.
Loading dose:
250 mL D$_5$W (5% dextrose in water) with 4 g MgSO$_4$ is administered over 20 minutes.
Maintenance dose:
Based on serum magnesium levels and deep tendon reflexes, 1–3 g/hr is administered (Berkowitz et al., 1981).

IM: Initial loading dose involves 10 g in 50% solution divided into two injections and administered into each buttock (deep IM) in conjunction with the 4 g IV loading dose just described.
Maintenance dose
5 g every 4 hours in 50% solution is administered if deep tendon reflexes, respirations, and urine output are satisfactory. This route is very painful and avoided whenever possible.

Maternal contraindications

Extreme care is necessary in administration to women with impaired renal function because the drug is eliminated by the kidneys and toxic magnesium levels may develop.

Maternal side effects

Sweating, flushing, depression or absence of reflexes, hypothermia, muscle weakness, oliguria, confusion, circulatory collapse, and respiratory paralysis are all possible side effects. Rapid administration of large doses may cause cardiac arrest.

Effects on fetus/neonate

The drug readily crosses the placenta. Hypermagnesemia in the newborn may have contributed to low Apgar scores and symptoms of lethargy, hypotonia, and weakness (Berkowitz et al., 1981).

NURSING CONSIDERATIONS

1. Monitor blood pressure continuously with IV administration and every 15 minutes with IM administration.

2. Monitor respirations closely. If the rate is less than 14–16/min, magnesium toxicity may be developing and further assessments are indicated.

3. Assess knee jerk (patellar tendon reflex) for evidence of diminished or absent reflexes.

4. Determine urinary output. Output less than 30 mL/hr may result in the accumulation of toxic levels of magnesium.

5. If the respirations or urinary output fall below specified levels or if the reflexes are diminished or absent, no further magnesium should be administered until these factors return to normal.

6. The antagonist of magnesium sulfate is calcium. Consequently an ampule of calcium gluconate should be available at the bedside. The usual dose is 10 mL of a 10% solution given IV by the physician over a period of about 3 minutes.

7. IM administration of MgSO$_4$ is painful and irritating. Therefore it is given deep into the gluteal muscle with 1% procaine to reduce the pain. The dose is divided between both buttocks and given Z-track with a long needle (Wheeler and Jones, 1981) or by circular rotation with the area massaged well afterwards.

8. Monitor fetal heart tones continuously with IV administration.

9. Continue MgSO$_4$ infusion for approximately 24 hours after delivery as prophylaxis against postpartum seizures.

considered. Delivery is the only known cure for PIH. The woman and her partner should be given careful explanation about the status of the woman and her fetus. Plans for delivery and further treatment must also be discussed with them.

Labor and delivery management The plan of care for the woman with PIH in labor depends on both maternal and fetal condition. The nurse attending the laboring woman with PIH must take all the precautions needed to assist normal labor as well as those required to manage PIH. The patient may receive intravenous oxytocin and MgSO$_4$ simultaneously. MgSO$_4$ has a depressant action on smooth muscles, and thus oxytocin may be necessary to augment labor. The woman is kept on her left side as much as possible, and signs of progressing labor are noted. Both the woman and her fetus are carefully monitored. The nurse must be alert for indications of worsening PIH, placental separation, pulmonary edema, circulatory renal failure, and fetal distress. During the second stage of labor, the woman should be encouraged to push while lying on her side. Delivery position should be Sims' or semi-sitting. If a lithotomy position is used, a wedge is placed under the patient's right buttocks to displace the uterus. Specialists (either a pediatrician or a neonatal nurse practitioner) should be available to care for the newborn in the delivery room.

Postpartum management   The woman with PIH usually improves rapidly after delivery, although seizures can still occur during the first 48 hours postpartum. For this reason, when the hypertension is severe, the patient may continue to receive hydralazine or magnesium sulfate postpartally.

The amount of vaginal bleeding is noted carefully. Because the woman with PIH is hypovolemic, even normal blood loss can be serious. The nurse assesses the vital signs regularly and instructs the woman to report any of the signs of severe preeclampsia. Ergot products are avoided because of their hypertensive effect.

Postpartal depression can develop after the long ordeal of the pregnancy. Emotional support should be provided and mother-infant contact encouraged.

(For a concise summary of care for the woman with PIH, see the Nursing Care Plan— Preeclampsia-Eclampsia).

Chronic Hypertensive Disease

Chronic hypertension exists when the blood pressure is 140/90 or higher before pregnancy or when a blood pressure of 140/90 or higher develops before the twentieth week of gestation and/or persists indefinitely following delivery (Gant and Worley, 1980). The cause of chronic hypertension has not been determined.

Chronic hypertension of long standing is usually associated with vascular changes such as arteriosclerosis, retinal hemorrhage, and renal disease. These conditions are seen most commonly in the older pregnant woman. *Chronic hypertensive vascular disease* is the name given to these changes.

Chronic hypertension with superimposed preeclampsia   Preeclampsia may develop in a woman previously found to have chronic hypertension. When elevations of systolic blood pressure 30 mm Hg or of diastolic blood pressure 15–20 mm Hg above the baseline are discovered on two occasions at least 6 hours apart, when proteinuria develops, or when edema occurs in the upper half of the body (Gant and Worley, 1980), the woman needs close monitoring and careful management. Her condition often progresses quickly to eclampsia, sometimes before 30 weeks of pregnancy.

Late or transient hypertension   Late hypertension, as defined by Gant and Worley (1980), exists when transient elevation of blood pressure occurs during labor or in the early postpartal period, returning to normal within 10 days postpartum.

Rh Sensitization

Rh sensitization results from an antigen-antibody immunologic reaction within the body. Sensitization most commonly occurs when an Rh-negative woman carries an Rh-positive fetus to term or when the pregnancy is terminated by spontaneous or induced abortion. It can also occur if an Rh-negative nonpregnant woman receives an Rh-positive blood transfusion.

The red blood cells from the fetus invade the maternal circulation, thereby stimulating the production of Rh antibodies. Because this usually occurs at delivery, the first offspring is not affected. However, in a subsequent pregnancy, Rh antibodies cross the placenta and enter the fetal circulation, causing severe hemolysis. The destruction of fetal red blood cells causing anemia in the fetus is proportional to the extent of maternal sensitization (Figure 10-3).

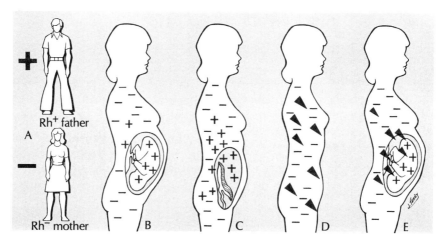

Figure 10-3

Rh isoimmunization sequence. **A**, Rh-positive father and Rh-negative mother. **B**, Pregnancy with Rh-positive fetus. Some Rh-positive blood enters the mother's blood. **C**, As placenta separates, further inoculation of mother by Rh-positive blood. **D**, Mother sensitized to Rh-positive blood; anti-Rh-positive antibodies are formed. **E**, With subsequent pregnancies with Rh-positive fetus, Rh-positive red blood cells are attacked by the anti–Rh-positive maternal antibodies, causing hemolysis of red blood cells in the fetus.

NURSING CARE PLAN
Preeclampsia-Eclampsia (PIH)

PATIENT ASSESSMENT

Nursing History

1. Complete assessment: patient and family
2. Identification of patient's predisposition to preeclampsia-eclampsia
   a. Primigravida
   b. Presence of diabetes mellitus
   c. Multiple pregnancy
   d. Hydramnios
   e. Hydatidiform mole
   f. Preexisting vascular or renal disease
   g. Adolescent or "elderly" gravida

Physical Examination

1. Blood pressure—if possible compare with baseline
2. Observe for edema—note weight gain > 1 kg/wk
3. Patient's weight—obtain weekly weight gain if possible
4. Evaluate for hyperreflexia
5. Assess presence of visual disturbances, headache, drowsiness, epigastric pain

Laboratory Evaluation

1. Urine for urinary protein: 1 g protein/24 hr = 1–2 +; 5 g protein/24 hr = 3–4 +
2. Hematocrit: Elevation of hematocrit implies hemoconcentration, which occurs as fluid leaves the intravascular space and enters the extravascular space
3. BUN: Not usually elevated except in patients with cardiovascular renal disease
4. Blood uric acid appears to correlate well with the severity of the preeclampsia-eclampsia (Note: Thiazide diuretics can cause significant increases in uric acid levels)

NURSING CARE PLAN (continued)
Preeclampsia-Eclampsia (PIH)

PLAN OF CARE

Nursing Priorities

1. Carefully monitor patient's vital signs, urinary output, hyperreflexia
2. Evaluate fetal status
3. Provide support to patient and family
4. Observe for signs of worsening condition:
   a. Increase in BP
   b. Decrease in hourly urine output $\leq$ 30 mL/hr
   c. Increased drowsiness
   d. Increased hyperreflexia
   e. Severe headache
   f. Visual disturbances
   g. Epigastric pain
   h. Convulsion

Client/Family Educational Focus

1. Discuss significance of PIH for the health of the woman and her fetus
2. Explain treatment modalities and their rationale
3. Explore possible long-term implications of PIH, such as need for frequent rest, the possible need to stop working if the woman is employed, and the possibility of hospitalization
4. Provide opportunities to discuss questions and individual concerns of the woman and her family

Problem	Nursing interventions and actions	Rationale
Water retention	Weigh patient daily; gain of 1 kg/wk or more in second trimester or ½ kg/wk or more in third trimester is suggestive of PIH	Weight gain and evidence of edema are due to sodium and water retention
	Assess edema (Danforth, 1982) +(1+) Minimal; slight edema of pedal and pretibial areas ++(2+) Marked edema of lower extremities +++(3+) Edema of hands, face, lower abdominal wall, and sacrum ++++(4+) Anasarca with ascites	Decreased renal plasma flow and glomerular filtration contribute to retention; actual mechanisms are not clear
	Maintain patient on bed rest Maintain normal salt intake (2.5–6 g/24 hr)	Bed rest produces an increase in GFR Normal salt intake is now advised, but excessive salt intake may cause the condition to become more severe
Hypertension	Assess BP every 1–4 hr, using same arm, with patient in same position	Blood pressure can fluctuate hourly; BP increases as a result of increased peripheral resistance due to peripheral vasoconstriction and arteriolar spasm Diastolic pressure is a better indicator of severity of condition
Proteinuria	Obtain clean urine specimen	Urine contaminated with vaginal discharge or red cells may test positive for protein
	Test urine for proteinuria, hourly and/or daily	Helps evaluate severity and progression of preeclampsia Proteinuria results from swelling of the endothelium of the glomerular capillaries Escape of protein is enhanced by vasospasm in afferent arterioles

NURSING CARE PLAN (continued)
Preeclampsia-Eclampsia

Problem	Nursing interventions and actions	Rationale
Decreased urine output	Insert indwelling catheter	Catheter facilitates hourly urine assessment Renal plasma flow and glomerular filtration are decreased
	Determine hourly urine output; notify physician if urine output ≤ 30 mL/hr	Increasing oliguria signifies a worsening condition
Inadequate protein intake	Provide adequate protein: 1.5 g/kg/24 hr for mild preeclampsia Patients with severe preeclampsia will be NPO ("nothing by mouth")	Plasma proteins affect movement of intravascular and extravascular fluids
Hyperreflexia	Assess knee, ankle, and biceps reflexes Determine presence of clonus Promote bed rest; allow patient to rest quietly in a darkened, quiet room Limit visitors	Assessing reflexes helps determine level of muscle and nerve irritability Rest reduces external stimuli
	Administer sedation as ordered (diazepam or phenobarbital orally or IM)	Sedation is frequently ordered
	Administer magnesium sulfate per physician order: 1. IM dose: 5–10 g of 50% solution every 4–6 hours 2. IV dose: 20 mL of 10% solution or as continuous infusion at a rate of 1 g/hr	Magnesium sulfate is cerebral depressant; it also reduces neuromuscular irritability and causes vasodilatation and drop in BP Therapeutic blood level is 4–7 mEq/L*
	Before administering subsequent doses of magnesium sulfate, check reflexes (knee, ankle, biceps)	Knee jerk disappears when magnesium sulfate blood levels are 8–10 mEq/L* Toxic signs and symptoms develop with increased blood levels; respiratory arrest can be associated with blood levels of 12 mEq/L or more* (Pritchard, MacDonald, and Gant, 1985)
	Check respirations and measure urine output Do not give magnesium sulfate if: 1. Reflexes are absent 2. Respirations are < 14–16/min 3. < 100 mL urine output in past 4 hours	Kidneys are only route for excretion of magnesium sulfate
	Have calcium gluconate available	Calcium gluconate is antidote for magnesium sulfate
Convulsions	Provide supportive care during convulsion: 1. Place tongue blade or airway in patient's mouth, if can be done without force 2. Suction nasopharynx as necessary 3. Administer oxygen 4. Note type of seizure and length of time it lasts	Acts to maintain airway and to prevent patient from biting tongue Removes mucus and secretions Promotes oxygenation
	After seizure, assess for uterine contractions Assess fetal status	Precipitous labor may start during seizures Continuous fetal monitoring is necessary to identify fetal stress
	Maintain seizure precautions: 1. Quiet, darkened room 2. Have emergency equipment available— O₂, suction, padded tongue blade 3. Pad side rails	Quiet reduces stimuli Padding protects patient

*Values may vary according to agency.

NURSING CARE PLAN (continued)
Preeclampsia-Eclampsia

Problem	Nursing interventions and actions	Rationale
Increased fetal morbidity and mortality	Assess fetal status; monitor fetal heart tones every 4 hours if patient has mild eclampsia Patient with severe preeclampsia-eclampsia requires continuous fetal monitoring	Evaluates fetal status
Increased risk of abruptio placentae	Assess for signs of abruptio placentae: 1. Vaginal bleeding 2. Uterine tenderness 3. Change in fetal activity 4. Change in fetal heart rate 5. Sustained abdominal pain	40%–60% of women with abruptio placentae have preeclampsia; in patients with severe preeclampsia-eclampsia, abruption occurs in 10%–15% of the cases (Danforth, 1982)

NURSING CARE EVALUATION

Infant delivered
Blood pressure within normal range
Absence of protein in urine
Symptoms of preeclampsia-eclampsia resolved or controlled
Woman independent in activities of daily living
Mother able to care for infant
Mother understands and can verbalize course of condition, diet and medication instructions, infant care, and symptoms to report to physician (Davidson et al., 1977)

NURSING DIAGNOSIS*	SUPPORTING DATA	NURSING ORDERS
Fluid volume excess; edema related to fluid shift to extravascular space	Edema—generalized and pitting Weight gain Increased blood pressure Decreased urine output	Monitor status of edema 1. Determine I and O 2. Weigh patient daily 3. Assess extent of edema Prevent injury to skin 1. Determine need for changes in skin care based on extent of edema 2. Encourage regular position change 3. Inspect skin for redness or blanching
Potential for injury related to possibility of convulsion	DTRs 3+ or 4+; clonus Headache Signs of CNS irritability Epigastric pain	Decrease external stimuli 1. Assign to room with minimal external noise and traffic 2. Limit visits to those by close support persons 3. Arrange interventions so there are frequent rest periods Protect from injury 1. Have emergency supplies available to treat convulsions (for example, O_2 equipment, suction, tongue blade and/or airway, emergency medications) 2. Educate other health care individuals regarding the possibility of convulsions and appropriate actions

*These are examples of nursing diagnoses that may be appropriate for a person with this condition. It is not an inclusive list and must be individualized for each woman.

Fetal-neonatal implications   In the presence of maternal Rh sensitization, the fetus develops a severe hemolytic syndrome known as **erythroblastosis fetalis**. If treatment for Rh sensitization is not begun, the resulting anemia can cause marked fetal edema, called **hydrops fetalis**. Congestive heart failure may result, as well as severe jaundice, which can lead to neurologic damage (*kernicterus*).

Prenatal assessment and interventions   Screening will identify the Rh-negative woman who may be carrying an Rh-positive fetus. An indirect Coombs' test or antibody screen is then done to determine if the woman is sensitized (has developed antibodies) to the Rh antigen. The indirect Coombs' test measures the number of antibodies in the maternal blood.

Negative antibody titers and a negative indirect Coombs' test can consistently identify the fetus *not* at risk. However, the titers cannot reliably point out the fetus in danger, since titer level does not correlate with the severity of the disease. Antibody titers are determined periodically throughout the pregnancy. If the maternal antibody titer is 1:16 or greater, an optical density (ΔOD) analysis of the amniotic fluid is performed. This optical density analysis measures the amount of pigment from the breakdown of red blood cells and can determine the severity of the hemolytic process.

Two primary interventions can help the fetus whose blood cells are being destroyed by maternal antibodies: early delivery and intrauterine transfusion, both of which carry risks. Ideally, delivery should be delayed until fetal maturity is confirmed at about 36–37 weeks. Only fetuses with a prognosis of death before 32 weeks as indicated by the ΔOD should be given intrauterine transfusion (Pritchard, MacDonald, and Gant, 1985).

Postpartal interventions The Rh-negative mother who has no antibody titer (indirect Coombs' negative, nonsensitized) and who has delivered an Rh-positive fetus (direct Coombs' negative) is given an intramuscular injection of RhoGAM, an anti-Rh$_o$ (D) gamma-globulin. She must receive RhoGAM within 72 hours of delivery so that she does not have time to produce antibodies to fetal cells that entered her bloodstream when the placenta separated. Administration of RhoGAM provides temporary passive immunity to the mother, which prevents the development of permanent active immunity (antibody formation).

When the woman is Rh-negative and not sensitized and the father is Rh-positive or unknown, RhoGAM is also given after each abortion, ectopic pregnancy, or amniocentesis. Many caregivers have recently begun administering RhoGAM at approximately 28 weeks' gestation. This seems to provide additional protection to the Rh-negative woman with an Rh-positive

fetus. RhoGAM is not given to the neonate or the father. It is not effective for and should not be administered to previously sensitized women. (See Essential Facts to Remember below.)

Rh sensitization and the resultant hemolytic disease of the newborn are less common today because of the development of RhoGAM. See Chapter 22 for treatment of the neonate.

Surgical Procedures During Pregnancy

A woman can generally undergo surgery during pregnancy without affecting its course or

ESSENTIAL FACTS TO REMEMBER

Rh Sensitization

When trying to work through Rh problems, the nurse should remember the following:

• A potential problem exists when an Rh$^-$ mother and an Rh$^+$ father conceive a child that is Rh$^+$.

• In this situation, the mother may become sensitized or produce antibodies to her fetus's Rh$^+$ blood.

The following tests are used to detect sensitization:

• Indirect Coombs' test—done on the mother's blood to measure the number of Rh$^+$ antibodies.

• Direct Coombs' test—done on the infant's blood to detect antibody-coated Rh$^+$ RBCs.

Based on the results of these tests, the following may be done:

• If the mother's indirect Coombs' test is negative and the infant's direct Coombs' test is negative, the mother is given RhoGAM within 72 hours of delivery.

• If the mother's indirect Coombs' test is positive and her Rh$^+$ infant has a positive direct Coombs' test, RhoGAM is *not* given; in this case, the infant is carefully monitored for hemolytic disease.

causing harm to the fetus. Although general preoperative and postoperative care is similar for pregnant and nonpregnant women, special considerations must be kept in mind whenever the surgical client is pregnant. The early part of the second trimester is the best time to operate because there is less risk of causing spontaneous abortion or early labor, and the uterus is not so large as to impinge on the abdominal field.

To prevent uterine compression of major blood vessels while the woman is supine, the caregiver must place a wedge under her right hip to tilt the uterus both during surgery and recovery. Because of the decreased intestinal motility and delayed gastric emptying that occurs in pregnancy, the risk of vomiting when anesthetics are given and during the postoperative period is increased. Thus, inserting a nasogastric tube is recommended before a pregnant woman has major surgery.

Caregivers must guard against maternal hypoxia. During surgery, uterine circulation is decreased, and fetal oxygenation may be reduced quickly. Fetal heart tones must be monitored electronically before, during, and after surgery. Blood loss is also closely monitored throughout the procedure and following it.

Accidents and Trauma

Accidents and injury are not uncommon during pregnancy. Fortunately, most accidents produce minor injuries, and the outcome of the pregnancy is seldom affected. Late in pregnancy, when balance and coordination are adversely affected, the woman may fall. Her protruding abdomen is vulnerable to a variety of minor injuries. The fetus is usually well protected by the amniotic fluid, which distributes the force of a blow equally in all directions, and by the muscle layers of the uterus and abdominal wall. In early pregnancy, while the uterus is still in the pelvis, it is shielded from blows by the surrounding pelvic organs, muscles, and bony structures.

Treatment of major injuries during pregnancy focuses initially on life-saving measures for the woman. Specifically, such measures include establishing an airway, controlling external bleeding, and administering intravenous fluid to alleviate shock. The patient must be kept on her left side to avoid further hypotension. Fetal heart tones are monitored. Exploratory surgery is necessary following abdominal trauma to determine the extent of injuries. If the fetus is near term and the uterus has been damaged, cesarean delivery is performed. If the fetus is still immature, the uterus can often be repaired, and the pregnancy continues until term.

Infections

A major factor predisposing to risk in pregnancy is the presence of maternal infection, whether contracted prior to conception or during the gestational period. Frequently, spontaneous abortion is the result of a severe maternal infection. If the pregnancy is carried to term in the presence of infection, the risk of fetal and maternal morbidity and mortality increases. In many instances of fetal risk due to infection, the woman presents few or no signs or symptoms. Therefore, it is essential to maternal and fetal health that diagnosis and treatment be prompt.

Urinary Tract Infections

Urinary tract infections affect 2%–10% of pregnant women. Stasis of urine, compression of ureters (especially the right ureter), decreased bactericidal capabilities of leukocytes in the urine, and vesicoureteral reflux (backward urine flow) make the pregnant woman more susceptible to urinary tract infection.

A woman who has had a urinary tract infection is more likely to get another urinary tract infection, either in the same or subsequent pregnancies, than a woman who has not. With acute urinary tract infection, especially with associated high temperatures, amniotic fluid infection may develop, and the growth of the placenta may be retarded. Increased risk of premature labor exists if the infection occurs near term.

If cystitis occurs early in pregnancy, oral sulfonamides, particularly sulfisoxazole (Gantrisan), are generally effective. These drugs are not used in the last few weeks of pregnancy because they interfere with protein binding of bilirubin in the fetus. Altered protein binding can lead to neonatal hyperbilirubinemia and kernicterus. Thus, late in pregnancy, cystitis is treated with ampicillin or nitrofurantoin (Furadantin).

Acute pyelonephritis, an upper urinary tract infection, is quite serious. The woman is hospitalized and started on intravenous antibiotic therapy as soon as pyelonephritis is diagnosed by symptoms and urine culture. She is kept in bed lying on her left side. With appropriate drug therapy, the patient shows marked improvement within a few days. Follow-up urinary cultures are needed to ensure that the infection has been eliminated completely.

The nurse should make sure the client is aware of good hygiene practices, since most bacteria enter through the urethra after having spread from the anal area. The nurse also reinforces instructions or answers questions regarding the prescribed antibiotic, the amount of liquids to take, and the reasons for treatments.

Sexually Transmitted Diseases

Sexually transmitted diseases (STDs), also called *venereal diseases*, are infectious disorders contracted primarily through intimate sexual contact, oral or genital, with another person. In this section, syphilis, gonorrhea and chlamydial infections are discussed. Herpesvirus type II and cytomegalovirus infections are also STDs but are discussed with the TORCH group.

Syphilis Syphilis is a chronic infection caused by the spirochete *Treponema pallidum*. Syphilis is primarily transmitted through sexual contact, although it can also occur from contact with open wounds or infected blood. The fetus can contract congenital syphilis through transplacental exposure. Because syphilis has significant effects on the fetus, serologic testing of every pregnant woman is recommended, and required by law in some states, at the initial prenatal screening and again during the third trimester.

Fetal-neonatal implications One of the following outcomes can occur in the presence of untreated maternal syphilis: (a) second trimester abortion, (b) a stillborn infant at term, (c) a congenitally infected infant born prematurely or at term, or (d) an uninfected live infant. The clinical manifestations and treatment of the syphilitic newborn are discussed in Chapter 22.

Interventions If testing of maternal serum is positive, treatment with penicillin should be started immediately. If the woman is allergic to penicillin, erythromycin (Ilotycin) can be given. The likelihood of fetal infection is almost nonexistent if the woman is treated before 18 weeks' gestation. If treatment is given later in pregnancy, congenital syphilis may have already developed.

Gonorrhea Gonorrhea is an infection caused by the bacteria *Neisseria gonorrhoeae*. The expectant woman can be screened for this infection during her prenatal examination by means of a cervical culture.

Fetal-neonatal implications No congenital anomalies are associated with gonorrhea. However, if untreated, gonorrhea can cause illness in the fetus and neonate if the membranes have been ruptured for a long time or as a result of vaginal delivery through an infected birth canal. An acute gonorrheal infection may also predispose to premature labor. For the fetus delivered through an infected birth canal, the result is a gonococcal eye infection known as *ophthalmia neonatorum*. Infections of the stomach, external ear canal, oropharynx, and anus can also occur.

Interventions Therapy consists of antibiotic treatment with penicillin. If the woman is allergic to penicillin, kanamycin sulfate (Kantrex) or erythromycin may be used. All sexual partners must also be treated, or the woman may be reinfected.

Chlamydial infections Nongonococcal urethritis (NGU) is becoming one of the most common STDs in the United States. *Chlamydia trachomatis* is the causative organism in 40%–50% of NGU cases. Chlamydial infection is difficult to identify in women because most women who harbor the organism are asymptomatic. Thus, women whose sexual partners have NGU should be treated (Osborne and Pratson, 1984).

Fetal-neonatal implications The infant is at risk for developing ophthalmia neonatorum and newborn chlamydial pneumonia.

Interventions The specific treatment for chlamydial infection is tetracycline. However, pregnant women should by given erythromycin instead. (See discussion of tetracycline in Chapter 8.) Ilotycin ophthalmic ointment, an erythromycin preparation, may be used for the newborn.

Vaginal Infections

Monilial (yeast) infections   The fungus *Candida albicans* normally is found in the intestinal tract. It can, however, invade the vagina, causing monilial infection. Monilial infection is present in about 20% of pregnant women. It is commonly seen at term in women with poorly controlled diabetes because the organism thrives in a high glucose environment. Women who are on antibiotic or steroid therapy are also susceptible because these drugs reduce the number of Döderlein's bacilli, which are normally present in flora.

Fetal-neonatal implications   If the infection is not cured before delivery, the fetus may contract thrush by direct contact with the organism in the birth canal.

Interventions   Monilial infection is usually treated with locally applied drugs. Two commonly prescribed medications include miconazole (Monistat) or clotrimazole cream (Mycelex) applied to the vulva and vaginal mucosa. Nystatin (Mycostatin) vaginal suppositories may be used. The sexual partner is also treated to prevent recurrence.

TORCH

The **TORCH** group of infectious diseases may cause serious harm to the embryo-fetus. These are toxoplasmosis, rubella, cytomegalovirus, and herpesvirus type 2. Some sources consider the O in TORCH to represent **o**ther infections.

Use of the TORCH label assists health team members to assess quickly the potential risk to each pregnant woman. Exposure of the woman during the first 12 weeks of gestation may cause developmental anomalies.

Toxoplasmosis   Toxoplasmosis is caused by the protozoan *Toxoplasma gondii*. It is innocuous in adults, but when contracted in pregnancy, it is transmitted to the fetus in half the cases (Danforth, 1982). The pregnant woman may contract the organism by eating raw or poorly cooked meat or by contact with the feces of infected animals. In the United States, the most common vehicle is cat feces. It is therefore strongly recommended that pregnant women avoid cat litter boxes.

If toxoplasmosis is diagnosed before 20 weeks of gestation, damage to the fetus is more severe than if the disease is acquired later. Therapeutic abortion may be considered.

The incidence of abortion, stillbirths, neonatal deaths, and severe congenital anomalies is increased in the affected fetus and neonate. In very mild cases, chorioretinitis may be the only recognizable damage, which may not appear until adolescence or young adulthood. Severe neonatal disorders associated with congenital infection are neurologic abnormalities, such as convulsions, coma, hypotonia, microcephaly, or hydrocephalus. Other conditions seen in the infant are ecchymosis, hepatosplenomegaly, intracranial calcifications, jaundice, microphthalmia, and pallor (anemia).

Rubella   The effects of rubella on the pregnant woman are the same as the effects on a nonpregnant woman of comparable age. But the effects of this infection on the fetus and neonate are great. Rubella causes a chronic infection that begins in the first trimester of pregnancy and may persist for months after birth.

Fetal-neonatal implications   The period of greatest risk for the teratogenic effects of rubella on the fetus is during the first trimester.

Clinical signs of congenital infection are congenital heart disease, IUGR, and cataracts. Cardiac involvements most often seen are patent ductus arteriosis and narrowing of peripheral pulmonary arteries. Other abnormalities may become evident in infancy, such as mental retardation or cerebral palsy. Conclusive diagnosis in the neonate can be made in the presence of these conditions and with an elevated rubella antibody titer at birth.

Interventions   The best therapy for rubella is prevention. Live attenuated vaccine is available and should be given to all children. It is recommended that women of childbearing age be tested for immunity and vaccinated if they are susceptible and *not pregnant*.

If a woman becomes infected during the first trimester, therapeutic abortion is an alternative. Nursing support and understanding are vital at this time because such a decision may initiate a crisis for a couple who has planned the pregnancy. They need objective data to understand the possible effects on the fetus and the prognosis for the child.

Cytomegalovirus   Cytomegalovirus (CMV) belongs to the herpesvirus group and causes both congenital and acquired infections referred to as *cytomegalic inclusion disease* (CID). Asymptomatic women can transmit this virus across the placenta to the fetus or by the vaginal route during delivery.

CID is probably the most prevalent infection in the TORCH group. Nearly half of adults have antibodies for the virus. The virus can be found in urine, saliva, cervical mucus, semen, and breast milk. It can be passed between humans by any close contact such as kissing, breast-feeding, and sexual intercourse. Asymptomatic CMV infection is particularly common in children and pregnant women.

Accurate diagnosis in the pregnant woman depends on the presence of CMV in the urine, a rise in IgM levels, and identification of the CMV antibodies within the serum IgM fraction. At present, none of the antiviral drugs has been effective in preventing CMV or in treating the congenital disease in the neonate.

For the fetus, this infection can result in extensive intrauterine tissue damage that is incompatible with life, in brain damage, or in no damage at all. Subclinical infections in the newborn are capable of producing mental retardation and auditory deficits, sometimes not recognized for several months. Learning disabilities may not appear until childhood. CMV may be the most common cause of mental retardation.

Herpesvirus type 2   Herpesvirus hominis (HVH) type 2 causes the disease herpes simplex, which affects the cervix, vagina, and external genitals and can be transmitted through sexual contact. Herpesvirus hominis type 1 is responsible for lip lesions (cold sores) and skin lesions usually found above the umbilicus. Primary lesions of HVH-2 (herpes genitalis) consist of multiple vesicles involving the vulva, vagina, and cervix. Couples engaging in oral sex may develop HVH-2 lesions of the lips and mouth. Conversely, genital lesions caused by HVH-1 are sometimes seen.

Control of the transmission of genital herpes simplex is difficult because viral shedding occurs in mild or asymptomatic cases and may continue after lesions have healed. The woman with only internal lesions may not be aware of them and can transmit the infection unknowingly.

Transmission of the HVH virus to the fetus almost always occurs after the membranes rupture, with the virus ascending from active lesions. It also occurs during vaginal delivery when the fetus comes in contact with genital lesions. Transplacental infection of the fetus is rare, apparently because the presence of circulating maternal antibodies to HVH-2 minimizes the risk (Noller, 1981b).

Fetal-neonatal implications   If active HVH infection occurs during the first trimester chorioamnionitis may occur and the rate of spontaneous abortion is 20%–50% (Oleske and Minnetor, 1981). Infection after the 20 weeks' gestation is related to increased incidence of premature birth but not to teratogenic defects.

Most perinatal infections are acquired during labor rather than earlier. Approximately 40%–50% of infants born vaginally when active maternal genital lesions are present develop some form of HVH infection (Grossman et al., 1981). There is no definitive treatment, and the infection is fatal to more than half of the infants acquiring it. Half or more of the survivors have permanent visual damage and impaired psychomotor and intellectual development.

Interventions   When HVH-2 is suspected in the pregnant woman, amniocentesis can be performed to determine if there is fetal involvement. The amniotic fluid is tested for the presence of herpesvirus antibodies. Traditionally, if no infection is present on amniotic fluid analysis, a cesarean birth is indicated to protect the fetus from possible infection from the birth canal. If antibodies are present, a cesarean delivery should not be performed; the presumably infected fetus should be delivered vaginally.

A new drug, acyclovir (Zovirax), does not cure the infection or prevent recurrence. However, acyclovir does reduce healing time of the initial attack and shortens the time that the live virus is in the lesions, thereby reducing the infectious period.

Nurses must be particularly concerned with client education for this fast-spreading disease. Clients must be informed of the association of genital herpes simplex with spontaneous abortion, neonatal mortality and morbidity, and the possibility of cesarean delivery. A client needs to inform her future health care providers of her infection. Clients also should know of the possible association of genital herpes with cervical cancer and the importance of a yearly Pap smear.

Drug Use and Abuse

Indiscriminate drug use during pregnancy, particularly in the first trimester, may adversely affect the growth and development of the fetus. As discussed in Chapter 7, drugs adversely affecting fetal growth and development are called *teratogens*. Table 10-4 identifies common addictive drugs and their effects on the fetus and neonate.

Drugs that are commonly misused include alcohol, amphetamines, barbiturates, hallucinogens, and heroin and other narcotics. Abuse of these drugs constitutes a major threat to the successful completion of pregnancy.

Table 10-4
Possible Effects of Selected Drugs of Abuse/Addiction on Fetus and Neonate

Maternal drug	Effect on fetus/neonate
I. Depressants	
A. Alcohol	Cardiac anomalies, IUGR, potential teratogenic effects, FAS
B. Narcotics	
1. Heroin	Withdrawal symptoms, convulsions, death, IUGR, respiratory alkalosis, hyperbilirubinemia
2. Methadone	Fetal distress, meconium aspiration; with abrupt termination of the drug, severe withdrawal symptoms, neonatal death
C. Barbiturates	Neonatal depression, increased anomalies; teratogenic effect(?); withdrawal symptoms, convulsions, hyperactivity, hyperreflexia, vasomotor instability
1. Phenobarbital	Bleeding (with excessive doses)
D. "T's and Blues" (combination of the following)	
1. Talwin (narcotic)	Safe for use in pregnancy; depresses respiration if taken close to time of birth
2. Amytal (barbiturate)	See barbiturates
E. Tranquilizers	
1. Phenothiazine derivatives	Withdrawal, extrapyramidal dysfunction, delayed respiratory onset, hyperbilirubinemia, hypotonia or hyperactivity, decreased platelet count
2. Diazepam (Valium)	Hypotonia, hypothermia, low Apgar score, respiratory depression, poor sucking reflex, possible cleft lip
F. Antianxiety drugs	
1. Lithium	Congenital anomalies; lethargy and cyanosis in the newborn
II. Stimulants	
A. Amphetamines	
1. Amphetamine sulfate (Benzedrine)	Generalized arthritis, learning disabilities, poor motor coordination, transposition of the great vessels, cleft palate
2. Dextroamphetamine sulfate (dexedrine sulfate)	Congenital heart defects, hyperbilirubinemia
B. Cocaine	Learning disabilities
C. Caffeine (more than 600 mg/day)	Spontaneous abortion, IUGR, increased incidence of cleft palate; other anomalies suspected
D. Nicotine (half to one pack cigarettes/day)	Increased rate of spontaneous abortion, increased incidence placental abruption, SGA, small head circumference, decreased length
III. Psychotropics	
A. PCP ("angel dust")	Flaccid appearance, poor head control, impaired neurologic development
B. LSD	Chromosomal breakage?
C. Marijuana	IUGR, potential impaired immunologic mechanisms

Drug Addiction

Maternal implications   Drug addiction has an adverse effect on the expectant woman. It affects her state of health, nutritional status, susceptibility to infection, and psychosocial condition. A majority of drug-abusing pregnant women are malnourished and receive little or no antepartal care. Heroin-addicted pregnant women have two to six times the risk of PIH, malpresentation, third trimester bleeding, and puerperal morbidity (Pritchard, MacDonald, and Gant, 1985). In addition, the risk of drug toxicity is present. In general, the woman's psychologic and physiologic ability to handle the stress of pregnancy is severely reduced.

Fetal-neonatal implications   The fetus of a pregnant addict is at increased risk for congenital malformations, IUGR, and premature birth. The newborn may also experience symptoms of withdrawal during the first days of life. (For a discussion of the effects of drug addiction on the newborn, see Chapter 22.)

Interventions   Antepartal care of the pregnant addict involves medical, socioeconomic, and legal considerations. A team approach allows the comprehensive management necessary to provide safe labor and delivery for woman and fetus. Care should be taken to maintain and improve the woman's general health and nutritional status. The woman should receive regular prenatal care and, if she is willing, support and counseling. "Cold turkey" withdrawal should be avoided because of the potential risk to the fetus.

The use of analgesics during labor and delivery should be avoided if possible. Immediate intensive care should be available for the newborn, who will probably be depressed, SGA, and premature.

Alcoholism

Maternal implications   Alcoholism has increased dramatically among women in the United States. The incidence is highest among women 20–40 years old; alcoholism is also seen in teenagers. Chronic abuse of alcohol can undermine maternal health by causing malnutrition (especially folic acid and thiamine deficiencies), bone marrow suppression, increased

incidence of infections, and liver disease. As a result of alcohol dependence, the woman may have withdrawal seizures in the intrapartal period as early as 12–48 hours after she stops drinking. Delirium tremens may occur in the postpartal period, and the neonate may suffer a withdrawal syndrome.

Fetal-neonatal implications   The effects of alcohol on the fetus may result in a group of signs referred to as *fetal alcohol syndrome (FAS)*. The syndrome has characteristic physical and mental abnormalities that vary in severity and combination. (The abnormalities and care of these infants are discussed in Chapter 22).

Interventions   There is no definitive answer to how much alcohol a woman can safely consume during pregnancy. The expectant woman should "play it safe" by avoiding alcohol completely during the early weeks of pregnancy when organogenesis is occurring. During the remainder of pregnancy, she may have an occasional drink, although none at all is safest.

The nursing staff in the maternity unit must be aware of the manifestations of alcohol abuse so that they can prepare for the client's special needs. The care regimen includes sedation to decrease irritability and tremors, seizure precautions, intravenous fluid therapy for hydration, and preparation for an addicted neonate. Although high doses of sedatives and analgesics may be necessary for the woman, caution is advised because these can cause fetal depression.

Breast-feeding generally is not contraindicated, although alcohol is excreted in breast milk. Excessive alcohol consumption may intoxicate the infant and inhibit maternal let-down reflex. Discharge planning for the alcohol-addicted mother and newborn should be correlated with the social service department of the hospital.

Summary

The diagnosis of high-risk pregnancy can be a shock to an expectant couple. The stress involved may lead to crisis unless appropriate nursing interventions are intitiated.

Nursing care should be planned individually and in depth, depending on each couple's specific needs. During assessment, the nurse should delineate the factors that place couples at high risk, identify their understanding of the specific disruption, evaluate their coping mechanisms, and anticipate the questions they need answered.

Specific nursing interventions include teaching and guidance related to necessary treatment and procedures; encouragement of communication among the couple, physician, and nurse; and support of the pregnant woman's self-esteem and body image. In addition, the nurse must support the physiologic function of the woman and her fetus as effectively as possible. Through these caring efforts, the nurse increases the chances that the high-risk pregnancy will result in a physiologically and psychologically healthy mother and child.

Resource Groups

HELP Program (The American Social Health Association, P.O. Box 100, Palo Alto, Calif. 94302).

References

Bernstine RS: Placenta abruptio. In: *Principles and Practice of Obstetrics and Perinatology*. Iffy L, Kaminetzky HA (editors). New York: Wiley, 1981.

Berkowitz RL, Couston DR, Mochizuki T: *Handbook for Prescribing Medication During Pregnancy*. Boston: Little, Brown, 1981.

Berkowitz RS, Goldstein DP: Complications of molar pregnancy. *Contemp OB/Gyn* August 1984; 24:57.

Borg S, Lasker J: *When Pregnancy Fails*. Boston: Beacon Press, 1981.

Burrow GN, Ferris GF: *Medical Complications During Pregnancy*, 2nd ed. Philadelphia: Saunders, 1982.

Criteria Committee of the New York Heart Association, Inc. *Nomenclature and Criteria for Diagnosis of Diseases of the Heart and Blood Vessels*, 5th ed. New York: The Association, 1955.

Danforth DN (editor): *Obstetrics and Gynecology*, 4th ed. Philadelphia: Harper & Row, 1982.

Davidson SV et al: *Nursing Care Evaluation*. St. Louis: Mosby, 1977.

Gant NF, Worley RJ: *Hypertension in Pregnancy: Concepts and Management*. New York: Appleton-Century-Crofts, 1980.

Grossman JH III et al: Management of genital herpes simplex virus infection during pregnancy. *Obstet Gynecol* 1981; 58(1):1.

Guthrie DW, Guthrie RA: *Nursing Management of Diabetes Mellitus*, 2nd ed. St. Louis: Mosby, 1982.

Jovanovic L, Peterson CM: Optimal insulin delivery for the pregnant diabetic patient. *Diabetes Care*. 5 May/June 1982; (Suppl. 1):24.

Leman RE et al: Heart disease and pregnancy. *South Med J* 1981; 74(8):944.

Moore DS, Bingham PE, Kessling O: Nursing care of the pregnant woman with diabetes mellitus. *J Obstet Gynecol Neonatal Nurs* 1981; 10(3):188.

National Diabetes Data Group: *Classification of Diabetes Mellitus and Other Categories of Glucose Intolerance*. Washington, DC: National Institutes of Health, 1979.

Noller KL: Heart disease in pregnancy. In: *Principles and Practice of Obstetrics and Perinatology*. Iffy L, Kaminetzky HA (editors). New York: Wiley, 1981a.

Noller KL: Sexually transmitted diseases in pregnancy. In *Principles and Practice of Obstetrics and Perinatology*. Iffy L, Kaminetzky HA (editors). New York: Wiley, 1981b.

Oleske SM, Minnetor AE: Herpes simplex infection during pregnancy. In: *Principles and Practice of Obstetrics and Perinatology*. Iffy L, Kaminetzky HA (editors). New York: Wiley, 1981.

Osborne NG, Pratson L: Sexually transmitted diseases and pregnancy. *J Obstet Gynecol Neonatal Nurs* 1984; 13(1):9.

Pritchard JA, MacDonald P, Gant NF: *Williams Obstetrics*, 17th ed. New York: Appleton-Century-Crofts, 1985.

Skyler J, Mintz D, O'Sullivan M: Management of diabetes and pregnancy. In: *Diabetes Mellitus*. Vol 5. Rifkin H, Raskin P (editors). Bowie, Md.: Brady, 1981.

Spellacy WN. Diabetes and pregnancy. In: *Gynecology and Obstetrics*. Vol. 2. Sciarri JJ (editor). Philadelphia: Harper & Row, 1984.

Weil SG: The unspoken needs of families during high-risk pregnancies. *Am J Nurs* 1981; 81(11):2047.

Wheeler L, Jones MB: Pregnancy-induced hypertension. *J Obstet Gynecol Neonatal Nurs* 1981: 10(3):212.

White P: Pregnancy and diabetes: Medical aspects. *Med Clin North Am* 1965; 49:1016.

Willis SE: Hypertension in pregnancy: Pathophysiology. *Am J Nurs* 1982; 82(5):792.

Zuspan FP: Toxemia of pregnancy. In: *Gynecology and Obstetrics*. Vol 2. Sciarri JJ (editor). Philadelphia: Harper & Row, 1984.

Additional Readings ————

Altchek A: Ectopic pregnancy in young patients. *Contemp Ob/Gyn* September 1984; 24(3):120.

Berkowitz RS, Goldstein DP: Complications of molar pregnancy. *Contemp Ob/Gyn* August 1984; 24(2):57.

Caudle MR, Scott JR: Rh disease: Why it's still a clinical problem. June 1983; *Contemp Ob/Gyn* 21:177.

DeVore NE, Jackson VM, Piening SL: TORCH infections. *Am J Nurs* December 1983; 83(12):1660.

Gilstrap LC et al: Renal infection and pregnancy outcome. *Am J Obstet Gynecol* 1981; 141(6):709.

Hammer RM, Bower EJ; Messina LJ: The prenatal use of Rh_o (D) Immune Globulin. *MCN* January/February 1984; 9:29.

Hoffmaster JE: Detecting and treating pregnancy-induced hypertension: A review. *MCN* November/December 1983; 8:398.

Morrison JC et al: Management of the pregnant patient with cardiovascular disease. *CVP* February/March 1981; 9:17.

Osborne NG, Pratson L: Sexually transmitted diseases and pregnancy. *J Obstet Gynecol Neonatal Nurs* January/February 1984; 13:9.

Willis SE, Sharp ES: Hypertension in pregnancy: Prenatal detection and management. *Am J Nurs* 1982; 82(5):798.

11
Diagnostic Assessment of Fetal Status

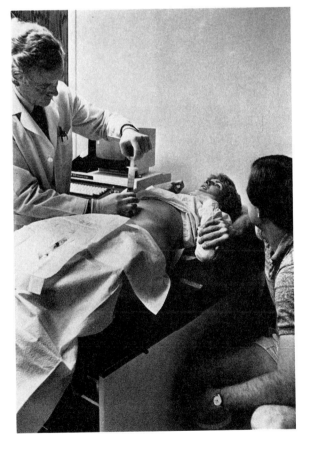

Chapter Contents

Objectives

- List indications for performing ultrasonic examinations.
- Compare the nonstress test (NST) and the contraction stress test (CST), giving indications, contraindications, and predictive value of each.

- Discuss the value of estriols as a measure of fetal well-being.

- Discuss the use of amniocentesis as a diagnostic tool.

- Describe the tests that may be done on amniotic fluid.

Key Terms

amniocentesis
amnioscopy
contraction stress
   test (CST)

fetoscopy
lecithin/sphingomye-
   lin (L/S) ratio
nonstress test (NST)

During the past 15–20 years, the problems of the high-risk pregnant woman and her baby have received increasing attention. This attention has been stimulated by the observation that conditions such as prematurity, congenital anomalies, mental retardation, and cerebral palsy seem to be associated with the presence of certain factors, such as maternal infections or diabetes mellitus, during pregnancy and delivery. In addition, it has been demonstrated that perinatal morbidity (sickness) and mortality (death) can be significantly reduced when there is early diagnosis of pregnancy and high-risk factors and ongoing prenatal care of the pregnant woman.

A variety of tests can be used to assess fetal well-being during the pregnancy. These tests include diagnostic ultrasound, measurements of specific hormones and enzymes in the maternal plasma and urine, amniocentesis for lung maturity studies, amnioscopy, and fetal stress tests.

Many of these tests pose risks to the fetus and possibly to the pregnant woman, and these risks should be considered before a particular test is done. One must be certain that the advantages outweigh the potential risks and the added expense. In addition, the diagnostic accuracy and applicability of these tests vary. Certainly, not all high-risk pregnancies require the same tests. Conditions that indicate a high-risk pregnancy include:

- Maternal age less than 16 years or more than 35 years

- Chronic maternal hypertension, preeclampsia, diabetes mellitus, or heart disease

- Presence of Rh isoimmunization

- A maternal history of previous unexplained stillbirth

- Suspected IUGR

- Pregnancy prolonged past 42 weeks

See Chapter 6 for further discussion of prenatal high-risk factors and Chapter 10 for descriptions of various conditions that may threaten the successful completion of pregnancy.

Ultrasound

Valuable information about the fetus may be obtained from pulsed echo ultrasound testing. Intermittent ultrasonic waves (high-frequency sound waves) are transmitted by an alternating current to a transducer, which is applied to the woman's abdomen. The ultrasonic waves deflect off tissues within the woman's abdomen, showing structures of varying densities.

The most common types of ultrasound are gray-scale and real-time scanning. Gray-scale ultrasound provides a static or fixed image. Various internal structures can be visualized in many shades of gray (Figure 11-1). This type of ultrasound is done in an x-ray or ultrasound department. In real-time scanning, a transducer produces a rapid sequence of fixed images, which are displayed on a small screen similar to a television screen. Real-time scanning allows the observer to detect movement, such as that of the beating fetal heart. The operator may "freeze" an image on the screen and photograph the image for a permanent record. Real-time ultrasound is particularly helpful in late pregnancy for assessing functions that can be detected through movement, such as fetal breathing, cardiac activity, and bladder function. Real-time ultrasound equipment is small and easily moved and need not be used in the x-ray department. Thus, it is frequently kept in labor and delivery units so a pregnant woman can have the procedure done without the inconvenience of a trip to a different department.

Although ultrasound testing can be beneficial, the NIH Consensus Development Confer-

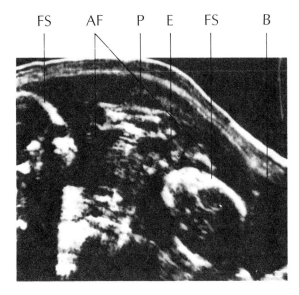

FS   AF   P   E   FS   B

Figure 11-1

Gray scale. Longitudinal scan demonstrating twin gestation, anterior placenta, fetal extremity. Both biparietal diameter (BPDs) correlate with approximately 25–26 weeks' gestation. (AF = amniotic fluid; FS = fetal skull; E = extremity; B = woman's urinary bladder; P = placenta.) (Courtesy Section of Diagnostic Ultrasound, Department of Diagnostic Radiology, Kansas University Medical Center.)

ence on Ultrasound Imaging in Pregnancy recommends that it not be routinely used on all pregnant women because its long-term effects are not fully known (Kremkau, 1984; Queenan, 1984).

Diagnostic ultrasound has several advantages. It is noninvasive, painless, nonradiating to both the woman and fetus, and has no known harmful effects to either. Serial studies (several ultrasound tests done over a span of time) may be done for assessment and comparison. Soft tissue masses can be differentiated. The practitioner obtains results immediately. Finally, ultrasound does not pose the same risk as other diagnostic or medical procedures, such as amniocentesis or intrauterine surgery, yet allows the clinician to "see" the fetus.

Procedure

The woman is usually scanned with a full bladder except when ultrasound is used to localize the placenta prior to amniocentesis. When the bladder is full, the examiner can then assess other structures, especially the vagina and

cervix, in relation to the bladder. This is particularly important when vaginal bleeding is noted and placenta previa is the suspected cause. The woman is advised to drink 1 quart of water approximately 2 hours before the examination, and she is asked to refrain from emptying her bladder. If the bladder is not sufficiently filled, she is asked to drink three to four 8-oz glasses of water and is rescanned 30–45 minutes later.

Mineral oil or a transmission gel is generously spread over the woman's abdomen, and the sonographer slowly moves a transducer over the abdomen to obtain a picture of the contents of the uterus. Ultrasound testing takes 20–30 minutes. The woman may feel discomfort due to pressure applied over a full bladder. In addition, the woman lies on her back during the test; this position may cause shortness of breath, which may be relieved by elevating her upper body during the test.

Clinical Application

Ultrasound testing can be of benefit in the following ways:

- Early identification of pregnancy. (Pregnancy may be detected as early as the fifth or sixth week following the LMP.)

- Identification of more than one fetus (Figure 11-1).

- Measurement of the biparietal diameter of the fetal head or the fetal femur length. These measurements help to determine the gestational age of the fetus and also to identify IUGR (Figure 11-2).

- Detection of fetal anomalies. Two major abnormalities that may be detected are anencephaly and hydrocephalus.

- Detection of hydramnios or oligohydramnios. The presence of more or less than normal amounts of amniotic fluid is frequently associated with fetal anomalies.

- Identification of amniotic fluid pockets. The presence of a pocket of amniotic fluid measuring at least 1 cm is associated with normal fetal status. The presence of one pocket measuring less than 1 cm or the absence of a pocket is abnormal. It is associated with increased risk of perinatal death (Manning, 1985).

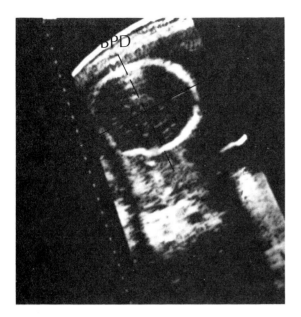

Figure 11-2
Transverse scan of the skull of a fetus of 25–26 weeks. BPD is measured perpendicular to midline echo (MLE). (Courtesy Section of Diagnostic Ultrasound, Department of Diagnostic Radiology, Kansas University Medical Center.)

- Location of the placenta. This is done prior to amniocentesis to avoid puncturing the placenta. Ultrasound is also used to determine the presence of placenta previa.

- Observation of fetal heart beat and respiration by real-time scanning. Respirations (fetal breathing movements, or FBM) have been observed as early as the eleventh week of gestation. Some researchers suggest that evaluation of fetal breathing movements may give information about the health of the fetus.

- Placental grading. As the fetus matures, the placenta calcifies. These changes can be visualized by ultrasound and graded according to the degree of calcification (grades 0 to III). Grade III placentas appear to be correlated with fetal lung maturity as determined by amniotic fluid analysis (Golde and Platt, 1984). Placental grading may be a way of determining fetal maturity when amniocentesis cannot be done.

- Detection of fetal death. Inability to visualize the fetal heart beating and the separation of the bones in the fetal head are signs of fetal death.

- Determination of fetal position and presentation. Ultrasound images give information about position and presentation.

Risks of Ultrasound

Ultrasound has been used clinically for 20 years, and to date no clinical studies verify harmful effects to the mother, fetus, or child. Several studies with animals suggest that ultrasound may retard fetal growth, cause cell damage, and impair the immune response, but the ultrasound levels used in these studies were higher than those levels used in medical diagnosis in pregnancy (Queenan, 1984; Shearer, 1984).

Maternal Assessment of Fetal Activity

The clinician may ask the expectant woman to count fetal movements during the third trimester as a screening test. Decreased fetal movements may indicate fetal stress and the need for further assessment. The woman can perform this test at her convenience and without any expense.

Fetal activity is affected by many factors, including sound, drugs, cigarette smoking, sleep states of the fetus, blood glucose levels, and time of day. The expectant mother's perception of fetal movements and the accuracy with which she documents them are also influenced by many factors, so this test is not always reliable.

Authorities differ on how many fetal movements indicate health in the fetus. Freeman and Garite (1981) report that two or more movements per hour are reassuring, while fewer than two should be reported to the clinician for evaluation with a nonstress test. Chez and Sadovsky (1984) recommend that beginning at 27 weeks the woman count fetal movements twice daily for 20–30 minutes. Five or six movements during each counting session is a reassuring sign. If fewer than three movements are noted in the session, the counting time is extended to one hour. If there are fewer than ten movements in a 12-hour period of counting, the clinician should be notified. The pregnant woman should be reassured that the fetus has rest-sleep states during which minimal or no movement may occur. Even though fetal movements may be a sign of fetal well-being, episodic absence of movement is characteristic of normal fetuses.

Nonstress Test

The **nonstress test (NST)** has become a widely accepted method of evaluating fetal status. The test involves observation of baseline variability and acceleration of the fetal heart rate (FHR) with fetal movement. FHR accelerations indicate intact central and autonomic nervous systems that are not being affected by intrauterine hypoxia (see the discussion of baseline variability and acceleration in Chapter 13).

The advantages of the NST are as follows:

- It is quick to perform.
- It permits easy interpretation.
- It is inexpensive.
- It can be done in office or clinic setting.
- There are no known side-effects.

The disadvantages of the NST include:

- It is sometimes difficult to obtain a suitable tracing.
- The woman has to lie relatively still for at least 20 minutes.

Procedure

An electronic fetal monitor is used to obtain a tracing of FHR and fetal movement (FM). The examiner puts two belts on the woman's abdomen. One belt holds a device that detects uterine or fetal movement. The other belt holds a device that detects the FHR. As the NST is done, each fetal movement is documented so that associated or simultaneous FHR changes may be evaluated.

Interpretation of NST Results

The NST is classified as follows (Lavery, 1982):

- *Reactive.* A reactive NST shows two accelerations of 15 beats/minute lasting 15 seconds, associated with fetal movement, over a 20-minute period (Figure 11-3).

- *Suspicious.* A suspicious NST shows fewer than two accelerations of 15 beats/minute lasting 15 seconds with fetal movement. Accelerations not accompanied by fetal movement are also suspicious.

- *Nonreactive.* The criteria for a reactive NST are not met.

- *Unsatisfactory.* The tracing yields uninterpretable or insufficient data.

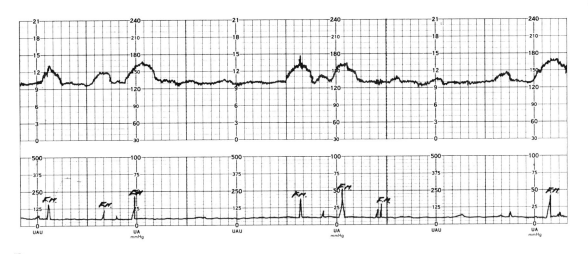

Figure 11-3

Example of a reactive nonstress test (NST). Accelerations of 15 beats/minute, lasting 15 seconds with each fetal movement (FM). (*Top of strip* = FHR; *bottom of strip* = uterine activity tracing.)

Note: The criteria for classifying NSTs vary among authors.

Prognostic Value

A reactive NST appears to be indicative of fetal well-being, and the test usually does not need to be repeated for 1 week. Any change in maternal or fetal status—such as decreased fetal movement, decreasing estriol levels (p. 237), vaginal bleeding, or deterioration of maternal condition—warrants more frequent testing.

A nonreactive NST indicates the need for further testing. Some authorities recommend rescheduling the NST again within 24 hours, while others believe a contraction stress test should be done immediately. (See Essential Facts to Remember—Nonstress Test.)

A new method of conducting an NST is currently being investigated. The new method is called an *acoustic stimulation test* and uses sound to stimulate the fetus. The test is evaluated in the same way as other NSTs (Serafini et al., 1984).

Fetal Biophysical Profile _____

The fetal biophysical profile is a collection of information regarding selected fetal measurements and assessments of the fetus and amniotic fluid. Ultrasound is used to determine fetal biparietal diameter, femur length, and abdominal circumference, and characteristics such as FBM, fetal tone, and amniotic fluid vol-

ume. Additional assessments include FHR reactivity and fetal movements, both of which may be assessed by a NST.

The fetal biophysical profile can be used to monitor fetal well-being. Some researchers suggest that it can be used to identify a fetus at risk for asphyxia (Manning, 1985). A detailed explanation of the fetal biophysical profile is beyond the scope of this book. (For further information, see Manning, 1985.)

Contraction Stress Test _____

The **contraction stress test (CST)** is a means of evaluating the respiratory function (oxygen and carbon dioxide exchange) of the placenta. It enables the health care team to identify the fetus at risk for intrauterine asphyxia by observing the response of the FHR to the stress of uterine contractions (spontaneous or induced). During contractions, intrauterine pressure increases. Blood flow to the intervillous space of the placenta is reduced momentarily, thereby decreasing oxygen transport to the fetus. A healthy fetus usually tolerates this reduction well. If the placental reserve is insufficient, fetal hypoxia, depression of the myocardium, and a decrease in FHR occur (Figure 11-4).

The CST is indicated when there is risk of placental insufficiency or fetal compromise because of the following:

- IUGR
- Diabetes mellitus
- Heart disease
- Chronic hypertension
- Preeclampsia-eclampsia (PIH)
- Sickle cell anemia
- Suspected postmaturity (more than 42 weeks' gestation)
- History of previous stillbirths
- Rh sensitization
- Abnormal estriol excretion
- Hyperthyroidism
- Renal disease
- Nonreactive NST

 ESSENTIAL FACTS TO REMEMBER

Nonstress Test

Diagnostic value: Demonstrates fetus's ability to respond to its environment by acceleration of FHR with movement

Results:

- Reactive test: Accelerations are present, indicating fetal well-being.
- Nonreactive test: Accelerations are not present, indicating that the fetus is sick or asleep.

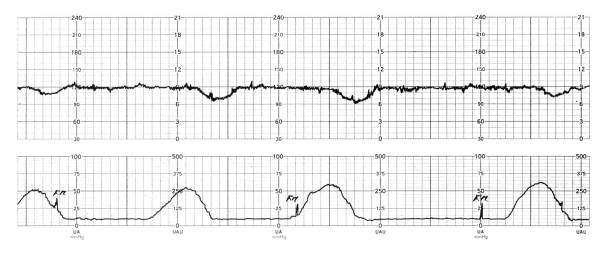

Figure 11-4

Example of a positive contraction stress test (CST). Repetitive late decelerations occur with each contraction. *Note:* There are no accelerations of FHR with three fetal movements (FM): Baseline FHR = 120 beats/minute. Uterine contractions (*bottom half of strip*) occurred three times in 8 minutes.

The CST is contraindicated if there is third trimester bleeding from placenta previa or marginal abruptio placenta; previous cesarean with classical uterine incision; risk of precipitating premature labor outweighing the advantage of the CST; premature rupture of the membranes; incompetent cervix; and multiple gestation (Collea and Holls, 1982).

The advantages of the CST are:

- The test provides information about how the fetus will react to the stress of uterine contractions.

- It can show that the fetal environment is deteriorating.

The disadvantages include:

- The test needs to be administered in a hospital setting.

- It is an invasive procedure if an intravenous line is used.

- It may initiate uterine contractions that precipitate labor.

Procedure

A necessary component of the CST is the presence of uterine contractions. They may occur spontaneously (which is unusual), or they may be induced (stimulated) with oxytocin. The most common method of stimulating uterine contractions for a CST is through intravenous administration of oxytocin (Pitocin). Consequently, the CST has been called oxytocin challenge test (OCT). Some facilities are using the newer breast self-stimulation test (BSST). This method is based on the knowledge that the body produces oxytocin in response to stimulation of the breasts or nipples.

The procedure, reasons for administering the test, equipment used, and normal variations in monitoring that occur during the test should be clearly explained to the woman prior to the test. A consent form is signed. The woman should empty her bladder before the CST is begun because she may be confined to bed for 1.5–2 hours.

The woman is placed in a semi-Fowler's position to avoid supine hypotension. An electronic monitor provides continuous data regarding FHR and uterine activity. The ultrasonic transducer (from the electronic fetal monitor) is placed on the woman's abdomen so that the FHR may be accurately recorded on the monitoring strip. To record uterine contractions, the examiner places a tocodynamometer (pressure transducer) over the uterine fundus. The ultrasonic transducer and tocodynamometer are secured in place with belts. A continuous recording from the electronic fetal monitor is begun. Maternal blood pressure and pulse are assessed as the recording is begun. After a 15-minute baseline recording of uterine activity and FHR, the tracing is evaluated for evidence of spontaneous contractions. If three spontaneous contractions of good quality and lasting 40–60 seconds occur in a 10-minute period, the results are evaluated, and the test is concluded. If no contractions occur or if they are insufficient for interpretation, oxytocin is administered intravenously or breast stimulation is done to produce contractions of good quality.

CST with intravenous oxytocin   An electrolyte solution such as lactated Ringer's solution is started as a primary infusion. A piggyback infusion of oxytocin in a similar solution is attached. An infusion pump is used so that the amount of oxytocin being infused can be measured accurately. The administration procedure is the same as for inducing labor through oxytocin administration. See Chapter 18 for further discussion. Oxytocin is administered until three uterine contractions lasting 40–60 seconds occur in a 10-minute period. If late decelerations are repetitive or occur more than three times, the oxytocin infusion should be discontinued.

Breast self-stimulation test   In BSST, the breasts are stimulated by applying warm washcloths and/or manually rolling one nipple. When the contractions are sufficient to allow interpretation, the test is concluded. Continued assessment is maintained until contractions subside. The results are reviewed, recorded, and explained to the woman. Breast stimulation is discontinued just as intravenous oxytocin administration is stopped in a CST, if late decelerations are repetitive or if they occur more than three times (Freeman, 1982; Huddleston et al., 1984; Lenke and Nemes, 1984).

Interpretation of CST Results

The CST is classified as follows:

- *Negative*. A negative CST shows three contractions of good quality lasting 40 or more seconds in 10 minutes without evidence of late decelerations.

- *Positive*. A positive CST shows repetitive persistent late decelerations with more than 50% of the contractions (Figure 11-4).

- *Hyperstimulation*. A hyperstimulation test is signalled by contractions occurring more frequently than every 2 minutes or lasting more than 90 seconds.

- *Suspicious*. A suspicious CST occurs when the tracing cannot be interpreted or when contractions are inadequate.

Clinical Application

CSTs are usually begun at approximately 32–34 weeks' gestation and are repeated at weekly intervals until intervention is necessary or the woman delivers.

A negative CST implies that placental support is adequate. In that case, the physician can avoid premature intervention and gain approximately 1 additional week of intrauterine life for the fetus. A negative test also suggests that the fetus is probably able to tolerate the stress of labor should it ensue within the week (Collea and Holls, 1982).

A positive CST may indicate a fetus who has compromised placental reserves. A positive CST, however, does not appear to be as reliable an indicator of fetal status as a negative one (Collea and Holls, 1982). Because false-positive results are not uncommon, a positive test requires further evaluation, as follows:

1. Does the monitor tracing show variability of the fetal heart beat? Good variability is usually associated with a healthy fetus. In addition, are FHR accelerations present? Accelerations with fetal movement are also a good sign. The absence of variability and accelerations is usually not seen with a healthy fetus and therefore is another sign of fetal problems.

2. Was the client's blood pressure maintained at baseline levels during the testing? If she lay flat on her back and became hypotensive, the test results may be misleading.

3. If intravenous oxytocin was used, were the contractions more intense than normally occurring contractions?

If the CST is positive, FHR variability is minimal, FHR accelerations do not occur with fetal movement, and the fetal lungs are mature (as demonstrated by L/S ratio or PG), the fetus must be delivered immediately. Whether the woman with a positive CST should have a cesarean delivery instead of a vaginal delivery depends on the speed with which the fetus must be delivered to avoid severe fetal distress, the adequacy of cervical dilatation and effacement at the time the decision is being made, and the woman's condition.

Nursing Implications

The nurse has an opportunity to provide support and information to the pregnant woman who has been scheduled for testing. The woman may not have anticipated that additional testing would be needed during the pregnancy. The knowledge that testing is needed increases her concern about the baby. Each scheduled test has the potential to provide information that indicates the baby is all right, but the test may also indicate that something is wrong. The nurse can help by listening to the woman as she vents her concerns. Providing information about the test, the equipment used, and the way results are determined may also relieve concern. The parents-to-be frequently receive only partial information, which only increases the stress they feel. Working with the same nurse during each scheduled test helps to form a trusting relationship that makes the couple feel free to ask their questions. The tests are usually done more than once, increasing the time away from a job or from the home. Paying attention to the woman's scheduling needs can help decrease the frustration she may feel (see Essential Facts to Remember—Contraction Stress Test).

Estriol Determinations ⸻

Estriol is a form of estrogen produced by the placenta. Its production depends on precursors from both the woman and fetus. For estrogen levels to be within normal limits, the mother, fetus, and placenta must be healthy, and all three must be functioning in harmony.

The amount of estriol in the maternal plasma or urine is an indication of the well-being of the maternal-fetal-placental unit. Estriol levels in both plasma and urine should increase as pregnancy advances, with significant amounts being produced in the third trimester. At term (40 weeks' gestation) the normal mean values of urine estriol are approximately 28 mg/24 hr and 14 ng/mL for plasma estriol. Conditions that affect one of the parts of the maternal-fetal-placenta unit can cause a decrease in the amount of estriol produced.

Determinations of estriol levels may be obtained by either a plasma (serum) test or urine. Plasma tests are gradually replacing urine estriols because they are easily obtained and accurate. Urinary estriols require a 24-hour, accurate collection, which is often inconvenient for the pregnant woman. Estriol level determinations are done serially (over time) in the management of high-risk maternity clients with hypertension, PIH, diabetes, renal disease, suspected placental insufficiency, IUGR, and postmaturity.

Interpretation of Findings

The range of normal values is broad, and various patterns are seen in both plasma and urinary estriol levels. A single estriol measurement in the normal range does not necessarily indicate fetal well-being. Of more significance than any specific single value is the general

 ESSENTIAL FACTS TO REMEMBER

Contraction Stress Test

Diagnostic value: Demonstrates reaction of FHR to stress of uterine contraction

Results:

- Negative test: Stress of uterine contraction does not cause a deceleration of the FHR.

- Positive test: Stress of uterine contraction is associated with a deceleration in the FHR.

trend in day-to-day or week-to-week values. Similar or gradually increasing estriol values are a sign of fetal well-being as long as the value stays above the critical level—12 ng/mL for plasma estriol and 12 mg/24 hrs for urinary estriol. Generally, a drop of 40% or more occurring on two consecutive tests may signify fetal distress (Kochenour, 1982). (See Essential Facts to Remember—Estriol Determinations.)

Amniotic Fluid Analysis

The analysis of amniotic fluid (**amniocentesis**) provides valuable information about fetal status. The amniotic fluid is withdrawn through a needle inserted through the abdominal wall into the uterus (Figure 11-5). Amniocentesis is a fairly simple procedure, although complications do occur rarely (less than 1% of cases). Procedure 11-1 describes the nursing interventions during amniocentesis.

A number of studies can be performed on amniotic fluid. These tests can provide genetic information about the fetus (see Chapter 3) as well as information about the health and maturity of the fetus. The remainder of the section describes amniotic fluid studies.

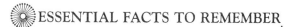
ESSENTIAL FACTS TO REMEMBER

Estriol Determinations

Diagnostic value: Indicates metabolic placental function and fetal jeopardy

Results: Plasma estriol of at least 12 ng/mL, urinary estriol of at least 12 mg/24 hrs are suggestive of fetal well-being.

If estriol levels are lower than expected, one of the following may be indicated:

- Normal fluctuation
- Gestation less advanced than expected
- Problem with placenta, or fetus, or maternal production
- Fetal anomalies; e.g., anencephaly, hydrocephalus
- Use of drugs; e.g., penicillin
- Laboratory error

If estriol levels are higher than expected, one of the following may be indicated:

- Gestation more advanced than expected
- More than one fetus
- Laboratory error

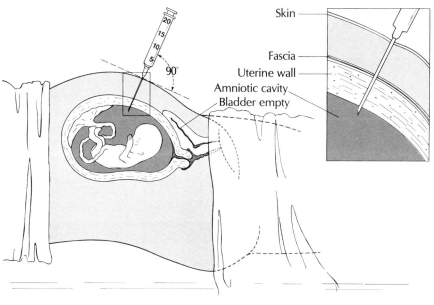

Figure 11-5

Amniocentesis. The woman is usually scanned by ultrasound to determine the placental site and to locate a pocket of amniotic fluid. When the needle is placed within the uterine cavity, amniotic fluid is withdrawn.

PROCEDURE 11-1
Amniocentesis

Objective	Nursing action	Rationale
Prepare client	Explain procedure Reassure client Have client sign consent form Have client empty bladder.	Anxiety will be decreased with information To indicate client's awareness of risks and consent to procedure To decrease risk of bladder perforation
Prepare equipment	Collect supplies: 3 mL syringe with 25-gauge needle Local anesthetic (1% procaine or 1% lidocaine) 3–6-inch 22-gauge spinal needle with stylet 10 mL syringe 20 mL syringe Three 10 mL test tubes with tops (amber-colored or covered with tape)	Amniotic fluid must be shielded from light to prevent breakdown of bilirubin
Monitor vital signs	Obtain baseline data on maternal BP, pulse, respiration, and FHR Monitor every 15 minutes	Status of client and fetus is assessed
Locate fetus and placenta	Provide assistance as physician palpates for fetal position Assist with real-time ultrasound	Real-time ultrasound is used to locate the placenta and various fetal parts.
Cleanse abdomen	Scrub abdomen with Betadine (or other cleansing agent)	Risk of infection is decreased
Collect specimen of amniotic fluid	Obtain test tubes from physician; provide correct identification; send to lab with appropriate lab slips	
Reassess vital signs	Determine client's BP, pulse, respirations, and FHR; palpate fundus to assess fetal and uterine activity; monitor client with external fetal monitor for 20–30 minutes after amniocentesis Have client rest on left side	Fetus may have been inadvertently punctured Uterine contractions may ensue following procedure; treatment course should be determined to counteract supine hypotension and to increase venous return and cardiac output
Complete client record	Record type of procedure done, date, time, name of physician performing test, client–fetal response, and disposition of specimen	Client records will be complete and current
Educate client	Reassure client; instruct her to report any of the following side effects: 1. Fetal hyperactivity or lack of fetal movement 2. Vaginal discharge—clear drainage or bleeding 3. Uterine contractions or abdominal pain 4. Fever or chills	Client will know how to recognize side-effects or conditions that warrant further treatment

Evaluation of Rh-Sensitized Pregnancies

When a sensitized Rh-negative woman produces an incompatible Rh-positive fetus, antibodies cross the placenta and cause hemolytic anemia in the fetus. Spectrophotometry shows concentrations of bilirubin and other breakdown products from destroyed red blood cells in the amniotic fluid. By plotting their concentration or optical density on a Liley curve, the physician can ascertain the degree to which the fetus is affected and the need for intervention, such as intrauterine transfusion.

Evaluation of Fetal Maturity

When managing a high-risk pregnancy, the caregiver is faced with the possibility of needing to deliver an infant before term and the onset of labor. Indications for early termination of pregnancy include premature rupture of membranes and developing amnionitis, severe pre-eclampsia or eclampsia, bleeding problems, and placental insufficiency. When an infant is delivered before the lungs are mature, the risk of such complications as respiratory distress syndrome is high.

Concentrations of certain substances in amniotic fluid reflect the pulmonary condition of the fetus. Because gestational age, birth weight, and the rate of development of organ systems do not necessarily correspond, amniotic fluid may be analyzed to determine the maturity of the fetal lungs.

Lecithin/sphingomyelin ratio   The alveoli of the lungs are lined with a substance called *surfactant*, which is composed of phospholipids. Surfactant lowers the surface tension of the alveoli when the newborn exhales. When a newborn with mature pulmonary function takes its first breath, a tremendously high pressure is needed to open the lungs. By lowering the alveolar surface tension, surfactant stabilizes the alveoli, and a certain amount of air always remains in the alveoli during expiration. Thus, when the infant exhales, the lungs do not collapse. An infant born before synthesis of surfactant is complete is unable to maintain lung stability. Each breath requires an effort similar to that of the first breath. This results in under-inflation of the lungs and development of respiratory distress syndrome (RDS).

Fetal lung maturity can be ascertained by determining the ratio of two components of surfactant—lecithin and sphingomyelin. Early in pregnancy, the sphingomyelin concentration in amniotic fluid is greater than the concentration of lecithin, and so the **lecithin/sphingomyelin (L/S)** ratio is low. At about 30–32 weeks' gestation, the amounts of the two substances become equal. The concentration of lecithin begins to exceed that of sphingomyelin, rising abruptly at about 35 weeks' gestation (Gluck, 1975; Cruikshank, 1982). At the same time, the sphingomyelin concentration begins to decrease. Fetal maturity is attained when the L/S ratio is 2:1 or greater; that is, when the amniotic fluid contains at least twice as much lecithin as sphingomyelin.

Under certain conditions of stress, the fetal lungs mature more rapidly. These situations include premature rupture of the membranes, acute placental infarction, placental insufficiency, chronic abruptio placentae, renal hypertensive disease due to degenerative forms of diabetes, cardiovascular hypertensive disease, and severe PIH. This accelerated maturation of the fetal lungs is thought to be a protective mechanism for the preterm fetus if delivery actually does occur (Cruikshank, 1982).

Delayed maturation is often seen in infants born to mothers with class A, B, and C diabetes, and in those born to mothers with nonhypertensive glomerulonephritis or hydrops fetalis (Cruikshank, 1982). In these instances, a higher L/S ratio (3:1) may be necessary to ensure adequate lung maturity.

Lung profile   The L/S ratio, which is determined from a sample of amniotic fluid, is the most widely used assay of functional pulmonary maturity in the fetus. However, problems can be incurred in this determination, including the following:

- High false-negative rate
- Unpredictability of a value that is borderline
- Unpredictability of blood-contaminated specimens
- Occasional false-positive values associated with such conditions as Rh disease, diabetes, and severe birth asphyxia

Some of these difficulties are overcome by using a lung profile of amniotic fluid to evaluate maturity. The lung profile looks for not only lecithin but also for two other phospholipids: phosphatidylglycerol (PG) and phosphatidylinositol (PI). PI increases in amniotic fluid after 26–30 weeks of gestation, peaks at 35–36 weeks, and then decreases gradually. PG appears after 35 weeks and continues to increase until term (Fletcher, 1984).

The lung profile is a useful adjunct to evaluating L/S ratio. It appears that lung maturity can be confirmed in most pregnancies if PG is present in conjunction with an L/S ratio of 2:1 (Gabbe, 1982). At this time, only large medical centers can perform analysis of PG and PI.

Shake test and foam stability index   The shake test was introduced by Clements et al. (1972). It is a quick, inexpensive way to predict fetal lung maturity. The shake test is based on the surfactant's property of forming bubbles or foaming in the presence of ethanol. The test requires about 15 minutes. Exact amounts of 95% ethanol, isotonic saline, and amniotic fluid are shaken together for 15 seconds. The persistence of a complete ring of bubbles on the surface of the liquid after 15 minutes is considered a positive shake test, indicating lung maturity. There is a high false-negative rate, but a low false-positive rate (Cruikshank, 1982).

The foam stability index (FSI) is similar to the shake test. In this test, 0.5 mL of amniotic fluid is added to variable amounts of 95% ethanol. The sample is shaken and observed for foam, which indicates maturity. This test seems as reliable as the L/S ratio in normal pregnancies and seems to have a lower false-positive rate than the shake test (Cruikshank, 1982).

Creatinine level   Amniotic creatinine progressively increases as pregnancy advances, apparently because of increasing fetal muscle mass and maturing fetal renal function. Creatinine levels of 2 mg/dL of amniotic fluid seem to correlate closely with a pregnancy of 37 weeks or more (Pitkin, 1975; Cruikshank, 1982). (See Essential Facts to Remember—Creatinine Level.)

Identification of Meconium Staining

Amniotic fluid is normally clear, but the presence of meconium makes the fluid greenish. Once meconium staining is identified, more assessments must be made to determine if the fetus is suffering ongoing episodes of hypoxia.

Amnioscopy ─────────────

The amniotic membranes can be seen by inserting an amnioscope in the vagina and placing the amnioscope against the fetal presenting

 ESSENTIAL FACTS TO REMEMBER

Creatinine Level

Diagnostic value: provides information to help determine fetal age

Results: 2 mg/dL correlates with 37 weeks' gestation

If creatinine values are lower than expected, one of the following may be indicated:

- Gestation less advanced than expected
- Fetus smaller than normal
- Fetal kidney abnormalities

If creatinine levels are higher than expected, one of the following may be indicated:

- Gestation more advanced than expected
- Fetus larger than normal
- Elevated maternal creatinine levels

part (**amnioscopy**). The purpose of this procedure is usually to evaluate if the fluid is stained with meconium.

Fetoscopy ─────────────

Fetoscopy, a technique for directly observing the fetus and obtaining a sample of fetal blood or skin, was developed in 1972. Real-time ultrasound is used to locate an area through which to insert a cannula and trocar into the uterus. Following insertion, an endoscope is inserted to the desired part of the fetus for viewing and sampling. Skin biopsies may be obtained as well as blood samples. These samples can be tested for the presence of different congenital diseases or disorders. At this time, only a few perinatal centers are equipped to do fetoscopy (Hobbins, 1982).

Summary ─────────────

Assessment of fetal status is difficult in many situations. Each woman must be treated individually in light of her specific circumstances.

In addition, no one system of care is appropriate for all high-risk clients. Clinical judgment by the attending physician, based on data obtained during the nursing assessment and coupled with appropriate tests of fetal well-being, helps to decide the outcome of the pregnancy.

The nurse is in a prime position to offer support and reassurance to the high-risk woman and to provide valuable input to those caring for her. The nurse can maintain the flow of information to and from the woman at risk, thus ensuring optimal care for both the woman and her unborn child. In addition, the establishment of regionalized centers for high-risk pregnant clients, with specialized teams of health care professionals and equipment for electronic, biophysical, and biochemical monitoring of the fetus, better the chances for a successful childbirth experience.

References

Chez RA, Sadovsky E: Teaching patients how to record fetal movements. *Contemp Ob/Gyn* October 1984; 24(4):85.

Clements JA et al: Assessment of the risk of respiratory distress syndrome by a rapid test for surfactant in amniotic fluid. *N Engl J Med* 1972; 286:1077.

Collea JV, Holls WM: The contraction stress test. *Clin Obstet Gynecol* December 1982; 25(4):707.

Cruikshank DP: Amniocentesis for determination of fetal maturity. *Clin Obstet Gynecol* 1982; 25(4):773.

Fletcher MA: Prematurity, chap 70. In: *Gynecology and Obstetrics*. Vol 3. Sciarra JJ (editor). Philadelphia: Harper & Row, 1984.

Freeman RK: Stress testing: Conceptual origin and current applications. Proceedings of Sixth International Symposium on Perinatal Medicine, 1982, Corometrics Medical Systems, Inc. Las Vegas, Nev.

Freeman RK, Garite TJ: *Fetal Heart Rate Monitoring*. Baltimore: Williams & Wilkins, 1981.

Gabbe SG: Amniotic fluid indices of maturity. In: *Protocols for High-Risk Pregnancies*, Queenan JT, Hobbins JC (editors). Oradell, N.J.: Medical Economics, 1982.

Golde SH, Platt LD: The use of ultrasound in the diagnosis of fetal lung maturity. *Clin Obstet Gynecol* June 1984; 27(2):391.

Gluck L: Fetal maturity and amniotic fluid surfactant determinations. In: *Management of the High-Risk Pregnancy*. Spellacy WN (editor). Baltimore: University Park Press, 1975.

Hobbins JC: Fetoscopy. In: *Protocols for High-Risk Pregnancies*. Queenan JT, Hobbins JE (editors). Oradell, N.J.: Medical Economics, 1982.

Huddleston JF, Sutliff F, Robinson D: Contraction stress test by intermittent nipple stimulation. *Obstet Gynecol* May 1984; 63(5):669.

Kochenour NK: Estrogen assay during pregnancy. *Clin Obstet Gynecol* December 1982; 25(4):659.

Kremkau FW: Safety and long-term effects of ultrasound: What to tell your patients. *Clin Obstet Gynecol* 1984; 27(2):269.

Lavery JP: Nonstress fetal heart rate testing. *Clin Obstet Gynecol* December 1982; 25(4):689.

Lenke RR, Nemes JM: Use of nipple stimulation to obtain contraction stress test. *Obstet Gynecol* March 1984; 63(3):345.

Manning FA: Fetal biophysical profile scoring predicts trouble—when it counts. *Contemp Ob/Gyn* January 1985; 25(1):126.

Pitkin RM: Fetal maturity: Nonlipid amniotic fluid assessment. In: *Managment of the High-Risk Pregnancy*. Spellacy WN (editor). Baltimore: University Park Press, 1975.

Queenan JT: The NIH consensus report: A closer look. *Contemp Ob/Gyn* May 1984; 23(5):164.

Serafini P, Lindsay MB, Nagey DA, et al: Antepartum fetal heart rate response to sound stimulation: The acoustic stimulation test. *Am J Obstet Gynecol* January 1984; 148(1):41.

Shearer MH: Revelations: A summary and analysis of the NIH consensus development conference on ultrasound imaging in pregnancy. *Birth* Spring 1984; 11(1):23.

Additional Readings

Alexander ES, Spitz HB, Clark RA: Sonography of polyhydramnios. *AJR* 1982; 138:343.

Beeson D, Douglas R: Prenatal diagnosis of fetal disorders. 1. Technological capabilities. *Birth* Winter, 1983; 10(4):227.

DeVore, GR: Fetal echocardiography: A new frontier. *Clin Obstet Gynecol* June 1984; 27(2):359.

Gottesfeld KR: The clinical role of placental imaging. *Clin Obstet Gynecol* June 1984; 27(2):327.

Graham D, Jacques S, Degeorges V: The role of ultrasound in the diagnosis and management of the obstetrical patient. *J Obstet Gynecol Neonatal Nurs* September/October 1983; 12(5):307.

Harrison MR: Hydronephronsis in utero. *Contemp Ob/Gyn* October 1983; 22(4):47.

Manning FA, Lange IR, Morrison MBI, et al: Treatment of the fetus in utero: Evolving concepts. *Clin Obstet Gynecol* June 1984; 27(2):378.

O'Brien GD: Fetal femur: A new dimension of growth. *Contemp Ob/Gyn* April 1983; 21(4):186.

Platt LD, DeVore GR: Detecting fetal malformations. *Contemp Ob/Gyn* January 1983; 21(1):203.

Queenan JT: When fetal growth lags. *Contemp Ob/Gyn* January 1983; 21(1):214.

Richardson BS: Fetal activity: Measure of well-being. *Contemp Ob/Gyn* August 1983; 22(3):211.

Vintzileos AM, Campbell WA, Nochimson DJ, et al: Congenital defects: Let ultrasound guide your delivery plan. *Contemp Ob/Gyn* August 1984; 24(2):46.

*For me. . .my nurse-midwife meant the support I'd hoped for. . .
when I thought I was really not holding up under the stress, she'd
say, "That was pretty intense," verifying that it was okay to be
"falling apart" and that I was doing great.*

THE NEW OUR BODIES, OUR SELVES
Boston Women's Health Book Collective
Simon and Schuster, 1984

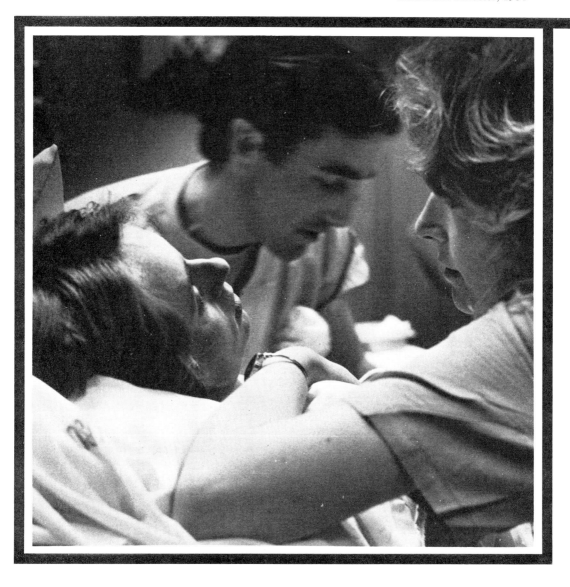

III

Labor and Delivery

12
Processes and Stages of Labor

Chapter Contents

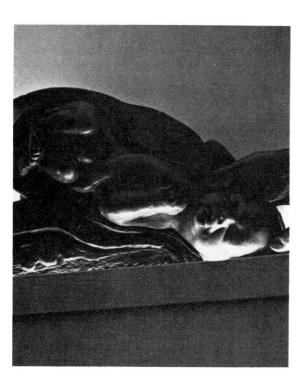

Maternal Systemic Response to Labor
    Cardiovascular System
    Blood Pressure
    Fluid and Electrolytes
    Gastrointestinal System
    Respiratory System
    Hemopoietic System
    Renal System
    Pain

Fetal Response to Labor

    Biochemical Changes
    Cardiac Changes
    Hemodynamic Changes
    Positional Changes

Objectives

- Discuss the significance of each type of pelvis to the birth process.

- Examine the factors that influence labor and the physiology of the mechanisms of labor.

- Describe the fetal positional changes that constitute the mechanisms of labor.

- Discuss the probable causes of labor onset and the premonitory signs of labor.

- Differentiate between false and true labor.

- Describe the physiologic and psychologic changes occurring in each of the stages of labor.

Key Terms

bloody show	frequency
cardinal movements	intensity
cervical dilatation	lightening
crowning	molding
duration	presentation
effacement	presenting part
engagement	rupture of mem-
fetal attitude	branes (ROM)
fetal lie	station
fetal position	sutures
fontanelles	

During the weeks of gestation, the fetus and the expectant woman prepare themselves for birth. The fetus progresses through various stages of growth and development in readiness for the independence of extrauterine life. The expectant woman undergoes various physiologic and psychologic adaptations during pregnancy that gradually prepare her for childbirth and the role of mother. The onset of labor marks a significant change in the relationship between the woman and the fetus.

Critical Factors in Labor

Four factors are important in the process of labor and delivery: the passage, the passenger, the powers, and the psyche. The "four Ps," as they are commonly known, are defined as follows:

1. Passage
   a. Size of the pelvis (diameters of the pelvic inlet, midpelvis, and outlet)
   b. Type of pelvis (gynecoid, android, anthropoid, or platypelloid)
   c. Ability of the cervix to dilate and efface, and ability of the vaginal canal and introitus to distend
2. Passenger
   a. Fetal head (size and presence of molding)
   b. Fetal attitude (flexion or extension of the fetal body and extremities)
   c. Fetal lie
   d. Fetal presentation (the part of the fetal body entering the pelvis in a single or multiple pregnancy)
   e. Fetal position (relationship of the presenting part to one of the four quadrants of the maternal pelvis)
   f. Placenta (implantation site)
3. Powers
   a. The frequency, duration, and intensity of uterine contractions as the passenger moves through the passage
   b. The duration of labor
4. Psyche
   a. Physical preparation for childbirth
   b. Sociocultural heritage

c. Previous childbirth experience
d. Support from significant others
e. Emotional integrity

The progress of labor is critically dependent on the complementary relationship of these four factors. Abnormalities of the passage, the passenger, the powers, or the psyche can alter the outcome of labor and jeopardize both the expectant woman and her baby. Complications involving the four Ps are discussed in Chapter 17.

The Passage _____

The true pelvis, which forms the bony canal through which the baby must pass, is divided into three sections: the inlet, the pelvic cavity (midpelvis), and the outlet. (*Note:* See Chapter 2 for discussion of each part of the pelvis and Chapter 6 for assessment techniques of the pelvis).

Pelvic Types

The Caldwell-Moloy classification of pelvic types is based on pertinent characteristics of both male and female pelves (Caldwell and Moloy, 1933). Although it is common for a particular pelvis to have characteristics of more than one type of pelvis, the four classic types are gynecoid, android, anthropoid, and platypelloid.

The *gynecoid* pelvis is often referred to as the "female" pelvis. Approximately 50% of women have this type of pelvis. All diameters of the gynecoid are adequate for childbirth.

The *android* pelvis is often referred to as the "male" pelvis. Approximately 20% of women have this type of pelvis. The diameters of the android pelvis are usually not adequate for vaginal delivery.

The *anthropoid* pelvis is narrowed from side to side and widened from front to back. The diameters are usually adequate for vaginal delivery.

The *platypelloid* pelvis is flattened (narrowed) from front to back and widened from side to side. Diameters are usually not adequate for vaginal delivery.

The Passenger _____

Fetal Head

The fetal head is composed of bony parts that can either hinder childbirth or make it easier. Once the head (the least compressible and largest part of the fetus) has been delivered, the birth of the rest of the body is rarely delayed.

The fetal skull has three major parts: the face, the base of the skull (cranium), and the vault of the cranium (roof). The bones of the face and cranial base are well fused and are basically fixed. The base of the cranium is composed of the two temporal bones, each with a sphenoid and ethmoid bone. The bones composing the vault are the two frontal bones, the two parietal bones, and the occipital bone (Figure 12-1). These bones are not fused, allowing this portion of the head to adjust in shape as the presenting part of the passenger passes through the narrow portions of the pelvis. The cranial bones overlap under pressure of the powers of labor and the demands of the unyielding pelvis. This overlapping is called **molding**.

The **sutures** of the fetal skull are membranous spaces between the cranial bones. The intersections of the cranial sutures are called **fontanelles**. These sutures allow for molding

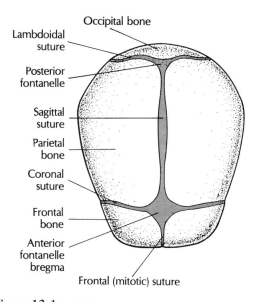

Lambdoidal suture
Occipital bone
Posterior fontanelle
Sagittal suture
Parietal bone
Coronal suture
Frontal bone
Anterior fontanelle bregma
Frontal (mitotic) suture

Figure 12-1 ▬▬▬▬▬▬
Superior view of the fetal skull.

of the passenger's head and help the examiner to identify the position of the fetal head during vaginal examination. The important sutures of the cranial vault are as follows (see Figure 12-1):

- *Mitotic suture*: Located between the two frontal bones; becomes the anterior continuation of the sagittal suture

- *Sagittal suture*: Located between the parietal bones; divides the skull into left and right halves; runs anteroposteriorly, connecting the two fontanelles

- *Coronal sutures*: Located between the frontal and parietal bones; extend transversely left and right from the anterior fontanelle

- *Lambdoidal suture*: Located between the two parietal bones and the occipital bone; extends transversely left and right from the posterior fontanelle

The anterior and posterior fontanelles are clinically useful in identifying the position of the fetal head in the pelvis and in assessing the status of the newborn after birth. The anterior fontanelle is diamond-shaped and measures 2 × 3 cm. It permits growth of the brain by remaining unossified for as long as 18 months. The posterior fontanelle is much smaller and closes within 8–12 weeks after birth. It is shaped like a small triangle and marks the meeting point of the sagittal suture and the lambdoidal suture (Oxorn, 1980).

Following are several important landmarks of the fetal skull (Figure 12-2):

- *Sinciput*: The anterior area known as the brow

- *Bregma*: The large diamond-shaped anterior fontanelle

- *Vertex*: The area between the anterior and posterior fontanelles

- *Posterior fontanelle*: The intersection between posterior cranial sutures

- *Occiput*: The area of the fetal skull occupied by the occipital bone, beneath the posterior fontanelle

- *Mentum*: The fetal chin

The diameters of the fetal skull vary considerably within normal limits. Some diameters

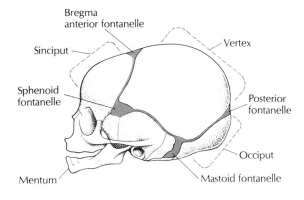

Figure 12-2
Lateral view of the fetal skull. The landmarks that have significance in obstetrics are identified.

shorten and others lengthen as the head is molded during labor. Fetal head diameters are measured between the various landmarks on the skull (Figure 12-3). The compound words used to designate the various diameters allow one to identify which measurement is actually being reported. For example, the suboccipito-bregmatic diameter is the distance from the undersurface of the occiput to the center of the bregma, or anterior fontanelle. Fetal skull measurements are given in Figure 12-3.

Much can be learned about the degree of extension or flexion of the fetal head from these diameters. Extension of the head results in a larger diameter presenting than if the head is strongly flexed. Alterations in flexion of the fetal head can cause problems during the process of labor. The fetus tries to accommodate its most favorable head diameters to the limited measurements of the bony pelvis.

Fetal Attitude

Fetal attitude refers to the relation of the fetal parts to one another. The normal attitude of the fetus is one of moderate flexion of the head, flexion of the arms onto the chest, and flexion of the legs onto the abdomen.

Changes in fetal attitude, particularly in the position of the head, cause the fetus to present larger diameters of the fetal head to the maternal pelvis. These deviations from a normal fetal attitude often contribute to difficult labor.

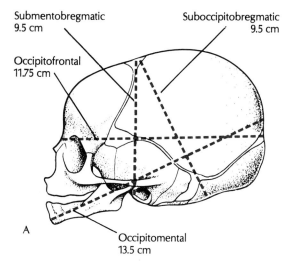

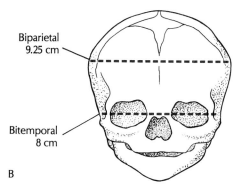

Figure 12-3

A, Anteroposterior diameters of the fetal skull. When the vertex of the fetus presents and the fetal head is flexed with the chin on the chest, the smallest anteroposterior diameter (suboccipitobregmatic) enters the birth canal. **B**, Transverse diameters of the fetal skull.

Fetal Lie

Fetal lie refers to the relationship of the cephalocaudal axis of the fetus to the cephalocaudal axis of the woman. The fetus may assume either a longitudinal or a transverse lie. A *longitudinal lie* occurs when the cephalocaudal axis of the fetus is parallel to the woman's spine. A *transverse lie* occurs when the cephalocaudal axis of the fetus is at right angles to the woman's spine.

Fetal Presentation

Fetal presentation is determined by fetal lie and by the body part of the fetus that enters the pelvic passageway first. This portion of the fetus is referred to as the **presenting part**. Fetal presentation may be either cephalic, breech, or shoulder.

Cephalic presentation   The fetal head presents itself to the passage in approximately 97% of term deliveries. The cephalic presentation can be further classified according to the degree of flexion or extension of the fetal head (attitude) (Figure 12-4).

Vertex presentation

- The fetal head is completely flexed on the chest.
- The smallest diameter of fetal head (suboccipitobregmatic) presents to the maternal pelvis.
- The occiput is the presenting part.
- The vertex is the most common type of presentation.

Military presentation

- The fetal head is neither flexed nor extended.
- The occipitofrontal diameter presents to the maternal pelvis.
- The vertex (see Figure 12-2) is the presenting part.

Brow presentation

- The fetal head is partially extended.
- The occipitomental diameter, the largest anteroposterior diameter, is presented to the maternal pelvis.
- The sinciput (see Figure 12-2) is the presenting part.

Face presentation

- The fetal head is hyperextended (complete extension).
- The submentobregmatic diameter presents to the maternal pelvis.
- The face is the presenting part.

Breech presentation   Breech presentations occur in 3% of term births. These presentations are classified according to the attitude of the fetus's hips and knees. In all variations of the breech presentation, the sacrum is the landmark to be noted.

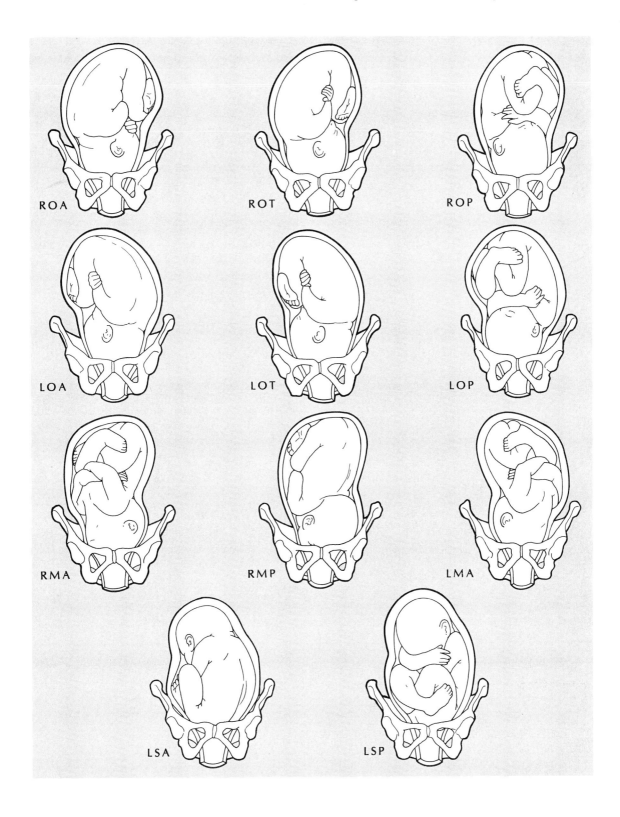

Figure 12-4
Categories of presentation. (Reprinted with permission of Ross Laboratories, Columbus, OH 43216. From Clinical Education Aide.)

Complete breech

- The fetal knees and hips are both flexed; the thighs are on the abdomen, and the calves are on the posterior aspect of the thighs.
- The buttocks and feet of the fetus present to the maternal pelvis.

Frank breech

- The fetal hips are flexed, and the knees are extended.
- The buttocks of the fetus present to the maternal pelvis.

Footling breech

- The fetal hips and legs are extended.
- The feet of the fetus present to the maternal pelvis.
- In a single footling, one foot presents; in a double footling, both feet present.

Shoulder presentation   A shoulder presentation is also called a *transverse lie*. Most frequently, the shoulder is the presenting part, and the acromion process of the scapula is the landmark to be noted. However, the fetal arm, back, abdomen, or side may present in a transverse lie.

Functional Relationships of Presenting Part and Passage

Engagement   Engagement of the presenting part occurs when the largest diameter of the presenting part reaches or passes through the pelvic inlet (Figure 12-5).

Engagement can be determined by vaginal examination. In primigravidas, engagement usually occurs 2 weeks before term. Multiparas, however, may experience engagement several weeks before the onset of labor or during the process of labor. Engagement confirms the adequacy of the pelvic inlet. Engagement does not indicate that the midpelvis and outlet are also adequate.

Station   Station refers to the relationship of the presenting part to an imaginary line

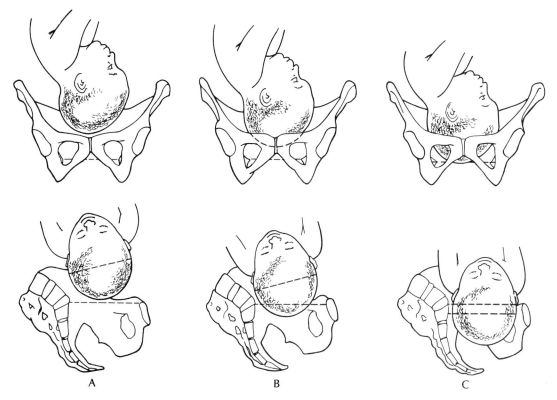

A   B   C

Figure 12-5

Process of engagement. **A**, Floating. **B**, Dipping. **C**, Engaged.

drawn between the ischial spines of the maternal pelvis. In a normal pelvis, the ischial spines mark the narrowest diameter through which the fetus must pass. These spines are not sharp protrusions that harm the fetus but rather blunted prominences at the midpelvis. The ischial spines as a landmark have been designated as zero station (Figure 12-6). If the presenting part is higher than the ischial spines, a negative number is assigned, noting centimeters above zero station. Station −5 is at the inlet, and station +4 is at the outlet. If the presenting part can be seen at the woman's perineum, delivery is imminent. During labor, the presenting part should move progressively from the negative stations to the midpelvis at zero station and into the positive stations. Failure of the presenting part to descend in the presence of strong contractions may be due to disproportion between the maternal pelvis and fetal presenting part, or to a short and/or entangled umbilical cord.

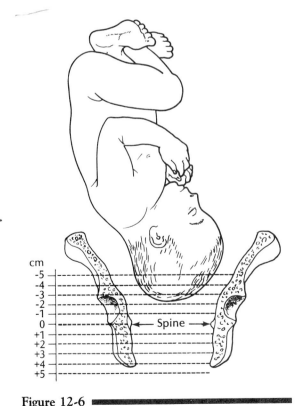

cm
-5
-4
-3
-2
-1
0   ← Spine →
+1
+2
+3
+4
+5

Figure 12-6 ▬▬▬▬▬▬▬▬▬

Measuring station of the fetal head while it is descending.

Fetal Position

Fetal position refers to the relationship of the landmark on the presenting fetal part to the front, sides, or back of the maternal pelvis. The landmark on the fetal presenting part is related to four imaginary quadrants of the pelvis: left anterior, right anterior, left posterior, and right posterior. These quadrants designate whether the presenting part is directed toward the front, back, left, or right of the passage. The landmark chosen for vertex presentations is the occiput, and the landmark for face presentations is the mentum. In breech presentations, the sacrum is the designated landmark, and the acromion process on the scapula is the landmark in shoulder presentations. If the landmark is directed toward the center of the side of the pelvis, fetal position is designated as *transverse*, rather than anterior or posterior.

Three notations are used to describe the fetal position:

1. Right (R) or left (L) side of the maternal pelvis

2. The landmark of the fetal presenting part: occiput (O), mentum (M), sacrum (S), or acromion process (A)

3. Anterior (A), posterior (P), or transverse (T), depending on whether the landmark is in the front, back, or side of the pelvis.

The abbreviations of these notations help the health care team communicate the fetal position. Thus, when the fetal occiput is directed toward the back and to the left of the passage, the abbreviation used is LOP (left-occiput-posterior). The term *dorsal* (D) is used when denoting the fetal position in a transverse lie; it refers to the fetal back. Thus the abbreviation RADA indicates that the acromion process of the scapula is directed toward the woman's right and the passenger's back is anterior.

Following is a list of the positions for various fetal presentations, some of which are illustrated in Figure 12-4.

Positions in vertex presentation:
ROA   Right-occiput-anterior
ROT   Right-occiput-transverse
ROP   Right-occiput-posterior
LOA   Left-occiput-anterior
LOT   Left-occiput-transverse
LOP   Left-occiput-posterior

Positions in face presentation:
RMA   Right-mentum-anterior
RMT   Right-mentum-transverse
RMP   Right-mentum-posterior
LMA   Left-mentum-anterior
LMT   Left-mentum-transverse
LMP   Left-mentum-posterior

Positions in breech presentation:
RSA   Right-sacrum-anterior
RST   Right-sacrum-transverse
RSP   Right-sacrum-posterior
LSA   Left-sacrum-anterior
LST   Left-sacrum-transverse
LSP   Left-sacrum-posterior

Positions in shoulder presentation:
RADA   Right-acromion-dorsal-anterior
RADP   Right-acromion-dorsal-posterior
LADA   Left-acromion-dorsal-anterior
LADP   Left-acromion-dorsal-posterior

The fetal position influences labor and delivery. For example, in a posterior position the fetal head presents a larger diameter than in an anterior position. A posterior position increases the pressure on the sacral nerves, causing the laboring woman backache and pelvic pressure and perhaps encouraging her to bear down or push earlier than normal. (See Chapter 17 for discussion of malpositions and their management.)

Assessment techniques to determine fetal position include inspection and palpation of the maternal abdomen, and vaginal examination (see Chapter 13 for further discussion of assessment of fetal position).

The Powers

Primary and secondary powers work together to deliver the fetus, the fetal membranes, and the placenta from the uterus into the external environment. The *primary power* is uterine muscular contractions, which cause the changes of the first stage of labor—complete effacement and dilatation of the cervix. The *secondary power* is the use of abdominal muscles to push during the second stage of labor. The pushing adds to the primary power after full dilatation has occurred.

In labor, uterine contractions are rhythmic but intermittent. Between contractions is a period of relaxation. This period of relaxation allows uterine muscles to rest and provides respite for the laboring woman. It also restores uteroplacental circulation, which is important to fetal oxygenation and adequate circulation in the uterine blood vessels.

Each contraction has three phases: (a) *increment*, the "building up" of the contraction (the longest phase); (b) *acme*, or the peak of the contraction; and (c) *decrement*, or the "letting up" of the contraction. When describing uterine contractions during labor, caregivers use the terms *frequency*, *duration*, and *intensity*. **Frequency** refers to the time between the beginning of one contraction and the beginning of the next contraction.

The **duration** of each contraction is measured from the beginning of the increment to the completion of decrement (Figure 12-7). In beginning labor, the duration is about 30 seconds. As labor continues, duration increases to

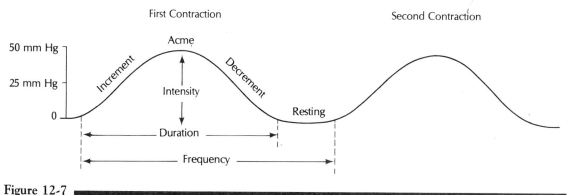

Figure 12-7
Characteristics of uterine contractions.

an average of 60 seconds with a range of 45–90 seconds (Varney, 1980).

Intensity refers to the strength of the uterine contraction during acme. In most instances, the intensity is estimated by palpating the contraction but it may be measured directly with an intrauterine catheter. When estimating intensity by palpation, the nurse determines whether it is mild, moderate, or strong by judging the amount of indentability of the uterine wall during the acme of a contraction. If the uterine wall can be indented easily, the contraction is considered mild. Strong intensity exists when the uterine wall cannot be indented. Moderate intensity falls between these two ranges. When intensity is measured with an intrauterine catheter, the normal resting tonus (between contractions) averages 10 mm Hg of pressure. During acme, the intensity ranges from 30–55 mm Hg of pressure (Cibils, 1981). (See discussion on stages of labor, p. 260, and Chapter 13 for further discussions of assessment techniques.)

At the beginning of labor, the contractions are usually mild, of short duration, and relatively infrequent. As labor progresses, duration of contractions lengthens, the intensity increases, and the frequency is every 2–3 minutes. Because the contractions are involuntary, the laboring woman cannot control their duration, frequency, or intensity.

The Psyche

Colman and Colman (1971) describe labor as a journey into the unknown that is uncertain, irrevocable, and uncontrollable. Every woman is uncertain about what her labor will be like: Nulliparas face a new experience, and multiparas cannot be certain what each new labor will bring. The woman does not know whether she will live up to her expectations of herself, whether she will be physically injured through laceration, episiotomy, or cesarean incision, or whether significant others will be as supportive as she imagines (Mercer, 1981). The woman faces an irrevocable event—the birth of a new family member and its consequences—change of life-style, relationships, and self-image. Finally, the woman must deal with concerns about her loss of control of bodily functions,

emotional responses to an unfamiliar situation, and reactions to the pain of labor.

Various factors influence a woman's reaction to the physical and emotional crisis of labor. Her accomplishment of the tasks of pregnancy, usual coping mechanisms in response to stressful life events, support system, preparation for childbirth, and cultural influences are all significant factors.

The coping mechanisms a woman uses during the pregnancy, labor, and delivery seem to be similar to those that she uses throughout her life. They are also influenced by the way that she perceives the event. Westbrook (1979) studied new mothers not only as individuals but also as members of a socioeconomic level (working, middle, or upper-middle level). In general, women in the upper-middle group tended to view childbearing as positive, were more likely to seek information about their situation, and tended to use coping styles such as confrontation, optimism, seeking interpersonal help, and control to meet their needs. Women in the working group tended to have a more negative view; feared physical harm, physical discomfort, and problems during labor; and used coping styles such as fatalism and avoidance.

The laboring woman's support system also influences the course of labor and delivery. The presence of the father and other significant persons, including the nurse, tends to have a positive effect.

Preparation for childbirth is another factor that influences a woman's reaction to childbirth. Much attention has been focused on preparation during pregnancy as a way of increasing the woman's ability to cope during childbirth; decreasing her stress, anxiety, and pain; and imparting satisfaction with the childbearing experience. Although opinions vary concerning whether the amount of pain or discomfort is actually decreased, there is agreement that preparation tends to increase perceived satisfaction. Humenick (1981) suggests that *mastery*, or control, of the childbearing experience is the key factor in perceived satisfaction. Childbirth education helps to increase positive reactions to the birth experience because education gives the laboring woman and her support persons greater opportunities to control the experience of labor.

Physiology of Labor ————————

Possible Causes of Labor Onset

For some reason, usually at the appropriate time for the uterus and the fetus, the process of labor begins. Although medical researchers have been conducting numerous studies to determine the exact cause, it still remains a mystery. Some widely accepted theories are discussed here.

Oxytocin stimulation theory   Oxytocin is produced by the maternal posterior pituitary. One of the effects of oxytocin is to stimulate contractions of the smooth muscle of the uterus. The uterus becomes increasingly sensitive (or responsive) to the effects of oxytocin as the pregnancy nears term (40 weeks). This increased responsiveness may be the result of increased production of oxytocin, and/or a change in the threshold of response.

Estrogen stimulation theory   Estrogen stimulates the smooth muscle of the uterus to contract. During pregnancy, the stimulatory effects of estrogen are counterbalanced by the relaxant effects of progesterone. The balance between these two hormones keeps the uterine muscles from contracting in a regular pattern during pregnancy. As term approaches, the balance changes because estrogen levels increase and progesterone levels decrease (Challis and Mitchell, 1981). This leads to increased irritability (a readiness to contract) of the uterine smooth muscle and the promotion of uterine contractions.

The stimulatory effect is increased further because estrogen promotes the synthesis of prostaglandin in the decidua and the fetal membranes (amnion and chorion). Prostaglandins also stimulate the smooth muscle of the uterus (Takahashi and Burd, 1980).

Progesterone withdrawal theory   Progesterone exerts a relaxant effect on the uterine smooth muscle by interfering with conduction of impulses from one cell to the next. The placenta produces progesterone, and toward the end of gestation, the amount or effectiveness of progesterone may decrease, contributing to increased uterine contractility.

Fetal cortisol theory   As the woman approaches term, the fetus produces more cortisol. Cortisol is thought to exert two effects: (a) It slows the production of progesterone by the placenta; and (b) it stimulates the precursors to prostaglandins. These two effects decrease the relaxant effect of progesterone on the uterus and increase the stimulatory effect of prostaglandins.

Uterine distention theory   The uterus slowly increases in size during the gestation, and its smooth muscle is stretched. Most smooth muscle contracts when stretched, but the uterine smooth muscle does not because of the effect of progesterone. As the woman approaches term, the decreased amount or effectiveness of progesterone increases uterine irritability and contractions. The irritability of the smooth muscle is enhanced by uterine distention, which stimulates the production of prostaglandins.

Prostaglandin theory   Although the exact relationship between prostaglandins and the onset of labor is not yet established, there is growing evidence that prostaglandin involvement is significant. Prostaglandin is known to stimulate smooth muscle contractions. It may also stimulate the production and release of oxytocin and lower the uterine threshold to oxytocin. The production of prostaglandins increases just before labor begins, most likely as a result of the interaction of such factors as increased estrogen and decreased progesterone, increased fetal cortisol, and increased distention of the uterus.

Myometrial Activity

Stretching of the cervix causes an increase in endogenous oxytocin, which increases myometrial activity. Pressures exerted by the contracting uterus vary from 20–60 mm Hg, with an average of 40 mm Hg.

In true labor, the uterus divides into two portions. This division is known as the *physiologic retraction ring*. The upper portion, which is the contractile segment, becomes progressively thicker as labor advances. The lower portion, which includes the lower uterine segment and cervix, is passive. As labor continues, the lower uterine segment expands and thins out.

With each contraction the muscles of the upper uterine segment shorten and exert a longitudinal traction on the cervix, causing effacement. **Effacement** is the taking up of the internal os and the cervical canal into the uterine side walls. The cervix changes progressively from a long, thick structure to a structure that is tissue-paper thin (Figure 12-8). In primigravidas, effacement usually precedes dilatation.

The uterus elongates with each contraction, decreasing the horizontal diameter. This elongation causes a straightening of the fetal body, pressing the upper pole against the fundus and thrusting the presenting part down toward the lower uterine segment and the cervix. The pressure exerted by the fetus is called the fetal axis pressure. As the uterus elongates, the longitudinal muscle fibers are pulled upward over the presenting part. This action, plus the hydrostatic pressure of the fetal membranes, causes **cervical dilatation**. The cervical os and cervical canal widen from less than a centimeter to approximately 10 cm, allowing delivery of the fetus. When the cervix is completely dilated and retracted up into the lower uterine segment, it can no longer be palpated.

The round ligament pulls the fundus forward, thus aligning the fetus with the bony pelvis.

Intraabdominal Pressure

After the cervix is completely dilated, the maternal abdominal muscles contract as the woman pushes. The pushing aids in expulsion of the fetus and placenta. If the cervix is not completely dilated, bearing down can cause cervical edema (which retards dilatation), possible tearing and bruising of the cervix, and maternal exhaustion.

Musculature Changes in the Pelvic Floor

The levator ani muscle and fascia of the pelvic floor draw the rectum and vagina upward and forward with each contraction, along the curve of the pelvic floor. As the fetal head descends to the pelvic floor, the pressure of the presenting part causes the perineal structure, which was once 5 cm in thickness, to change to a structure of less than a centimeter. A normal physiologic anesthesia is produced as a result of the decreased blood supply to the area. The anus everts, exposing the interior rectal wall as the fetal head descends forward (Pritchard, MacDonald, and Gant, 1985).

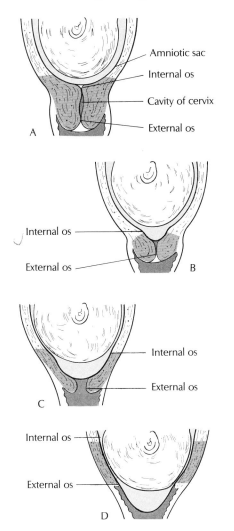

Figure 12-8 ▬▬▬▬▬▬▬▬▬
Effacement of the cervix in the primigravida. **A,** At the beginning of labor, there is no cervical effacement or dilatation. **B,** Beginning cervical effacement. **C,** Cervix is about one-half effaced and slightly dilated. **D,** Complete effacement and dilatation.

Premonitory Signs of Labor ▬▬▬▬▬▬▬▬▬▬▬▬▬▬▬

Most primigravidas and many multiparas experience the following signs and symptoms of impending labor.

Lightening

Lightening occurs because the fetus begins to settle into the pelvic inlet (engagement). With its descent, the uterus moves downward, and the fundus no longer presses on the diaphragm.

The woman can breathe more easily after lightening. With increased downward pressure of the presenting part, however, the woman may notice the following:

- Leg cramps or pains due to pressure on the nerves that course through the obturator foramen in the pelvis
- Increased pelvic pressure
- Increased venous stasis leading to dependent edema
- Increased vaginal secretions resulting from congestion of the vaginal mucous membranes

Braxton Hicks Contractions

Prior to the onset of labor, Braxton Hicks contractions, the irregular, intermittent contractions that have been occurring throughout the pregnancy may become uncomfortable. The pain seems to be in the abdomen and groin but may feel like the "drawing" sensations experienced by some with dysmenorrhea. When these contractions are strong enough for the woman to believe she is in labor, she is said to be in false labor. False labor is uncomfortable and may be exhausting as the woman wonders if "this is it." Since the contractions can be fairly regular, she has no way of knowing if they are the beginning of true labor. She may come to the hospital for a vaginal examination to determine if cervical dilatation is occurring. Frequent episodes of false labor and trips back and forth to the physician's office or hospital may frustrate or embarrass the woman, who feels that she should know when she is really in labor. Reassurance by nursing staff can ease embarrassment.

Cervical Changes

For some time, the softening (also called *ripening*) of the cervix was thought to be caused by increasing intensity of Braxton Hicks contractions. Liggins (1978) suggests that softening of the cervix begins in the second half of pregnancy. A few days before the onset of labor, the cervix becomes even more soft and begins to efface and dilate slightly. The mechanism for this ripening is biochemical and is the result of changes in the connective tissue of the cervix.

Bloody Show

The mucous plug is accumulated cervical secretions that have closed off the opening of the uterine cavity. With softening and effacement of the cervix, the mucous plug is often expelled, resulting in a small amount of blood loss from the exposed cervical capillaries. The resulting pink-tinged secretions are called **bloody show**.

Bloody show is considered a sign of imminent labor, which usually begins within 24–48 hours. Vaginal examination with manipulation of the cervix may also result in a blood-tinged discharge, which may be confused with bloody show.

Rupture of Membranes

In approximately 12% of women, the amniotic membranes rupture before the onset of labor. This is called **rupture of membranes (ROM)**. Labor usually begins within 24 hours for 80% of these women. Frequently, when labor does not begin within 12–24 hours after ROM it is induced if the pregnancy is near term (40 weeks).

When the membranes rupture, the amniotic fluid may be expelled in large amounts. If engagement has not occurred, the danger of the umbilical cord washing out with the fluid (called *prolapsed cord*) exists. In addition, the open pathway into the uterus causes danger of infection. Because of these threats, the woman is advised to notify her physician or nurse-midwife and proceed to the hospital. In some instances, the fluid is expelled in small amounts and may be confused with episodes of urinary incontinence associated with urinary urgency, coughing, or sneezing. The discharge should be checked to ascertain its source and to determine further action. (See Chapter 13 for assessment techniques.)

Sudden Burst of Energy

Some women report a sudden burst of energy approximately 24–48 hours before labor. They may do their spring housecleaning or rearrange all the furniture; these activities are often referred to as the *nesting instinct*. The cause of the energy spurt is unknown. The nurse in prenatal teaching should warn prospective mothers not to overexert themselves at this time so that they will not be excessively tired when labor begins.

Other Signs

Other premonitory signs include:

- Weight loss of 1–3 pounds resulting from fluid loss and electrolyte shifts produced by changes in estrogen and progesterone levels
- Increased backache and sacroiliac pressure from the influence of relaxin hormone on the pelvic joints
- Diarrhea, indigestion, or nausea and vomiting just prior to the onset of labor

The causes of these signs are unknown.

Differences Between True and False Labor

The contractions of true labor produce progressive dilatation and effacement of the cervix. They occur regularly and increase in frequency, duration, and intensity. The discomfort of true labor contractions usually starts in the back and radiates around to the abdomen. The pain is not relieved by ambulation (in fact, walking may intensify the pain).

The contractions of false labor do not produce progressive cervical effacement and dilatation. Classically, they are irregular and do not increase in frequency, duration, and intensity. The contractions may be perceived as a hardening or "balling up" without discomfort, or discomfort may occur mainly in the lower abdomen and groin. The discomfort may be relieved by ambulation.

The woman will find it helpful to know the characteristics of true labor contractions as well as the premonitory signs of ensuing labor. However, many times the only way to differentiate accurately between true and false labor is to assess dilatation. The woman must feel free to come in for accurate assessment of labor and should never be allowed to feel foolish if the labor is false. The nurse must reassure the woman that false labor is common and that it often cannot be distinguished from true labor except by vaginal examination. (See Essential Facts to Remember—Comparison of True and False Labor.)

Stages of Labor and Delivery

There are three stages of labor. The first stage begins with the beginning of true labor and ends when the cervix is completely dilated at 10 cm. The second stage begins with complete dilatation and ends with the birth of the infant.

 ESSENTIAL FACTS TO REMEMBER

Comparison of True and False Labor

True labor	False labor
Contractions are at regular intervals	Contractions are irregular
Intervals between contractions gradually shorten	Usually no change
Contractions increase in duration and intensity	Usually no change
Discomfort begins in back and radiates around to abdomen	Discomfort is usually in abdomen
Intensity usually increases with walking	Walking has no effect or lessens contractions
Cervical dilatation and effacement are progressive	No change

The third stage begins with the expulsion of the infant and ends with the delivery of the placenta.

Some clinicians identify a fourth stage of labor. During this stage, which lasts 1–4 hours after delivery of the placenta, the uterus effectively contracts to control bleeding at the placental site (Pritchard, MacDonald, and Gant, 1985).

The management of the laboring woman is discussed in Chapter 13.

First Stage

The first stage of labor is divided into the *latent* and the *active* phase. Friedman (1978) further divides the active phase into three stages according to cervical dilatation: acceleration phase, phase of maximum slope, and deceleration phase. In addition, Friedman distinguishes among three physiologic objectives of labor, calling them preparatory, dilatational, and pelvic divisions. The preparatory division includes the latent and acceleration phase. The dilatational division includes the phase of maximum slope. The pelvic division begins with the deceleration phase. Each phase of labor is characterized by physical and psychologic changes (Figure 12-9).

Latent phase   The latent phase begins with the onset of regular contractions. It can be graphed as a flat slope of cervical dilatation to about 3–4 cm. As the cervix begins to dilate, it also effaces, although little or no fetal descent is evident. For nulliparas, the latent phase averages 8.6 hours but should not exceed 20 hours. The latent phase in multiparas averages 5.3 hours but should not exceed 14 hours.

Uterine contractions become established during the latent phase and increase in frequency, duration, and intensity. They may start as mild contractions lasting 15–30 seconds with a frequency of 15–30 minutes and progress to moderate ones lasting 30–40 seconds with a frequency of 5–7 minutes. They average 40 mm Hg during acme from a baseline tonus of 10 mm Hg.

In the early or latent phase of the first stage of labor, contractions are usually mild. The client feels able to cope with the discomfort. She may be relieved that labor has finally started. Although she may be anxious, she is able to recognize and express those feelings of anx-

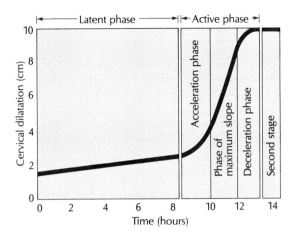

Figure 12-9

Composite of the average dilatation curve for nulliparous labor based on analysis of the date derived from the patterns traced by a large, nearly consecutive series of gravidas. The first stage is divided into a relatively flat latent phase and a rapidly progressive active phase. The active phase has three identifiable component parts—an acceleration phase, a linear phase of maximum slope, and a deceleration phase. (From Friedman, E. A. 1978. *Labor: Clinical evaluation and management*, 2nd ed. New York: Appleton-Century-Crofts, p. 33, Figure 3.)

iety. The woman is often talkative and smiling and is eager to talk about herself and answer questions. Excitement is high, and her partner or other support person is often as elated as the client.

Active phase   During the active phase, the cervix dilates from about 3–4 cm to 10 cm (complete dilatation). Fetal descent is progressive.

The active period begins with the *acceleration phase* as cervical dilatation changes from a flat slope (as in the latent phase) to an upward curve. The *phase of maximum slope* covers the period when cervical dilatation progresses from approximately 3–4 cm to 8 cm. The cervical dilatation should be at least 1.2 cm/hr in nulliparas, and 1.5 cm/hr in multiparas (Friedman, 1978).

The *deceleration phase* is the last part of the active phase. Cervical dilatation slows as it progresses from 8–10 cm and the rate of fetal descent increases. The average rate of descent is at least 1 cm/hr in nulliparas, and 2 cm/hr in multiparas. The deceleration phase should not be longer than 3 hours for nulliparas and 1 hour for multiparas (Friedman, 1978). The deceleration phase may be referred to as *transition*.

During the active phase, contractions become more frequent, are longer in duration, and increase in intensity. By the end of the active phase, contraction frequency is usually every 2–3 minutes. Contraction duration averages 60 seconds. The intensity is moderate or strong.

As the woman enters the early active phase, her anxiety tends to increase as she senses the fairly constant intensification of contractions and pain. She begins to fear a loss of control and may use coping mechanisms to maintain control. Some women exhibit decreased ability to cope and a sense of helplessness. Clients who have support persons available, particularly fathers, experience greater satisfaction and less anxiety throughout the birth process than those without these supports (Doering et al., 1980).

When the woman enters the deceleration (transition) phase, she may demonstrate significant anxiety. She becomes acutely aware of the increasing force and intensity of the contractions. She may become restless, frequently changing position. Because the most commonly expressed fear at this time is that of abandonment, it is crucial that the nurse be available as backup and relief for the support person. By the time the woman enters the active phase, she is inner-directed and, often, tired. At the same time, the support person may be feeling the need for a break. The woman should be reassured that she will not be left alone and should always be told where her support people are if they leave the room and where her nurse is should she need her.

The woman may also fear that she will be "torn open" or "split apart" by the force of the contractions (Kopp, 1971). Many clients experience a sensation of pressure so great with the peak of a contraction that it seems to them that their abdomens will burst open with the force. The woman should be informed that this is a normal sensation and reassured that such bursting will not happen.

By the time the woman reaches the deceleration phase (transition), she will most likely be withdrawn and inner-focused. Increasingly she may doubt her ability to cope with her labor. During the deceleration or transition phase, the woman may become apprehensive and irritable. The woman is often terrified of being left alone but also does not want anyone to talk to or touch her. However, with the next contraction, she may ask for verbal and physical support. Other characteristics may accompany this phase:

- Hyperventilation as the woman increases her breathing rate
- Restlessness
- Difficulty understanding directions
- A sense of bewilderment and anger at the contractions
- Statements that she "can't take it anymore"
- Requests for medication
- Hiccupping, belching, nausea, or vomiting
- Beads of perspiration on the upper lip
- Increasing rectal pressure

The woman in this phase is anxious to "get it over with." She may be amnesic and sleep between her now-frequent contractions. Her support persons may start to feel helpless and may turn to the nurse for increased participation as their efforts to alleviate her discomfort seem less effective.

As dilatation approaches completion, increased rectal pressure and uncontrollable desire to bear down, increased amount of bloody show, and rupture of membranes may occur.

Amniotic membranes   At the beginning of labor, the amniotic membranes bulge through the cervix in the shape of a cone. ROM generally occurs at the height of an intense contraction with a gush of the fluid out the introitus.

Second Stage

The second stage of labor (also called the expulsive stage) begins when the cervix is completely dilated (10 cm) and ends with delivery of the infant. The second stage should be completed within an hour after the cervix becomes fully dilated for primigravidas (multiparas average 15 minutes). Contractions are 60–90 seconds in duration, are strong in intensity, and have a frequency of 2–3 minutes. Descent of the fetal presenting part continues until it reaches the perineal floor.

As the fetal head descends, the woman has the urge to push because of pressure of the fetal head on the sacral and obturator nerves. As she pushes, intraabdominal pressure is exerted from contraction of the maternal abdominal muscles. As the fetal head continues its descent, the perineum begins to bulge, flatten, and move anteriorly. The amount of bloody show may increase. The labia begin to part with each contraction. Between contractions the fetal head appears to recede. With succeeding contractions and maternal pushing effort, the fetal head descends farther. **Crowning** occurs when the fetal head is encircled by the introitus and means delivery is imminent.

Usually, a childbirth-prepared woman feels relieved that the acute pain she felt during the transition phase is over (see Essential Facts to Remember—Characteristics of Labor). She also may be relieved that the delivery is near and she can now push. Some women feel a sense of control now that they can be actively involved. Others, particularly those without childbirth preparation, may become frightened. They tend to fight each contraction and any attempt of others to persuade them to push with contractions. Such behavior may be frightening and disconcerting to her support persons. The woman may feel she has lost control and become embarrassed and apologetic or she may demonstrate extreme irritability toward the staff or her supporters in an attempt to regain control over external forces against which she feels helpless.

Some women feel acute and increasingly severe pain as the perineum distends.

Spontaneous delivery (vertex presentation)   As the head distends the vulva with each contraction, the perineum becomes extremely thin and the anus stretches and protrudes. With assistance from the physician or nurse-midwife, the head is delivered slowly under the symphysis pubis, with the face sliding over the perineum. (See Chapter 14 for medical and nursing interventions to facilitate the delivery process.) After delivery of the head, restitution and external rotation of the head occurs. (See the discussion of fetal movement on p. 268.) When the anterior shoulder meets the underside of the symphysis pubis, gentle traction applied to the infant's head aids in delivery. The body then follows.

Delivery of infants in other than vertex presentations is discussed in Chapter 17.

Third Stage

Placental separation   After the infant is delivered, the uterus contracts firmly, diminishing its capacity and the surface area of placental attachment. The placenta begins to separate because of this decrease in surface area. As this separation occurs, bleeding results in the formation of a hematoma between the placental tissue and the remaining decidua. This hematoma accelerates the separation process. The membranes are the last to separate. They are

---

✷ ESSENTIAL FACTS TO REMEMBER

Characteristics of Labor

	First stage		Second stage
	LATENT PHASE	ACTIVE PHASE	
Nullipara	8½ hours	6 hours	1 hour
Multipara	5 hours	4½ hours	15 minutes
Cervical Dilatation	0 to 3–4 cm	4 to 10 cm	
Contractions Frequency	Every 15–30 minutes at the beginning and progressing to every 5–7 minutes	Every 4–5 minutes progressing to every 2–3 minutes	Every 2–3 minutes
Duration	30–45 seconds	60 seconds	60–90 seconds
Intensity	Begin as mild and progress to moderate	Begin as moderate and progress to strong	Strong

peeled off the uterine wall as the placenta extrudes into the vagina.

Signs of placental separation usually appear around 5 minutes after delivery of the infant. These signs are (a) a globular-shaped uterus, (b) a rise of the fundus in the abdomen, (c) a sudden gush or trickle of blood, and (d) further protrusion of the umbilical cord out of the introitus.

Placental delivery   When the signs of placental separation appear, the woman may bear down to aid in placental expulsion. If this fails and the clinician has ascertained that the fundus is firm, gentle traction may be applied to the cord while pressure is exerted on the fundus. The weight of the placenta as it is guided into the placental pan aids in the removal of the membranes from the uterine wall. A placenta is considered to be *retained* if 30 minutes have elapsed from completion of the second stage of labor.

If the placenta separates from the inside to the outer margins, it is delivered with the fetal or shiny side presenting (Figure 12-10). This is known as the *Schultze mechanism* of placental delivery, or more commonly *shiny Schultze*. If the placenta separates from the outer margins inward, it will roll up and present sideways with the maternal surface delivering first. This is known as the *Duncan mechanism* of placental delivery and is commonly called *dirty Duncan* because the placental surface is rough.

Nursing and medical interventions during the third stage of labor are discussed in detail in Chapter 13.

Fourth Stage

The fourth stage of labor is the time from 1–4 hours after delivery, in which physiologic readjustment of the mother's body begins. With the delivery, hemodynamic changes occur. Blood loss at delivery may be up to 500 mL. With this blood loss, and the lifting of the weight of the gravid uterus from surrounding vessels, blood is redistributed into venous beds. This results in a moderate drop in both systolic and diastolic blood pressure, increased pulse pressure, and moderate tachycardia (Cibils, 1981).

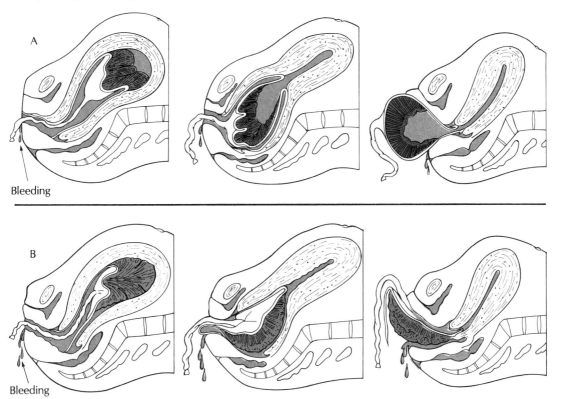

Figure 12-10

Placental separation and delivery. **A**, Schultze mechanism. **B**, Duncan mechanism.

The cerebrospinal fluid pressure, which increased during labor, now drops and rapidly returns to normal values (Cibils, 1981).

The uterus remains contracted and is in the midline of the abdomen. The fundus is usually midway between the symphysis pubis and umbilicus. Its contracted state constricts the vessels at the site of placental implantation. Immediately after delivery of the placenta, the cervix is widely spread and thick.

Nausea and vomiting usually cease. The woman may be thirsty and hungry. She may experience a shaking chill, which is thought to be associated with the ending of the physical exertion of labor. The bladder is often hypotonic due to trauma during the second stage and/or the administration of anesthetics that may decrease sensations. Hypotonic bladder leads to urinary retention. Management of this stage is discussed in Chapter 13.

Maternal Systemic Response to Labor

Cardiovascular System

A strong contraction greatly diminishes or completely stops the blood flow in the branches of the uterine artery, which supplies the intervillous space. This leads to a redistribution of the blood flow to the peripheral circulation and an increase in peripheral resistance. Increase of the systolic and diastolic blood pressure and a slowing of the pulse rate result. Changes in maternal blood pressure and pulse also depend on the woman's position.

Cardiac output is increased by 10%–15% during rest periods between contractions in early labor and by 30%–50% in the second stage (Albright, 1978). Additional increases and decreases in cardiac output mirror the changes in uterine pressure; that is, cardiac output increases as the contraction builds and peaks and slowly returns to precontraction levels as the contraction diminishes.

Immediately after delivery, cardiac output peaks with an 80% increase over prelabor values, and then in the first 10 minutes decreases by 20%–25%. Cardiac output further decreases by 20%–25% in the first hour after delivery (Albright, 1978).

Blood Pressure

As a result of increased cardiac output, systolic blood pressure rises during uterine contractions. In the immediate postpartal period, the arterial pressure remains essentially normal even though the cardiac output increases due to peripheral vasodilatation.

Approximately 10%–15% of women demonstrate clinical symptoms (hypotension, tachycardia) of vena cava syndrome. Some women with this syndrome are asymptomatic due to compensatory mechanisms. These women are at risk because even though they are initially asymptomatic, blood flow to the placenta is slowly compromised by vasoconstriction of the peripheral arteries (Albright, 1978).

Women with the highest risk of developing supine hypotensive syndrome are nulliparas with strong abdominal muscles and tightly drawn abdominal skin, gravidas with hydramnios and/or multiple pregnancy, and obese women. Other predisposing factors include hypovolemia, dehydration, hemorrhage, metabolic acidosis, administration of narcotics (which results in vasodilatation and inhibits compensatory mechanisms), and administration of regional anesthetics that results in *sympathetic blockade* (blocking of the sympathetic nervous system, which results in vasodilatation and hypotension).

Fluid and Electrolyte Balance

Profuse perspiration (diaphoresis) occurs during labor. Hyperventilation also occurs, altering electrolyte and fluid balance from insensible water loss. The muscle activity elevates the body temperature, which increases sweating and evaporation from the skin. As the woman responds to the work of labor the rise in the respiratory rate increases the evaporative water volume, since each breath of air must be warmed to the body temperature and humidified. With the increased evaporative water volume, giving parenteral fluids during labor to ensure adequate hydration becomes increasingly important.

Gastrointestinal System

During labor, gastric motility and absorption of solid food are reduced. Gastric-emptying time is prolonged. It is not uncommon for a laboring woman to vomit food she ate up to 12 hours earlier.

Respiratory System

Oxygen consumption, which increased approximately 20% during pregnancy, is further increased during labor. During the early first stage of labor, oxygen consumption increases 40%, with a further increase to 100% during the second stage.

Minute ventilation increases to 20–25 L/min (normal 10 L/min), and in the unprepared and unmedicated client it may reach 35 L/min or more. This hyperventilation results in a rise in the maternal pH in early labor, followed by a return to normal toward the end of the first stage. If the first stage is prolonged, the woman may develop acidosis (Albright, 1978).

Hemopoietic System

Leukocyte levels may reach 25,000/mm³ or more during labor. Although the precise cause of the leukocytosis is unknown, it may be due to the strenuous exercise and stress response of labor (Pritchard, MacDonald, and Gant, 1985). Blood glucose levels may decrease, as a result of increased activity of uterine and skeletal muscles (Varney, 1980).

Renal System

The base of the bladder is pushed forward and upward when engagement occurs. The pressure from the presenting part may impair blood and lymph drainage from the base of the bladder, leading to edema of the tissues (Pritchard, MacDonald, and Gant, 1985).

Approximately one-third to one-half of all laboring women have slight proteinuria of 1+ as a result of muscle breakdown from exercise. An increase to 2+ or above is indicative of pathology (Varney, 1980).

Pain

Theories of pain According to the *gate-control theory* (Melzack, 1973), pain results from activity in several interacting specialized neural systems. The gate-control theory proposes that a mechanism in the dorsal horn of the spinal column serves as a valve or gate that increases or decreases the flow of nerve impulses from the periphery to the central nervous system. The gate mechanism is influenced by the size of the transmitting fibers and by the nerve impulses that descend from the brain. Psychologic processes such as past experiences, attention, and emotion may influence pain perception and response by activating the gate mechanism. The gates may be opened or closed by central nervous system activities, such as anxiety or excitement, or through selective localized activity (Melzack, 1973).

The gate-control theory has two important implications for obstetrics: Pain may be controlled by tactile stimulation and can be modified by activities controlled by the central nervous system. These include suggestion, distraction, and conditioning.

Causes of pain during labor The pain associated with the first stage of labor is unique in that it accompanies a normal physiologic process. Even though perception of the pain of childbirth may vary among women, there is a physiologic basis for discomfort during labor. Pain during the first stage of labor arises from (a) dilatation of the cervix, which is the primary source of pain; (b) hypoxia of the uterine muscle cells during contraction; (c) stretching of the lower uterine segment; and (d) pressure on adjacent structures. The areas of pain include the lower abdominal wall and the areas over the lower lumbar region and the upper sacrum (Figure 12-11).

During the second stage of labor, discomfort is due to (a) hypoxia of the contracting uterine muscle cells, (b) distention of the vagina and perineum, and (c) pressure on adjacent structures. The area of pain increases as shown in Figures 12-12 and 12-13.

Pain during the third stage results from uterine contractions and cervical dilatation as the placenta is expelled. This stage of labor is short, and after this phase of labor, anesthesia is needed primarily for episiotomy repair.

Factors affecting response to pain Many factors affect the individual's perception of pain impulses. Individuals tend to respond to painful stimuli in the way that is acceptable in their culture. When assessing a client's need for assistance, the nurse must remember that there are many ways to respond to pain. The absence of

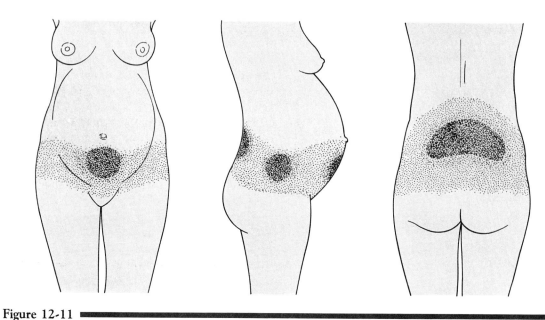

Figure 12-11

Area of reference of labor pain during the first stage. Density of stippling indicates intensity of pain. (From Bonica, J. J. 1972. *Principles and practice of obstetric* *analgesia and anesthesia*. Philadelphia: F. A. Davis Co., p. 108.)

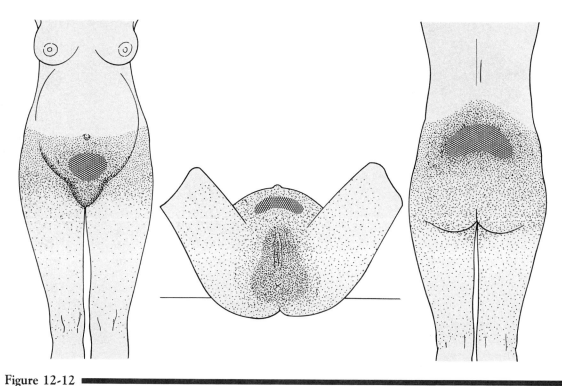

Figure 12-12

Distribution of labor pain during the later phase of the first stage and early phase of the second stage. Crosshatched areas indicate location of the most intense pain; dense stippling, moderate pain; and light stippling, mild pain. Note that the uterine con- tractions, which at this stage are very strong, produce intense pain. (From Bonica, J. J. 1972. *Principles and practice of obstetric analgesia and anesthesia*. Phil- adelphia: F. A. Davis Co., p. 109.)

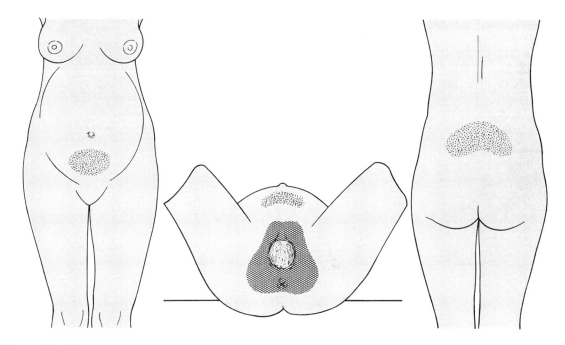

Figure 12-13

Distribution of labor pain during the later phase of the second stage and actual delivery. The perineal component is the main cause of discomfort. Uterine contractions contribute much less. (From Bonica, J. J. 1972. *Principles and practice of obstetric analgesia and anesthesia*. Philadelphia: F. A. Davis Co., p. 109.)

crying and moaning does not necessarily mean that pain is absent, nor does the presence of crying and moaning necessarily mean that pain relief is desired at that moment. In some cultures, it is natural to communicate pain, no matter how mild, while members of other cultures stoically accept pain out of fear or because it is expected.

Another factor that may influence response to pain is *fatigue and sleep deprivation*. The fatigued woman has less energy and ability to use such strategies as distraction or imagination to deal with pain. As a result, the fatigued woman may choose analgesics or other medications to relieve the discomfort.

The woman's *previous experience* with pain also affects her ability to manage current and future pain. Those who have had experience with pain seem more sensitive to painful stimuli than those who have not.

Anxiety can affect a woman's response to pain. Unfamiliar surroundings and events can increase anxiety as does separation from family and loved ones. Anticipation of discomfort and questions about whether she can cope with the contractions can also increase anxiety.

Fetal Response to Labor

When the fetus is normal, the mechanical and hemodynamic changes of normal labor have no adverse effects.

Biomechanical Changes

High pressures are exerted on the fetal head during contractions and to an even greater extent after ROM. During labor's second stage, the pressures may rise as high as 200 mm Hg (Aladjem, 1980).

Cardiac Changes

Fetal heart rate decelerations can occur with intracranial pressures of 40–55 mm Hg. The currently accepted explanation of this deceleration is hypoxic depression of the central nervous system, which is under vagal control. The absence of these head compression decelerations in some fetuses during labor is explained by the existence of a threshold that is reached more gradually in the presence of intact membranes and lack of maternal resistance. These changes are harmless in the normal fetus (Aladjem, 1980).

Hemodynamic Changes

The adequate exchange of nutrients and gases in the fetal capillaries and intervillous spaces depends in part on the fetal blood pressure. Fetal blood pressure is a protective mechanism for the normal fetus during the anoxic periods caused by the contracting uterus during labor. The fetal and placental reserve is enough to see the fetus through these anoxic periods unharmed (Aladjem, 1980).

Positional Changes

For the fetus to pass through the birth canal, the fetal head and body must adjust to the passage by certain positional changes. These changes, called **cardinal movments** or *mechanisms of labor*, are described in the order in which they occur (Figure 12-14).

Descent   Descent is thought to occur because of four forces: (a) pressure of the amniotic fluid, (b) direct pressure of the fundus on the breech, (c) contraction of the abdominal muscles, and (d) extension and straightening of the fetal body. The head enters the inlet in the occiput transverse or oblique position because the pelvic inlet is widest from side to side. The sagittal suture is an equal distance from the maternal symphysis pubis and sacral promontory.

Flexion   Flexion occurs as the fetal head descends and meets resistance from the soft tissues of the pelvis, the muscles of the pelvic floor, and the cervix.

Internal rotation   The fetal head must rotate to fit the diameter of the pelvic cavity, which is widest in the anteroposterior diameter. As the occiput of the fetal head meets resistance from the levator ani muscles and their fascia, the occiput rotates from left to right and the sagittal suture aligns in the anteroposterior pelvic diameter.

Extension   The resistance of the pelvic floor and the mechanical movement of the vulva opening anteriorly and forward assist with extension of the fetal head as it passes under the symphysis pubis. With this positional change, the occiput, then brow and face, emerge from the introitus.

Restitution   The shoulders of the infant enter the pelvis obliquely and remain oblique

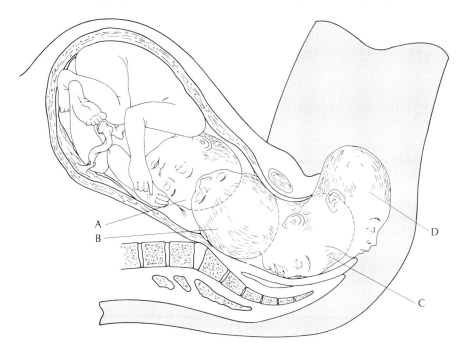

Figure 12-14 ▬▬▬▬▬▬▬▬▬▬▬▬▬▬▬▬▬▬▬▬▬▬▬▬▬▬▬▬▬▬▬▬▬▬▬
Mechanism of labor. **A**, Descent. **B**, Flexion. **C**, Internal rotation. **D**, Extension. (External rotation not shown.)

when the head rotates to the anteroposterior diameter through internal rotation. Because of this rotation, the neck becomes twisted. Once the head delivers and is free of pelvic resistance, the neck untwists, turning the head to one side (restitution), and aligns with the position of the back in the birth canal.

External rotation   As the shoulders rotate to the anteroposterior position in the pelvis, the head is turned farther to one side (external rotation).

Expulsion   After the external rotation and through the pushing efforts of the laboring woman, the anterior shoulder meets the undersurface of the symphysis pubis and slips under it. As lateral flexion of the shoulder and head occurs, the anterior shoulder is born before the posterior shoulder. The body follows quickly (Oxorn, 1980).

The adaptations of the newborn to extrauterine life are discussed in Chapter 19.

Summary ───────────────────

The wonderful phenomenon of labor—the process of birth—is a period of transition for the pregnant woman. Delivery is the climax. A competent maternity nurse must understand the physiologic and psychologic changes during normal labor and delivery to support the childbearing family and intervene appropriately.

References ───────────────────

Aladjem S: *Obstetric Practice*. St. Louis: Mosby, 1980.

Albright GA: *Anesthesia in Obstetrics: Maternal, Fetal and Neonatal Aspects*. Menlo Park, Calif.: Addison-Wesley, 1978.

Caldwell WE, Moloy HC: Anatomical variations in the female pelvis and their effect on labor with a suggested classification. *Am J Obstet Gynecol* 1933; 26:479.

Challis JR, Mitchell BF: Hormonal control of preterm and term parturition. *Semin Perinatol* July 1981; 5:192.

Cibils LA: *Electronic Fetal-Neonatal Monitoring*. Boston: PSG, Inc, 1981.

Colman AD, Colman LL: *Pregnancy: The Psychological Experience*. New York: Herder & Herder, 1971.

Danforth D (editor): *Textbook of Obstetrics and Gynecology*, 4th ed. Philadelphia: Harper & Row, 1982.

Doering SG, Entwisle DR: Preparation during pregnancy and ability to cope with labor and delivery. *Am J Orthopsychiatry* 1975; 45:825.

Doering SG et al: Modeling the quality of women's birth experience. *J Health Social Behavior* March 1980; 21:12.

Friedman EA: *Labor: Clinical Evaluation and Management*, 2nd ed. New York: Appleton-Century-Crofts, 1978.

Humenick SS: Mastery: The key to childbirth satisfaction? A review. *Birth Fam J* Summer 1981; 8:79.

Kopp LM: Ordeal or ideal—the second stage of labor. *Am J Nurs* 1971; 71:1140.

Liggins GC: Fetal influences on myometrial contractility. *Clin Obstet Gynecol* 1978; 16:148.

Melzack R: *The Puzzle of Pain*. New York: Basic Books, 1973.

Mercer RA: A theoretical framework for studying factors that impact on the maternal role. *Nurs Res* March/April 1981; 30:73.

Oxorn H: *Human Labor and Birth*. New York: Appleton-Century-Crofts, 1980.

Pritchard J, MacDonald PC, Gant NF: *Williams Obstetrics*, 17th ed. New York: Appleton-Century-Crofts, 1985.

Takahashi K, Burd L: Initiation of labor. In: *Gynecology and Obstetrics*. Sciarri JJ (editor). Philadelphia: Harper & Row, 1980.

Varney H: *Nurse-Midwifery*. Boston: Blackwell Scientific Publications, 1980.

Westbrook MT: Socioeconomic differences in coping with childbearing. *Am J Community Psychol* 1979; 7:397.

Additional Readings ───────────

Davis JA: The place of birth. *Arch Dis Child* June 1982; 57:406.

Fullerton JDT: Choice of in-hospital or alternative birth environment as related to the concept of control. *J Nurse Midwifery*, March/April 1982; 27:17.

Garfield RE et al: Appearance of gap junctions in the myometrium of women during labor. *Am J Obstet Gynecol* June 1981; 140:154.

Goodlin RC et al: Determinants of maternal temperature during labor. *Am J Obstet Gynecol* May 1982; 143:97.

Griffith S: Childbearing and the concept of culture. *J Obstet Gynecol Neonatal Nurs* May/June 1982; 11:181.

Huszar G et al: Biochemistry and pharmacology of the myometrium and labor: Regulation at the cellular and molecular levels. *Am J Obstet Gynecol* January 1982; 142:225.

Lavery JP et al: The effect of labor on the rheologic response of chorioamniotic membranes. *Obstet Gynecol* July 1982; 60:87.

McKay S: Maternity care in China; Report of a 1982 tour of Chinese medical facilities. *Birth* Summer 1982; 9:105.

Murata Y: Advances on the horizon. *Clin Perinatol* June 1982; 9:433.

Okita JR et al: Initiation of human parturition. *Am J Obstet Gynecol* February 1982; 142:432.

Richardson P: Significant relationships and their impact on childbearing: A review. *Matern Child Nurs J* Spring 1982; 11:17.

Scott-Palmer J et al: Pain during childbirth and menstruation: A study of locus of control. *J Psychosom Res* 1981; 25:151.

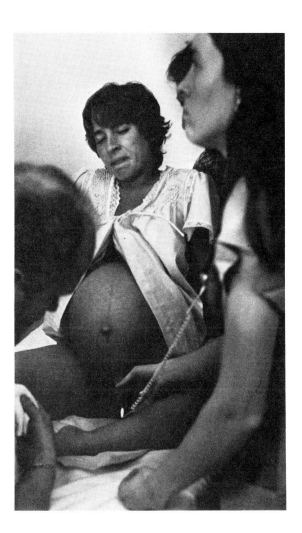

13

Intrapartal Nursing ━━━ Assessment

Chapter Contents ▰

Maternal Assessment
   History
   Intrapartal High-Risk Screening
   Intrapartal Physical Assessment
   Intrapartal Psychologic Assessment
   Methods of Evaluating Labor Progress

Fetal Assessment
   Fetal Position
   Evaluation of Fetal Status During Labor

Objectives ▰

- Discuss intrapartal physical and psychologic assessment.

- Identify the methods used to evaluate the progress of labor.

- Describe the procedure for performing Leopold's maneuvers and the information that may be obtained.

- Differentiate between baseline and periodic changes and describe the appearance of each and their significance.

- Outline steps to be performed in the systematic evaluation of fetal heart rate tracings.

- Identify nonreassuring fetal heart rate patterns and nursing interventions that should be carried out in the management of fetal distress.

- Discuss the indications for fetal blood sampling and state related pH values.

- Discuss psychologic reactions to electronic fetal monitoring.

Key Terms ▬▬▬▬▬

acceleration	fetal bradycardia
baseline rate	fetal tachycardia
baseline variability	Leopold's maneuvers
deceleration	sinusoidal pattern
fetal blood sampling	

The physiologic events that occur during labor call for many adaptations by the mother and fetus. Accurate and frequent assessment is crucial because the changes are rapid and involve two individuals, mother and child.

The number and effectiveness of intrapartal assessment techniques have increased over the years. In the past, observation, palpation, and auscultation were the only assessment techniques available. In current practice, these techniques are enhanced by the use of ultrasound and electronic monitoring. These tools can provide more detailed information and assessment.

Maternal Assessment ▬▬▬▬

History

A brief history is obtained from the woman when she is admitted to the labor and delivery area. Each agency has its own admission form but the following information is usually obtained:

- Woman's name and age

- Attending physician or certified nurse-midwife

- Personal data: blood type; Rh factor; results of serology testing; prepregnant and present weight; allergies to medications, foods, or substances; and medications taken during pregnancy

- History of previous illness, such as tuberculosis, heart disease, diabetes, convulsive disorders, thyroid disorders

- Problems in the prenatal period, such as elevated blood pressure, bleeding problems, recurrent urinary tract infection

- Pregnancy data: gravida, para, abortions, neonatal deaths

- The method the woman has chosen for infant feeding

- Attendance at prenatal education classes

- Woman's requests regarding labor and delivery, such as no enema, no analgesics or anesthetics, or the presence of the father in the delivery room

Intrapartal High-Risk Screening

Screening for intrapartal high-risk factors is an integral part of assessing the normal laboring woman. As the history is obtained, the nurse notes the presence of any factors that may be associated with a high-risk condition. For example, the woman who reports intermittent bleeding needs further assessment before the admission process continues. In addition to identifying the presence of a high-risk condition, the nurse must recognize the implications of the condition for the laboring woman and her fetus. A partial list of intrapartal risk factors is presented in Table 13-1. The factors precede the Intrapartal Physical Assessment Guide because they must be kept in mind during the assessment.

Intrapartal Physical Assessment

A physical examination is part of the admission procedure and part of the ongoing care of the client. Although the intrapartal physical assessment is not as complete and thorough as the initial prenatal physical examination (Chapter 6), the former involves assessment of some body systems and the actual labor process. The accompanying Intrapartal Physical Assessment Guide provides a framework the maternity nurse can use when examining the laboring woman.

The guide includes assessments performed immediately on admission and on an ongoing basis. Critical assessments include vital signs, labor status, fetal status, laboratory findings, and psychologic status. These assessments are continued throughout the labor process (see the Intrapartal Physical Assessment Guide, p. 274).

Table 13-1
Intrapartal High-Risk Factors

Factor	Maternal implication	Fetal/neonatal implication
Abnormal presentation	↑ Risk cesarean delivery ↑ Risk prolonged labor	Cesarean delivery Prematurity ↑ Risk congenital abnormality Neonatal physical trauma
Multiple gestation	↑ Uterine distention→ ↑ risk postpartum hemorrhage ↑ Risk premature labor	Low birth weight Prematurity Fetus to fetus transfusion
Hydramnios	↑ Discomfort ↑ Distention	↑ Risk esophageal or other high alimentary tract atresias ↑ Risk CNS anomalies (myelocele)
Oligohydramnios	Maternal fear of "dry birth"	↑ Risk congenital anomalies ↑ Risk renal lesions Postmaturity
Meconium staining of amniotic fluid	↑ Psychologic stress due to fear for fetus	Fetal asphyxia ↑ Risk meconium aspiration ↑ Risk pneumonia due to aspiration of meconium
Premature rupture of membranes (48 hours)	↑ Risk infection (amnionitis)	↑ Risk infection Prematurity
Premature labor	Fear for baby	Prematurity Respiratory distress syndrome Prolonged hospitalization
Induction-tetanic contractions	↑ Risk hypercontractility of uterus ↑ Risk uterine rupture	Prematurity if gestational age not assessed correctly Hypoxia
Abruptio placentae-placenta previa	Hemorrhage ↓ Uterine contractions after delivery	Fetal asphyxia Fetal exsanguination ↑ Perinatal mortality
Prolonged labor	Maternal exhaustion	Fetal asphyxia Intracranial birth injury
Precipitous labor (<3 hr)	Perineal lacerations	Tentorial tears Neonatal asphyxia
Prolapse of umbilical cord	↑ Fear for fetus	Fetal asphyxia
Fetal heart aberrations	↑ Fear for fetus	Tachycardia, acute asphyxic insult, bradycardia Chronic asphyxia Congenital heart disease
Uterine rupture	Hemorrhage Death	Fetal asphyxia Fetal hemorrhage Fetal death

Text continued on p. 279.

INTRAPARTAL PHYSICAL ASSESSMENT GUIDE: FIRST STAGE OF LABOR

Assess/Normal findings	Alterations and possible causes of alterations*	Nursing responses to data base†
VITAL SIGNS Blood pressure: 90–140/60–90 or no more than 15–20 mm Hg rise over baseline BP during early pregnancy	High blood pressure (essential hypertension, preeclampsia, renal disease, apprehension or anxiety) Low blood pressure (supine hypotension)	Evaluate history of preexisting disorders and check for presence of other signs of preeclampsia Turn woman on her side and recheck blood pressure Do not assess during contractions; implement measures to decrease anxiety and then reassess
Pulse: 60–90 beats/min	Increased pulse rate (excitement or anxiety, cardiac disorders)	Evaluate cause, reassess to see if rate continues; report to physician
Respirations: 6–24/min (or pulse rate divided by 4)	Marked tachypnea (respiratory disease) Hyperventilation (anxiety)	Assess between contractions; if marked tachypnea continues, assess for signs of respiratory disease Encourage slow breaths if woman is hyperventilating
Temperature: 36.2–37.6C (98–99.6F)	Elevated temperature (infection, dehydration)	Assess for other signs of infection or dehydration
WEIGHT 15–30 lb greater than pre-pregnant weight	Weight gain > 30 lb (fluid retention, obesity, large infant, hypertension of pregnancy)	Assess for signs of edema
FUNDUS At 40 weeks' gestation, located just below xyphoid process	Uterine size not compatible with estimated delivery time (SGA, hydramnios, multiple pregnancy)	Reevaluate history regarding pregnancy dating. Refer to physician for additional assessment
EDEMA Slight amount of dependent edema	Pitting edema of face, legs, abdomen (preeclampsia)	Check deep tendon reflexes for hyperactivity, check for clonus; refer to physician
HYDRATION Normal skin turgor	Poor skin turgor (dehydration)	Assess skin turgor; refer to physician for deviations
PERINEUM Tissues smooth, pink color (see Prenatal Initial Physical Assessment Guide, Chapter 9)	Varicose veins of vulva	Exercise care while doing a perineal prep; note on client record need for follow-up in postpartal period; reassess after delivery
Clear mucus	Profuse, purulent drainage	Suspect gonorrhea; report to physician; initiate care to newborn's eyes; notify neonatal nursing staff and pediatrician

*Possible causes of alterations are placed in parentheses.
†This column provides guidelines for further assessment and initial nursing interventions.

INTRAPARTAL PHYSICAL ASSESSMENT GUIDE (continued)

Assess/Normal findings	Alterations and possible causes of alterations*	Nursing responses to data base†
Presence of small amount of bloody show that gradually increases with further cervical dilatation	Hemorrhage	Assess BP and pulse, pallor, diaphoresis; report any marked changes (Note: Gaping of vagina and/or anus and bulging of perineum are suggestive signs of second stage of labor)
LABOR STATUS Uterine contractions: Regular pattern	Failure to establish a regular pattern, prolonged latent phase Hypertonicity Hypotonicity	Evaluate whether client is in true labor; ambulate if in early labor Evaluate client status and contractile pattern
Cervical dilatation: Progressive cervical dilatation from size of fingertip to 10 cm (Procedure 13-1, p. 277)	Rigidity of cervix (frequent cervical infections, scar tissue, failure of presenting part to descend)	Evaluate contractions, fetal engagement, position, and cervical dilatation. Inform client of progress
Cervical effacement: Progressive thinning of cervix (Procedure 13-1)	Failure to efface (rigidity of cervix, failure of presenting part to engage); cervical edema (pushing effort by woman before cervix is fully dilated and effaced, trapped cervix)	Evaluate contractions, fetal engagement, and position Notify physician/nurse-midwife if cervix is becoming edematous; work with client to prevent pushing until cervix is completely dilated
Fetal descent: Progressive descent of fetal presenting part from station −5 to +4 (see Figure 13-2)	Failure of descent (abnormal fetal position or presentation, macrosomic fetus, inadequate pelvic measurement)	Evaluate fetal position, presentation, and size Evaluate maternal pelvic measurements
Membranes: May rupture before or during labor	Rupture of membranes more than 12–24 hours before initiation of labor	Assess for ruptured membranes using Nitrazine test tape before doing vaginal exam Instruct clients with ruptured membranes to remain on bed rest if presenting part is not engaged Keep vaginal exams to a minimum to prevent infection
Findings on Nitrazine test tape: Membranes probably intact yellow pH 5.0 olive pH 5.5 olive green pH 6.0 Membranes probably ruptured blue-green pH 6.5 blue-gray pH 7.0 deep blue pH 7.5	False-positive results may be obtained if large amount of bloody show is present or if previous vaginal examination has been done using lubricant	Assess fluid for consistency, amount, odor; assess FHR frequently. Assess fluid at regular intervals for presence of meconium staining

*Possible causes of alterations are placed in parentheses.
†This column provides guidelines for further assessment and initial nursing interventions.

INTRAPARTAL PHYSICAL ASSESSMENT GUIDE (continued)

Assess/Normal findings	Alterations and possible causes of alterations*	Nursing responses to data base†
Amniotic fluid clear, no odor	Greenish amniotic fluid (fetal distress)	Assess FHR; do vaginal exam to evaluate for prolapsed cord; apply fetal monitor for continuous data; report to physician
	Strong odor (amnionitis)	Take client's temperature and report to physician
FETAL STATUS FHR: 120–160 beats/min	<120 or >160 beats/min (fetal distress); abnormal patterns on fetal monitor: decreased variability, late decelerations, variable decelerations (p. 286)	Initiate interventions based on particular FHR pattern (p. 290)
Presentation: Cephalic, 97% Breech, 3%	Face or brow presentation	Report to physician; after presentation is confirmed as face or brow, client may be prepared for cesarean delivery
Position: LOA most common	Persistent occipital-posterior position; transverse arrest	Carefully monitor maternal and fetal status
Activity: Fetal movement	Hyperactivity (may precede fetal hypoxia)	Carefully evaluate FHR; may apply fetal monitor
	Complete lack of movement (fetal distress or fetal demise)	Carefully evaluate FHR; may apply fetal monitor
LABORATORY EVALUATION Hematologic tests Hemoglobin: 12–16 g/dL	< 12 g (anemia, hemorrhage)	Evaluate woman for problems due to decreased oxygen-carrying capacity caused by lowered hemoglobin
CBC Hematocrit: 38%–47% RBC: 4.2–5.4 million/µL WBC: 4,500–11,000/µL although leukocytosis to 20,000/µL is not unusual	Presence of infection or blood dyscrasias	Evaluate for other signs of infection or for petechia, bruising, or unusual bleeding
Serologic testing STS or VDRL test: Nonreactive	Positive reaction (see Chapter 6, Initial Prenatal Physical Assessment Guide)	For reactive test, notify newborn nursery and pediatrician
Urinalysis Glucose: Negative	Glycosuria (low renal threshold for glucose, diabetes mellitus)	Assess blood glucose; test urine for ketones; ketonuria and glycosuria require further assessment of blood sugars‡
Ketones: Negative	Ketonuria (starvation ketosis)	

*Possible causes of alterations are placed in parentheses.
†This column provides guidelines for further assessment and initial nursing interventions.
‡Glycosuria should not be discounted. The presence of glycosuria necessitates follow-up.

INTRAPARTAL PHYSICAL ASSESSMENT GUIDE (continued)

Assess/Normal findings	Alterations and possible causes of alterations*	Nursing responses to data base†
Proteins: Negative	Proteinuria (urine specimen contaminated with vaginal secretions, fever, kidney disease); proteinuria of 2+ or greater found in uncontaminated urine may be a sign of ensuing preeclampsia	Instruct client in collection technique; incidence of contamination from vaginal discharge is common
Red blood cells: Negative	Blood in urine (calculi, cystitis, glomerulonephritis, neoplasm)	Assess collection technique
White blood cells: Negative	Presence of white blood cells (infection in genitourinary tract)	Assess for signs of urinary tract infection
Casts: None	Presence of casts (nephrotic syndrome)	

*Possible causes of alterations are placed in parentheses.
†This column provides guidelines for further assessment and initial nursing interventions.

PROCEDURE 13-1
Intrapartal Vaginal Examination

Objective	Nursing action	Rationale
Prepare client	Explain procedure, indications for carrying out procedure, and information being obtained	Explanation of procedure decreases anxiety and increases relaxation
	Position client with thighs flexed and abducted; instruct her to put heels of feet together	Prevents contamination of area during examination and allows for visualization of external signs of labor progress
	Drape so that only the perineum is exposed	Provides as much privacy as possible
	Encourage her to relax her muscles and legs during procedure	
Assemble and prepare equipment	Have following equipment easily accessible: • Sterile disposable gloves • Lubricant • Nitrazine tape test prior to first examination	Examination is facilitated and can be done quickly
Use aseptic technique during examination	If leakage of fluid has been noted or if client reports leakage of fluid, use Nitrazine test tape before doing vaginal exam	Nitrazine test tape registers a change in pH if amniotic fluid is present (unless a lubricant has already been used)
	Put on both gloves; using thumb and forefinger of left hand, spread labia widely, insert well-lubricated second and index fingers of right hand into vagina until they touch the cervix	Avoid contaminating hand by contact with anus; positioning of hand with wrist straight and elbow tilted downward allows fingertips to point toward umbilicus and find cervix

Continued

PROCEDURE 13-1 (continued)
Intrapartal Vaginal Examination

Objective	Nursing action	Rationale
Determine status of fetal membranes	Palpate for movable bulging sac through the cervix; observe for expression of amniotic fluid during exam	If intact, bag of waters feels like a bulge
Determine status of labor progress during and after contractions	Carry out vaginal examination during and between contractions	Examination varies
Identify degree of: 1. Cervical dilatation	Palpate for opening or what appears as a depression in the cervix	Estimation of the diameter of the depression identifies degree of dilatation
	Estimate diameter of cervical opening in centimeters (0–10cm)	One finger represents approximately 1.5–2 cm cervical dilatation
2. Cervical effacement	Palpate the thickness of the surrounding circular ridge of tissue; estimate degree of thinning in percentages	Degree of thinning determines the amount of lower uterine segment that has been taken up into the fundal area
Determine presentation and position of presenting part	As cervix opens, palpate for presenting part and identify its relationship to the maternal pelvis (Figures 13-1 and 13-2)	Presenting part is easier to palpate through a dilated cervix and differentiation of landmarks is easier
Determine station	Locate lowest portion of presenting part	Identification of station provides information as to degree of descent
Inform client about progress in labor	Discuss with client findings of the vaginal examination and correlate them to her progress in labor	Assists the client in identifying progress and reinforces need for frequency of procedure Information is reassuring and supportive for client and family

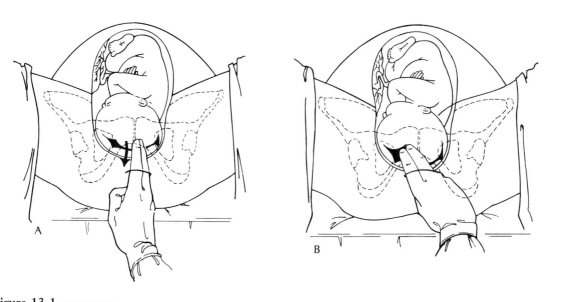

Figure 13-1

Assessment of fetal position and station. **A,** Palpate sagittal suture and assess station. **B,** Identify anterior fontanelle.

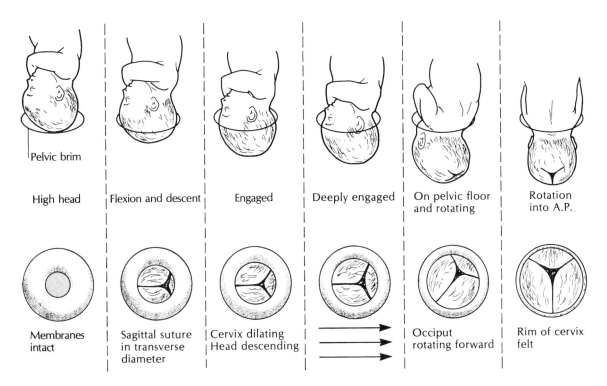

High head	Flexion and descent	Engaged	Deeply engaged	On pelvic floor and rotating	Rotation into A.P.
Pelvic brim					
Membranes intact	Sagittal suture in transverse diameter	Cervix dilating Head descending		Occiput rotating forward	Rim of cervix felt

Figure 13-2

Top, the fetal head progressing through the pelvis. *Bottom*, the changes that the nurse will detect on palpation of the occiput through the cervix while doing a vaginal examination. (From Myles MF: *Textbook for Midwives*. Edinburgh, Scotland: Churchill Livingstone, 1975, p. 246.)

Intrapartal Psychologic Assessment

Assessing the laboring woman's psychologic status is an important part of the total assessment. The woman has previous ideas, knowledge, and fears about childbearing. By assessing her psychologic status, the nurse can meet the woman's needs for information and support.

The nurse can support the woman and her partner or, in the absence of a partner, the nurse may become the support person. See the accompanying Intrapartal Psychologic Assessment Guide.

INTRAPARTAL PSYCHOLOGIC ASSESSMENT GUIDE

Assess/Normal findings	Alterations and possible causes of alterations*	Nursing response to data base†
SUPPORT SYSTEM Physical intimacy of mother-father (or mother-support relationship): Care-taking activities such as soothing conversation, touching	Limited physical contact or continual clinging together (may reflect normal pattern for this couple or their attempt to cope with this situation)	Encourage care-taking activities that appear to comfort the woman; encourage support to the woman; if support is limited, the nurse may take a more active role

*Possible causes of alterations are placed in parentheses.
†This column provides guidelines for further assessment and nursing interventions.

INTRAPARTAL PSYCHOLOGIC ASSESSMENT GUIDE (continued)

Assess/Normal findings	Alterations and possible causes of alterations*	Nursing response to data base†
Support person stays in close proximity	Maintaining a distance from woman for prolonged periods (may be normal pattern for this couple or may indicate strained relationship or anxiety due to labor)	Encourage support person to stay close (if this seems appropriate)
Relationship of mother-father (or support person): Involved interaction	Limited interaction (may reflect normal interaction pattern or strained relationship)	Support interactions; if interaction is limited, the nurse may provide more information and support
ANXIETY Some anxiety and apprehension is within normal limits	Rapid breathing, nervous tremors, frowning, grimacing or clenching of teeth, thrashing movements, crying, increased pulse and blood pressure (anxiety, apprehension)	Provide support and encouragement
PREPARATION FOR CHILDBIRTH Client has some information regarding process of normal labor and delivery	Insufficient information	Add to present information base
Client has breathing and/or relaxation techniques to use during labor	No breathing or relaxation techniques (insufficient information)	Support breathing and relaxation techniques that client is using; provide information if needed
RESPONSE TO LABOR Latent phase: relaxed, excited, anxious for labor to be well established	Inability to cope with contractions (fear, anxiety, lack of education)	Provide support and encouragement; establish trusting relationship
Active phase: becomes more intense, begins to tire		
Transitional phase: feels tired, may feel unable to cope, needs frequent coaching to maintain breathing patterns		Provide support and coaching if needed
Coping mechanisms: Ability to cope with labor through utilization of support system, breathing, relaxation techniques	Marked anxiety, apprehension (insufficient coping mechanisms)	Support coping mechanisms if they are working for the client; provide information and support if client is exhibiting anxiety or needs additional alternatives to present coping methods

*Possible causes of alterations are placed in parentheses.
†This column provides guidelines for further assessment and initial nursing interventions.

Methods of Evaluating Labor Progress

Contraction assessment   Uterine contractions may be assessed by palpation and/or continuous electronic monitoring.

Palpation   Contractions are assessed for frequency, duration, and intensity by placing one hand on the uterine fundus. The hand is kept relatively still because excessive movement may stimulate contractions or cause discomfort. To determine contraction duration, the nurse notes the time when tensing of the fundus is first felt (beginning of contraction) and again as relaxation occurs (end of contraction). During the acme of the contraction, intensity can be evaluated by estimating the indentability of the fundus. At least three successive contractions should be assessed to provide enough data to determine the contraction pattern. Frequency is determined by noting the time from the beginning of one contraction to the beginning of the next. Thus, if contractions are noted at 7:00, 7:04, and 7:08, their frequency is every 4 minutes.

Electronic monitoring   Electronic monitoring of the uterine contractions provides continuous data. In many agencies, electronic monitoring is routine for all high-risk clients and women who are having oxytocin-induced labor.

External monitoring with tocodynamometer   The tocodynamometer provides an indirect method of monitoring uterine activity. This instrument contains a flexible disk that responds to pressure. This disk is strapped to the woman's abdomen directly over the fundus, which is the area of greatest contractility. The disk records the external tension exerted by contractions (Figure 13-3). The pressure is amplified and recorded on graph paper.

The advantages of this method are: (a) it may be used prior to ROM antepartally and intrapartally, and (b) it provides a continuous recording of the duration and frequency of contractions. The disadvantages are: (a) this method does not record the magnitude or intensity of a contraction, and (b) the woman may be bothered by the strap, which requires frequent readjustment when she changes position.

Internal monitoring of uterine pressure during labor is discussed on page 286.

Cervical assessment   Cervical dilatation and effacement are evaluated directly by sterile vaginal examination (see Procedure 13-1, Intrapartal Vaginal Examination). The vaginal examination can also provide information about membrane status, fetal position, and station of the presenting part.

Using the Friedman graph   Evaluation of the intensity, frequency, and duration of contractions does not present the entire labor picture. Nurses can document labor progress objectively by using the Friedman graph, which evaluates uterine activity, cervical dilatation, and fetal descent.

To use the Friedman graph, one needs special graph paper and skill in determining cervical dilatation and fetal descent. The numbers at the bottom of the graph in Figure 13-4 are hours of labor from 1 to 16. Vertically, at the

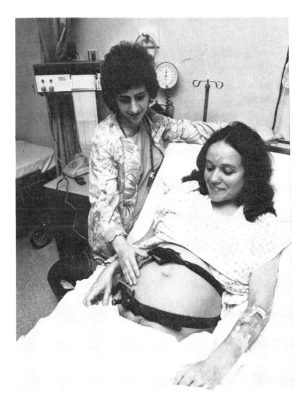

Figure 13-3
Client with external monitor applied.

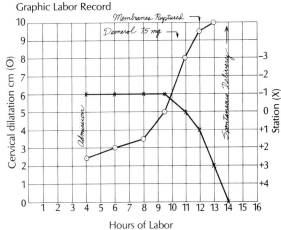

Figure 13-4
Example of charting labor progress on a Friedman graph. (Modified with permission; Friedman, Emanuel A., "An Objective Method of Evaluating Labor," *Hospital Practice* 5:7 1970. Chart by Albert Miller.)

left, cervical dilatation is measured from 0 to 10 cm. The vertical line on the right indicates fetal station in centimeters, from −5 to +5 (Friedman, 1970). When one plots cervical dilatation and descent on the basic graph, a characteristic pattern emerges: An S curve represents dilatation and an inverse S curve represents descent.

To determine the appropriate point to begin plotting data, the nurse must know how many hours the woman has been having regular contractions. When the laboring woman enters the hospital, she is asked at what time regular contractions began. A sterile vaginal examination determines cervical dilatation and the station of the presenting part of the fetus. This information is plotted on the graph. In the example shown in Figure 13-4, on admission the cervix was dilated 2–3 cm after 4 hours of labor, and the station was −1. Later examinations are noted on the graph. When the client was in the eleventh hour of labor, the graph indicates that cervical dilatation was 8 cm and the station was zero. At 14 hours of labor, she delivered spontaneously, as the graph shows.

The progress of cervical dilatation (in centimeters) per hour (or maximum slope of active dilatation) can be calculated as follows: Divide the difference between two consecutive observations by the intervening time interval to obtain the value for the slope in centimeters per hour. For example, in the case illustrated in Figure 13-4, at 9½ hours of labor, the cervix dilated to 5 cm. At 11 hours of labor, the cervix dilated to 8 cm. The difference is 3 cm. Divide the difference by the intervening time interval, which is 1½ hours: 3 cm ÷ 1½ = 2 cm/hr.

Evaluating labor progress by using the Friedman graph helps the health care team identify normal and abnormal labor patterns.

Fetal Assessment

Fetal Postition

Fetal position is determined in several ways. The woman's abdomen is inspected and palpated to determine fetal position; also, auscultation of fetal heart tones helps determine fetal position. A vaginal examination may be done to determine the presenting part, and ultrasound examination may be used.

Inspection   The nurse should observe the woman's abdomen for size and shape. The lie of the fetus should be assessed by noting whether the uterus projects up and down (longitudinal lie) or left to right (transverse lie).

Palpation   Leopold's maneuvers are a systematic way to evaluate the maternal abdomen. Frequent practice increases the examiner's skill in determining fetal position by palpation. Leopold's maneuvers may be difficult to perform on an obese woman or on a woman who has excessive amniotic fluid (hydramnios).

Before performing Leopold's maneuvers:

1. Have the woman empty her bladder.
2. Have the woman lie on her back with her feet on the bed and her knees bent.

First manuever   Face the client. Palpate the upper abdomen with both hands. Note the shape, consistency, and mobility of the palpated part. The fetal head is firm, hard, and round and moves independently of the trunk. The breech (buttocks) feels softer and it moves with the trunk.

Second manuever   Moving the hands down toward the pelvis, palpate the abdomen with gentle but deep pressure. The fetal back, on one side of the abdomen, feels smooth, and the fetal arms, legs, and feet, on the other side, feel knobby and bumpy.

Third manuever   Place one hand just above the symphysis. Note whether the part palpated feels like the fetal head or the breech and whether the presenting part is engaged.

Fourth maneuver   Face the client's feet. Place both hands on the lower abdomen, and move the fingers of both hands gently down the sides of the uterus toward the pubis. Note the cephalic prominence or brow (Figure 13-5).

Vaginal   examination   and   ultrasound Other assessment techniques to determine fetal position and presentation include vaginal examination and the use of ultrasound. During the vaginal examination, the examiner can palpate the presenting part if the cervix is dilated. Information about the position of the fetus and the degree of flexion of its head (in cephalic presentations) also can be obtained.

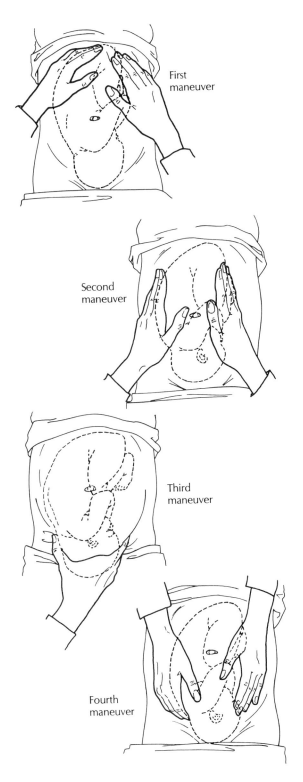

First
maneuver

Second
maneuver

Third
maneuver

Fourth
maneuver

Figure 13-5

Leopold's maneuvers for determining fetal position and presentation.

Ultrasound is used when the fetus's position cannot be determined by abdominal palpation (see Chapter 11 for an indepth discussion of ultrasound).

Evaluation of Fetal Status During Labor

Auscultation of FHR   The fetoscope, which is used to detect fetal heart rate (FHR), is a primary means of assessing the status of the fetus antepartally and during labor. (See Procedure 13-2.) Assessment by fetoscope yields subjective findings, but they can be most helpful when interpreted along with other findings.

Instead of listening haphazardly over the client's abdomen for FHR, the nurse may choose to perform Leopold's maneuvers first. Leopold's maneuvers not only indicate the probable location of FHR but also help to determine the presence of multiple fetuses, fetal lie, and fetal presentation. FHR is heard most clearly at the fetal back (Figure 13-6). Thus, in a cephalic presentation, FHR is best heard in the lower quadrant of the maternal abdomen. In a breech presentation, it is heard at or above the level of the maternal umbilicus. In a transverse lie, FHR may be heard best just above or just below the umbilicus. As the presenting part descends and rotates through the pelvic structure during labor, the location of the FHR tends to descend and move toward the midline.

After FHR is located, it is counted for 15 seconds and multiplied by 4 to obtain the number of beats per minute. The nurse should occasionally listen for 1 full minute through a contraction to detect any abnormal heart rate especially if tachycardia, bradycardia, or irregular beats are heard. If the FHR is irregular or has changed markedly from the last assessment, the nurse should listen for 1 full minute. The FHR should be auscultated every 30–60 minutes in early labor, every 15 minutes during active labor, and every 5 minutes during second stage of labor. If decelerations (see p. 287) are noted, the woman should be electronically monitored to rule out abnormalities in the FHR.

Only gross changes in FHR may be detected with the fetoscope. Subtle changes that occur in response to contractions may not be heard because it is difficult to hear the FHR during the

PROCEDURE 13-2
Auscultation of Fetal Heart Tones

Objective	Nursing action	Rationale
Assemble equipment	Obtain a fetoscope	Fetoscope is a special type of stethoscope that amplifies sound
Prepare client	Explain the procedure, indications for the procedure, and the information that will be obtained	Explanation of the procedure decreases anxiety and increases relaxation
	Uncover client's abdomen	
	Place the metal band of the fetoscope on your head; the diaphragm should extend out from your forehead	The metal band conducts sound
	Place the diaphragm on the client's abdomen halfway between the umbilicus and symphysis and in the midline	The FHR is most likely to be heard in this area
	Without touching the fetoscope, listen carefully for the FHR	
	Check the woman's pulse against the sounds heard; if rates are not similar, count FHR	Ensures the FHR, not the woman's pulse, is being heard
	If FHR not found, move fetoscope out from this area in a circle	
Report and record findings	Tell the parents what the FHR is; offer to help them listen if they would like	
	Record the FHR on the client's chart	Provides permanent record

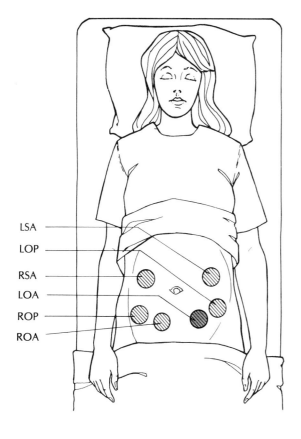

LSA
LOP
RSA
LOA
ROP
ROA

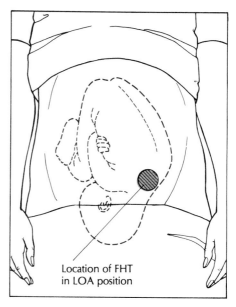

Location of FHT
in LOA position

Figure 13-6

Location of FHR in relation to the more commonly seen fetal positions.

peak of a contraction. Consequently, transient accelerations or decelerations in the FHR may be missed. In addition, occasional counting errors are inevitable. The ausculated FHR is an average measurement.

Electronic monitoring   There are two methods of assessing FHR during labor: indirect (external) and direct (internal). The indirect method may be accomplished using a fetoscope, fetal electrocardiography, and Doppler ultrasound (intermittent or continuous). Direct monitoring provides continuous information about the FHR from a scalp electrode. Uterine contractions may be monitored externally with a tocodynamometer or internally with an intrauterine pressure catheter.

When the FHR is monitored electronically, the interval between two successive fetal heart beats is measured and the rate is displayed as if the beats occurred at the same interval for 60 seconds. For example, if the interval between two beats is 0.5 seconds, the rate for one full minute would be 120 beats per minute. This measurement is called the instantaneous rate. The instantaneous rate provides documentation that the normal FHR varies from one moment to the next. Figure 13-7 compares instantaneous rates with those averaged by auscultation.

Electronic monitoring has major advantages over auscultation with the fetoscope. Electronic monitoring is a more reliable measure of fetal well-being. Fetal distress can be detected by observing the continuous FHR and the periodic changes that occur during and after uterine con-

tractions. Interventions can be timely and thus more effective.

Indications for electronic monitoring   If one or more of the following factors are present, the woman should be monitored electronically:

1. Previous history of a stillborn at 38 or more weeks of gestation
2. Complication of pregnancy (for example, PIH, placenta previa)
3. Induction of labor
4. Preterm labor
5. Fetal distress
6. Meconium staining of amniotic fluid

Methods   of   electronic   monitoring External monitoring of the fetus is usually accomplished by the use of ultrasound. A transducer, which emits continuous sound waves, is placed on the maternal abdomen. When placed correctly, the sound waves bounce off the fetal heart and are picked up by the electronic monitor. The actual moment-by-moment FHR is displayed graphically on a screen.

Internal monitoring requires an internal spiral electrode and intrauterine pressure catheter. These conditions must be present for internal monitoring to be possible: The cervix must be dilated at least 2 cm, the fetal position and presenting part must be known, the presenting fetal part must be accessible by vaginal examination, and the amniotic membranes must have ruptured. After cleansing the perineum, the caregiver inserts a sterile internal electrode into

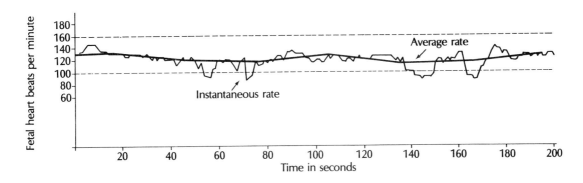

Figure 13-7

Comparison of instantaneous and average FHRs. The average FHR illustrates a more constant rate, while the instantaneous rate illustrates the normal variation of the FHR. (From Hon E: *An Introduction to Fetal* *Heart Rate Monitoring*, 2nd ed. Los Angeles: University of Southern California School of Medicine, 1976, p. 9.)

the vagina and places it against the fetal presenting part. The electrode is rotated clockwise until it is attached to the presenting part. Wires that extend from the electrode are attached to a leg plate (which is placed on the woman's thigh) and then attached to the monitor. This method of monitoring the FHR provides more accurate continuous data than external monitoring provides.

Uterine contractions can be monitored with an internal pressure catheter. The sterile catheter is introduced into the uterus, connected to a strain gauge (a transducer that interprets pressure changes), and then attached to the monitor. The uterine contractions can be evaluated by the intrauterine pressure that is present both during contractions and between contractions.

The FHR tracing at the top of Figure 13-8 was obtained by internal monitoring, and the uterine contraction tracing at the bottom of the figure by external monitoring. Note the FHR is variable (the tracing moves up and down instead of in a straight line), and the tracing stays close to the line numbered 150. If the graph paper moves through the monitor at 3 cm/min, each vertical dark line represents 1 minute. The frequency of the uterine contractions is every

2½–3 minutes. The duration of the contractions is 50–60 seconds.

FHR   FHR is evaluated by assessing an electronic monitor tracing for baseline and periodic changes. These changes are described in this section. Normal FHR ranges from 120–160 beats/min. The **baseline rate** refers to the average FHR observed during a 10-minute period of monitoring. *Baseline changes* in FHR are defined in terms of 10-minute periods. These changes are tachycardia, bradycardia, and beat-to-beat variability of the FHR.

Fetal tachycardia is defined as a rate of 160 beats/min or more during a 10-minute period. Moderate tachycardia is 160–179 beats/min, and severe tachycardia is 180 beats/min or more. Causes of fetal tachycardia include:

- Prematurity of the fetus
- Insufficient oxygenation of the fetus
- Fetal infection
- Fetal anemia
- Maternal fever or anxiety

Fetal bradycardia is defined as a rate less than 120 beats/min during a 10-minute period. Mild bradycardia ranges from 100–119 beats/

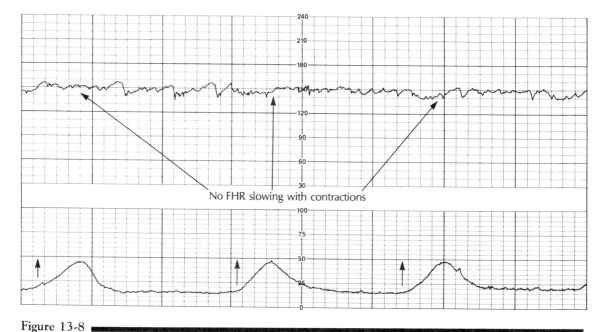

Figure 13-8

Normal fetal heart rate pattern utilizing internal monitoring. Note normal FHR, 140–158 beats/min, presence of long- and short-term variability, and absence of deceleration with adequate contractions.

min and is considered benign. Moderate bradycardia is a FHR less than 100 beats/min, and severe bradycardia is a FHR rate of less than 70 beats/min. Causes of fetal bradycardia include:

- Fetal hypoxia
- Prolapse or prolonged compression of the umbilical cord
- Fetal arrhythmias as seen with congenital heart block

Baseline variability is a measure of the interplay (the "push-pull" effect) between the sympathetic and parasympathetic nervous systems. There are two types of fetal heart variability—short term and long term. Short-term variability is the beat-to-beat irregularity. Long-term variability is the waviness or rhythmic fluctuations of the FHR tracing, which occur from 2–6 times per minute. Variability can be classified as none, minimal, average, moderate, or marked (Figure 13-9). As long as the FHR has average variability, it can be assumed that the sympathetic and parasympathetic systems are intact (Freeman and Garite, 1981).

Causes of decreased variability include:

- Deep fetal sleep
- Fetal congenital anomalies
- Fetal hypoxia and acidosis
- Fetus of less than 32 weeks' gestation
- Administration of certain drugs (hypnotics, analgesics, magnesium sulfate, atropine) to the woman.

Causes of increased variability include:

- Maternal activity
- Abdominal palpation
- Strong uterine contractions

Periodic changes   Periodic changes are transient decelerations or accelerations of the FHR from the baseline. They usually occur in response to uterine contractions and fetal movement.

Accelerations are transient increases in the FHR normally caused by fetal movement. When the fetus moves, its heart rate increases, just as the heart rates of adults increase during exercise. Often, accelerations accompany uterine contractions, usually due to fetal movement

in response to the pressure of the contractions. Accelerations of this type are thought to be a sign of fetal well-being and adequate oxygen reserve.

Decelerations are periodic decreases in FHR from the normal baseline. Hon and Quilligan (1967) categorize them into three types—early, late, and variable—according to the time of their occurrence in the contraction cycle and to their waveform (Figure 13-10).

When the fetal head is compressed, cerebral blood flow is decreased, which leads to central vagal stimulation and results in *early deceleration*. The onset of early deceleration occurs before the onset of the uterine contraction. This type of deceleration is of uniform shape, is usually considered benign, and does not require intervention.

Late deceleration is due to uteroplacental insufficiency resulting from decreased blood flow and oxygen transfer to the fetus through the intervillous spaces during uterine contractions. The onset of the deceleration occurs after the onset of the uterine contraction and is of uniform shape that tends to reflect associated uterine contractions. The late deceleration pattern is considered an ominous sign but does not necessarily require immediate delivery.

Variable decelerations occur if the umbilical cord becomes compressed, thus reducing blood flow between the placenta and fetus. The resulting increase in peripheral resistance in the fetal circulation causes fetal hypertension. The fetal hypertension stimulates the baroreceptors in the aortic arch and carotid sinuses, which slow the FHR. The onset of variable decelerations varies in timing with the onset of the contraction and they are variable in shape. This pattern requires further assessment.

Nursing interventions for periodic changes in FHR are presented in Table 13-2.

Sinusoidal pattern appears similar to a wave form. Long-term variability is present, but there is no short-term variability. The baseline FHR usually ranges from 110–115 beats/min. Fetal activity may be minimal or absent, and accelerations of FHR are not seen. The cause of the pattern is not clearly known, although it seems to "imply severe fetal jeopardy and impending death" (Modanlou and Freeman, 1982).

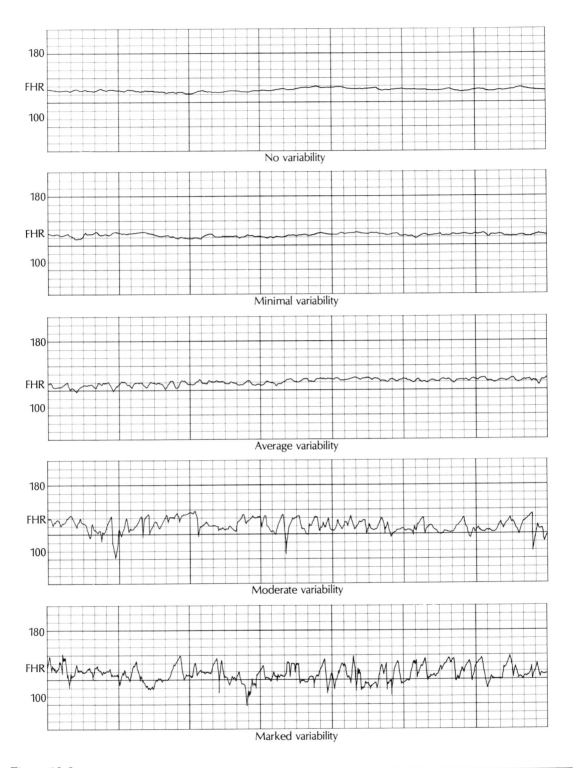

Figure 13-9

Types of variability. No variability = 0–2 beats/min; minimal variability = 3–5 beats/min; average variability = 6–10 beats/min; moderate variability = 11–25 beats/min; marked variability = more than 25 beats/min. (From Hon E: *An Introduction to Fetal Heart Monitoring*, 2nd ed. Los Angeles: University of Southern California School of Medicine, 1976, p. 41.)

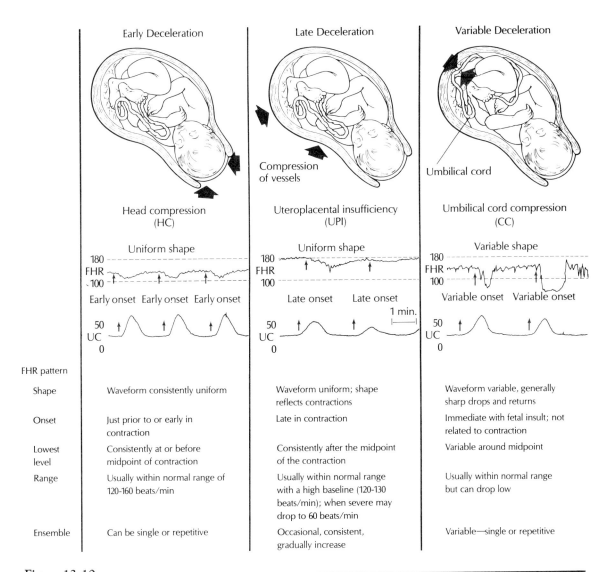

Figure 13-10
Types and characteristics of early, late, and variable decelerations. (From Hon E. *An Introduction to Fetal Heart Rate Monitoring*, 2nd ed. Los Angeles: University of Southern California School of Medicine, 1976, p. 29.)

Reassuring and nonreassuring FHR patterns FHR patterns must be assessed for evidence that shows whether they are reassuring or nonreassuring. Reassuring patterns indicate that the fetus is at no risk and labor can continue. Nonreassuring patterns indicate that the fetus may be at risk and intervention is required. The characteristics of both types of patterns are presented in Table 13-3.

Psychologic reactions to electronic monitoring Women have many different reactions

to electronic monitoring. Many women have little knowledge of monitoring unless they have attended a prenatal class that dealt with this subject. Some women react to electronic monitoring positively, viewing it as a reassurance that "the baby is OK." They may also feel that the monitor will help identify problems that develop in labor. Other women may feel negatively about the monitor. They may think that the monitor is interfering with a natural process, and they do not want the intrusion. They may resent the time and attention that the monitor

Table 13-2
General Principles of Management of FHR Patterns

Pattern	Therapeutic intervention
Normal	Evaluate maternal vital signs Follow labor by means of vaginal examination at appropriate intervals Observe and assess quality of labor and FHR patterns Document data and assessment of findings Ensure adequate hydration Change maternal position when indicated Decrease or discontinue oxytocin when indicated Administer oxygen when needed Maintain communication
Tachycardia	Assess maternal temperature Reconfirm EDC Monitor for changes in FHR pattern
Bradycardia	Monitor for changes in FHR pattern
Early decelerations	Monitor for changes in FHR pattern

Variable decelerations
  Isolated or occasional
  Severe
	Monitor for changes in FHR pattern
	Change maternal position to one in which FHR pattern is most improved
	Discontinue oxytocin if it is being administered
	Perform vaginal examination to assess for prolapsed cord or imminent delivery
	Administer 100% oxygen by tight face mask
	Monitor FHR continuously to assess current status and further changes in FHR pattern

If variable decelerations are severe and uncorrectable and client is in
  Early labor
  Second stage labor
	
	Cesarean delivery should be performed
	Vaginal delivery should be permitted unless baseline variability is decreasing or FHR is progressively rising, then cesarean delivery

Late decelerations occasional with good or increased variability	Monitor for further FHR changes Maintain client in side-lying position Maintain good hydration Discontinue oxytocin if it is being administered Administer oxygen Monitor maternal blood pressure and pulse for signs of hypotension Treat hypotension
Late decelerations persistent with good variability	Maintain side-lying position Administer oxygen Discontinue oxytocin if it is being administered Assess maternal blood pressure and pulse Begin intravenous fluids to maintain volume and hydration Assess labor progress Perform fetal blood sampling; if pH stays above 7.25, continue monitoring and resample as needed; if pH shows downward trend (between 7.25 and 7.20) resample in 10–15 minutes; if pH is below 7.20, deliver the infant immediately
Ominous patterns	Delivery should occur without delay. If delivery is not in progress, cesarean delivery is performed Supportive care while waiting for delivery includes: administer O_2; maintain side-lying or any position in which FHR is most improved; assess FHR continuously; assess maternal blood pressure and pulse; correct maternal hypotension

requires, time that could otherwise be spent providing nursing care. Some women may find

that the equipment, wires, and sounds increase their anxiety. The discomfort of lying in one

Table 13-3
Reassuring and Nonreassuring Patterns

Reassuring Patterns

No periodic changes

Early decelerations

Variable decelerations that do not exceed the following limits:

- Decelerations lasting less than 45 seconds
- Abrupt return to baseline
- Baseline not increasing
- Baseline variability not decreasing

FHR accelerations
- With contractions
- With fetal movement

Nonreassuring Patterns

Intermittent late decelerations with good FHR variability

Variable decelerations that exceed criteria (in reassuring patterns) with respect to duration and/or rate of return but with good FHR variability and no rising baseline

Total loss of FHR variability with decelerations

Prolonged deceleration due to:

- Paracervical block
- Epidural block
- Supine hypotension
- After vaginal examination or manipulation

Ominous Patterns

Persistent, uncorrectable late decelerations with loss of FHR variability with or without fetal tachycardia

Variable decelerations accompanied by:

- Loss of FHR variability
- Fetal tachycardia
- Prolonged "overshoot" (accelerations of FHR over the baseline as FHR deceleration ends)
- Blunted shape (which indicates rapid deceleration)

Sinusoidal FHR pattern

From Freeman RK, Garite TJ: *Fetal Heart Rate Monitoring.* Baltimore: Williams & Wilkins, 1981.

position and fear of injury to the baby are other objections (Shields, 1978; Molfese et al., 1982).

Nursing responsibilities Before applying the monitor, the nurse should fully explain the reason for its use and the information that it can provide. After the monitor is applied, basic information should be recorded on a label attached to the monitor strip. The data included are the date, client's name, physician, hospital number, age, gravida, para, EDC, membrane sta-

tus, and maternal vital signs. As the monitor strip continues to run and care is provided, occurrences during labor should be recorded not only in the medical record but also on the fetal monitoring tracing. This information helps the health care team assess current status and evaluate the tracing.

The following information should be included on the tracing:

1. Vaginal examination (dilatation, effacement, station, and position)
2. Amniotomy
3. Maternal vital signs
4. Maternal position changes
5. Application of internal monitor
6. Medications
7. Oxygen administration
8. Maternal behaviors (emesis, coughing, hiccups)
9. Fetal blood sampling

The tracing is considered to be a legal part of the woman's medical record and is submissible as evidence in court.

Interpretation of FHR tracings The nurse needs to use a systematic approach in evaluating FHR tracings to avoid interpreting findings on the basis of inadequate or erroneous data. With a systematic approach, the nurse can make a more accurate and rapid assessment, communicate data to the woman, clinician and staff easily, and have a systematic, universal language for documenting the client's record.

In assessing tracings, the nurse should first identify the uterine contractions. The contractions should be in evidence on the tracing at or even before the time the woman actually feels them. If not, adjustments are needed. The contraction pattern (frequency, duration, intensity, and baseline resting tone between contractions) is assessed. Next, the fetal response to the uterine contractions is assessed. Baseline FHR and changes are evaluated. What is the FHR? Is it increasing? Is it decreasing? Is the variability increasing or decreasing? Finally, the nurse looks at periodic changes. Are there accelerations with fetal movement? Are there decelerations? What are the characteristics of decelerations?

Under current standards of practice the nurse must be able to recognize FHR patterns and to communicate an accurate assessment of fetal status so that appropriate intervention can be made. Unless nurses are able to distinguish between nonreassuring and reassuring patterns and can take responsibility for evaluating the status of labor, they cannot detect impending problems.

Fetal blood sampling When nonreassuring or confusing FHR patterns are noted, additional information regarding the acid-base status of the fetus must be sought. This may be accomplished by the physician obtaining a **fetal blood sample**. The blood sample is usually drawn from the fetal scalp, but may be obtained from the fetus in the breech position.

Indications for fetal blood sampling are as follows (Freeman, 1982):

1. Persistent uncorrectable late decelerations with good variability in a woman who is expected to deliver in less than 2 hours
2. Confusing FHR patterns with possibly ominous elements
3. Total loss of FHR variability but no deceleration pattern

Before fetal blood can be sampled, the membranes must be ruptured, the cervix must be dilated at least 2–3 cm, and the presenting part must not be above −2 station. Sampling is not done when FHR patterns are ominous. It is contraindicated in acute emergencies and in cases of vaginal bleeding. In these instances, delivery by the most expeditious means is indicated.

Normal fetal pH values during labor are at or above 7.25, with 7.20–7.24 considered preacidotic. Values below 7.20 indicate serious acidosis (Petrie and Pollack, 1976).

Intervention based on fetal pH is recommended as follows:

1. If pH is greater than 7.25, allow labor to continue and resample as needed.
2. If pH is between 7.20 and 7.25, resample in 10–15 minutes.
3. If pH is less than 7.20, resample immediately. If low pH is confirmed, deliver the infant immediately (Monheit and Cousins, 1981).

The more information available about FHR monitoring, the less need for taking a fetal blood sample. Only when FHR patterns are uninterpretable, worsening, or suggestive of high risk is this adjunctive procedure indicated. Fetal blood sampling may prevent unnecessary cesarean delivery. Fetal blood sampling and electronic fetal monitoring are complementary tools. They give the physician the knowledge to make appropriate decisions about intervention or nonintervention.

Summary

To make an effective and thorough assessment of both woman and fetus during the intrapartal period, the nurse must have an understanding of normal and abnormal physiology as well as risk factors. The nurse must know how to use monitoring techniques and have specific assessment skills. Finally, the nurse must be knowledgeable about intervention techniques and be a committed member of the health care team.

References

Freeman RK: Fetal distress: Diagnosis and management. Presented at the Sixth International Symposium on Perinatal Medicine, April 1982; Las Vegas, Nevada.

Freeman RK, Garite TJ: *Fetal Heart Rate Monitoring*. Baltimore: Williams & Wilkins, 1981.

Friedman EA: An objective method of evaluating labor. *Hosp Pract* 1970; 5:82.

Hon E, Quilligan EJ: The classification of fetal heart rate: II. A revised working classification. *Conn Med* 1967; 31:779.

Molfese V, Sunshine P, Bennett A: Reactions of women to intrapartum fetal monitoring. *Obstet Gynecol* 1982; 59(6):705.

Mondanlou HD, Freeman RK: Sinusoidal fetal heart rate pattern: Its definition and clinical significance. *Am J Obstet Gynecol* 1982; 142(8):1033.

Monheit A, Cousins L: When do you measure scalp and blood pH? *Contemp Ob/Gyn* August 1981.

Petrie R, Pollack KJ: Intrapartum fetal biochemical monitoring by fetal blood sampling. *J Obstet Gynecol Neonatal Nurs* 1976; (Suppl) 5(5):52s.

Shields D: Maternal reactions to fetal monitoring. *Am J Nurs* December 1978; 78:2110.

Additional Readings ————————

Banta HD, Thacker SB: Assessing the costs and benefits of electronic fetal monitoring. *Obstet Gynecol Surv* 1979; 34(8):627.

Butnarescu GF, Tillotson DM, Villarreal PP: Assessment of reproductive risk. In: *Perinatal Nursing.* Vol 2. New York: Wiley, 1980.

Cranston CS: Obstetrical nurses' attitudes toward fetal monitoring. *J Obstet Gynecol Neonatal Nurs* 1980; 9(6):344.

Hon EH, Zannini D, Quilligan EJ: The neonatal value of fetal monitoring. *Am J Obstet Gynecol* 1975; 122(4):508.

McDonough M, Sheriff D, Simmel P: Parents' responses to fetal monitoring. *MCN* 1981; 6:32.

NAACOG Technical Bulletin. The nurses' role in electronic fetal monitoring. 1980; no. 7.

Perez RH: Fetal monitoring. In: *Protocols for Perinatal Nursing Practice.* St. Louis: Mosby, 1981.

Tucker SM: Electronic monitoring. In: *Fetal Monitoring and Fetal Assessment in High-Risk Pregnancy.* St. Louis: Mosby, 1978.

14

The Family in Childbirth: Needs and Care

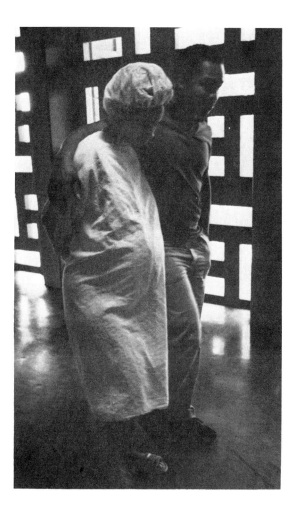

Chapter Contents

Objectives

- Identify the data base to be obtained when a woman is admitted to the labor and delivery area and the nursing care that is given at that time.

- Discuss nursing interventions to meet the psychologic and physiologic needs of the woman during each stage of labor and delivery.

- Identify the immediate needs of the newborn following delivery.

- Discuss management of a delivery in less-than-ideal situations.

- Discuss management of a delivery in less-than-ideal situations.

Key Terms

Apgar score   prep
birthing room

It is time for a child to be born. The waiting is over; labor has begun. The dreams and wishes of the past months fade as the expectant parents face the reality of the tasks of childbearing and childrearing that are ahead.

The couple is about to undergo one of the most meaningful and stressful events in their life together. The adequacy of their preparation for childbirth will now be tested. The coping mechanisms, communication, and support systems that they have established as a couple will be put to the test. In particular, the childbearing woman may feel that her psychologic and physical limits are about to be challenged.

The couple has also been involved in collecting information and making decisions regarding the setting for childbirth. Not many years ago, the only choice was an in-hospital labor unit with separate labor room, delivery room and recovery area. This type of unit is still available in some hospitals. However, many hospitals have changed their labor and delivery units to more closely reflect changing philosophies of family-centered childbirth. Many have single purpose units, which means that the woman stays in the same room for labor, delivery, recovery and possibly the postpartal period. These rooms may be called LDRPP (meaning labor, delivery, recovery and postpartum), or LDR (meaning labor, delivery and recovery). Some labor and delivery units use the term "alternative birthing room" or "birthing room" instead of LDR or LDRPP.

Maternity nursing has also kept pace with the changing philosophy of childbirth. In the past, much of the maternity nurse's role involved doing what she was told to do by the physician and then informing parents of what would happen to them. However, the maternity nursing role has developed it's own identity. Today's maternity nurse in the labor and delivery setting uses the full spectrum of nursing skills in working with childbearing families. Maternity nurses assess clients; gather information; provide information and teaching so that couples can make informed choices; function as a patient advocate; collaborate with other health care professionals; ensure that they function within current nursing standards of care; and communicate with physicians and certified nurse-midwives. Maternity nurses have become an integral part of family-centered care as they provide support, encouragement, and safe, caring nursing care.

Nursing Management of Admission

The woman is instructed during her prenatal visits to come to the hospital if any of the following occurs:

- ROM
- Uterine contractions (nullipara, 8–12 minutes apart; multiparas, 10–15 minutes apart)
- Vaginal bleeding

Early admission means less discomfort for the laboring woman when traveling to the hospital and more time to prepare for the delivery. Sometimes the labor is advanced and delivery is imminent, but usually the woman is in early labor at admission.

The woman may be facing a number of unfamiliar procedures that are routine for health care providers. It is important to remember that all women have the right to determine what happens to their bodies. *The woman's informed consent should be obtained prior to any procedure that involves touching her body.*

The manner in which the woman and her partner are greeted by the maternity nurse influences the course of her hospital stay. The sudden environmental change and the sometimes impersonal and technical aspects of admission can produce additional stress. If women are greeted in a brusque, harried manner, they are less likely to look to the nurse for support. A calm, pleasant manner indicates to the woman that she is an important person. It helps instill in the couple a sense of confidence in the staff's ability to provide quality care during this critical time.

Following the initial greeting, the woman is taken into the labor or birthing room. Some couples prefer to remain together during the admission process, and others prefer to have the partner wait outside. As the nurse helps the woman undress and get into a hospital gown, the nurse can begin conversing with her to develop rapport and establish the nursing data base. The experienced labor and delivery nurse can obtain essential information regarding the woman and her pregnancy within a few minutes after admission, initiate any immediate interventions needed, and establish individualized priorities. The nurse is then able to make effective nursing decisions regarding intrapartal care:

- Will a "prep" and/or enema be given?
- Should ambulation or bed rest be encouraged?
- Is more frequent monitoring needed?
- What does the woman want during her labor and delivery?
- Is a support person available?

A major challenge for nurses is the formulation of realistic objectives for laboring women. Each woman has different coping mechanisms and support systems. The single nullipara 14-year-old who has had no prenatal care and comes to the hospital alone does not have the same coping mechanisms as the couple who planned the pregnancy and attended prepared childbirth classes. The nurse may be the 14-year-old girl's only support, but the couple may need the nurse's support only minimally.

If indicated, the woman is assisted into bed. A side-lying or semi-Fowler's position rather than a supine position is most comfortable and avoids supine hypotensive syndrome (vena caval syndrome).

After obtaining the essential information from the woman and her records, the nurse begins the intrapartal assessment. (Chapter 13 considers intrapartal maternal assessment in depth.)

The nurse auscultates the FHR. (Detailed information on monitoring FHR is presented in Chapter 13.) The woman's blood pressure, pulse, respiration, and oral temperature are determined. Contraction frequency, duration, and intensity are assessed; this may be done as other data are gathered. Before the sterile vaginal examination, the woman should be informed about the procedure and its purpose. Afterward the nurse tells the woman about the findings. If there are signs of advanced labor (frequent contractions, an urge to bear down, and so on), a vaginal examination must be done quickly. If there are signs of excessive bleeding or if the woman reports episodes of bleeding in the last trimester, a vaginal examination should *not* be done.

Results of FHR assessment, uterine contraction evaluation, and the vaginal examination help determine whether the rest of the admission process can proceed at a more leisurely pace or whether additional interventions have higher priority. For example, a FHR of 110 beats/min on auscultation indicates that a fetal monitor should be applied immediately to obtain additional data. The woman's vital signs can be assessed after this is done.

Admission Procedures

After admission data are obtained, a clean-voided mid-stream urine specimen is collected. The woman with intact membranes may walk to the bathroom. If the membranes are ruptured and the presenting part is not engaged, the woman is generally asked to remain in bed to avoid prolapse of the umbilical cord. The advisability of ambulation when membranes are ruptured depends on the woman's desires, clinician requests, or agency policy.

The nurse can test the woman's urine for the presence of protein, ketones, and glucose by using a dipstick before sending the sample to the laboratory. This procedure is especially important if edema or elevated blood pressure is noted on admission. Proteinuria of 2+ or more may be a sign of impending preeclampsia. Ketonuria is a good index of starvation ketosis. Glycosuria is found frequently in pregnant women because of the increased glomerular filtration rate in the proximal tubules and the inability of these tubules to increase reabsorption of glucose. However, it may also be associated with latent diabetes and should not be discounted.

While the woman is collecting the urine specimen, the nurse can prepare the equipment for shaving the pubic area (the shaving is referred to as the **prep**) and for the enema if one is to be given. Prep orders vary, but many clinicians leave standing orders for prep measures. The use of preps is a controversial issue. Some clinicians believe that this form of skin preparation facilitates their work during the delivery, makes perineal repair easier and prevents infection (Mahan and McKay, 1983). Many women question the need for a prep and request that it be omitted. The nurse needs to ascertain the woman's wishes in this matter. Women who do not want a prep probably have discussed this with the physician/nurse-midwife during the prenatal period.

If a prep is to be done, the perineal hair below the vaginal opening is either shaved or clipped with a pair of sterile scissors.

The administration of an enema is also controversial. Proponents say the purposes of an enema are to (a) evacuate the lower bowel so that labor will not be impeded, (b) stimulate uterine contractions, (c) avoid embarrassment if bowel contents are expelled during pushing efforts, and (d) prevent contamination of the sterile field during delivery. Those who question the routine use of an enema on admission suggest that labor is impeded only by a severe bowel impaction, question whether labor is stimulated, and find that feces still may be expelled during pushing efforts. They also note that the enema may be uncomfortable.

After determining the woman's wishes regarding an enema, the nurse notifies the clinician. Some factors contraindicate the enema. They are vaginal bleeding, unengaged presenting part, rapid labor progress, and imminent delivery. These factors need to be identified. If an enema is to be given, the reasons and the procedure are explained to the woman. Then the enema is administered while she is on her left side.

If the membranes are intact and labor is not far advanced, the woman may expel the enema in the bathroom. Otherwise she is positioned on a bedpan in bed. The side rails of the bed should be raised for safety. They also support the woman as she positions herself over the bedpan.

Before leaving the labor area, the nurse must be sure that the woman knows how to operate the call system so that she can obtain help if she needs it. After the enema is expelled, the nurse monitors the FHR again to assess any changes. If the woman's partner has been out of the labor room, the couple is reunited as soon as possible.

Laboratory tests are also carried out during admission. Hemoglobin and hematocrit values help determine the oxygen-carrying capacity of the circulatory system and the ability of the woman to withstand blood loss at delivery. Elevation of the hematocrit indicates hemoconcentration of blood, which occurs with edema or dehydration. A low hemoglobin, in the absence of other evidence of bleeding, suggests anemia. Blood may be typed and crossmatched if the woman is in a high-risk category. A serology test for syphilis is obtained if one has not been done in the last 3 months or if an antepartal serology result was positive.

In many hospitals, the admission process also includes signing a delivery permit, fingerprinting the woman for the infant records, and fastening an identification bracelet to her wrist.

Depending on how rapidly labor is progressing, the nurse notifies the clinician before or after completing the admission procedures. The report should include the following information: cervical dilatation and effacement, station, presenting part, status of the membranes, contraction pattern, FHR, vital signs that are not in the normal range, the woman's wishes, and her reaction to labor.

Nursing management of labor is influenced by the physical, psychologic, and cultural data obtained during admission.

Nursing Management of the First and Second Stages of Labor

Cultural Considerations

Knowledge of values, customs, and practices of different cultures is as important during labor as it is in the prenatal period. Without this knowledge, a nurse is less likely to understand a woman's behavior and may impose personal values and beliefs upon a woman. As cultural sensitivity increases, so does the likelihood of providing high-quality care.

Modesty Modesty is important for Oriental, American Indians, and Mexican-American women. In these three cultures pregnancy is often viewed as "female business" (Chung, 1977). Some Oriental women are not accustomed to male physicians and attendants and may prefer female physicians and attendants. Modesty is of great concern to these women, and exposure of as little of the woman's body as possible is strongly recommended (Abril, 1977).

Pain expression Orientals, Blacks, and Mexican Americans vary in the way they express pain. The laboring Oriental woman may not express pain outwardly for fear of shaming herself and her family (Hollingsworth et al., 1980). Black women may also appear rather stoic in an effort to avoid showing weakness or calling undue attention to themselves (Carrington, 1978). Mexican-American women, by contrast, may be more expressive during labor. One way they may express pain and suffering is through groaning and moaning (Murillo-Rohde, 1979). Another behavior of laboring Mexican-American women is to keep their mouths closed for fear of making the uterus rise. They are to yell only when they exhale (Kay, 1978).

The Adolescent During Labor and Delivery

Each adolescent in labor is different. The nurse must assess what each client brings to the experience by asking the following questions:

- Has the young woman received prenatal care?

- What are her attitudes and feelings about the pregnancy?

- Who will attend the birth and what is the person's relationship to her?

- What preparation has she had for the experience?

- What are her expectations and fears regarding labor and delivery?

- How has her culture influenced her?

- What are her usual coping mechanisms?

- Does she plan to keep the newborn?

Any adolescent who has not had prenatal care requires close observation during labor. Fetal well-being is established by fetal monitoring. Adolescent women are at highest risk for pregnancy and labor complications and must be monitored intensively (Mercer, 1979).

The nurse should be alert to any physiologic complications of labor in the adolescent. The young woman's prenatal record is carefully reviewed for risks. The adolescent is screened for PIH, CPD, anemia, drugs ingested during pregnancy, sexually transmitted disease, and size-date discrepancies.

The support role of the nurse depends on the woman's support system during labor. The young woman may not be accompanied by someone who will stay with her during childbirth. Whether she has a support person or not, it is important for the nurse to establish a trusting relationship with the young woman. In this way, the nurse can help her maintain control and understand what is happening to her. Establishing rapport without recrimination for possible inappropriate behavior is essential. The adolescent who is given positive reinforcement for "work well done" will leave the experience with increased self-esteem, despite the emotional problems that may accompany her situation.

If a support person did accompany the adolescent, that person also needs the nurse's encouragement and support. The nurse must explain changes in the young woman's behavior and substantiate her wishes. Hospital rules that exclude people under age 16 years may be waived to allow a young father-to-be to remain with the adolescent woman. The nursing staff should reinforce the adolescents' feelings that they are wanted and important.

The adolescent who has taken childbirth education classes is generally better prepared than the adolescent who has had no preparation. The nurse must keep in mind, however, that the younger the adolescent, the less she may be able to participate actively in the process.

The very young adolescent (under age 14) has fewer coping mechanisms and less experience to draw on than her older counterparts have. Because her cognitive development is incomplete, the younger adolescent may have fewer problem-solving capabilities. Her ego integrity may be more threatened by the experience, and she may be more vulnerable to stress and discomfort.

The very young woman needs someone to rely on at all times during labor. She may be more childlike and dependent than older teens. The nurse must be sure that instructions and explanations are simple and concrete. During the transition phase, the young teenager may become withdrawn and unable to express her need to be nurtured. Touch, soothing encouragement, and measures to maintain her comfort help her maintain control and meet her needs for dependence. During the second stage of labor, the young adolescent may feel as if she is losing control and may reach out to those around her. By remaining calm and giving directions, the nurse helps her control feelings of helplessness.

The middle adolescent (age 14–16 years) often attempts to remain calm and unflinching during labor. If unable to break through the teenager's stoic barrier, the nurse needs to rise above frustration and realize that a caring attitude will still affect the young woman.

Many older adolescents feel that they "know it all," but they may be no more prepared for childbirth than younger counterparts. The nurse's reinforcement and nonjudgmental manner will help them save face. If the adolescent has not taken classes, she may require preparation and explanations. The older teenager's response to the stresses of labor, however, is similar to that of the adult woman.

Even if the adolescent is planning to relinquish her newborn, she should be given the option of seeing and holding the infant. She may be reluctant to do this at first, but the grieving process is facilitated if the mother sees the infant. However, seeing or holding the newborn should be the young woman's choice. (See Chapter 26 for further discussion of the relinquishing mother and the adolescent parent.)

Comfort Measures

Assessment   The first step in planning care for the woman is to identify factors that may contribute to discomfort in labor. These factors include the woman's position, diaphoresis, continual leaking of amniotic fluid, a full bladder, a dry mouth, anxiety, and fear. Nursing interventions can minimize the effects of these factors. These are described later in this section.

There are eight types of behavioral responses to pain (McCaffery, 1979):

- Physiologic manifestations
- Body movement
- Facial expression
- Verbal statements
- Vocal behavior
- Physical contact
- Response to environment
- Patterns of handling pain

Many of these behaviors occur simultaneously. The most frequent physiologic manifestations are increased pulse and respiratory rates, dilated pupils, and increased blood pressure and muscle tension. In labor, these reactions are transitory because the pain is intermittent. Increased muscle tension is most significant because it may impede the progress of labor. Women in labor frequently tighten skeletal muscles voluntarily during a contraction and remain motionless. Grimacing is also common. Verbal statements relating to pain and requests for intervention usually mean that the woman has reached her tolerance level. Vocalization may take many forms during the first stage of labor. A grunting sound typically accompanies the bearing-down effort during the second stage of labor.

Some women desire body contact during a contraction and may reach out to grasp the supporting person. As the intensity of the contractions increases with the progress of labor, the woman is less aware of the environment and may have difficulty hearing verbal instructions. The pattern of coping with labor contractions varies from the use of highly structured breathing techniques to loud vocalizations. Irritability and refusal of touch are common responses to the discomfort of the second stage of labor. The tense and frightened woman is more likely to lose control during any stage of labor.

Intervention   A decrease in the intensity of discomfort is one of the goals of nursing support during labor. Nursing measures used to decrease pain include:

- Ensuring general comfort
- Decreasing anxiety
- Providing information
- Using specific supportive relaxation techniques
- Administering pharmacologic agents as ordered by the physician

General comfort   General comfort measures are of utmost importance throughout labor. By relieving minor discomforts the nurse helps the woman use her coping mechanisms to deal with pain.

The woman should be encouraged to assume any position that she finds the most comfortable. A side-lying position is generally the most advantageous for the laboring woman, although frequent position changes seem to achieve more efficient contractions (Roberts et al., 1983). Care should be taken that all body parts are supported, with the joints slightly flexed. If the woman is more comfortable on her back, the head of the bed should be elevated to relieve the pressure of the uterus on the vena cava. Back rubs and frequent change of position contribute to comfort and relaxation.

Diaphoresis and the constant leaking of amniotic fluid can dampen the woman's gown and bed linen. Fresh, smooth, dry bed linen promotes comfort. To avoid having to change the bottom sheet following rupture of the membranes, the nurse may replace chux at frequent intervals. The perineal area should be kept as clean and dry as possible to promote comfort as well as to prevent infection. A full bladder adds to the discomfort during a contraction and may prolong labor by interfering with the descent of the fetus. The bladder should be kept as empty as possible. Even though the woman is voiding, urine may be retained because of the pressure of the fetal presenting part. A full bladder can be detected by palpation directly over the symphysis pubis. Some of the regional procedures for analgesia during labor contribute to the inability to void, and catheterization may be necessary.

The woman may experience dryness of the oral mucous membranes. A lemon glycerine swab, popsicles, ice chips, or a wet 4-by-4 sponge may relieve the discomfort. Some prepared childbirth programs advise the woman to bring suckers to help combat the dryness that occurs with some of the breathing patterns.

Handling anxiety   The anxiety experienced by women entering labor is related to a combination of factors inherent to the process. A moderate amount of anxiety about the pain enhances the woman's ability to deal with the pain. An excessive degree of anxiety decreases her ability to cope with the pain.

Two ways to decrease anxiety that is not related to pain are to give information, which eases fear of the unknown, and to establish rapport with the couple, which helps them preserve their personal integrity. In addition to being a good listener, the nurse must demonstrate genuine concern for the laboring woman. Remaining with the woman as much as possible conveys a caring attitude and dispels fears of abandonment. Praise for correct breathing, relaxation efforts, and pushing efforts not only encourages repetition of the behavior but also decreases anxiety about the ability to cope with labor (Stephany, 1983).

Client teaching   Providing information about the nature of the discomfort that will occur during labor is important. Stressing the intermittent nature and maximum duration of the contractions can be most helpful. The woman can cope with pain better when she knows that a period of relief will follow. Describing the type of discomfort and specific sensations that will occur as labor progresses helps the woman recognize these sensations as normal and expected when she does experience them.

During the second stage, the woman may interpret rectal pressure as a need to move her bowels. The instinctive response is to tighten muscles rather than bear down (push). A sensation of splitting apart also occurs in the latter part of the second stage, and the woman may be afraid to bear down. The woman who expects these sensations and understands that bearing down contributes to progress at this stage is more likely to do so.

Descriptions of sensations should be accompanied with information on specific comfort measures (Simkin, 1982). Some women experience the urge to push during transition when the cervix is not fully dilated and effaced. This sensation can be controlled by panting, and instructions should be given prior to the time that panting is required.

A thorough explanation of surroundings, procedures and equipment being used also decreases anxiety, thereby reducing pain (Frink and Chally, 1984). Attachment to an electronic monitor can produce fear, because equipment of this type is associated with critically ill patients. The beeps, clicks, and other strange noises should be explained, and a simplified explanation of the monitor strip should be given. The nurse can emphasize that the use of the monitor provides a more accurate way to assess the well-being of the fetus during the course of labor. In addition, the nurse can show the woman and her coach how the monitor can help them use controlled breathing techniques to relieve pain. The monitor may indicate the beginning of a contraction just seconds before the woman feels it. The woman and coach can learn how to read the tracing to identify the beginning of the contraction.

Supportive relaxation techniques   Tense muscles increase resistance to the descent of the fetus and contribute to maternal fatigue. This fatigue increases pain perception and decreases the woman's ability to cope with the pain. Comfort measures, massage, techniques for decreasing anxiety, and client teaching can contribute to relaxation. Other factors are adequate sleep and rest. The laboring woman needs to be encouraged to use the periods between contractions for rest and relaxation. A prolonged prodromal phase of labor may have prohibited sleeping. An aura of excitement naturally accompanies the onset of labor, making it difficult for the woman to sleep although the contractions are mild and infrequent.

Distraction is another method of increasing relaxation and coping with discomfort. During early labor, conversation or activities such as light reading, cards, or other games serve as distractions. One technique that is effective for relieving moderate pain is to have the woman concentrate on a pleasant experience she has had in the past.

Touch is another type of distraction. Although some women regard touching as an invasion of privacy or threat to their independence, others want to touch and be touched during a painful experience. Nurses can make themselves available to the woman who desires touch. The nurse can place a hand on the side of the bed within the woman's reach. The person who needs touch will reach out for contact, and the nurse can pick up and follow through with this behavioral cue (Figure 14-1).

Visualization techniques enhance relaxation; with this method the woman visualizes her body relaxing, or the perineum relaxing (Morton, 1983).

Mild to moderate abdominal discomfort during contractions may be relieved or lessened by effleurage. Back pain associated with labor may be relieved more effectively by firm pressure on the lower back or sacral area. To apply firm pressure, the nurse places her hand or a rolled, warmed towel or blanket in the small of the woman's back.

In addition to the measures just described, the nurse can enhance the woman's relaxation by providing encouragement and support for her controlled breathing techniques.

Controlled breathing   Controlled breathing may help the laboring woman. Used correctly, it increases the woman's pain threshold, permits relaxation, enhances the woman's ability to cope with the uterine contractions, and allows the uterus to function more efficiently.

Women usually learn Lamaze breathing in prenatal classes and practice it a number of weeks before delivery. If the woman has not learned Lamaze or another controlled breathing technique, teaching her may be difficult when she is admitted in active labor. In this instance, the nurse can teach abdominal and pant-pant-blow breathing. In abdominal breathing, the woman moves the abdominal wall upward as she inhales and downward as she exhales. This method tends to lift the abdominal wall off the contracting uterus and thus may provide some pain relief. The breathing is deep and rhythmical. As transition approaches, the woman may

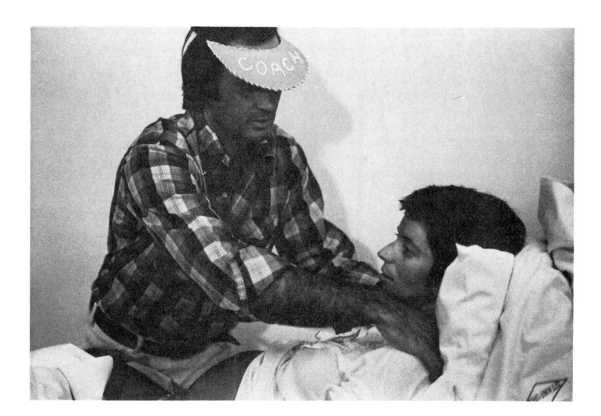

Figure 14-1

The woman's partner provides support and encouragement during labor. (Photo by Suzanne Arms.)

feel the need to breathe more rapidly. To avoid hyperventilation, which may occur with deep abdominal breathing, the woman can use the pant-pant-blow breathing pattern.

As the woman uses her breathing technique, the nurse can assess and support the interaction between the woman and her coach or support person. In the absence of a coach, the nurse helps the laboring woman by helping to identify the beginning of each contraction and encouraging her as she breathes through each contraction. Continued encouragement and support with each contraction throughout labor have immeasurable benefits.

Hyperventilation may occur when a woman breathes very rapidly over a prolonged period of time. Hyperventilation is the result of an imbalance of oxygen and carbon dioxide (that is, too much carbon dioxide is exhaled, and too much oxygen remains in the body). The signs and symptoms of hyperventilation are tingling or numbness in the tip of nose, lips, fingers, or toes; dizziness; spots before the eyes; or spasms of the hands or feet (carpal-pedal spasms). If hyperventilation occurs, the woman should be encouraged to slow her breathing rate and to take shallow breaths. With instruction and encouragement, many women are able to change their breathing to correct the problem. Encouraging the woman to relax and counting out loud for her so she can pace her breathing during contractions are also helpful. If the signs and symptoms continue or become more severe (that is, if they progress from numbness to spasms), the woman can breathe into a paper surgical mask or a paper bag until symptoms abate. Breathing into a mask or bag causes rebreathing of carbon dioxide. The nurse should remain with the woman to reassure her.

In some instances, analgesics and/or regional anesthetic blocks may be used to enhance comfort and relaxation during labor. See Chapter 16 for a discussion of analgesia and anesthesia. Table 14-1 summarizes labor progress, possible responses of the laboring woman, and support measures.

Table 14-1

Normal Progress, Psychologic Characteristics, and Nursing Support During First and Second Stage of Labor

Phase	Cervical dilatation	Uterine contractions	Client response	Support measures
Stage 1				
Latent phase	1-4 cm	Every 15-30 min, 15-30 sec duration Mild intensity	Usually happy, talkative, and eager to be in labor Exhibits need for independence by taking care of own bodily needs and seeking information	Get acquainted with client (and partner, if present) and ascertain her preparation and needs; initiate discharge planning; instruct her in breathing techniques if she has not had prenatal classes Orient family to equipment, monitors, procedures; allow client to participate in care Provide needed information
Active phase	4-7 cm	Every 3-5 min, 30-60 sec duration Moderate intensity	May experience feelings of helplessness; exhibits increased fatigue and may begin to feel restless and anxious as contractions become stronger; expresses fear of abandonment Becomes more dependent as she is less able to meet her needs	Encourage to maintain breathing patterns; provide quiet environment to reduce external stimuli and reassure Inform couple of labor progress Anticipate needs; allow client to assist in her care as she desires or is able to
Transition	8-10 cm	Every 2-3 min, 45-90 sec duration Strong intensity	Tires and may exhibit increased restlessness and irritability; may feel she cannot keep up with labor process and is out of control Physical discomforts Fear of being left alone May fear tearing open or splitting apart with contractions	Encourage client to rest between contractions; if she sleeps between contractions, wake her at increment of contraction so she can begin breathing pattern; this measure decreases feelings of being out of control Praise couple's efforts and inform them of progress Encourage continued participation of supports and provide support
Stage 2	Complete		May feel out of control; helpless; panicky	Gentle but firm directions to couple; maintain good eye contact with client; encourage inclusion and participation of support person

First Stage

After the admission process is completed, the nurse can help the laboring woman and her partner to become comfortable with the surroundings. The nurse can also assess their individual needs and plans for this experience. As long as there are no contraindications (such as vaginal bleeding or ROM with the fetus unengaged), the woman may be encouraged to ambulate. Many women feel much more at ease and comfortable if they can move around and do not have to remain in bed. In addition, ambulation may decrease the need for analgesics, shorten labor, and decrease the incidence of FHR abnormalities (Carr, 1980; McKay, 1980).

The nurse will need to assess physical parameters of the woman and her fetus. Maternal temperature is assessed every 4 hours unless the temperature is over 37.5C (99.6F); if it is, it must be taken every 2 hours. Blood pressure, pulse, and respirations are assessed every hour. If the woman's blood presssure is over 140/90 mm Hg or her pulse is more than 100, the physician or nurse-midwife must be notified. The blood pressure and pulse are then reassessed more frequently. Uterine contractions are assessed for frequency, intensity, and duration. The FHR is assessed every 30–60 minutes as long as it remains between 120–160 beats/min. The FHR should be assessed throughout one contraction and for about 15 seconds after the contraction to assure that there are no decelerations. If the FHR is not in the 120–160 range and/or decelerations are heard, continuous electronic monitoring is recommended.

The laboring woman may be feeling some discomfort during contractions. The nurse can assist with diversions or by repositioning the woman. The woman may begin to use her breathing method during contractions (see the preceding discussion of management of pain).

The nurse should offer fluids in the form of clear liquids and/or ice chips at frequent intervals. Because gastric-emptying time is prolonged during labor, solid foods are usually avoided.

Active phase   During this phase, the contractions have a frequency of 3–5 minutes, a duration of 30–60 seconds and a moderate intensity. Contractions need to be assessed every 15–30 minutes. As the contractions become more frequent and intense, vaginal exams are done to assess cervical dilatation and effacement and fetal station and position. During the active phase, the cervix dilates from 4–7 cm, and vaginal discharge and bloody show increase. Maternal blood pressure, pulse, and respirations should be assessed every hour (unless elevated as previously noted). The FHR is assessed every 15 minutes.

A woman who has been ambulatory up to this point may now wish to sit in a chair or on a bed. If the woman wants to lie on the bed, she is encouraged to assume a side-lying position. The nurse can assist her to a position of comfort and may place pillows to support her body. To increase comfort, the nurse can give back rubs or effleurage, or place a cool cloth on the woman's forehead or across her neck. Because vaginal discharge increases, the nurse needs to change the chux frequently. Washing the perineum with warm soap and water removes secretions and increases comfort.

If the amniotic membranes have not ruptured previously, they may during this phase. When the membranes rupture, the nurse notes the color and odor of the amniotic fluid and the time of rupture, and immediately auscultates the FHR. The fluid should be clear with no odor. Fetal stress leads to intestinal and anal sphincter relaxation, and meconium may be released into the amniotic fluid. Meconium turns the fluid greenish-brown. Whenever the nurse notes meconium-stained fluid, an electronic monitor is applied to continuously assess the FHR. The time of rupture is noted because current practice suggests that delivery should occur within 24 hours of ROM. An additional concern is prolapse of the umbilical cord that occurs when membranes rupture and the fetus is not engaged. The concern is that the amniotic fluid coming through the cervix will propel the umbilical cord through the cervix (prolapsed cord). The FHR is auscultated because a drop in the rate might indicate an undetected prolapsed cord. Immediate intervention is necessary to remove pressure on a prolapsed umbilical cord (see Chapter 17). See Table 14-2 for additional deviations from normal.

Transition (deceleration phase)   During transition, the contraction frequency is every 2–3 minutes, duration is 45–90 seconds, and intensity is strong. Cervical dilatation increases from 8 to 10 cm, effacement is complete (100%), and there is usually a heavy amount of bloody show. Contractions are assessed at least every 15 minutes. Sterile vaginal examinations are done more frequently because this stage of labor usually is accompanied by rapid change. Maternal blood pressure, pulse, and respirations are assessed at least every 30 minutes, and FHR is assessed every 15 minutes.

Comfort measures become very important in this phase of labor, but continual assessment is required to intervene appropriately. The woman may rapidly change from wanting a back rub and other "hands-on" care to wanting to be left completely alone. The support person and the nurse need to follow her cues and change interventions as needed. Because the woman is breathing more rapidly, the nurse can increase her comfort by offering small spoons of ice chips to moisten her mouth or applying petroleum jelly to dry lips. The nurse can encourage

Table 14-2
Deviations from Normal Labor Process Requiring Immediate Intervention

Problem	Immediate action	Problem	Immediate action
Client admitted with vaginal bleeding or history of painless vaginal bleeding	1. Do not perform vaginal examination 2. Assess FHR 3. Evaluate amount of blood loss 4. Evaluate labor pattern 5. Notify clinician immediately	Prolapse of umbilical cord	1. Relieve pressure on cord manually 2. Continuously monitor FHR; watch for changes in FHR pattern 3. Notify physician

Presence of greenish amniotic fluid	1. Continuously monitor FHR
	2. Evaluate dilatation status of cervix and determine whether umbilical cord is prolapsed
	3. Maintain client on complete bed rest
	4. Notify physician immediately
		Client admitted in advanced labor; delivery imminent	1. Proceed directly to delivery room
			2. Obtain necessary information:
			  a. Physician's name
			  b. Bleeding problems
			  c. Obstetric problems
			  d. FHR and maternal vital signs, if possible
			  e. Length of labor and last time she ate
			3. Direct ancillary personnel to telephone physician
			Do not leave client alone
			4. Provide support to couple

Absence of FHR and fetal movement	1. Notify physician 2. Provide emotional support to laboring couple (client has an idea that "something is wrong")		

the woman to rest between contractions. If analgesics have been administered, a quiet environment enhances the quality of rest between contractions. The nurse can awaken the woman just before another contraction begins so that she can begin her breathing.

Some women have difficulty maintaining control during this time and need help with their breathing. Either the support person or the nurse can breathe along with the woman during each contraction to help her maintain her pattern. It is helpful to encourage her and assure her that she is doing a good job. The woman will begin to feel increased rectal pressure as the fetal presenting part moves down the birth canal. The nurse encourages the woman to refrain from pushing until the cervix is completely dilated. This measure helps prevent cervical edema.

Second Stage (Expulsion Phase)

The second stage is reached when the cervix is completely dilated (10 cm). The uterine contractions continue as in the transition phase. Frequent sterile vaginal examinations are done to assess progress. Maternal pulse, blood pressure, and FHR are assessed every 5–15 minutes; some protocols recommend assessment after each contraction. The woman feels an uncontrollable urge to push (bear down). The nurse can help by encouraging her and by assisting with positioning (see Figure 14-2). The woman can be propped up with pillows to a semireclining position.

When the contraction begins, the nurse tells the woman to take two short breaths, then to take a third breath and hold it while pulling back on her knees and pushing down with her abdominal muscles. Some women prefer to exhale slightly, called *exhale breathing*, while pushing to avoid the physiologic effects of the Valsalva maneuver. With this method, the woman takes several deep breaths and then holds her breath for 5–6 seconds. Then, through slightly pursed lips, she exhales slowly every 5–6 seconds while continuing to hold her breath. The woman takes another breath and continues exhale breathing and pushing during the contraction (McKay, 1981).

A nullipara is usually prepared for delivery when perineal bulging is noted. A multipara usually progresses much more quickly, so she

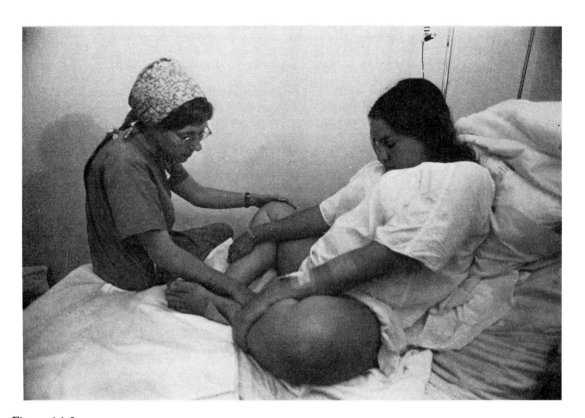

Figure 14-2
Nurse provides support during pushing efforts. (Photo by Suzanne Arms.)

may be prepared for delivery when the cervix is dilated 7–8 cm. As delivery approaches, the woman's partner or support person also prepares for delivery. In most facilities, this necessitates putting on a scrub suit and perhaps disposable boots, cap, and mask. (See Essential Facts to Remember—Indications of Delivery.)

✳ **ESSENTIAL FACTS TO REMEMBER**

Indications of Imminent Delivery

Delivery is imminent if the woman shows the following changes:
   Bulging of the perineum
   Uncontrollable urge to bear down
   Increased bloody show

Management of Spontaneous Delivery

Birthing Room

Couples often choose the **birthing room** or labor delivery recovery room (LDR) for labor and delivery because of the more relaxed atmosphere maintained there. Consequently, the birthing room (LDR) should be prepared for delivery before it is imminent. A delivery pack and instrument set can be placed on a small table close to the labor bed. Essentials for the immediate care of the newborn are prepared, and emergency resuscitation equipment is available somewhere in the room. Often, birthing rooms have a bed that can be adapted for delivery by removing a small section near the foot. Many of the same interventions described in the following section apply. After delivery, the newborn is given to the mother or couple, and their interaction is not interrupted.

Delivery Room

The instrument table, which is set up under surgical asepsis, has the instruments and drapes that will be used during the delivery. Warmed sterile water is usually available for various procedures. A radiant warmer or similar heated bed is prepared for the newborn. Emergency equipment for resuscitating the newborn or for dealing with unexpected maternal complications should also be on hand.

Nursing interventions   The woman is usually positioned for delivery on a bed, birthing chair, or delivery table. In some facilities the woman may choose a squatting or side-lying position. The position that the woman assumes is determined not only by her individual wishes but also by the physician/nurse-midwife.

Stirrups, if used, are padded to alleviate pressure, and both legs shold be lifted simultaneously to avoid strain on abdominal and perineal muscles. The stirrups should be adjusted to fit the woman's legs. The feet are supported in the stirrup holders. The height and angle of the stirrups are adjusted so there is no pressure on the back of the knees or the calf, which might cause discomfort and postpartal vascular problems. The delivery table or bed is elevated about 30–60° to help the woman bear down, and handles are provided so she may pull back on them.

Cleansing the perineum   The woman's vulvar and perineal area is prepared in the following manner. After thoroughly washing her hands, the nurse opens the sterile prep tray, dons sterile gloves and cleans the vulva and perineum with the cleansing solution (Figure 14-3). Some agency policy dictates the area be rinsed with sterile water. Beginning with the mons, the area is cleansed up to the lower abdomen. The second sponge is used to cleanse the inner groin and thigh of one leg, and the third one is used to cleanse the other leg, moving outward to avoid carrying material from surrounding areas to the vaginal outlet. The last three sponges are used to cleanse the labia and vestibule with one downward sweep each. The used sponges are then discarded.

The labor coach is given a stool to sit on if desired. Both the woman and the coach are kept informed of procedures and progress and are supported throughout the delivery. In some

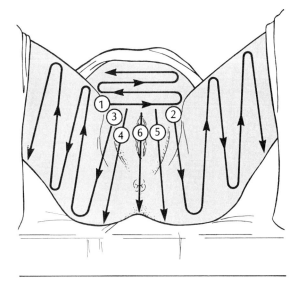

Figure 14-3

Cleansing the perineum prior to delivery. The nurse follows the numbered diagram, using a new sponge for each area.

delivery rooms, there is a mirror that can be adjusted so that the couple may watch the delivery.

The woman's blood pressure and the FHR are monitored between contractions, and the contractions are palpated until delivery. The nurse continues to assist the woman in her pushing efforts.

In addition to assisting the woman and her partner, the nurse also assists the physician or nurse-midwife in preparing for the delivery. The physician or nurse-midwife dons a sterile gown and gloves and places sterile drapes over the woman's abdomen and legs. An episiotomy may be done just before delivery if there is a need for one. See the discussion of episiotomy in Chapter 18.

The woman is encouraged to push with the contractions until the fetal chin clears the perineum. Then she is asked to pant to avoid too rapid a delivery of the fetal head. While supporting the fetal head, the physician or nurse-midwife assesses whether the umbilical cord is around the fetal neck and removes it if it is, and then suctions the nose and mouth with a bulb syringe. The woman is encouraged to push again as the rest of the body is born. Figures 14-4 to 14-13 depict the labor and delivery experience of one family.

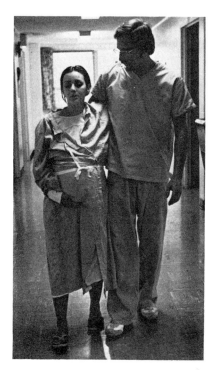

Figure 14-4
Woman and her husband walking in the hospital during labor.*

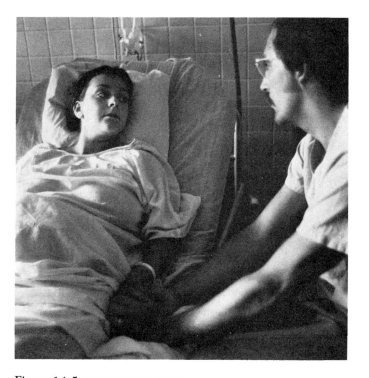

Figure 14-5
The husband coaches his wife during a contraction.

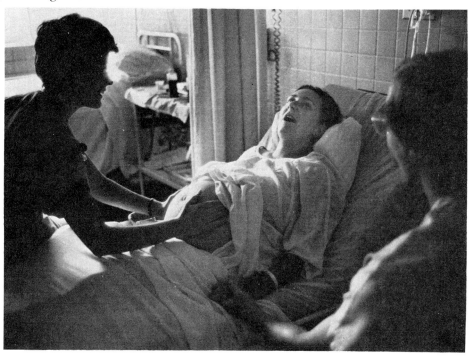

Figure 14-6
The attending nurse-midwife assesses a contraction.

*Figures 14-4 to 14-13: photos by Suzanne Arms.

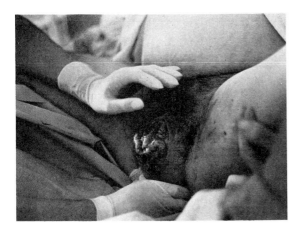

Figure 14-7
The baby's head is crowning.

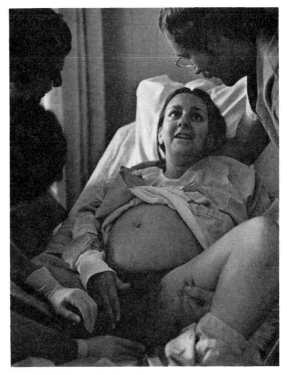

Figure 14-8
The mother can feel her baby's head crowning.

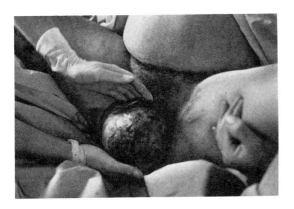

Figure 14-9
The nurse-midwife holds the baby's head as it is delivered.

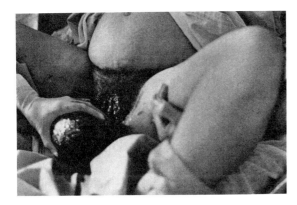

Figure 14-10
The baby's head is delivered.

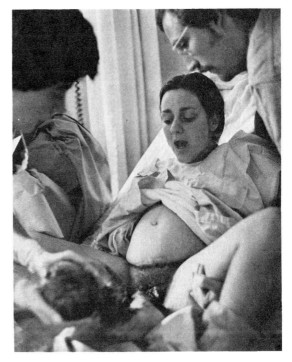

Figure 14-11
The rest of the baby's body is quickly delivered.

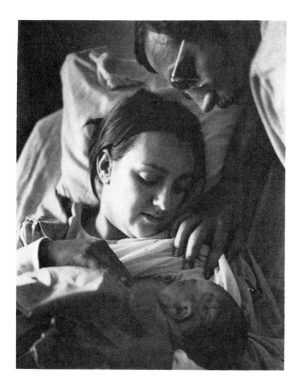

Figure 14-12
The new family.

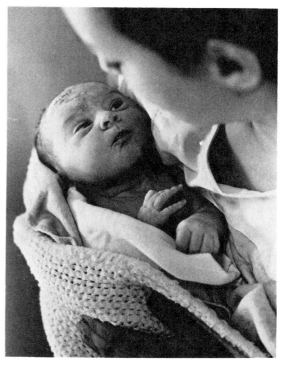

Figure 14-13
The baby gets acquainted with his mother.

Immediate Care of the Newborn

The physician/nurse-midwife places the newborn on the mother's abdomen or in the radiant heated unit. The newborn is maintained in a modified Trendelenburg position. This position aids drainage of mucus from the nasopharynx and trachea by gravity. The newborn is dried immediately. Warmth can be maintained by placing warmed blankets over the newborn or placing the newborn in skin-to-skin contact with the mother. If the newborn is in a radiant heated unit, he or she is dried, placed on a dry blanket, and left uncovered under the radiant heat. Because radiant heat warms the outer surface of objects, a newborn wrapped in blankets will receive no benefit from radiant heat.

The newborn's nose and mouth are suctioned with a bulb syringe as needed.

Most immediate care of the newborn can be accomplished while the newborn is in the parent's arms or in the radiant heated unit.

Apgar scoring system   The Apgar scoring system (Table 14-3) was designed in 1952 by Dr. Virginia Apgar, an anesthesiologist. The pur-

pose of the **Apgar score** is to evaluate the physical condition of the newborn at birth and the immediate need for resuscitation. The newborn is rated 1 minute after birth and again at 5 minutes and receives a total score ranging from 0 to 10 based on the following criteria:

1. The *heart rate* is auscultated or palpated at the junction of the umbilical cord and skin. This is the most important assessment. A newborn heart rate of less than 100 beats/min indicates the need for immediate resuscitation.

2. The *respiratory effort* is the second most important Apgar assessment. Complete absence of respirations is termed *apnea*. A vigorous cry indicates good respirations.

3. The *muscle tone* is determined by evaluating the degree of flexion and resistance to straightening of the extremities. A normal newborn's elbows and hips are flexed, with the knees positioned up toward the abdomen.

4. The *reflex irritability* is evaluated by flicking the soles of the feet or by inserting a nasal catheter in the nose. A cry merits a full score of 2. A grimace is 1 point, and no response is 0.

Table 14-3
The Apgar Scoring System*

Sign	Score		
	0	1	2
Heart rate	Absent	Slow — below 100	Above 100
Respiratory effort	Absent	Slow — irregular	Good crying
Muscle tone	Flaccid	Some flexion of extremities	Active motion
Reflex irritability	None	Grimace	Vigorous cry
Color	Pale blue	Body pink, blue extremities	Completely pink

*From Apgar, V. Aug. 1966. The newborn (Apgar) scoring system, reflections and advice. *Pediatr. Clin. North Am.* 13:645.

5. The *skin color* is inspected for cyanosis and pallor. Generally, newborns have blue extremities, and the rest of the body is pink, which merits a score of 1. This condition is termed *acrocyanosis* and is present in 85% of normal newborns at 1 minute after birth. A completely pink newborn scores a 2 and a totally cyanotic, pale infant is scored 0. Newborns with darker skin pigmentation will not be pink in color. Their skin color is assessed for pallor and acrocyanosis, and a score is selected based on the assessment.

A score of 8–10 indicates a newborn in good condition who requires only nasopharyngeal suctioning and perhaps some oxygen near the face. If the Apgar score is below 8, resuscitative measures may need to be instituted. See the discussion in Chapter 22.

Care of umbilical cord   If the clinician has not placed a cord clamp (Figure 14-14) on the newborn's umbilical cord, it is the responsibility of the nurse to do so. Before applying the cord clamp, the nurse examines the cut end for the presence of two arteries and one vein. The umbilical vein is the largest vessel, and the arteries are seen as smaller vessels. The number of vessels is recorded on the delivery room and newborn records. The cord is clamped approximately ½–1 inch from the abdomen to allow room between the abdomen and clamp as the cord dries. Abdominal skin must not be clamped, as this will cause necrosis of the tissue.

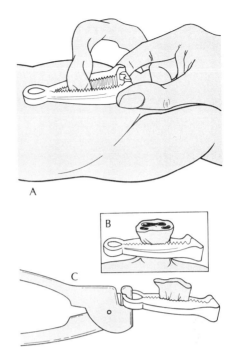

Figure 14-14
Hollister cord clamp. **A**, Clamp is positioned ½–1 inch from the abdomen and then secured. **B**, Cut cord. **C**, Plastic device for removing clamp after cord has dried.

The Hollister clamp is removed in the newborn nursery approximately 24 hours after the cord has dried.

Physical assessment of newborn by delivery room nurse   An abbreviated systematic physical assessment is performed by the nurse in the delivery room to detect any abnormalities (Figure 14-15). First, the size of the newborn and the contour and size of the head in relationship to the rest of the body are noted. The newborn's posture and movements indicate tone and neurologic functioning.

The skin is inspected for discoloration, presence of vernix caseosa and lanugo, and evidence of trauma and desquamation. Vernix caseosa is a white, cheesy substance found normally on newborns. It is absorbed within 24 hours after delivery. Vernix is abundant on preterm infants and absent on postterm newborns. A large quantity of fine hair (lanugo) is often seen on preterm newborns, especially on their shoulders, foreheads, backs, and cheeks. Desquamation of the skin is seen in postterm newborns.

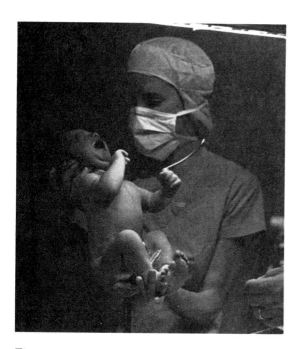

Figure 14-15
The delivery room nurse assesses the newborn. Notice the urine bag on the infant. (In most institutions, urine is not collected in the delivery room.)

The nares are observed for flaring. As the newborn cries, the palate can be inspected for cleft palate. The presence of mucus in the nose and mouth can be assessed and removed with the bulb syringe as needed. The chest is inspected for respiratory rate and the presence of retractions. If retractions are present, the newborn is assessed for grunting or stridor. A normal respiratory rate is 30–40 per minute. The lungs may be auscultated bilaterally for breath sounds. Absence of breath sounds on one side could mean pneumothorax. Rales may be heard immediately after birth because a small amount of fluid may remain in the lungs; this fluid will be absorbed. Rhonchi indicate aspiration of oral secretions. If there is excessive mucus or respiratory distress, the nurse suctions the newborn with a DeLee suction. (See Procedure 14-1, DeLee Suction.)

The elimination of urine or meconium is noted and recorded on the newborn record.

Newborn identification To ensure correct identification, the nurse gives the mother and the newborn matching identification bands in the delivery room. One bracelet is placed on the mother's wrist. Two bracelets are placed on the newborn—one on the wrist and one on the ankle. The newborn bands must be applied snugly to prevent their loss.

Most hospitals footprint the newborn and fingerprint the mother for further identification purposes. To prepare the newborn for footprinting, the nurse wipes the soles of both the newborn's feet to remove any vernix caseosa.

Management of the Third and Fourth Stages of Labor

Third Stage

After delivery, the physician or nurse-midwife prepares for the delivery of the placenta. The following signs suggest placental separation (see Chapter 13):

1. The uterus rises upward in the abdomen because the placenta settles into the lower uterine segment.

2. As the placenta moves downward, the umbilical cord lengthens.

3. A sudden trickle or spurt of blood appears.

4. The shape of the uterus changes from a disk to a globe.

While waiting for these signs, the nurse palpates the uterus to check for ballooning of the uterus caused by uterine relaxation and subsequent bleeding into the uterine cavity.

After the placenta has separated, the woman may be asked to bear down to aid delivery of the placenta.

Oxytocics are frequently given at the time of the delivery of the placenta, so the uterus will contract and bleeding will be minimized. Oxytocin (Pitocin), 10 units, may be added to an intravenous infusion or given by slow intravenous push. Some physicians may order methylergonovine maleate (Methergine), 0.2 mg, intramuscularly. In addition to administering the ordered medications, the nurse assesses and records maternal blood pressure before and after administration of oxytocics. (For further information, refer to the Drug Guides—Oxytocin in Chapter 18 and Methylergonovine maleate in Chapter 25.)

PROCEDURE 14-1
DeLee Suction

Objective	Nursing action	Rationale
Clear secretions from newborn's nose and/or oropharynx	Tighten the lid on the DeLee mucus trap collection bottle (Figure 14-16)	Avoids spillage of secretions and prevents air from leaking out of lid
	Place the whistle tip in your mouth; insert other end of tubing in newborn's nose or mouth approximately 3–5 in.; provide suction by sucking on whistle tip	Provides suction Clears nasopharynx Gives gentle suction
	Continue suction as tube is removed	Avoids redepositing secretions in newborn's nasopharynx
	Continue reinserting tube and providing suction for as long as:	Facilitates removal of secretions
	1. Secretions are being removed	
	2. Newborn continues to have depressed respirations	
	3. Movement of secretion can be heard with respiratory effort by ausculation of lungs	If meconium was present in amniotic fluid the baby may have swallowed some
	Occasionally the tube may be passed into the newborn's stomach to remove secretions or meconium that was swallowed before birth; if this action is needed, insert tube into newborn's mouth and then into the stomach	Secretions and/or meconium aspirate may be removed from newborn's stomach to decrease incidence of aspiration of stomach contents
	Provide suction and continue suction as tube is removed	

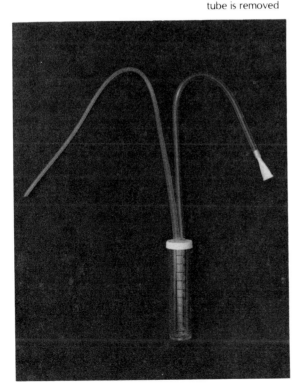

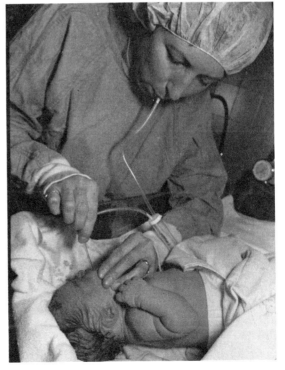

Figure 14-16
DeLee suction trap.

Fourth Stage

After the delivery of the placenta, the physician or nurse-midwife inspects the placental membranes to make sure they are intact and that all cotyledons are present. This inspection is especially important with Duncan placentas. If there is a defect or a part missing from the placenta, a manual uterine examination is done.

The time of delivery of the placenta and the mechanism (Schultze or Duncan) are noted on the delivery record.

The vagina and cervix are inspected for lacerations, and any necessary repairs are made. The episiotomy may be repaired now if it has not been done previously. (See further discussion of episiotomy in Chapter 18.) The fundus of the uterus is palpated; normal position is at the midline and below the umbilicus. A displaced fundus may be caused by a full bladder or blood collected in the uterus. The uterus may be emptied of blood by grasping it anteriorly and posteriorly and squeezing.

The uterine fundus is palpated at frequent intervals to ensure that it remains firmly contracted. The maternal blood pressure is monitored at 5–15-minute intervals to detect any changes. An increase in blood pressure may be due to oxytocic drugs. A decrease may be associated with excessive blood loss.

The nurse washes the woman's perineum with gauze squares and warmed solution and dries the area with a sterile towel before placing the maternity pads. The woman's legs are removed from the stirrups at the same time to avoid muscle strain. The legs may be bicycled to help circulation return. The woman is transferred to a recovery room bed, and the nurse helps her don a clean gown. The mother may feel cold and begin shivering. She can be covered with a warmed bath blanket and a second blanket. If the mother has not had a chance to hold her infant, she may do so before she leaves the delivery room. The nurse ensures that the mother, father, and newborn are provided with time to begin the attachment process. (See Chapter 24 for further discussion of attachment.)

The woman remains in the recovery room for 1–2 hours and is monitored closely. Deviations from normal in vital signs require frequent checking. Blood pressure should return to the prelabor level due to an increased volume of blood returning to the maternal circulation from the uteroplacental shunt. Pulse rate should be slightly lower than it was during labor. Baroreceptors cause a vagal response, which slows the pulse. A rise in the blood pressure may be a response to oxytocic drugs or may be caused by toxemia. Blood loss may be reflected by a lowered blood pressure and a rising pulse rate.

The fundus should be firm at the umbilicus or lower and in the midline. It is palpated (Figure 14-17) but not massaged unless it is soft (boggy). If it becomes boggy or appears to rise in the abdomen, the fundus is massaged until firm; then with one hand supporting the uterus at the symphysis, the nurse exerts firm pressure on the fundus in an attempt to express retained clots. Overmassaging of the fundus causes an increased tendency toward uterine relaxation due to muscle exhaustion.

The nurse inspects the bloody vaginal discharge for amount and charts it as minimal, moderate, or heavy and with or without clots. This discharge, or *lochia rubra*, should be

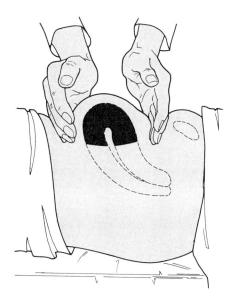

Figure 14-17
Suggested method of palpating the fundus of the uterus during the fourth stage. The left hand is placed just above the symphysis pubis, and gentle downward pressure is exerted. The right hand is cupped around the uterine fundus.

bright red. A soaked perineal pad contains approximately 100 mL of blood. If the perineal pad becomes soaked in a 15-minute period or if blood pools under the buttocks, continuous observation is necessary. When the fundus is firm, a continuous trickle of blood may signal laceration of the vagina or cervix, or an unligated vessel in the episiotomy. See Essential Facts to Remember—Immediate Postdelivery Danger Signs.

If the fundus rises and displaces to the right, the nurse palpates the bladder to determine whether it is distended. The bladder fills rapidly with the extra fluid volume returned from the uteroplacental circulation (and with fluid received intravenously, if given during labor and delivery). The postpartal woman may not realize that her bladder is full because trauma to the bladder and urethra during childbirth decreases bladder tone and the urge to void.

All measures should be taken to enable the mother to void. A warm towel placed across the lower abdomen or warm water poured over the perineum may relax the urinary sphincter and thus facilitate voiding. If the woman is unable to void, catheterization is necessary.

The perineum is inspected for edema and hematoma formation. An ice pack often reduces the swelling and alleviates the discomfort of an episiotomy.

Frequently women have tremors in the immediate postpartal period. This shivering response may be caused by a difference in internal and external body temperatures (higher temperature inside the body than on the outside). Another theory is that the woman is reacting to the fetal cells that have entered the maternal circulation at the placental site. A heated bath blanket placed next to the woman tends to alleviate the problem.

The couple may be tired, hungry, and thirsty. Some hospitals serve the couple a meal. The tired mother will probably drift off into a welcomed sleep. The father should also be encouraged to rest, since his supporting role is tiring physically and mentally. The mother is usually transferred from the delivery unit to the postpartal floor after 2 hours or more depending on agency policy and if the following criteria are met:

- Stable vital signs
- No bleeding
- Nondistended bladder
- Firm fundus
- Sensations fully recovered from any anesthetic agent received during delivery

Enhancing Attachment

Dramatic evidence indicates that the first few hours and even minutes after birth are an important period for the attachment of mother and infant (Klaus and Kennell, 1982). Separation during this period not only delays attachment but may affect maternal and child behavior over a much longer period.

Klaus and Kennell (1982) believe the bonding experience can be enhanced by at least 30–60 minutes of early contact in privacy. If this period of contact can occur during the first hour after birth, the newborn will be in the quiet state and able to interact with parents by looking at them. Newborns also turn their heads in response to a spoken voice. (See Chapter 20 for further discussion of newborn states.)

The first parent–newborn contact may be brief (a few minutes) to be followed by a more extended contact after uncomfortable procedures (delivery of the placenta and suturing of the episiotomy) are completed. When the newborn is returned to the mother, she can be assisted to begin breast-feeding if she so desires. The nurse can help the mother to a more comfortable position for holding the infant and

---

✳ **ESSENTIAL FACTS TO REMEMBER**

Immediate Postdelivery Danger Signs

In the immediate postdelivery recovery period, the following conditions should be reported to the physician or nurse-midwife:

Hypotension
Tachycardia
Uterine atony
Excessive bleeding

breast-feeding. Even if the newborn does not actively nurse, he or she can lick, taste, and smell the mother's skin. This activity by the newborn stimulates the maternal release of prolactin, which promotes the onset of lactation.

Darkening the delivery room by turning out most of the lights causes newborns to open their eyes and gaze around. This in turn enhances eye-to-eye contact with the parents. (*Note:* if the physician or nurse-midwife needs a light source, the spotlight can be left on.) Treatment of the newborn's eyes may also be delayed. Many parents who establish eye contact with the newborn are content to quietly gaze at their infant. Others may show more active involvement by touching and/or inspecting the newborn. Some mothers talk to their babies in a high-pitched voice, which seems to be soothing to newborns. Some couples verbally express amazement and pride when they see they have produced a beautiful, healthy baby. Their verbalization enhances feel-

ings of accomplishment and ecstasy. Figure 14-18 shows a new parent establishing bonds with his newborn son.

Both parents need to be encouraged to do whatever they feel most comfortable doing. Some parents prefer only limited contact with the newborn in the delivery room and instead desire private time together in a more quiet environment, such as the recovery room or postpartal area. In spite of the current zeal for providing immediate attachment opportunities, nursing personnel need to be aware of parents' wishes. The desire to delay interaction with the newborn does not necessarily imply a decreased ability of the parents to bond to their newborn (see Chapter 23 for further discussion of parent–newborn attachment).

CASE STUDY

Allison and Scott Jones are expecting their first child. During the pregnancy, they attended prenatal classes and made special preparations in anticipation of using the birthing room at their local hospital. The pregnancy has proceeded without difficulty or problems.

When labor begins, they go to the hospital and are greeted by Marie Carlson, a nurse in the labor and delivery department. Ms. Carlson helps Allison and Scott get settled and completes the admission process. Allison is having contractions every 2–3 minutes and lasting 45 seconds, and cervical dilatation is 5 cm. She is breathing with the contractions and is excited that the delivery day is at hand.

Ms. Carlson works to provide a comfortable, unhurried atmosphere. She is already acquainted with the Joneses because they have attended the prenatal classes that she teaches. She is familiar with their level of knowledge and will now work to support them as labor progresses. She notes that Allison and Scott are working well together in timing contractions and using relaxation techniques and breathing methods. Ms. Carlson completes her physical assessment, then talks with the couple about the progress. Ms. Carlson leaves, letting the Joneses know she is available whenever they need her. She has found that parents who use the birthing room are well prepared and that she may not

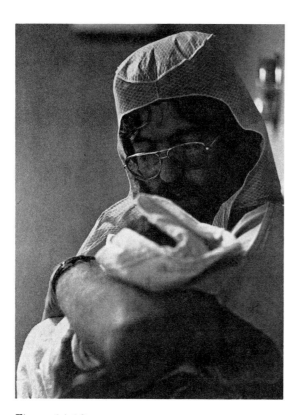

Figure 14-18 ▬▬▬
A father holds his newborn son.

need to stay quite so close. She returns periodically to assess progress and to see how the Joneses are coping with the labor. As long as all is going well, she allows the couple privacy. She has notified the physician, who is now on the way to the hospital, of Allison's admission and labor status.

As Allison proceeds into transition, Ms. Carlson notes that the Joneses need more encouragement and support, so she stays in constant attendance. She assesses maternal, fetal, and labor status and keeps the Joneses informed of their progress.

Dr. J. G. Grey comes in to see the Joneses and stays close by because the labor is progressing rapidly. Toward the end of the transition, Ms. Carlson prepares the equipment to be used during delivery. She assists Allison in her pushing efforts when the cervix has completely dilated. During the delivery, she assists Allison, Scott, and Dr. Grey. The delivery is managed in the same unhurried manner. Ms. Carlson assesses the physical parameters and offers continuing support as Allison delivers a baby girl of healthy appearance. Ms. Carlson assessses the newborn quickly and then places her in her mother's arms.

The postdelivery recovery period is monitored closely so that any problems can be identified. Allison is recovering without problems and is eager to learn more about her new daughter. Ms. Carlson talks to the Joneses to assess their level of knowledge and provides information that is needed. She does a physical assessment of the newborn and explains the findings to the Joneses. She assists Allison as she breast-feeds her baby for the first time. After the feeding, the nurse assists Scott in giving the baby her first bath. Ms. Carlson has found that the bath time provides opportunities to talk and share information.

During the recovery period, she provides quiet time for the new family to be together and get acquainted.

A few hours after delivery, Ms. Carlson assists the Joneses as they prepare for dismissal. She will be making a visit to the Joneses' home the next morning to assess the mother and newborn and to provide information and continued support.

Early Discharge

More hospitals are offering new mothers—whether they deliver in a conventional labor and delivery setting, a birthing room, or an in-hospital birth center—the option of early discharge. Early discharge is any discharge occurring from 2–24 hours postpartally. Most institutions have written policies and criteria about the mother and the newborn eligible for early discharge. Criteria for the mother may include any or all of the following:

- No antepartal or intrapartal complications
- A labor no longer than 30 hours for a primipara or 24 hours for a multipara
- An episiotomy or no greater than a third-degree laceration with no vaginal or cervical lacerations
- A spontaneous or low-forceps delivery
- Stable vital signs
- A firm uterine fundus
- Voiding without difficulty
- Ability to ambulate and provide care for herself and her newborn
- Help at home for 1–3 days
- Demonstrated understanding of home-care instructions

Early discharge criteria for the newborn may include:

- Stable vital signs
- Normal physical examination
- An hematocrit level of 45%–65% and a Dextrostix result of greater than 45%
- At least one feeding

The desired practice is to follow up early discharges with home visits by labor and delivery, postpartum, or public health nurses. The early discharge option offers both financial benefits, by reducing the costs of obstetric care, and psychologic benefits, by reuniting families in their homes more quickly. The most frequent neonatal problem requiring readmission to the hospital is hyperbilirubinemia. Research suggests readmission may be due to the high percentage of breast-feeding mothers who are discharged early, the trend toward late cord clamping in the birth experiences of this group, and the thorough assessments of nurses making home visits (Barton et al., 1980).

Delivery in Less-Than-Ideal Circumstances

Precipitous Delivery

Occasionally labor progresses so rapidly that the maternity nurse is faced with the task of delivering the baby. This is called a *precipitous delivery*. The attending maternity nurse has the primary responsibility for providing a physically and psychologically safe experience for the woman and her baby.

A woman whose physician or nurse-midwife is not present may feel disappointed, frightened, and abandoned, especially if she is not prepared through childbirth education. Fear is an inhibiting factor in childbirth; therefore, the nurse can support the woman by keeping her informed about the labor progress and assuring the woman that the nurse will stay with her. If delivery is imminent, the nurse must not leave the mother alone. Auxiliary personnel can be directed to contact the physician or nurse-midwife and to retrieve the emergency delivery pack ("precip pack"). An emergency delivery pack should be readily accessible to the labor rooms. A typical pack contains the following items:

1. A small drape that can be placed under the woman's buttocks to provide a sterile field

2. Several 4-by-4 gauze pads for wiping off the newborn's face and removing secretions from the mouth

3. A bulb syringe to clear mucus from the newborn's mouth

4. Two sterile clamps (Kelly or Rochester) to clamp the umbilical cord before applying a cord clamp

5. Sterile scissors to cut the umbilical cord

6. A sterile umbilical cord clamp, either Hesseltine or Hollister

7. A baby blanket to wrap the newborn in after delivery

8. A package of sterile gloves

As the materials are being gathered, the nurse must remain calm. The woman is reassured by the composure of the nurse and feels that the nurse is competent.

Delivery of Infant in Vertex Presentation

The nurse who manages precipitous delivery in the hospital conducts it as follows. The woman is encouraged to assume a comfortable position. If time permits, the nurse scrubs her hands with soap and water and puts on sterile gloves. Sterile drapes are placed under the woman's buttocks.

At all times during the delivery, the nurse gives clear instructions to the woman, supports her efforts, and provides reassurance.

When the infant's head crowns, the nurse instructs the woman to pant, which decreases her urge to push. The nurse checks whether the amniotic sac is intact. If it is, the nurse tears the sac so the newborn will not breathe in amniotic fluid with the first breath.

The nurse may place an index finger inside the lower portion of the vagina and the thumb on the outer portion of the perineum and gently massage the area to aid in stretching of perineal tissues and to help prevent perineal lacerations. This is called "ironing the perineum."

With one hand, the nurse applies gentle pressure against the fetal head to prevent it from popping out rapidly. *The nurse does not hold the head back forcibly*. Rapid delivery of the head may result in tears in the woman's perineal tissues. In the fetus the rapid change in pressure within the fetal head may cause subdural or dural tears. The nurse supports the perineum with the other hand and allows the head to be delivered between contractions.

As the woman continues to pant, the nurse inserts one or two fingers along the back of the fetal head to check for the umbilical cord. If the cord is around the neck, the nurse bends her fingers like a fish hook, grasps the cord, and pulls it over the baby's head. It is important to check that the cord is not wrapped around more than one time. If the cord is tightly looped and cannot be slipped over the baby's head, two clamps are placed on the cord, the cord is cut between the clamps, and the cord is unwound.

Immediately after delivery of the head, the mouth, throat, and nasal passages are suctioned. The nurse places one hand on each side of the head and exerts gentle downward traction until the anterior shoulder passes under the symphysis pubis. At this time, gentle upward traction helps delivery of the posterior shoulder. The nurse then instructs the woman to push gently so that the rest of the body can be delivered quickly. The newborn must be supported as it emerges.

The newborn is held at the level of the uterus to facilitate blood flow through the umbilical cord. The combination of amniotic fluid and vernix makes the newborn very slippery, so the nurse must be careful to avoid dropping the newborn. The nose and mouth of the newborn are suctioned again, using a bulb syringe. The nurse then dries the newborn to prevent heat loss.

As soon as the nurse determines that the newborn's respirations are adequate, the infant can be placed on the mother's abdomen. The newborn's head should be slightly lower than the body to aid drainage of fluid and mucus. The weight of the newborn on the mother's abdomen stimulates uterine contractions, which aid in placental separation. The umbilical cord should not be pulled.

The nurse is alert for signs of placental separation (slight gush of dark blood from the vagina, lengthening of the cord, or a change in uterine shape from discoid to globular). When these signs are present, the mother is instructed to push so that the placenta can be delivered. The nurse inspects the placenta to determine whether it is intact.

The nurse checks the firmness of the uterus. The fundus may be gently massaged to stimulate contractions and to decrease bleeding. Putting the newborn to breast also stimulates uterine contractions through release of oxytocin from the pituitary gland.

The umbilical cord may now be cut. Two sterile clamps are placed approximately 2–4 inches from the newborn's abdomen. The cord is cut between them with sterile scissors. A sterile cord clamp (Hollister or Hesseltine) can be placed adjacent to the clamp on the newborn's cord, between the clamp and the newborn's abdomen. The clamp *must not* be placed snugly against the abdomen, because the cord will dry and shrink.

The area under the mother's buttocks is cleaned, and her perineum is inspected for lacerations. Bleeding from lacerations may be controlled by pressing a clean perineal pad against the perineum and instructing the woman to keep her thighs together.

If the physician's arrival is delayed or if the newborn is having respiratory distress, the newborn should be transported immediately to the nursery. *The newborn must be properly identified before he or she leaves the delivery area.*

Record keeping   The following information is noted and placed on a delivery record:

1. Position of fetus at delivery
2. Presence of cord around neck or shoulder (nuchal cord)
3. Time of delivery
4. Apgar scores at 1 and 5 minutes after birth
5. Sex of newborn
6. Time of delivery of placenta
7. Method of placental expulsion
8. Appearance and intactness of placenta
9. Mother's condition
10. Any medications that were given to mother or newborn (per agency protocol)

Postdelivery interventions   Postdelivery implications are the same as those on p. 312.

Summary

Labor and delivery can be a time of anxious or eager anticipation. The nurse must remember that the care given to the woman and family at this time has an impact not only on the woman's feelings about and reactions to this labor and delivery but also on future childbearing plans and expectations.

The nurse must be adept at intrapartal assessment and must be aware of the physiologic changes that are occurring and the wide range of emotional reactions to labor and delivery. The nurse uses this knowledge to devise the plan of care for meeting the needs of the childbearing couple.

The first hour after delivery is critical for both mother and newborn from both a physiologic and psychologic viewpoint. Continued knowledgeable and caring nursing management is indispensable during this period.

References

Abril IF: Mexican-American folk beliefs: How they affect health care. *MCN* May/June 1977; 2:168.

Apgar V: The newborn (Apgar) scoring system: Reflections and advice. *Pediatr Clin North Am* August 1966; 13:645.

Barton J et al: Alternative birthing center: Experience in a teaching obstetric service. *Am J Obstet Gynecol* 1980; 137:377.

Burrow GN, Ferris T: *Medical Complications During Pregnancy*. Philadelphia: Saunders, 1982.

Carr KC: Obstetric practices which protect against neonatal morbidity: Focus on maternal position in labor and birth. *Birth Fam J* Winter 1980; 7:249.

Carrington BW: The Afro American. In: *Culture Childbearing Health Professionals*. Clark AL (editor). Philadelphia: Davis, 1978.

Chung JJ: Understanding the Oriental maternity patient. *Nurs Clin North Am* March 1977; 12:67.

Frink BB, Chally P: Managing pain responses to cesarean childbirth. *MCN* July/August 1984; 9(4):270.

Hollingsworth AO et al: The refugees and childbearing: What to expect. *RN* November 1980; 43:45.

Kay MA: The Mexican American. In: *Culture Childbearing Health Professionals*. Clark AL (editor). Philadelphia: Davis, 1978.

Klaus MH, Kennell JH: *Parent-Infant Bonding*. 2nd ed. St. Louis: Mosby, 1982.

Mahan CS, McKay S: Preps and enemas: Keep or discard? *Contemp Ob/Gyn* November 1983; 22(5):241.

McCaffery M: *Nursing Management of the Patient with Pain*. 2nd ed. Philadelphia: Lippincott, 1979.

McKay SR: Maternal position during labor and birth: A reassessment. *J Obstet Gynecol Neonatal Nurs* 1980; 9:288.

McKay SR: Second stage labor: Has tradition replaced safety? *Am J Nurs* 1981; 81:1061.

Mercer R: *Perspectives on Adolescent Health Care*. New York: Lippincott, 1979.

Morton K: Beyond "choice" in childbirth. *Birth* Fall 1983; 10(3):179.

Murillo-Rohde I: Cultural sensitivity in the care of the Hispanic patient. *Wash State J Nurs* 1979; (Special Suppl):25.

Roberts JE, Mendez-Bauer C, Wodell DA: The effects of maternal position on uterine contractility and efficiency. *Birth* Winter 1983; 10(4):243.

Simkin P: Preparing parents for second stage. *Birth* Winter 1982; 9(4):229.

Stephany T: Supporting the mother of a patient in labor. *J Obstet Gynecol Neonatal Nurs* September/October 1983; 12(5):345.

Additional Readings

Anderson CJ: Enhancing reciprocity between mother and neonate. *Nurs Res* March/April 1981; 30:89.

Bramptom B et al: Initial mothering patterns of low-income black primiparas. *J Obstet Gynecol Neonatal Nurs* May/June 1981; 10:174.

Brown MS: A cross-cultural look at pregnancy, labor, and delivery. *J Obstet Gynecol Neonatal Nurs* October 1976; 5:35.

Campbell A, Worthington EL: Teaching expectant fathers how to be better childbirth coaches. *MCN* January/February 1982; 7:28.

Dean PG et al: Making baby's acquaintance: A unique attachment strategy. *MCN* January/February 1982; 7:37.

Dunn DM, White DG: Interactions of mothers with their newborns in the first half-hour of life. *J Adv Nurs* 1981; 6:271.

Griffith S: Childbearing and the concept of culture. *J Obstet Gynecol Neonatal Nurs* May/June 1982; 11:181.

Howley C: The older primipara: Implications for nurses. *J Obstet Gynecol Neonatal Nurs* May/June 1981; 10:182.

Worthington EL et al: Which prepared-childbirth coping strategies are effective? *J Obstet Gynecol Neonatal Nurs* January/February 1982; 11:45.

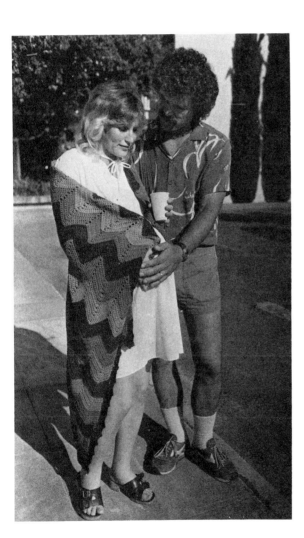

15
Birthing Options

Chapter Contents

Siblings at Birth

Alternative Positions

The Leboyer Method

Free-Standing Birth Centers

Home Births
Indications for Hospitalization

Objectives

- Discuss sibling attendance at birth.

- Examine alternative birthing positions and settings for labor and delivery.

- Describe early discharge programs and subsequent postpartal assessment.

- Explore philosophy, preparation, and management of home birth.

Key Terms

birth center   Leboyer method

    Many expectant parents consider birth a highly personal and significant life event, one over which they should have significant control. Consequently, the desires of expectant parents frequently include the following requests:

- That labor and delivery be performed in a supportive, quiet, and relaxed environment

- That an enema and perineal shave not be given at admission

- That the father be allowed to participate as much as the couple desires

- That medications and treatments be administered only with the couple's permission and only after a complete explanation about their actions and possible side-effects has been given
- That invasive fetal monitoring be avoided
- That forceps and anesthetics not be used unless medically indicated
- That the woman may labor and deliver in the same room and bed
- That an episiotomy not be performed
- That the baby be delivered in a dimly lighted room and handled gently
- That the parents be allowed maximal interaction with their child or that the infant be allowed to nurse immediately after delivery
- That the baby be allowed to remain with his or her parents
- That the labor and delivery be shared by persons significant to the couple

Some hospitals are not equipped to meet some of these requests. Others refuse because they believe that certain procedures are necessary to maintain maternal and fetal well-being. Other hospitals refuse because they resist change to new ideas and methods. In any case, many expectant families are frustrated in their attempt to make decisions about the kind of childbearing experience they want. As a result, they are seeking alternative modes of maternity care and health care providers who are more responsive to their desires.

In this chapter, we will discuss some of the more common alternative birth options and the role of the nurse in helping expectant parents fulfill their desires.

Siblings at Birth

More couples are choosing to extend the "family-centered" concept beyond mother, father, and newborn by including their other children in the birth experience. Many hospitals have yet to develop programs that allow siblings to visit the baby; having siblings attend a birth is an even rarer option. However, families who strongly wish their children to attend will prob-

ably find a way, even if they must create their own birthing situation.

The decision to have children present at birth is a personal and individual one. Children who will attend a birth can be prepared through books, audiovisual materials, models, and parental discussion. Nurses can assist parents with sibling preparation by helping them understand the stressors a child may experience. For example, the child may feel left out when there is a new child to love, or a brother may come when a sister was expected (MacLaughlin and Johnston, 1984). (For further discussion of sibling preparation, see Chapter 9.)

It is highly recommended that the child have his or her own support person or coach whose sole responsibility is tending to the needs of the child. The support person should be well known to the child, warm, sensitive, flexible, knowledgeable about the birth process, and comfortable with sexuality and birth. This person must be prepared to interpret what is happening to the child and intervene when necessary.

The child should be given the option of relating to the birth in whatever manner he or she chooses as long as it is not disruptive. Children should understand that it is their own option to be there and that they may stay or leave the room as they choose. To help the child meet his or her goal, the nurse may wish to elicit from the child exactly what he or she expects from the experience. The child needs to feel free to ask questions and express feelings (Daniels, 1983).

Many agencies are concerned about neonatal infection when siblings are present. Parents are requested not to bring children who are obviously ill. Children are requested to perform an antiseptic scrub and put on a cover gown. In agencies that allow siblings to visit only after the birth, infection has not been an issue.

In general, the presence of siblings at birth engenders feelings of interest and the desire to nurture "our" baby, as opposed to jealousy and rivalry directed at "Mom's" baby. The mother does not disappear mysteriously to the hospital, leaving the children at home, and return from the hospital with a demanding outsider. Instead, the family attending delivery together finds a new opportunity for closeness and growth by sharing in the birth of a new member.

Alternative Positions

An upright posture (squatting, kneeling, standing, or sitting) for labor and delivery was ·considered normal in most societies until modern times. Only within the last 200 years has the recumbent position for labor become more usual in the Western world. Its use in this century has been reinforced because of the convenience of applying new technology when the woman is recumbent. The lithotomy position has thus become the conventional manner in which North American women give birth in hospitals. In searching for alternative positions, consumers and professionals alike are refocusing on the comfort of the laboring woman rather than on the convenience of the birth attendant (Figures 15-1, 15-2, 15-3). Table 15-1 discusses advantages and disadvantages of various positions.

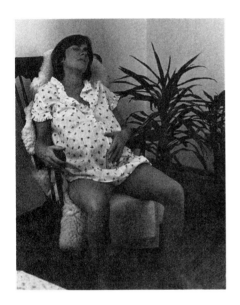
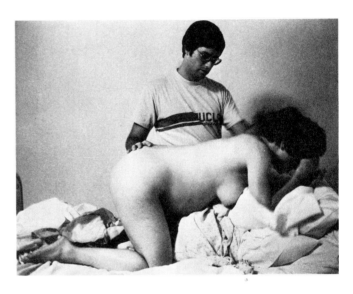
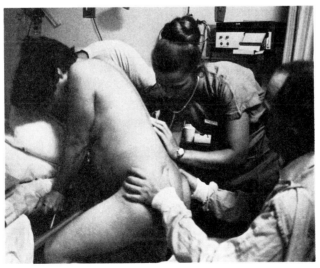

Figure 15-1
As long as no contraindications exist, the laboring woman is encouraged to choose a position of comfort. The nurse modifies her assessments and interventions as necessary. (Photos by Suzanne Arms.)

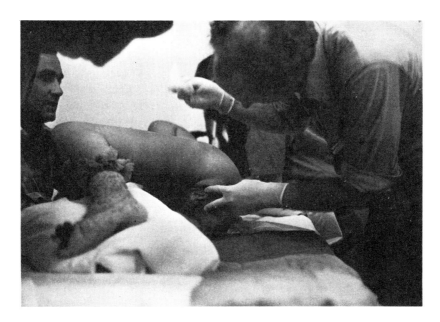

Figure 15-2
Side-lying delivery. Note that the woman's upper leg is supported by her partner. (Photo by Suzanne Arms.)

Table 15-1
Birthing Positions

Position	Advantages	Disadvantages	Nursing implications
Sitting in birthing chair	Gravity aids descent and expulsion of infant Does not compromise venous return from lower extremities Chair can be tilted to various degrees	If woman is short, sitting with legs spread may increase tension on perineum, which may lead to lacerations Position of body, legs, and feet cannot be altered	Encourage woman to tilt the chair to increase her comfort Assess for pressure points on legs
Semi-Fowler's	Does not compromise venous return from lower extremities Woman can view birth process	If legs are positioned widely apart, relaxation of perineal tissues is decreased	Assess that upper torso is evenly supported Increase support of body by changing position of bed or using pillows as props
Left Lateral Sims'	Does not compromise venous return from lower extremities Increased perineal relaxation and decreased need for episiotomy Appears to prevent rapid descent	It is difficult for woman to see the birth if she desires	Position the upper leg so that it is adequately supported
Squatting	Size of pelvic outlet is increased Gravity aids descent and expulsion of newborn Second stage may be shortened (McKay, 1984)	May be difficult to maintain balance while squatting	Help woman maintain balance

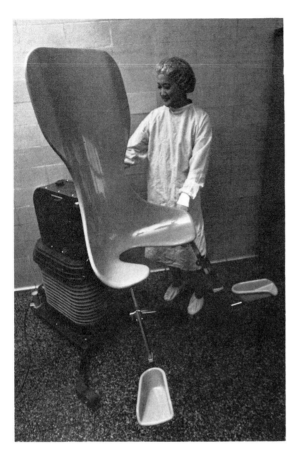

Figure 15-3
Birthing chair. Chair is contoured to provide optimum support. The chair can be tilted to various positions.

The Leboyer Method

In a conventional delivery, the newborn is subjected to extreme changes in sensory input—bright lights, voices, suctioning, and being quickly dried and placed in blankets. In 1975 Leboyer introduced a birthing technique that eases the newborn's transition to extrauterine life.

In the **Leboyer method**, the lights in the delivery room are dimmed, and the noise level, including talking, is kept to a minimum. After delivery the newborn is placed on his or her stomach on the mother's bare abdomen. The mother is encouraged to gently stroke and touch the newborn in a massaging motion.

Clamping of the umbilical cord is delayed until all pulsations have ceased out of respect

for the innate rhythms of the new life. Leboyer (1976) believes that this delay helps the newborn's initial respiratory efforts and shelters the newborn from anoxia at the time of birth. After the umbilical cord is clamped, the newborn is gently and slowly placed in a water bath that has been warmed to 98–99F. The newborn remains in the bath until he or she is completely relaxed. The warm water recreates the temperature and weightlessness of the womb. Following the bath the infant is carefully and gently dried and wrapped in layers of warm blankets.

Critics of the Leboyer method question the ability of the birth attendant to quickly assess maternal and/or neonatal complications or calculate Apgar scores in a dimly lit room. Traditional practitioners have expressed concern about the possibility of high neonatal bilirubin levels when cord clamping is delayed. Hypothermia as a result of the bath is also cited as a risk of the Leboyer method. On the other hand, proponents and couples themselves cite the advantages as increased participation by the father in the birth—particularly when he gives the bath—and the serenity of the birth experience (Crystle et al., 1980).

Free-Standing Birth Centers

Care in free-standing birth centers is given by certified nurse-midwives, labor and delivery nurses, nurse practitioners, physicians, nonmedical assistants, public health nurses, families themselves, or any combination of these. **Birth centers** require families to take more responsibility for the birth experience than usual while at the same time providing a more flexible and less costly way to give birth.

Birth centers strive for a warm, homelike atmosphere, with birthing rooms similar to typical bedrooms. The room is generally furnished with a bed, in which the woman labors and delivers, comfortable chairs for the father and other relatives or friends, a cradle, and a private bath and/or shower. Some free-standing centers also have play rooms for siblings, kitchens where families may keep food or beverages, and other amenities. Most free-standing centers encourage children to participate to whatever extent they choose; hospital-based centers are somewhat more reluctant to allow total participation by siblings.

Birth centers are generally equipped for emergencies with oxygen, suction, and resuscitation equipment. Rapid transport to more traditional settings is usually available.

In keeping with the concept of birth as a normal event, most birth center settings are set up for nurse-midwife management of labor and delivery rather than for obstetric technology and treatment. Therefore, these centers are not appropriate for high-risk deliveries. Couples intending to use the centers are screened during pregnancy for high-risk factors (see Chapter 6). The presence of any one factor does not automatically exclude the woman from delivering in a birth center, but it does mean that careful and continuous assessment is needed.

Each center also has policies about various circumstances that would require the woman to be transferred to a hospital labor and delivery setting. These may include, but are not limited to, the following:

- An increase in maternal temperature to over 100.4F (37.8C)
- A significant change in blood pressure
- Meconium stained amniotic fluid
- Prolonged true labor
- Significant vaginal bleeding
- Prolonged second stage of labor (more than 2 hours for a nullipara and more than 1 hour for a multipara)
- Indications of fetal distress

The couple is usually required to attend prenatal classes to prepare for their childbirth. They are also encouraged to meet birthing center personnel and to discuss their desires and preferences.

Traditional obstetric procedures frequently are not used. Episiotomies are not routine, forceps are not used, and in many centers the woman may deliver in the position of her choice. After delivery, physical contact between the parents and newborn is encouraged. The mother may breast-feed immediately. Siblings and accompanying support persons are also encouraged to interact with the newborn as they choose.

In most instances, rooming-in is immediate, and healthy newborns and their families are never separated. The initial pediatric examination is conducted in the presence of the family. The mother and newborn are monitored for a minimum of 2–24 hours after delivery and then are discharged. In birth centers in the hospital setting, women who do not wish to be discharged early are transferred to the postpartal unit.

Birth center personnel usually perform a home visit after discharge. The home visit provides an opportunity to see the family in their home setting, to make assessments of the mother and newborn, to answer questions, and to provide information and support.

Home Births

Another alternative to the traditional hospital delivery is home birth. Couples who choose home birth generally have strong beliefs about their rights to make their own birth choices. Couples choosing home births believe that the responsibility for the birth outcome is theirs. Furthermore, they do not believe the hospital is necessarily the safest place to give birth, and they see standard medical practice as frequently involving unnecessary trauma and intervention. Some women may feel that hospital routines and expectations will not allow them to conform to their cultural norms for childbearing behavior (Brackbill et al., 1984).

Therefore, in making the choice between home and hospital birth, medical risk is only one issue. The effect on the family unit is another issue. Parents who take responsibility for a home delivery find that it is a warm, close, loving experience under their control. The newborn is immediately incorporated into the family, and the continuous contact between the newborn and the family helps to bond the family as a unit. Siblings present during delivery are able to welcome the newborn into the family and are participants in an exciting and beautiful experience.

The safety of any home birth is maximized by thorough planning, careful prenatal care and screening, skilled physicians or nurse-midwives, and an organized and tested transport system to a facility where accepting caregivers are available. However, adequate medical back-up care is frequently unobtainable. Obstetricians as a group are particularly vocal opponents of home birth. Their opposition is often based on memories of serious emergencies they have witnessed at the time of birth. Therefore, they usually view home birth as a backward step in maternal child care. Despite their opposition, the trend toward home births seems to be growing rather than slowing.

However, a side-effect of physician opposition has been to make home births, when they do occur, even less safe (Zimmerman, 1980). Physicians may refuse to supervise the prenatal care of a couple planning a home birth or may refuse to attend one. Many physicians also refuse to act as back-up caregivers for the nurse-midwife attending a home birth. Hospital personnel in general also tend to oppose home birth. They may manifest this disapproval through punishing attitudes when couples unable to complete birth at home come to the hospital.

Home deliveries may be attended by a lay midwife, certified nurse-midwife (contingent upon the laws of respective states), or physician. Lay midwives rarely have an established educational program or state certification.

Certified nurse-midwives are well-educated, skilled practitioners whose scope of practice is closely regulated by state nurse practice acts.

Indications for Hospitalization

In many instances, home birth is a trouble-free, satisfying experience for the family. However, if a woman who has planned a home birth suddenly finds it necessary to seek hospital care, she is at risk both physiologically and psychologically. Either she, her fetus, or both are probably in distress if hospitalization is deemed necessary. Moreover, she is also vulnerable to disapproval, ridicule, and anger on the part of many hospital personnel. Her control over the birth process, which may have been a major factor in her decision to select home birth, is now almost totally gone. She must deal with her fears and concerns regarding the birth outcome, her guilt and responsibilities should the outcome be poor, and the unfamiliarity of her surroundings at this critical time.

Factors that may necessitate moving a planned home birth to the hospital include the following:

- Hard labor for longer than 8 hours without fetal descent
- The onset of true labor prior to 36 weeks' gestation
- Marked meconium staining
- An abnormal fetal heart rate or pattern
- Significant vaginal bleeding intrapartally or postpartally

The nurse who has initial contact with the family must be careful to remain nonjudgmental in attitude or remarks. All care and procedures and the rationales for them should be carefully explained. No required procedure should be presented in a punitive way. Depending on the circumstances, it may be appropriate for the nurse to reassure the couple that their choice of birth location did not cause the current problem. Every effort should be made to give them any control and options possible in the new situation.

Summary

Expectant parents are requesting and in some instances demanding alternatives to traditional maternity care. Many hospitals are now providing a variety of birthing experiences. Other couples are choosing to forego any institutional contact, opting instead for a free-standing birth center or home births. The maternity nurse needs to be informed of all birthing methods and their advantages and disadvantages. The functions of assessment and teaching play an even more important role because contact with the woman may be brief.

With sound nursing and medical care, consumers of maternity care are probably best served by making available a wide variety of birth options. In this way, society has its best chance of extending a satisfying and safe birth experience to every couple.

References _____

Brackbill Y, Woodward L, McManus KA et al: Characteristics related to drug consumption of women choosing between nontraditional birth alternatives—A comparison. *J Nurs Midwifery* May/June 1984; 29(3):177.

Crystle CD et al: The Leboyer method of delivery: An assessment of risk. *J Reprod Med* 1980; 25:267.

Daniels MB: The birth experience for the sibling: Description and evaluation of a program. *J Nurs Midwifery* September/October 1983; 28(5):15.

Leboyer F: *Birth Without Violence*. New York: Knopf, 1976.

MacLaughlin SM, Johnston KB: The preparation of young children for the birth of a sibling. *J Nurs Midwifery* November/December 1984; 29(6):371.

McKay SR: Squatting: An alternate position for the second stage of labor. *MCN* May/June 1984; 8(3):181.

Zimmerman E: Home birth safety. *J Obstet Gynecol Neonatal Nurs* 1980; 9:191.

Additional Readings _____

Arms S: *Immaculate Deception*. Boston: Houghton Mifflin, 1975.

Brody H, Thompson JR: The maximum strategy in modern obstetrics. *J Fam Pract* 1981; 12:977.

Haire D: *The Cultural Warping of Childbirth*. Seattle, Wash.: International Childbirth Education Association, 1972.

McKay SR: Second stage labor: Has tradition replaced safety? *Am J Nurs* 1981; 81:1016.

May IM: *Spiritual Midwifery*. Summertown, Tenn.: The Book Publishing Company, 1978.

Sagov SE, Feinbloom RI, Spindel P: *Home Birth: A Practitioner's Guide to Birth Outside the Hospital*. Rockville, Maryland: Aspen, 1984.

Roberts JF, Kriz DM: Delivery positions and perineal outcome. *J Nurs Midwifery* May/June 1984; 29(3)186.

Young D: *Changing Childbirth: Family Birth in the Hospital*. Rochester, New York: Childbirth Graphics LTD, 1982.

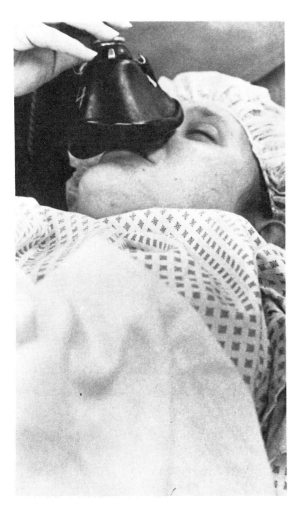

16

Obstetric Analgesia and Anesthesia

Chapter Contents

Systemic Drugs
    Nursing Considerations
    Analgesics
    Narcotic Antagonists
    Ataractics
    Sedatives

Regional Anesthesia
    Regional Anesthetic Agents
    Paracervical Block
    Lumbar Epidural Block
    Caudal Block
    Subarachnoid Block (Spinal, Low Spinal)
    Pudendal Block

Local Infiltration Anesthesia

General Anesthesia
    Inhalation Anesthetics
    Intravenous Anesthetics
    Balanced Anesthesia
    Complications of General Anesthesia

Objectives

- Describe the use of systemic drugs to promote pain relief during labor.

- Identify the major types of regional analgesia and anesthesia, including area affected, advantages, disadvantages, techniques, and nursing implications.

- Discuss the complications of regional anesthesia that may occur.

- Describe the major inhalation and intravenous anesthetics used to provide general anesthesia.

- Describe the major complications of general anesthesia.

Key Terms

caudal block   pudendal block
epidural block   regional anesthesia
local infiltration   spinal block
paracervical block

The management of pain during childbirth is an important aspect in the health care of the childbearing woman. Pain relief measures vary from breathing techniques, effleurage, and positive reinforcement (discussed in Chapter 14), to regional nerve blocks. The type of analgesics and anesthetics used during each woman's labor and delivery will depend on the preferences of the woman and the physician or nurse-midwife as well as the physical condition of the mother and fetus.

Systemic Drugs

The goal of pharmacologic pain relief during labor is to provide maximal analgesia at minimal risk for the mother and fetus. To reach this goal, clinicians must consider a number of factors:

- All systemic drugs used for pain relief during labor cross the placental barrier by simple diffusion, but some drugs cross more readily than others.
- Drug action in the body depends on the rate at which the substance is metabolized by liver enzymes and excreted by the kidneys.
- High drug doses remain in the fetus for long periods because the fetal liver enzymes and kidney excretion are inadequate to metabolize analgesic agents.

Nursing Considerations

Nursing interventions directed toward pain relief begin with nonpharmacologic measures such as providing information, support, and physical comfort. Back rubs, the application of cool cloths, and encouragement as the woman practices breathing techniques are examples of comfort measures. Some laboring women need no further interventions. However, for other women, the progression of labor brings increasing discomfort that interferes with her ability to perform breathing techniques and maintain a sense of control. In this instance, pharmacologic analgesics may be used to decrease discomfort, increase relaxation, and reestablish the woman's sense of control.

Because analgesic drugs affect the woman, fetus, and contraction pattern, the nurse must assess the following areas before administering medication:

Maternal assessment

- The woman is willing to receive medication.
- Vital signs are stable.

Fetal assessment

- The FHR is between 120–160 beats/minute, and no decelerations are present.
- The fetus exhibits normal movement.
- The fetus is at term.
- Meconium staining is not present.

Assessment of labor

- Contraction pattern is well established.
- The cervix is dilated at least 5–6 cm in nulliparas and 3–4 cm in multiparas.
- The fetal presenting part is engaged.
- There is progressive descent of the fetal presenting part. No complications are present.

If these normal parameters are not present further assessment will be necessary.

The general principles for administering analgesic drugs are as follows:

1. The woman is in an individual labor room.

2. The environment is free from sensory stimuli, such as bright lights, noise, and irrelevant conversation, to allow the woman to focus on the drug action.

3. An explanation of the effects of the medication is given, including how long the effects will last and how the drug will make the woman feel. See Essential Facts to Remember—What Women Need to Know About Pain Relief Medication.

What Women Need to Know About Pain Relief Medications

Before receiving medications, the woman should understand:

- Type of medication administered
- Route of administration
- Expected effects of medication
- Implications for fetus/neonate
- Safety measures needed (for example, remain in bed with side rails up)

4. The woman is encouraged to empty her bladder prior to administration of the drug.

5. The baseline FHR and maternal vital signs are recorded prior to administration.

6. The physician's written order is checked, and the medication prepared and signed out on the narcotic or control sheet.

7. The woman is asked again if she is allergic to any medication and her arm band checked for identification.

8. The drug is administered by the route ordered, using correct technique.

9. The side rails are pulled up for safety, and the reasons explained to the woman.

10. The medication, dosage, time, route, and site of administration are charted on the nurse's notes and on the monitor strip.

11. The FHR is monitored to assess the effects of the medication on the fetus, and the woman is evaluated for signs that the analgesic agent is having the desired effect.

12. The woman is not left alone. If no family member is present and it is necessary for the nurse to leave, the woman should be given a short explanation and assurances that the nurse will return.

There is no completely safe and satisfactory method of pain relief. Analgesia, when judiciously used, can be beneficial to the laboring woman and do little harm to the fetus. The woman who is free from fear and who has confidence in the medical and nursing personnel usually has a relatively comfortable first stage of labor and requires a minimum of medication. A positive, supportive, caring attitude on the part of the professional nurse and the expectant parents is an essential aspect of pain relief.

Analgesics

Meperidine hydrochloride   Meperidine hydrochloride (Demerol) is a narcotic analgesic frequently used for obstetric analgesia. See the Drug Guide—Meperidine Hydrochloride for further discussion.

Butorphanol tartrate   Butorphanol tartrate (Stadol) is a synthetic analgesic. It effectively relieves moderate to severe pain. The exact mechanism of the drug is unknown, but it is thought to act on the subcortical portion of the central nervous system.

The recommended initial dose is 2 mg intramuscularly every 3–4 hours. If it is given intravenously, however, the dosage is reduced.

Butorphanol tartrate has limited respiratory depressant effects, but, in patients with respiratory diseases, the respiratory depression may be pronounced. Other side-effects include sedation, nausea, dizziness, and a clammy, sweaty sensation.

It has a potential to elevate cerebrospinal fluid pressure. Because butorphanol has a weak narcotic antagonistic activity, it may cause withdrawal symptoms in patients who have been receiving opiates.

The specific antidote is naloxone (Narcan), which may be given intravenously, intramuscularly, or subcutaneously.

Narcotic Antagonists

Narcotic antagonists counteract the respiratory depressant effects of the opiate-type narcotics. The most commonly used narcotic antagonists include levallarphan tartrate (Lorfan) and naloxone.

Levallarphan   The narcotic antagonist levallarphan tartrate is effective only against neonatal respiratory depression caused by narcotic analgesics. This antagonist acts by competing with narcotics in the respiratory center receptors and by displacing the narcotic molecules from the receptor sites. If the receptors are not

DRUG GUIDE
Meperidine Hydrochloride (Demerol)

OVERVIEW OF OBSTETRICAL ACTION

Meperidine hydrochloride is a narcotic analgesic that interferes with pain impulses at the subcortical level of the brain. In addition, it enhances analgesia by altering the physiologic response to pain, suppressing anxiety and apprehension, and creating a euphoric feeling. Meperidine hydrochloride is used during labor to provide analgesia. Peak analgesia occurs in 40–60 minutes with intramuscular and in 5–7 minutes with intravenous administration. Duration is 2–4 hours.

Administration after labor has reached the active phase does not appear to delay labor or to decrease uterine contraction frequency or duration. Meperidine HCl crosses the placental barrier and appears in the fetus within 1–2 minutes after maternal intravenous injection (Roberts et al., 1984).

Route, dosage, frequency

IM: 50–100 mg every 3–4 hours
IV: 25–50 mg by slow intravenous push every 3–4 hours

Maternal contraindications

Hypersensitivity to meperidine, asthma
CNS depression
Respiratory depression
Fetal distress
Preterm labor if delivery is imminent
Hypotension
Respirations <12 per minute
Concurrent use with anticonvulsants may increase depressant effects

Maternal side effects

Respiratory depression
Nausea and vomiting, dry mouth

Drowsiness, dizziness, flushing
Transient hypotension
Bradycardia, palpitations
May precipitate or aggravate seizures in clients prone to convulsive activity (Giacoia and Yaffee, 1982)

Effect on fetus/neonate

Neonatal respiratory depression may occur if meperidine HCl is administered within 2–4 hours of delivery
Neonatal hypotonia, lethargy, interference of thermoregulatory response
Neurologic and behavioral alterations for up to 72 hours after delivery. Presence of meperidine in neonatal urine up to 3 days following delivery (Morrison et al., 1982)

NURSING CONSIDERATIONS

Assess client history, labor and fetal status, maternal blood pressure and respirations to identify contraindications to administration
Intramuscular doses should be injected deeply to avoid irritation to subcutaneous tissue
Intravenous doses should be diluted and administered slowly
Provide for client safety by instructing her to remain on bed rest, by keeping side rails up and placing call bell within reach
Evaluate effect of drug
Observe for maternal side effects
Observe newborn for respiratory depression, be prepared to initiate resuscitative measures and administer antagonist naloxone if needed

occupied solely by narcotics, this antagonist agent produces respiratory depression by occupying these sites. Therefore, levallarphan increases depression caused by barbiturates, tranquilizers, and other sedative drugs.

When a narcotic antagonist is needed, levallarphan 1 mg may be administered to the laboring woman intravenously, 5–10 minutes before delivery to prevent respiratory depression of the newborn.

Naloxone   Naloxone exhibits little pharmacologic activity in the absence of narcotics. Although it is an antagonist, naloxone has little or no agonistic effect. Naloxone is effective against neonatal depression due to narcosis. Unlike levallarphan, naloxone does not increase respiratory depression due to barbiturates, tranquilizers, or other sedatives. To determine neonatal dose, see Drug Guide—Naloxone in Chapter 22.

Ataractics

Ataractic drugs do not relieve pain but do decrease apprehension and anxiety, relieve nausea, and enhance the effects of narcotics. Ataractics frequently used in labor include promethazine hydrochloride (Phenergan), hydroxyzine hydrochloride (Vistaril), and diazepam (Valium).

Sedatives

The principal use of barbiturates in current obstetric practice is in false labor or in the early stages of beginning labor. An oral dose of secobarbital (Seconal) or pentobarbital (Nembutal) promotes relaxation and allows the woman to sleep a few hours. The woman can then enter the active phase of labor in a more relaxed and rested state.

Regional Anesthesia _____

Regional anesthesia is achieved by injecting local anesthetic agents so that they come into direct contact with nervous tissue. The methods most commonly used in labor are paracervical block, peridural block (lumbar epidural and caudal), subarachnoid block (spinal for cesarean birth, low spinal for vaginal delivery—also known as *saddle block*), pudendal block, and local infiltration. The nerve blocks are accomplished by a single injection or continuously by means of an indwelling plastic catheter.

Regional anesthesia has gained widespread popularity in recent years and is particularly compatible with the goals of psychoprophylactic preparation for childbirth. In general, the advantages of a regional anesthesia are as follows:

1. Relief from discomfort is complete in the area blocked.

2. Depression of maternal vital signs rarely occurs.

3. Aspiration of gastric contents is virtually eliminated if no additional sedative was administered.

4. Administration at the optimal time does not significantly alter the course of labor.

5. The woman remains alert and able to participate in the birth.

The disadvantages include:

1. A high degree of skill is required for proper administration of most regional anesthetics.

2. Failures such as no effect or unilateral or incomplete anesthesia can occur even when the agents are administered by experienced clinicians.

3. Some agents have side-effects.

4. Systemic toxic reactions to these agents are more common than to agents used for general anesthesia.

Prerequisites for the administration of regional anesthetics are knowledge of the anatomy and physiology of pertinent structures, techniques of administration, the pharmacology of local anesthetics, and potential complications. With the exception of nurse anesthetists and nurse-midwives, who may perform procedures for which they have been trained, nurses in the United States may *not* legally administer anesthetic agents. This restriction applies to the reinjection of agents through indwelling catheters. However, the nurse must have an adequate knowledge of all aspects of regional anesthesia to provide support and to give appropriate reinforcing explanations to the woman. The nurse who has a thorough understanding of the techniques and agents can also provide more efficient assistance to the administrator. Client safety is increased when the nurse recognizes complications and immediately initiates appropriate intervention.

Pain associated with the first stage of labor can be relieved by blocking the sensory nerves supplying the uterus with the techniques of paracervical and peridural (lumbar epidural, and caudal) blocks. Pain associated with the second stage and delivery can be alleviated with pudendal, peridural, and subarachnoid (spinal, low spinal, and saddle) blocks (Figure 16-1).

Regional Anesthetic Agents

Two types of local anesthetic agents are currently available—the ester and amide types. The ester type includes procaine hydrochloride (Novocain), chloroprocaine hydrochloride (Nesacaine), and tetracaine hydrochloride (Pentocaine). Esters are rapidly metabolized; therefore, toxic maternal levels are not as likely to be reached, and placental transfer to the fetus is prevented. Amide types include lidocaine hydrochloride (Xylocaine), mepivacaine hydrochloride (Carbocaine), and bupivacaine hydrochloride (Marcaine). Amide types are more powerful and longer-acting agents. They readily cross the placenta, can be measured in the fetal circulation, and affect the fetus for a prolonged period.

Regional anesthetic agents block the conduction of nerve impulses from the periphery to the central nervous system. Although the mechanism of their action is not fully understood, the smaller the fiber, the more sensitive it is to local anesthetics. The small fibers that conduct the sensations of pain, temperature, pressure, and touch can be blocked without affecting the large, heavily myelinated fibers that continue to maintain muscle tone, position sense, and motor function (Bonica, 1972).

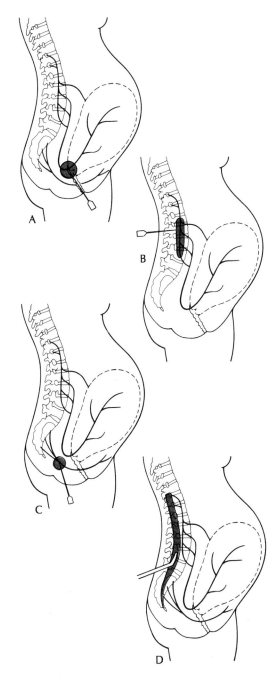

Figure 16-1 ▬▬▬▬▬
Schematic diagram showing pain pathways and sites of interruption. **A**, Paracervical block: Relief of uterine pain only. **B**, Lumbar sympathetic block: Relief of uterine pain only. **C**, Pudendal block: Relief of perineal pain. **D**, Lumbar epidural block: Dark area demonstrates peridural space and nerves affected, and white tube represents continuous plastic catheter. (From Bonica JJ: *Principles and Practice of Obstetric Analgesia and Anesthesia*. Philadelphia: Davis, 1972, pp. 492, 512, 521, and 614.)

Absorption of local anesthetics depends primarily on the vascularity of the area of injection. The agents also contribute to increased blood flow by causing vasomotor paralysis. Higher concentration of drugs causes greater vasodilatation. Good maternal physical condition or a high metabolic rate aids absorption. Malnutrition, dehydration, electrolyte imbalance, and cardiovascular and pulmonary problems lower the threshold for toxic effects. The pH of tissues affects the rate of absorption, which has implications for fetal complications. The addition of vasoconstrictors such as epinephrine delays absorption and prolongs the anesthetic effect. Recent studies have demonstrated that epinephrine decreases uteroplacental blood flow, making it an undesirable additive in many situations. The breakdown of local anesthetics in the body is accomplished by the liver and plasma esterase, with the resulting substance being eliminated by the kidneys (Santos, 1983).

The weakest concentration and the smallest amount necessary to produce the desired results are advocated.

Adverse maternal reactions   Reactions to local anesthetic agents range from mild symptoms to cardiovascular collapse. Mild reactions include palpitations, vertigo, tinnitus, apprehension, confusion, headache, and a metallic taste in the mouth. Moderate reactions include more severe degrees of mild symptoms plus nausea and vomiting, hypotension, and muscle twitching, which may progress to convulsions and loss of consciousness. The severe reactions are sudden loss of consciousness, coma, severe hypotension, bradycardia, respiratory depression, and cardiac arrest. Local toxic effects on tissues may also result with high concentrations of the agents. Because of the possibility of adverse reactions, especially hypotension, anesthetic agents should not be used unless an intravenous line is in place.

Paracervical Block

A **paracervical block** is the result of a local anesthetic agent injected transvaginally adjacent to the outer rim of the cervix. The agent may be administered during the acceleration phase of labor. This measure relieves the pain of cervical dilatation but does not anesthetize the lower vagina or perineum (Figure 16-2).

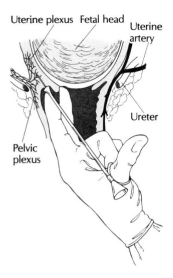

Figure 16-2
Technique for paracervical block from needle in place at appropriate distance beyond guide. (From Bonica JJ: *Principles and Practice of Obstetric Analgesia and Anesthesia.* Philadelphia: Davis, 1972, p. 515.)

Paracervical block has several disadvantages. The vascularity of the injection area increases the possibility of rapid absorption, with resulting systemic toxic reaction. Hematomas may occur as a result of uterine vessel damage. In addition, fetal bradycardia frequently occurs.

Nursing implications   Prior to the procedure, the maternal vital signs should be assessed to provide a baseline. The FHR is also assessed. An electronic fetal monitor is usually applied to provide a continuous assessment of the FHR. The procedure and expected results are explained to the woman, and any questions are answered. The nurse helps the woman into a dorsal recumbent position with her knees flexed so the agent can be administered. As the injection is given, the nurse provides support by maintaining communication, eye contact, or physical contact.

The FHR is continuously assessed. If bradycardia occurs, the woman is turned on her side and oxygen is administered. The bladder is assessed at frequent intervals because the woman may not be aware of the need to void. The amount of cervical dilatation is monitored because the paracervical block affects only the cervix and upper vagina. It is not sufficient for

pain relief during delivery and episiotomy repair.

Lumbar Epidural Block

A lumbar **epidural block** provides regional anesthesia during the first and second stages of labor. The area of the body affected depends on the amount of anesthetic that is injected.

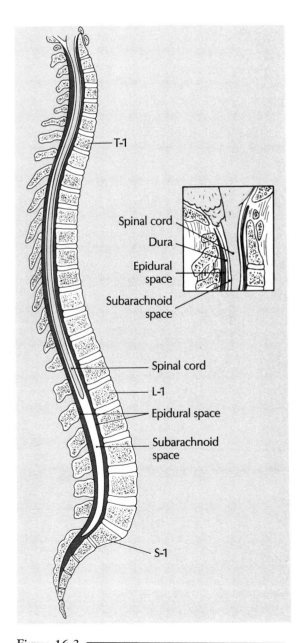

Figure 16-3
Epidural space.

The epidural (peridural) space is a potential space between the ligamentum flavum and the dura mater. The space extends from the base of the skull to the end of the sacral canal (Figure 16-3). Access to the space may be through the lumbar or caudal area. A lumbar epidural block is most frequently continuous, providing analgesia and anesthesia from active labor through episiotomy repair (Figure 16-4).

Once a woman is in active labor, a small amount of local anesthetic agent injected in the lumbar epidural space will relieve the discomfort of uterine contractions. A larger dose is given late in the first stage to extend anesthesia to the vagina, relieving the pain caused by the descent of the fetus. An additional dose may be given to provide anesthesia in the perineum during delivery.

The lumbar epidural block has several disadvantages:

1. Considerable skill is required to administer epidural blocks.
2. Pain relief is slower than with other methods.
3. A larger amount of anesthetic agent is required.

4. The dura mater may be punctured resulting in inadvertent spinal anesthesia.
5. Maternal hypotension and resulting FHR decelerations may occur.
6. Perineal relaxation interferes with fetal rotation and the ability to bear down, and a forceps delivery may be needed.

Epidural anesthesia is contraindicated when maternal hemorrhage is present or likely to occur; when there is local infection at the site of injection (such as pilonidal cyst); and when there is central nervous system, cardiac, or pulmonary disease.

Nursing implications   The nurse assesses the maternal vital signs and the FHR for a baseline. The procedure and expected results are explained, and the woman's questions are answered. The woman is positioned on her left side, shoulders parallel, with her legs slightly flexed. Maternal blood pressure and pulse must be taken every 1–2 minutes during the first 15 minutes after the injection and every 10–15 minutes thereafter until they are stable. The most common side-effect of epidural anesthesia is hypotension. Some clinicians attempt to prevent

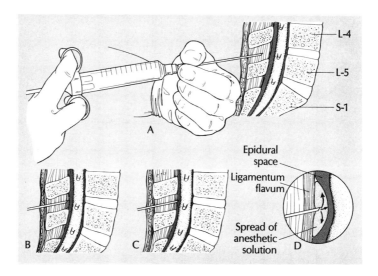

Figure 16-4

Technique of epidural block. **A**, Proper position of insertion. **B**, Needle in the ligamentum flavum. **C**, Tip of needle in epidural space. **D**, Force of injection pushing dura away from tip of needle. (From Bonica JJ: *Principles and Practice of Obstetric Analgesia and Anesthesia*. Philadelphia: Davis, 1972, p. 631.)

hypotension by infusing 500–1000 mL of solution intravenously at a rapid rate. If hypotension occurs, the nurse assists with corrective measures such as positioning the woman in a left side-lying position, increasing the flow rate of the intravenous infusion, and administering oxygen. The FHR should be assessed continuously during any hypotensive episode.

The bladder is assessed at frequent intervals because the epidural block lessens the urge to urinate. During the second stage of labor, the woman may also require more assistance with pushing, since she cannot feel her contractions and does not experience the urge to push.

Headache (as occurs with spinal blocks) is *not* a side-effect of epidural anesthesia, because the dura mater of the spinal canal has not been penetrated and there is no leakage of spinal fluid. Therefore, lying flat for a prescribed number of hours after delivery is not required. Ambulation should be delayed, however, until the anesthesia has worn off. This may take several hours, depending on the agent and the total dose. Motor control of the legs is weak but not totally absent after delivery. Return of complete sensation and the ability to control the legs are essential before ambulation is attempted. The woman must also be able to maintain blood pressure in a sitting or standing position. See Nursing Care Plan—Regional Anesthesia, for further nursing actions.

Text continues on p. 341.

NURSING CARE PLAN
Regional Anesthesia

PATIENT ASSESSMENT

History

1. Maternal information
   a. Allergies to drugs (specifically anesthetic agents)
   b. Psychologic status
      (1) What type anesthesia does the woman want and what kind will she accept?
      (2) Does the woman understand the procedure?
      (3) What does she expect it to accomplish?
      (4) Is the woman able to cope with the labor process and can she follow directions?
   c. Prenatal preparation and education
   d. Presence of other disease states, such as cardiovascular, pulmonary, and CNS disorders, and metabolic diseases
   e. Time of woman's last meal
2. Fetal assessment
   a. Gestational age
   b. Status
   c. Stability of FHR

Physical Examination

1. Determine whether site to be used for injection is free from infection

2. Determine whether hemorrhage is present or imminent
3. Evaluate blood pressure for evidence of hypotension
4. Note evidence of upper respiratory infection, which is a contraindication for general anesthesia

Laboratory Evaluation

1. No specific tests required for woman
2. Fetal scalp samples may be obtained in presence of fetal distress

PLAN OF CARE

Nursing Priorities

1. Maintain a safe environment for woman and fetus
2. Continuously monitor maternal status to recognize and to treat potential problems
3. Monitor fetal status
4. Promote thorough understanding of procedure through education of both parents

Client/Family Educational Focus

1. Discuss the purpose, expected effect, and possible side effects of anesthetic block
2. Discuss the procedure and the expected nursing care associated with regional anesthesia
3. Provide opportunities to discuss questions and individual concerns of the woman and her family

Problem	Nursing interventions and actions	Rationale
Woman's fear and anxiety	Thoroughly explain procedure, its effects, and its value to woman and significant other	Regional anesthesia frequently is poorly understood and frightening for women Thorough explanation during procedure ensures cooperation

NURSING CARE PLAN (continued)
Regional Anesthesia

Problem	Nursing interventions and actions	Rationale
	Provide an opportunity for questions and discussion Utilize charts and other teaching aids as necessary Evaluate emotional significance of regional anesthesia to the woman and intervene appropriately	
Adequate preparation for procedure	Have legal consents signed; have woman empty bladder Begin intravenous fluids	Regional anesthesia interferes with woman's urge to void Intravenous fluids maintain adequate hydration and provide systemic access in the event of untoward reactions or severe hypotension Women receiving subarachnoid or peridural block are to be overhydrated for 5 min prior to the procedure Increased intravenous fluid intake decreases the possibility of maternal hypotension
	Position woman correctly for procedure (see text for proper positioning for individual procedures) Assess maternal status: 1. Obtain baseline vital signs before any anesthetic agent is given 2. Monitor blood pressure every 5 min for 30 min following administration of anesthetic agent 3. Monitor pulse and respiration	Baseline reading allows more complete evaluation of maternal status Hypotension is a frequent complication of regional anesthesia Pulse may slow following spinal anesthesia due to decreased venous return, decreased venous pressure, and decreased right heart pressure Respiratory paralysis is a potential complication of regional anesthesia
	Assess fetal status: 1. Utilize fetal monitoring to establish a baseline reading of FHR and FHTs 2. Monitor FHR continuously Observe, record, and report complications of anesthesia, including hypotension, fetal distress, respiratory paralysis, changes in uterine contractility, decrease in voluntary muscle effort, trauma to extremities, nausea and vomiting, loss of bladder tone, and spinal headache	Maternal hypotension may interfere with fetal oxygenation and is evidenced by fetal bradycardia
Hypotension	Observe, record, and report symptoms of hypotension, including systolic pressure <100 mm Hg or a 25% fall in systolic pressure, apprehension, restlessness, dizziness, tinnitus, headache Institute treatment measures: 1. Place woman with head flat and foot of bed elevated	Gravity increases venous filling of the heart and the pulmonary blood volume; the result is an increase in stroke volume and cardiac output with a rise in blood pressure

NURSING CARE PLAN (continued)
Regional Anesthesia

Problem	Nursing interventions and actions	Rationale
	2. Increase IV fluid rate	Blood volume increases and circulation improves
	3. Administer O_2 by face mask	Oxygen content of circulating blood increases
	4. Administer vasopressors as ordered	Vasoconstriction occurs; vasopressors are not used in pregnant women unless absolutely necessary because they may further compromise the fetus
	Specific interventions for treatment of hypotension following peridural anesthesia: 1. Raise knee gatch on bed 2. Manually displace uterus laterally to left	Increases venous return (vena cava is usually to the right)
	3. Administer O_2 by face mask at 4–7 L/min	Face mask is method of choice, because woman in labor breathes through her mouth
	4. Increase rate of IV fluids 5. Keep woman supine for 5–10 min following administration of block to allow drug to diffuse bilaterally; after 5–10 min position woman on side	
	Specific interventions for hypotension following spinal anesthesia: 1. Administer O_2 by face mask at 4–7 L/min	BP drops following spinal anesthesia, probably because of paralysis of the sympathetic vasoconstrictor fibers to blood vessels
	2. Manually displace uterus to left 3. Increase rate of IV fluids 4. Place legs in stirrups	Increases venous return
Fetal distress	Observe, record, and report fetal bradycardia (FHR < 120/min) and loss of beat-to-beat variability Institute treatment measures for maternal hypotension (Note: Paracervical blocks commonly cause a drop in FHR for a short period of time)	Maternal hypotension causes decreased blood circulation to fetus and results in fetal hypoxia Amide group of anesthetic agents (bupivacaine, mepivacaine, and lidocaine) have potential to produce direct fetal myocardial depression, bradycardia may be caused by reduced placental blood flow
Respiratory paralysis and spinal blockade	Monitor respirations; if respiratory function is compromised, woman exhibits restlessness, dizziness, drowsiness, dyspnea, and an inability to speak; lapse into unconsciousness, hypotension, and apnea quickly follows Immediate treatment includes following: 1. Support of ventilation 2. Increase in IV fluid rate 3. Preparation for cardiac resuscitation	Respiratory paralysis may occur with total spinal blockade and results from too concentrated a dose (for example, injected during a contraction) or too large a dose
Change in uterine contractility	Monitor uterine contractions manually or electronically; if uterine contractions cease, oxytocic agent may be administered	Anesthetic agents generally decrease uterine contractility (although increased contractility occasionally occurs); this decrease frequently prolongs labor for the woman

NURSING CARE PLAN (continued)
Regional Anesthesia

Problem	Nursing interventions and actions	Rationale
Decrease in voluntary muscle effort	Monitor contractions; coordinate woman's pushing effort with pressure of uterine contraction; delivery by forceps may be necessary	Loss of muscle control results in loss of ability to push Woman does not have sensation of having contractions Pushing without contractions decreases effectiveness and tires the woman
Trauma to extremities	Support extremity during movement Position legs securely so they cannot fall off stirrups or delivery table Move legs slowly	Regional block anesthesia produces vasomotor paralysis Sudden movement in client with vasomotor paralysis may precipitate hypotensive episode
Nausea and vomiting	Protect woman from aspiration of vomitus Move woman slowly and gently	Nausea and vomiting may accompany hypotension and are related to hypoxia and excessive rise in BP following administration of vasopressor Nausea and vomiting are often related to sudden changes in position
Loss of bladder tone	Evaluate bladder distention Insert Foley catheter if distention is present	Regional anesthesia reduces feeling and control of sphincter muscles Full bladder during second stage of labor increases chance of bladder trauma
Spinal headache	1. Preventive measures include: 　a. Use of small (25–26) gauge needle 　b. Maintenance of recumbent position for 6–12 hr following delivery 　c. Adequate hydration—IV fluids during labor and delivery, oral fluids following delivery 2. Administer analgesics as ordered 3. Use of "blood patch" for severe and incapacitating headache	Spinal headache is related to the leakage of spinal fluid; a small needle permits less fluid loss Headache, which commonly occurs when the woman is upright, is related to decreased intracranial pressure Aids in fluid replacement

NURSING CARE EVALUATION

Client has not suffered injury
Client's BP, pulse, and respiration are within her normal limits

Fetus has not been compromised, FHTs remained fairly stable
Client understands type of regional block administered and possible side effects

NURSING DIAGNOSIS*	SUPPORTING DATA	NURSING ORDERS
Anxiety and/or fear related to invasive, unfamiliar procedure	Lack of knowledge about regional anesthesia Preconceived notions, fears	Explain the procedure and answer questions; refer questions to physician or anesthesiologist as needed
Potential for maternal injury	Respiratory paralysis Maternal hypotension	Assist anesthesiologist by identifying the beginning of each uterine contraction Assess maternal blood pressure to identify maternal hypotension

*These are a few examples of nursing diagnoses that may be appropriate for a woman receiving regional anesthesia. It is not an inclusive list and must be individualized for each woman.

Caudal Block

A **caudal block** is achieved by injecting a local anesthetic into the epidural space. The resulting anesthesia relieves the discomfort of uterine contractions. There is also loss of sensation in the cervix, lower vagina, and the perineal area (Figure 16-5).

Nursing implications   The nursing implications of the caudal block are much the same as those of the lumbar epidural block. The exception is that the woman is placed in a lateral Sims position for administration of the agent.

Subarachnoid Block (Spinal, Low Spinal)

In a subarachnoid block (**spinal block**), a local anesthetic agent is injected directly into the spinal fluid in the spinal canal to provide anesthesia for vaginal delivery and cesarean birth. A subarachnoid block is given late in the second stage, when the fetal head is on the perineum. The technique of administration varies depending on whether the block is being given for a cesarean or vaginal delivery (see Figure 16-6).

The disadvantages include a fairly high incidence of hypotension after the block, the need for the woman to remain flat for 6–12 hours after the block, and possible headache afterward.

Contraindications for subarachnoid block include severe hypovolemia, central nervous system disease, infection at the site of puncture, and severe hypotension or hypertension. In addition, the woman may not wish to have the spinal procedure.

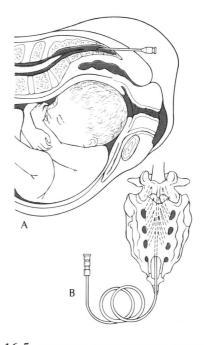

Figure 16-5

Caudal technique. **A**, Placement of needle in caudal canal. **B**, Plastic catheter in caudal canal. (Reprinted with permission of Ross Laboratories, Columbus, OH 43216. From Clinical Education Aid No. 17.)

Nursing implications   The nurse assesses maternal vital signs and the FHR to establish a baseline. The procedure and expected effect are explained to the woman, and any questions are answered. Before this block is given, the woman must sign a consent form. Because this block is given late in the second stage, the woman will be on the delivery bed. The nurse helps the woman sit on the side of the bed and put her feet on a stool. The woman places her arms

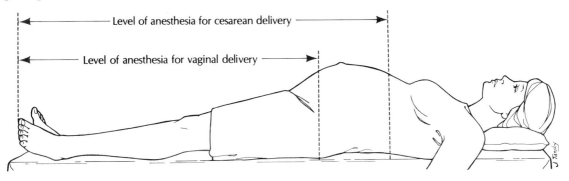

Figure 16-6

Levels of anesthesia for vaginal and cesarean deliveries. (Reprinted with permission of Ross Laboratories, Columbus, OH 43216. From Clinical Education Aid No. 17.)

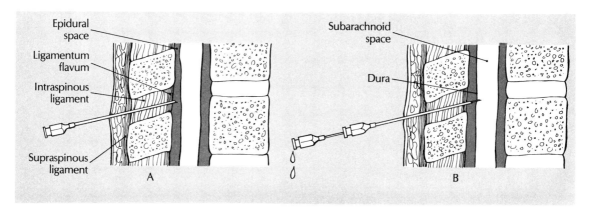

Figure 16-7

Double needle technique for spinal injection. **A**, Large needle in epidural space. **B**, 25–26 gauge needle in larger needle entering the spinal canal. (From Bonica JJ: *Principles and Practice of Obstetric Analgesia and Anesthesia*. Philadelphia: Davis, 1972, p. 563.)

between her knees, bows her head, and arches her back to widen the intervertebral spaces. The nurse supports the woman in this position and palpates the uterus to identify the beginning of uterine contractions. The clinician injects the anesthetic agent between contractions. If the anesthetic agent is injected during a contraction, the anesthesia is greater and may compromise respiration. After the woman returns to a lying position, the nurse places a rolled towel under her right hip so that the uterus is displaced slightly to the left. Maternal blood pressure, pulse, and FHR are assessed every 2–5 minutes until the woman is stable. In the absence of maternal hypotension or toxic reaction, the subarachnoid block has no direct effect on the fetus (Figure 16-7).

The nurse continues to monitor uterine contractions and instructs the woman to bear down because she will not experience the urge to do so. After delivery, motor paralysis of the woman's legs is not uncommon. The nurse exercises great care when moving the woman from the delivery bed to protect her from injury. The woman remains flat in bed for 6–12 hours following the block.

Pudendal Block

A **pudendal block**, administered by a transvaginal or transperineal method, intercepts signals to the pudendal nerve. The pudendal block provides perineal anesthesia for the latter part of the first stage, the second stage of labor, delivery, and episiotomy repair. The pudendal block stops the pain of perineal distention but not the discomfort of uterine contractions (Figure 16-8).

The disadvantages of the pudendal block include possible broad ligament hematoma, perforation of the rectum, and trauma to the sciatic nerve.

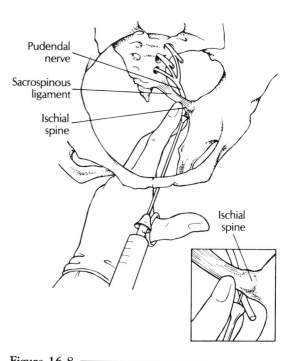

Figure 16-8

Technique for pudendal block. Inset shows needle extending beyond guide. (Modified from Bonica JJ: *Principles and Practice of Obstetric Analgesia and Anesthesia*. Philadelphia: Davis, 1972, p. 495.)

Nursing implications   The nurse explains the procedure and the expected effect and answers any questions. Pudendal block does not alter maternal vital signs or FHR; thus, additional assessments are not necessary.

Local Infiltration Anesthesia

Local infiltration of perineal tissues is achieved by injecting an anesthetic agent into the subcutaneous tissue in a fanlike pattern (Figure 16-9). Local anesthetics are generally used at the time of delivery for episiotomy repair.

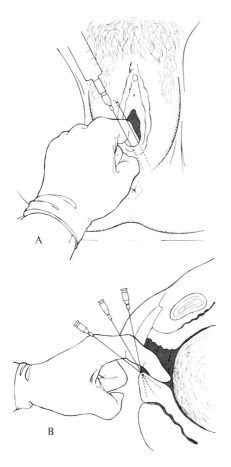

Figure 16-9

Local infiltration anesthesia. **A**, Technique of local infiltration for episiotomy and repair. **B**, Technique of local infiltration showing fan pattern for the fascial planes. (From Bonica JJ: *Principles and Practice of Obstetric Analgesia and Anesthesia*. Philadelphia: Davis, 1972, p. 505.)

A disadvantage of local infiltration is that large amounts of local anesthetic must be used.

Nursing implications   The nurse explains the procedure and the expected effect and answers any questions. Local anesthetic agents have no effect on maternal vital signs or FHR; thus, additional assessments are unnecessary.

General Anesthesia

General anesthetics, if given, are usually administered at the time of delivery. General anesthesia may be induced by intravenous injection or by inhalation.

Inhalation Anesthetics

Nitrous oxide   Nitrous oxide is the oldest analgesic and anesthetic gaseous agent. Induction is rapid and pleasant; it is nonirritating and nonexplosive and disturbs physiologic functioning less than any other agent (Bonica, 1972). The main obstetric uses of nitrous oxide are as an analgesic during the second stage of labor, as an induction agent or supplement to more potent inhalation anesthetics, and as a part of balanced anesthesia.

Halothane (fluothane)   Halothane is frequently used as a general anesthetic. Induction with this agent is smooth, rapid, safe, and predictable. It does cause depression of respiration and irritability of cardiac tissue, resulting in arrhythmias. Only a moderate degree of muscle relaxation is produced. Halothane increases blood flow to the uterus and does not contribute to uterine relaxation when used in low doses.

Intravenous Anesthetics

Thiopental sodium (Pentothal Sodium) is an ultrashort-acting barbiturate, which means that it exerts its effect rapidly and has a brief duration of action (Julien, 1984). Thiopental sodium produces narcosis within 30 seconds after intravenous administration. Induction and emergence from its effects are smooth, pleasant, and with little incidence of nausea and vomiting.

Thiopental sodium is most frequently used for induction and as an adjunct to other more potent anesthetics.

Balanced Anesthesia

A trend in the management of a vaginal delivery requiring anesthetic or cesarean birth is *balanced anesthesia*. Balanced anesthesia is induced by several different agents administered through different routes. Since no single anesthetic agent is suitable for all people in all situations, the combined use of several agents and techniques increases effectiveness and client safety. In this way, each agent is used for a specific purpose. Furthermore, because of the combined effect, much smaller amounts of the agents can be given than if they were used alone.

An example of balanced anesthesia is the use of an intravenous barbiturate (thiopental sodium) for sedation and rapid pleasant induction, then (Halothane or other general anesthetic agent) and oxygen inhaled through a face mask for analgesia and anesthesia. Intravenous succinylcholine chloride may be given to produce muscle relaxation. The purpose of balanced anesthesia is to obtain the maximum benefit from each agent and technique with a minimum of side effects for the woman and newborn.

Complications of General Anesthesia

The primary dangers of general anesthesia are as follows:

Fetal depression   Most general anesthetic agents reach the fetus in about 2 minutes. The depression in the fetus is directly proportional to the depth and duration of the anesthesia. The long-term significance of fetal depression in a normal delivery has not been determined. The poor fetal metabolism of general anesthetic agents is similar to that of analgesic agents administered during labor. General anesthesia is not advocated when the fetus is considered to be at high risk, particularly in premature delivery.

Uterine relaxation   The majority of general anesthetic agents cause some degree of uterine relaxation. The incidence of cesarean and forceps delivery as well as postpartal uterine atony is thus increased.

Vomiting and aspiration   Pregnancy results in decreased gastric motility, and the onset of labor halts the process almost entirely. Food eaten hours earlier may remain undigested in the stomach. The nurse must find out when the laboring woman last ate and record this information on the client's chart and on her anesthesia record.

Even when food and fluids have been withheld, the gastric juice produced during fasting is highly acidic and can produce chemical pneumonitis if aspirated. Such pneumonitis is known as Mendelson's syndrome. The signs and symptoms are chest pain, respiratory embarrassment, cyanosis, fever, and tachycardia. It has become common procedure to administer an antacid during labor to neutralize the gastric contents.

Vomiting and aspiration of undigested food or acidic gastric juice occurs most frequently during emergence from general anesthesia. Sellick's maneuver of applying cricoid pressure to compress the esophagus, thereby occluding the lumen to avoid regurgitation of stomach contents into the pharynx and trachea, is frequently practiced. Every nurse in the labor and delivery unit should be trained in the proper technique for applying cricoid pressure. All delivery room suites should have emergency equipment available to deal with complications such as aspiration.

Summary

The complications that may occur during obstetric anesthesia are serious. Anyone who performs anesthetic procedures should be proficient in preventing, detecting, and managing all possible complications. Nursing personnel in labor and delivery suites must have a thorough understanding of anesthetic techniques, since nurses provide continual and direct care to clients. In addition, the early detection of an incipient complication contributes to the success of medical management.

The use of regional anesthetic procedures for delivery and episiotomy repair has increased. The regional techniques pose certain maternal and fetal hazards, however.

References

Bonica JJ: *Principles and Practice of Obstetric Analgesia and Anesthesia.* Philadelphia: Davis, 1972.

Giacoia GP, Yaffe S: Perinatal pharmacology. In: *Gynecology and Obstetrics.* Vol 3. Sciarri JJ (editor). Philadelphia: Harper & Row, 1982.

Julien RM: *Understanding Anesthesia.* Menlo Park: Addison-Wesley, 1984.

Morrison JC et al: Meperidine metabolism in the parturient. *Obstet Gynecol* 1982; 59:359.

Roberts WE, Norman PF, Morrison J: Pros and cons of meperidine for intrapartum analgesia. *Contemp Ob/Gyn* April 1984; 23(4):69.

Santos AC: Obstetric use of local anesthetics. *Contemp Ob/Gyn* December 1983; 22(6):46.

Additional Readings

Horsley JA, Crane J: *Pain: Deliberative Nursing Intervention.* New York: Grune & Stratton, 1982.

Mateo-Woodburn CV: Choosing anesthesia for high-risk ob patients. *Contemp Ob/Gyn* August 1983; 22(3):75.

17
Complications of Labor and Delivery

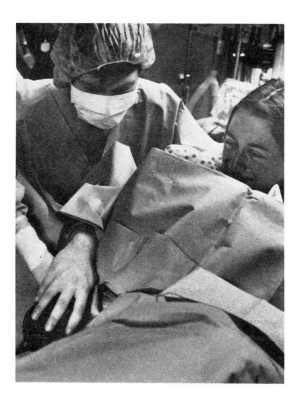

Chapter Contents

Complications Involving the Psyche

Complications Involving the Powers
Hypertonic Labor Patterns
Hypotonic Labor Patterns
Prolonged Labor
Precipitous Labor
Premature Rupture of Membranes
Preterm Labor
Ruptured Uterus

Complications Involving the Passenger
Fetal Malposition (Occiput-Posterior)
Malpresentations
Developmental Abnormalities
Multiple Gestation
Fetal Distress
Intrauterine Fetal Death
Placental Problems
Problems Associated with the Umbilical Cord
Problems Associated with Amniotic Fluid

Complications Involving the Passage
Contractures of the Inlet
Contractures of the Midpelvis
Contractures of the Outlet
Implications of Pelvic Contractures

Complications of Third and Fourth Stages
Postpartal Hemorrhage
Genital Tract Trauma

Complicated Childbirth: Effects on the Family

Objectives

• Describe the psychologic factors that may contribute to complications during labor and delivery.

- Discuss dysfunctional labor patterns.

- Describe various types of fetal malposition and malpresentation and possible associated problems.

- Compare abruptio placentae and placenta previa.

- Discuss the nursing care that is indicated in the event of fetal distress.

- Discuss intrauterine fetal death including etiology, diagnosis, management, and the nurse's role in assisting the family.

- Identify variations that may occur in the umbilical cord and insertion into the placenta.

- Discuss the implications of pelvic contractures on labor and delivery.

- Discuss complications of the third and fourth stages.

- Discuss the effects of complications in childbirth on the family.

Key Terms

abruptio placentae	placenta previa
amniotic fluid	precipitous labor
embolus	premature rupture
dystocia	of membranes
hydramnios	(PROM)
macrosomia	preterm labor
oligohydramnios	prolonged labor

The successful completion of the 40-week gestational period requires the harmonious functioning of four components: the psyche, powers, passenger, and passage. (These components are described in depth in Chapter 12.) The psyche is the intellectual and emotional processes of the pregnant woman as influenced by heredity and environment and includes her feelings about pregnancy and motherhood. The powers are the myometrial forces of the contracting uterus. The passenger includes all the products of conception: the fetus, placenta, cord, membranes, and amniotic fluid. The passage comprises the vagina, introitus, and bony pelvis. Disruptions in any of the four compo-

nents may affect the others and cause **dystocia** (abnormal or difficult labor).

Complications Involving the Psyche

The anxiety, fear, and pain associated with labor may lead to a vicious cycle of increased fear and anxiety because of continued central pain perception. This enhances catecholamine release, which in turn increases physical distress and results in myometrial dysfunction. Ineffectual labor may occur, especially when epinephrine is the predominant substance released.

Nursing research demonstrates that education is effective in minimizing the stress accompanying labor. Generally, research findings indicate that women who participate in prenatal classes benefit by maintaining better control in labor, decreasing their use of ataractics and analgesics, manifesting more positive attitudes, and experiencing feelings of anticipation rather than fear (Genest, 1981; Sasmor and Grossman, 1981; Zacharias, 1981).

Interventions Antepartal classes provide education about the developmental and psychologic changes that can be expected during childbirth. Couples learn coping mechanisms in the form of physical and emotional comfort measures, controlled breathing exercises, and relaxation techniques.

Unprepared couples can be taught many of these activities at the time of admission to the delivery room, especially if active labor has not begun. Information about the labor process, medical procedures, the surroundings, simple breathing exercises, and relaxation techniques can be given, thereby relieving some apprehension and fear. Even a woman in active labor who has had no prior preparation can derive a good deal of relaxation from physical comfort measures, touch, constant attendance, therapeutic interaction, and possibly pharmacologic support.

If the laboring woman is suffering from complications, the nurse should try to determine whether fear and stress are causative or contributing factors. In either case, support measures to alleviate the psychologic distress will help relieve the physical distress.

Complications Involving the Powers

Complications of the powers—the uterine contractions—can involve alterations in the frequency, duration, and/or intensity of the contractions. The resting tone of the uterus between contractions may also be altered. These alterations from normal can become dysfunctional and are associated with additional complications, such as maternal exhaustion, dehydration, increased risk of infection, and fetal complications.

Hypertonic Labor Patterns

In hypertonic labor patterns, ineffectual uterine contractions of poor quality occur in the latent phase of labor, and the resting tone of the myometrium rises. Contractions usually become more frequent, but their intensity may decrease (Figure 17-1, *B*). The contractions are painful but ineffective in dilating and effacing the cervix, and a prolonged latent phase may result.

Maternal implications

- Increased discomfort due to uterine muscle cell anoxia
- Fatigue as pattern continues and no labor progress results
- Dehydration and increased incidence of infection if labor is prolonged
- Stress on coping abilities

Fetal-neonatal implications

- Early fetal distress because contractions and increased resting tone interfere with the uteroplacental exchange
- Prolonged pressure on the fetal head, which may result in cephalhematoma, caput succedaneum, or excessive molding (Figure 17-2, Chapter 20).

Interventions Management of hypertonic labor may include bed rest and sedation to promote relaxation and to reduce pain. Oxytocin is not administered to a woman suffering from hypertonic uterine activity because it is likely to accentuate the abnormal labor pattern

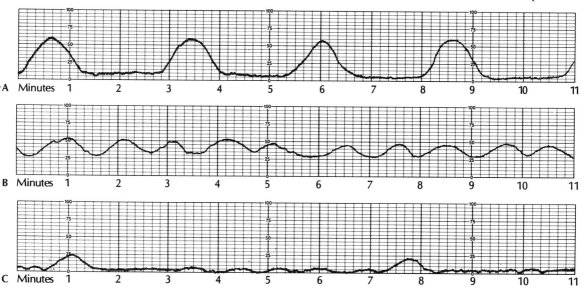

Figure 17-1

Comparison of labor patterns. **A**, Normal uterine contraction pattern. Note contraction frequency is every 3 minutes, duration is 60 seconds. The baseline resting tone is below 10 mm Hg, and the intensity of the contractions is approximately 50 mm Hg. **B**, Hypertonic uterine pattern. Note in this example, the contraction frequency is every 1 minute, duration is 50 seconds (which allows only a 10-second rest between contractions), intensity increases approximately 25 mm Hg during the contraction, and the resting tone of the uterus is increased. **C**, Hypotonic uterine contraction pattern. Note in this example, the contraction frequency is every 7 minutes with some uterine activity between contractions, duration is 50 seconds, and intensity increases approximately 25 mm Hg during contractions.

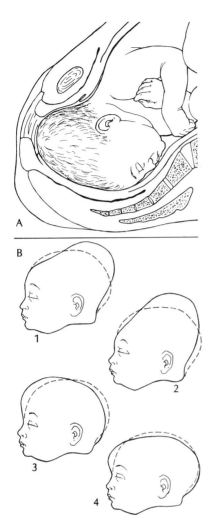

Figure 17-2

Effects of labor on the fetal head. **A**, Caput succedaneum formation. The presenting portion of the scalp area is encircled by the cervix during labor, causing swelling of the soft tissue. **B**, Molding of the fetal head in cephalic presentations: **1**, occiput anterior; **2**, occiput posterior; **3**, brow; **4**, face.

(Pritchard, MacDonald, and Gant, 1985). If the hypertonic pattern continues and develops into prolonged latent phase, the physician may use oxytocin infusion and/or amniotomy as treatment methods (see Chapter 18). These methods are instituted only after CPD and fetal malpresentation have been ruled out.

Nursing measures include identifying and reporting a hypertonic labor pattern, providing information to the laboring woman and her family, providing an environment conducive to relaxation if sedation is ordered, and imple-menting any supportive technique that the nurse can devise. The nurse may wish to try a change of position for the woman (a lateral position may correct the hypertonic pattern) or provide mouth care, effleurage, back rub, and change of linens. In addition, the labor coach may need assistance in helping the woman to cope.

Fluid balance is assessed by recording intake and output and obtaining urine hourly to test for ketones.

Nursing measures in the event of fetal-neonatal distress are given in the Nursing Care Plan on p. 350.

Hypotonic Labor Patterns

A hypotonic labor pattern usually occurs in the active phase of labor, although it may occur in the latent phase. When this pattern occurs in the active phase, it usually develops after labor has been well established. Hypotonic labor is characterized by fewer than two to three contractions in a 10-minute period (Figure 17-1,*C*).

Hypotonic labor may occur when the uterus is overstretched from a twin gestation or in the presence of a large fetus, hydramnios, and grandmultiparity. Bladder or bowel distention and CPD may also be associated with this pattern.

Maternal implications

- Intrauterine infection if labor is prolonged
- Postpartal hemorrhage from insufficient uterine contractions following delivery
- Maternal exhaustion
- Stress on coping abilities

Fetal-neonatal implications

- Fetal distress, due to prolonged labor pattern
- Fetal sepsis from maternal pathogens that ascend from the birth canal

Interventions After CPD and fetal malpresentation have been ruled out, oxytocin may be given intravenously in a controlled infusion to improve the uterine contractions. Additional intravenous fluids may be given if the woman is dehydrated or to prevent dehydration. Maternal exhaustion may be treated by administering a sedative or analgesic to increase her ability to rest between contractions. An amniotomy may

Text continued on p. 353.

NURSING CARE PLAN
Fetal Distress

PATIENT ASSESSMENT

History

Assess client for presence of predisposing factors:
1. Preexisting maternal diseases
2. Maternal hypotension, bleeding
3. Placental abnormalities

Physical Examination

Asphyxia is suggested when one or more of the following are present:
1. FHR decelerations, decreased variability, tachycardia followed by bradycardia
2. Presence of meconium in amniotic fluid
3. Fetal scalp blood pH determination ≤ 7.20

Laboratory Evaluation

Maternal hemoglobin and hematocrit
Urinalysis

PLAN OF CARE

Nursing Priorities

1. Evaluate maternal and fetal status for variations requiring immediate intervention
2. Identify and correct interferences with transplacental gas exchange
3. Identify and report FHR decelerations and lack of baseline variability
4. In presence of fetal asphyxia, prepare woman for immediate delivery (either vaginally or by cesarean)

Client/Family Educational Focus

1. Discuss the problems that are occurring
2. Explain the treatment methods
3. Provide opportunities to discuss questions and individual concerns of the client and her family

Problem	Nursing interventions and actions	Rationale
Fetal asphyxia	Observe and record the signs of fetal asphyxia:	Fetal asphyxia implies hypoxia (reduction in PO_2), hypercapnia (elevation of PCO_2), and acidosis (lowering of blood pH)
		Anaerobic glycolysis (breakdown of glycogen) takes place in the presence of hypoxia, and the end product of this process is lactic acid, resulting in metabolic acidosis
	1. Presence of meconium in amniotic fluid	Fetal hypoxic episode leads to increased intestinal peristalsis and anal sphincter relaxation resulting in meconium release
	2. Decelerations in FHR	Vagal stimulation elicited through hypoxic brain tissues causes bradycardia
	3. Fetal hyperactivity	Fetus may initially become hyperactive in an attempt to increase circulation
	Initiate following interventions:	
	1. Administer O_2 to the woman with tight face mask at 4–7 L/min, per physician order	Administration of O_2 may increase amount of oxygen available for transport to fetus Tight face mask is used because laboring woman tends to breathe through her mouth
	2. Change maternal position (lateral, left side preferred)	Changed maternal position may relieve compression of the maternal vena cava and the cord, thereby facilitating O_2 exchange
	3. Prepare equipment for fetal blood sampling	Evaluate fetal acidotic state. Hypoxia causes increase in lactic acid and results in acidosis, which causes a drop in the pH of the fetal blood (normal pH is 7.25–7.30); other tests that may be done on fetal blood sample are O_2 pressure (normal 18–22 mm Hg), CO_2 pressure (normal 48–50 mm Hg), base deficit (normal 0–10 mg/L)
	4. Prepare patient for immediate delivery (may be vaginal or cesarean delivery)	

NURSING CARE PLAN (continued)
Fetal Distress

Problem	Nursing interventions and actions	Rationale
	5. Correct maternal hypotension if present: a. Administer IV fluids b. Assess any maternal bleeding; if present, replace circulatory fluids	Lowered maternal blood pressure or circulating blood volume affects O_2 exchange gradient of maternal–placental–fetal unit
	6. Decrease uterine contractions; if oxytocin is infusing, decrease infusion rate or discontinue oxytocin	Increased uterine tone decreases exchange at placental site and decreases fetal recovery time following contractions
Impaired blood flow through umbilical cord Cord compression	Observe and note variable decelerations of FHR If bradycardia lasts longer than 30 sec, change maternal position; if necessary, follow interventions listed under fetal asphyxia	Umbilical vessels may be partially or completely occluded by compression of the cord; cord may prolapse through cervix and vagina, or compression may occur when the cord is trapped between a fetal part and the bony pelvis; transient episodes of compression are reflected by variable decelerations (decelerations that are unrelated to uterine contractions)
Prolapsed cord	Evaluate for presence of predisposing factors: 1. Abnormalities in presentation: breech, shoulder, transverse lie 2. Rupture of membranes 3. Multiple gestation Observe for prolapse of the cord externally through vaginal introitus While doing vaginal exam, evaluate for presence of cord, which feels like rope and pulsates	Occult or obvious prolapse of the cord may cause complete depletion of fetal oxygen within 2½ min if compression is not relieved
	Institute emergency measures for prolapse of cord:	Emergency measures for a prolapsed cord are aimed at immediately relieving compression and reestablishing fetal–neonatal blood/oxygen circulation
	1. Manually exert pressure on the presenting part; this must be done continuously; patient may be maintained in supine position, Trendelenburg position, knee-chest position, or on her side with a pillow to elevate her hips 2. If occult prolapse is suspected, change maternal position to side-lying position 3. Notify physician immediately	
Impaired transplacental gas exchange	Assess woman for conditions that produce maternal hypoxia: 1. Severe pneumonia, maternal hypotension of any cause,	Antepartal hypoxic insults influence the fetal response to labor and delivery by affecting O_2 exchange at placental site Severe maternal disorders, such as abruptio

NURSING CARE PLAN (continued)
Fetal Distress

Problem	Nursing interventions and actions	Rationale
	congestive heart failure with diminished blood flow to maternal organs 2. Disturbed O_2 carrying ability of hemoglobin 3. Low environmental oxygen tension at high altitudes, preeclampsia-eclampsia, apnea with convulsions, vena caval syndrome	placentae, seriously jeopardize the fetus, but the effects may be more pronounced in a fetus who has had antepartal stress because O_2 exchange has been compromised and fetal reserve has decreased Maternal hypoxia reduces O_2 tension in the blood that perfuses the placenta; fetal O_2 deprivation follows as the maternal–fetal Po_2 gradient is reduced or eliminated
	Assess client for placental problems (placenta previa, abruptio placentae) Maintain maternal blood pressure Maintain adequate maternal oxygenation by positioning (avoid supine position to prevent vena caval syndrome) and administration of O_2 as necessary	These maternal conditions reduce placental gas exchange by reducing surface area available for oxygen diffusion
	Replace circulating blood volume in presence of hemorrhage	Maternal blood loss may cause hypotension and impair perfusion of the intact portion of the placenta

NURSING CARE EVALUATION

Maternal conditions that produced maternal hypoxia are corrected or controlled
A live birth is accomplished with no signs of permanent damage from fetal asphyxia
Maternal blood volume is restored

NURSING DIAGNOSIS*	SUPPORTING DATA	NURSING ORDERS
Impaired fetal gas exchange related to prolapsed cord, cord compression, placental problems, or maternal hypoxia	Presence of meconium in amniotic fluid Decelerations of fetal heart rate, late or severe variable Fetal hyperactivity or hypoactivity Decreasing variability or loss of variability Fetal blood sampling results of less than 7.20	Monitor fetal status Assess for signs of fetal distress such as those listed under supporting data Increase placental perfusion 1. Assist woman to side lying position 2. Administer O_2 at 4–7 L/min by tight face mask 3. Discontinue oxytocin infusion 4. Increase IV fluid infusion rate if woman is hypotensive 5. Change maternal position if there is no improvement of fetal status 6. Continuously monitor fetal and maternal status
Fear related to knowledge of fetal distress	Anxiety Expressed concerns	Explain what is happening and each treatment Give correct, honest information Answer questions honestly, do not give false information or false hope

*These are a few examples of nursing diagnoses that may be appropriate for this condition. It is not an inclusive list and must be individualized for each woman.

be done to increase the pressure of the fetal presenting part on the cervix and to help dilate the cervix.

Nursing measures include assessing contractions and monitoring the maternal vital signs and FHR frequently. Maternal hydration may be assessed by maintaining intake and output records. The woman is encouraged to void every 2 hours, and her bladder is checked for distention. Because her labor may be prolonged, the woman is observed for signs of infection (elevated temperature, chills, and changes in characteristics of the amniotic fluid). Vaginal examinations should be kept to a minimum. Nursing concerns during oxytocin infusion are presented in Drug Guide—Oxytocin in Chapter 18.

Prolonged Labor

Labor lasting more than 24 hours is termed **prolonged labor**. In these cases, the latent and/or active phase is prolonged.

Prolonged labor is more common in women who have never had children (nulliparas). The principal causes are CPD, malpresentations, malpositions, uterine contraction dysfunction, and cervical dystocia. Other influencing factors are overuse of analgesics, anesthetics, and sedatives in the latent phase of labor.

Maternal implications

- Exhaustion
- Intrauterine infection
- Third stage and postpartum bleeding from inadequate uterine contractions

Fetal-neonatal implications

- Fetal distress
- Increased risk of infection
- Prolapse of the cord after ROM if presenting part is not well engaged
- Cephalhematoma and/or caput succedaneum (Chapter 20).

Interventions Management of prolonged labor begins with identification of any causal factors. Treatment depends on these factors and may include stimulating labor through the intravenous administration of oxytocin and/or performing an amniotomy. Hydration is maintained with intravenous fluids. Sedatives or analgesics may be given to increase rest and relaxation and to decrease anxiety. In the event of serious maternal or fetal distress or CPD, a cesarean delivery is usually done.

Nursing measures include monitoring maternal-fetus status. FHR patterns are assessed for any signs of distress, such as late decelerations and decreasing variability. Amniotic fluid is observed for meconium staining and signs of infection. The nurse analyzes labor progress by collecting data on the pattern of the labor contractions, the degree of cervical dilatation and effacement, the station of descent, and the fetal presentation. If the fetus is in a vertex presentation, the nurse may evaluate the amount of pressure on the fetal head by the presence or absence of a caput succedaneum and/or molding. The nurse calculates fluid intake and output and checks urine for presence of ketones to gain information about the maternal hydration state. If the woman is receiving oxytocin therapy, the nurse should implement appropriate measures to ensure the safety of the woman and fetus.

Helping the woman and her partner deal with the anxiety and frustration associated with prolonged labor is another important nursing responsibility. The nurse offers support, encouragement, and information as appropriate. Comfort measures such as helping the woman change position, providing for oral hygiene and skin care, or applying cool washcloths to the forehead may help the woman relax. The involvement of the woman's partner in her care may reduce her anxiety, and the nurse encourages this involvement.

Following delivery, the mother should be closely monitored for signs and symptoms of hemorrhage, shock, and infection. The fetus should be observed for signs of sepsis, cerebral trauma, and cephalhematoma. Nursing actions for fetal distress are given in the Nursing Care Plan—Fetal Distress.

Precipitous Labor

Precipitous labor is labor that lasts for less than 3 hours. The most common cause is the lack of resistance of the maternal tissues to the passage of the fetus (Oxorn, 1980). The other primary cause is intense uterine contractions.

Precipitous labor and precipitous delivery are not the same. A *precipitous delivery* is an unexpected, sudden, and often unattended birth. See Chapter 14 for discussion of emergency delivery.

Maternal implications

- Increased risk of uterine rupture from intense contractions

- Loss of coping abilities

- Lacerations of the cervix, vagina, and perineum due to rapid descent and delivery of the fetus

- Postpartal hemorrhage due to undetected lacerations and/or inadequate uterine contractions after delivery

Fetal-neonatal implications

- Fetal distress and/or hypoxia from decreased uteroplacental circulation due to intense uterine contractions

- Cerebral trauma from rapid descent through birth canal

Interventions   During the intrapartal nursing assessment, the nurse can identify a woman at increased risk of precipitous labor (for example, a previous history of precipitous or short labor places a woman at risk). During the labor the presence of one or both of the following factors may indicate potential problems:

- Accelerated cervical dilatation and fetal descent

- Intense uterine contractions with little uterine relaxation between contractions

If the woman has a history of precipitous labor, she is closely monitored, and an emergency delivery pack is kept at hand. The physician is informed of any unusual findings on the Friedman graph (Chapter 13). The nurse stays in constant attendance if at all possible. Comfort and rest may be promoted by assisting the woman to a comfortable position, providing a quiet environment, and administering sedatives as needed. Information and support are given before and after the delivery.

To avoid hyperstimulation of the uterus and possible precipitous labor during oxytocin administration, the nurse should be alert to the dangers of oxytocin overdosage (see Drug Guide—Oxytocin, p. 387). If the woman who is receiving oxytocin develops an accelerated labor pattern, the oxytocin is discontinued immediately, and the woman is turned on her left side to improve uterine perfusion. Oxygen may be started to increase the available oxygen in the maternal circulating blood; this increases the amount available for exchange at the placental site.

Premature Rupture of Membranes

Premature rupture of membranes (PROM) is spontaneous rupture of the membranes and leakage of amniotic fluid prior to the onset of labor. Preterm PROM is defined as rupture of membranes less than 259 days (37 weeks) from the start of the last menstrual period. PROM is associated with maternal age of 35 years or greater, multiparity, incompetent cervix, damage to the cervix by surgical instrumentation, and low weight gain (Flood and Naeye, 1984).

Maternal implications

- Intrauterine infection due to ascending pathogens

- Increased stress regarding the condition of the child if rupture occurs prior to term

- Prolonged hospitalization if the fetal gestational age is less than 37 weeks

Fetal-neonatal implications

- Fetal sepsis due to ascending pathogens

- Malpresentation

- Prolapse of the umbilical cord

- Increased perinatal morbidity and mortality

Interventions   Gestational age of the fetus and the presence or absence of maternal infection determine the management of PROM. After confirming with Nitrazine paper that the membranes have ruptured, the nurse calculates the gestational age. Single or combination methods of calculation may be used, including Nägele's rule, ultrasound to obtain fetal measurements, and amniocentesis to identify lung maturity. If maternal signs and symptoms of infection are evident, antibiotic therapy (usually by intravenous infusion) is initiated immediately, and the fetus is delivered vaginally or by cesarean birth regardless of the gestational age. Upon admission to the nursery, the neonate is assessed for sepsis and placed on antibiotics. Chapter 22 provides further information about the neonate with sepsis.

Management of PROM when maternal infection is not present may include induction of labor if gestation is more than 34 weeks (Oxorn, 1980). The induction may be delayed for 24 hours in the 34-to-36-week gestation. This delay is thought to permit elevation of maternal-fetal blood corticosteroids, thereby contributing to fetal lung maturity. If the gestation is less than 34 weeks, efforts are directed at maintaining the pregnancy. If the gestation is between 28 and 32 weeks and spontaneous labor is not present, the use of betamethasone (Celestone) may be considered. If labor is spontaneous and cervical dilatation is less than 4 cm, betamethasone may be given. The woman is given tocolytics in an attempt to delay the labor and delivery long enough to accelerate the development of fetal lung maturity sufficiently. See Drug Guide—Betamethasone. Management of the preterm neonate is discussed in Chapter 22.

Nursing actions should focus on the woman, her partner, and the fetus. The time the woman's membranes ruptured and the time of labor onset are recorded. The nurse observes the woman for signs and symptoms of infection by frequently monitoring her vital signs (especially temperature and pulse), describing the character of the amniotic fluid, and reporting elevated white blood cell counts (WBC) to the clinician. Uterine activity and fetal response to the labor are evaluated. Comfort measures may help promote rest and relaxation. Additionally, the nurse must ensure that hydration is maintained, particularly if the woman's temperature is elevated.

DRUG GUIDE
Betamethasone (Celestone Solupan®)

OVERVIEW OF OBSTETRIC/FETAL ACTION

"Betamethasone is a glucocorticoid which acts to accelerate fetal lung maturation and prevent hyaline membrane disease by inhibiting cell mitosis, increasing cell differentiation, promoting selected enzymatic actions, and participating in the storage and secretion of surfactant" (Bishop, 1981). The best results are obtained when the fetus is between 30–32 weeks' gestation. However, some researchers have noted beneficial effects as early as 28 weeks and as late as 34 weeks. To obtain optimal results, delivery should be delayed for at least 24 hours after the end of treatment. If delivery does not occur, the effect of the drug disappears in about week. A female fetus seems more likely than a male to obtain the most prophylactic effect (Giacoia and Yaffe, 1982).

Route, dosage, frequency

Prenatal maternal intramuscular administration of 12 mg of betamethasone is given once a day for 2 days. Repeated treatment will be needed on a weekly basis until 34 weeks of gestation (unless delivery occurs).

Contraindications

Inability to delay birth for 48 hours

Adequate L:S ratio

Presence of a condition which necessitates immediate delivery (e.g., maternal bleeding)

Presence of maternal infection, diabetes mellitus, hypertension

Concomitant use of tocolytic agents may increase risk of maternal pulmonary edema (Bishop, 1981)

Gestational age greater than 34 weeks

Maternal side effects

Bishop (1981) reports that suspected maternal risks include (a) initiation of lactation; (b) increased risk of infection; (c) augmentation of placental insufficiency in hypertensive clients; (d) gastrointestinal bleeding; (e) inability to use estriol levels to assess fetal status; (f) pulmonary edema when used concurrently with tocolytics (such as ritodrine)

May cause Na^+ retention, K^+ loss, weight gain, edema, indigestion

Effects on fetus/neonate

Lowered cortisol levels between 1 and 8 days following delivery (Giacoia and Yaffe, 1982)

Possible suppression of aldosterone levels up to 2 weeks following delivery (Giacoia and Yaffe, 1982)

Hypoglycemia

NURSING CONSIDERATIONS

Assess client for presence of contraindications

Client education regarding possible side effects

Administer deep into gluteal muscle, avoid injection into deltoid (high incidence of local atrophy)

Periodic evaluation of BP, pulse, weight, and edema

Assess lab data for electrolytes

Providing psychologic support for the couple is critical. The nurse may reduce anxiety by listening empathetically, relaying accurate information, and providing explanations of procedures. Preparing the couple for a cesarean birth, a preterm neonate, and the possibility of fetal or neonatal death may be necessary.

Preterm Labor

Labor that occurs between 20 and 38 weeks of pregnancy is referred to as **preterm labor**. Approximately 8% of all pregnancies end in preterm labor. Maternal factors associated with preterm labor include PIH, diabetes, infection, uterine anomalies, maternal age of less than 16 or more than 40 years, and height of less than 5 feet (Creasy, 1984).

Maternal implications

- Increased stress regarding status of the child
- Stress of unplanned hospitalization
- Administration of additional medications

Fetal-neonatal implications

- Increased morbidity and mortality
- Increased risk of trauma during delivery
- Immature organ systems that may be incompatible with life

Interventions   Women who are at risk for preterm labor are taught to recognize the symptoms associated with preterm labor. These symptoms may include menstrual-like cramps, rhythmic backache, rhythmic pelvic pressure, an increase or change in vaginal discharge, and intestinal cramping with or without diarrhea (Creasy, 1984). If any of these symptoms are present, she is encouraged to notify her physician immediately. Immediate diagnosis is necessary to stop preterm labor before it advances to a stage at which intervention will be ineffective. Diagnosis of preterm labor is confirmed by two contractions lasting at least 30 seconds in a 15-minute period and by cervical dilatation and effacement.

Labor is not interrupted if one or more of the following conditions are present:

- Active labor with cervical dilatation of 4 cm or more

- Presence of severe PIH, which creates risk for the woman if the pregnancy continues
- Fetal complications (isoimmunization, gross anomalies)
- Prolonged rupture of membranes
- Hemorrhage
- Fetal death

The drugs currently in use to arrest preterm labor are ritodrine (Yutopar), isoxsuprine hydrochloride (Vasodilan), terbutaline sulfate (Brethine), and intravenously administered magnesium sulfate. See Drug Guide—Ritodrine, p. 357.

Supportive treatment of the woman in preterm labor consists of providing for bed rest, monitoring vital signs (especially blood pressure and respirations), measuring intake and output, and continuous monitoring of FHR and uterine contractions. Placing the woman on her left side aids maternal-fetal circulation. Vaginal examinations are kept to a minimum (Boehm and Acker, 1984).

An additional treatment may be recommended. Administration of glucocorticoids helps the lungs of the preterm infant to mature. If glucocorticoids are given more than 24 hours before delivery, the incidence of respiratory distress syndrome is reduced. Dexamethasone (Decadron) or betamethasone may be administered intramuscularly to the woman, and delivery is delayed at least 24 hours if possible.

When labor cannot be arrested, plans for delivery are made. A cesarean delivery is usually performed to protect the fetal head from excessive trauma during delivery and to minimize the role of intraventricular hemorrhage. Qualified personnel who can assist the respiratory effort of the preterm infant should be present at delivery.

Emotional support for the woman and her partner during preterm labor and delivery is imperative. Common behavioral responses include feelings of anxiety and guilt about the possibility that the pregnancy will terminate early. The nurse can encourage the couple to express these feelings, thereby helping them to identify and implement coping mechanisms. The nurse also keeps the couple informed about the labor progress, the treatment regimen, and

DRUG GUIDE
Ritodrine (Yutopar)

Overview of obstetric action

Ritodrine is a sympathomimetic β_2-adrenergic agonist. It exerts its effect on β_2-receptors which "are involved in glycogenolysis and relaxation of the smooth muscle of arterioles, the bronchi, and the uterus" (Lipshitz and Schneider, 1980). Ritodrine is FDA-approved for use in treatment of preterm labor.

Route, dosage, frequency

150 mg of ritodrine is added to 500 mL IV fluid and administered as a piggy-back to a primary IV. Using an infusion pump, the infusion is started at 20 mL/hr. Rate may be increased by 10 mL/hr every 10 minutes until contractions cease. Maximum dosage is 70 mL/hr. When contractions cease, the infusion rate may be decreased by 10 mL/hr. The infusion may be maintained at a low rate for a period of hours to assure the contractions do not begin again. Before the intravenous infusion is discontinued, IM or PO administration is begun. Although protocols may differ in various clinical facilities, Foster (1981) reports that after labor ceases, ritodrine is administered by IM or PO route in the amount of 10 mg every 2 hours during the first 24 hours. This dosage can be administered safely to a maximum of 120 mg in four to six divided doses over 24 hours. The length of therapy varies.

Maternal contraindications

Preterm labor accompanied by cervical dilatation greater than 4 cm, chorioamniotitis, severe preeclampsia-eclampsia, severe bleeding, fetal death, significant IUGR contraindicate use of ritodrine, as do any of the following:
Hypovolemia, bleeding, uncontrolled hypertension
Pulmonary hypertension, thyroid dysfunction
Cardiac disease, arrhythmias
Diabetes mellitus (use with caution)
Use with caution in clients receiving concurrent therapy with glucocorticoids
Gestation less than 20 weeks
History of migraine headaches (Katz et al., 1983)

Maternal side effects

Tachycardia, occasionally premature ventricular contractions (PVCs), increased stroke volume, increased systolic pressure, palpitations, tremors, nervousness, nausea and vomiting, headache, erythema
Decreased peripheral vascular resistance, which lowers diastolic pressure $\rightarrow$ widening of pulse pressure

Hyperglycemia
Metabolic acidosis
Hypotension
Hypokalemia (causes internal redistribution)
Pulmonary edema in clients treated concurrently with glucocorticoids, and who have fluid overload
Increased concentration of lactate and free fatty acids
Increase in plasma volume as indicated by decreases in hemoglobin, hematocrit, and serum albumin levels (Philipsen et al., 1981)

Effects on fetus/neonate

Fetal tachycardia
Increased serum glucose concentration
Fetal acidosis
Fetal hypoxia
Neonatal hypoglycemia, hypocalcemia
Neonatal paralytic ileus
Neonatal hypotension at birth
May decrease incidence of neonatal respiratory distress syndrome (Lipshitz, 1981)

Nursing considerations

Assess client history and maternal and fetal status to determine contraindications to treatment with ritodrine
Explain procedure to client
Position woman in left lateral position to decrease incidence of hypotension and increase placental perfusion
Apply fetal monitor for continuous fetal and uterine contraction assessment
Assess contraction status, maternal blood pressure, pulse, and presence of maternal side effects prior to each increase in flow rate
Assess respiratory status for rate, rales, rhonchi
Assess fluid intake and output
Assess lab data on electrolytes, blood glucose
Weigh patient daily
Check urine for ketones daily
Have β-blocking agent available for emergency use
Notify physician if maternal pulse >120 beats/min and/or FHR >180 beats/min
If symptoms of side effects are severe, discontinue ritodrine infusion
To ensure continued uterine relaxation, encourage patient to take PO dosages on time to provide adequate drug levels
At delivery assess newborn for side effects

the status of the fetus to elicit their full cooperation. In the event of imminent vaginal or cesarean delivery, the couple should be offered brief but ongoing explanations to prepare them for the birth and the events following it.

Ruptured Uterus

A ruptured uterus is the tearing of previously intact uterine muscles or of an old uterine scar. The rupture can be caused by a weakened cesarean scar, usually from a "classic" incision;

obstetric trauma; mismanagement of oxytocin induction or augmentation; CPD; and congenital defects of the birth canal.

The signs and symptoms of a complete rupture include excruciating pain and cessation of contractions. Vaginal hemorrhage may occur, but vaginal bleeding is usually not profuse. Massive intraperitoneal hemorrhage and hematomas of the broad ligament are hidden sources of bleeding and may account for the scant vaginal bleeding. The woman exhibits signs of hypovolemic shock, and the fetal heart stops beating.

Maternal implications

- Development of profound shock and risk of maternal death
- Abdominal surgery and possibly hysterectomy
- Prolonged hospitalization for intensive care and recuperation
- Loss of the expected baby

Fetal-neonatal implications

- Fetal asphyxia and death

Interventions   The nurse may be the one to identify the signs of uterine rupture. The nurse monitors vital signs, evaluates maternal hemorrhage, and quickly mobilizes the staff for an emergency laparotomy or cesarean delivery. When the physiologic needs of the woman are met, the nurse can focus on the emotional needs of the family. The family must have a clear understanding of the procedure and its implications for future childbearing. In addition, if fetal death has occurred, the couple should be given an opportunity to grieve and allowed to see their infant if they desire.

Complications Involving the Passenger

Complications involving the passenger include any abnormality of the fetus (including position, presentation, fetal size, and developmental anomalies) and multiple gestation; the placenta (problems of implantation and separation of the placenta); the umbilical cord (length and attachment of the cord to the placenta); and the amniotic fluid (amount).

Fetal Malposition (Occiput-Posterior)

Persistent occiput-posterior position of the fetus is probably one of the most common complications encountered during childbirth. If the fetus is in this position, the occiput of the fetal head is directed toward the back of the maternal pelvis. The fetus may remain in this position throughout labor and delivery, or it may rotate (or change) to an occiput-anterior position during delivery. Signs and symptoms of a persistent occiput-posterior position include a dysfunctional labor pattern and complaints of intense back pain by the laboring woman. The changes in labor occur because the occiput pulls the cervix posterior, and the uterine contractions are not as effective. The back pain is caused by the fetal occiput compressing the woman's sacral nerves.

Assessment   FHTs will be heard far laterally on the maternal abdomen. When the cervix is examined by sterile vaginal examination, the diamond-shaped anterior fontanelle will be in the anterior portion of the pelvis. This fontanelle may be difficult to feel because of molding of the fetal head. Labor progress may be prolonged, and the woman may complain of severe back discomfort.

Interventions   The nurse helps the laboring woman to maintain a comfortable position during labor. Some researchers report that having the woman position herself on her hands and knees is helpful in rotating the fetus to an anterior position (Andrews and Andrews, 1983). The nurse or other support person can provide sacral pressure or back rubs to relieve the back discomfort.

As long as the second stage is within normal limits (less than 1 hour for multiparas and less than 2 hours for nulliparas) the fetus may remain in the posterior position for delivery. As the fetal head is delivered, the occiput distends the lower portion of the vagina and perineum and may cause lacerations and/or extensions of the episiotomy if one has been done. If the second stage is prolonged or fetal distress develops, an episiotomy is done, and the fetus is rotated to an anterior position, either manually or by forceps (Scanzoni's maneuver).

Malpresentations

Fetal malpresentations include brow, face, breech, shoulder (transverse lie), and compound presentation.

Brow presentation   In a brow presentation, the forehead of the fetus becomes the presenting part. The fetal neck is hyperextended instead of flexed, with the result that the fetal head enters the birth canal with the widest diameter of the head (occipitomental) foremost.

The brow presentation occurs more often in the multipara than the nullipara and is thought to be due to lax abdominal and pelvic musculature.

Maternal implications

• Cesarean birth in the presence of CPD

• Cesarean birth if the brow presentation does not convert to an occiput presentation

Fetal-neonatal implications

• Increased risk of fetal mortality from infection due to prolonged labor and/or injuries received during vaginal delivery

• Possibility of trauma during a vaginal birth, including tentorial tears, cerebral and neck compression, and damage to the trachea and larynx

Interventions   As long as dilatation and descent are occurring, active interference is not necessary. In the presence of labor problems but no CPD, a manual conversion may be attempted. In the presence of failed conversions, CPD, or secondary arrest of labor, cesarean birth is the management of choice.

In the case of brow presentation and face presentation that follows, the nurse observes the woman closely for labor problems and monitors the fetus for signs of distress. The nurse may need to explain the fetal presentation to the laboring couple or to interpret what the physician has told them. The nurse should stay close at hand to reassure the couple, inform them of any changes, and assist them with labor-coping mechanisms.

At the time of delivery, adequate resuscitation equipment and pediatric assistance should be available.

In face and brow presentations, the facial appearance of the infant may be affected. For this reason, the couple may need help beginning the attachment process. After the infant is inspected for gross abnormalities, the pediatrician and nurse can assure the couple that the facial edema and excessive molding are only temporary and will subside in 3 or 4 days.

Face presentation   In a face presentation, the face of the fetus is the presenting part. The fetal head is hyperextended even more than in the brow presentation. Face presentation occurs most frequently in multiparas, in preterm delivery, and in the presence of anencephaly.

When performing Leopold's maneuvers, the nurse finds that the back of the fetus is difficult to outline. A deep furrow can be palpated between the hard occiput and the fetal back (see Figure 17-3). FHTs may be heard on the side where the fetal feet are palpated. It may be difficult to determine by vaginal examination whether the presentation is breech or face, especially if facial edema is already present. During the vaginal examination, the nurse attempts

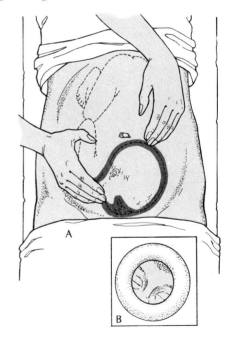

Figure 17-3

Face presentation. **A,** Palpation of the maternal abdomen with the fetus in right mentum posterior (RMP). **B,** Vaginal examination may permit palpation of facial features of the fetus.

to palpate the saddle of the nose and the gums. When assessing engagement, the nurse must remember that the face has to be deep within the pelvis before the biparietal diameters have entered the inlet.

Maternal implications

- Increased risk of CPD and prolonged labor
- With prolonged labor, increased risk of infection

Fetal-neonatal implications

- Postdelivery edema, giving the newborn a distorted appearance
- As in the brow presentation, possible swelling of the neck and internal structures due to trauma during descent

Interventions   If no CPD is present, if the chin (mentum) is anterior, and if the labor pattern is effective, the woman may deliver vaginally (Figure 17-4). Mentum posteriors can become wedged on the anterior surface of the sacrum (Figure 17-5). In this case, as well as in the presence of CPD, cesarean birth is the management of choice.

Breech presentations   The exact cause of breech presentation (Figure 17-6) is unknown. This malpresentation occurs in 3%–4% of all pregnancies and is associated with preterm birth, placenta previa, hydramnios, multiple pregnancies, grandmultiparity, hydrocephalus, and anencephaly. The most critical problem of this presentation is that the largest part of the infant (the head) is delivered last. In the presence of cephalopelvic disproportion, pelvic adequacy is not really tested until it is virtually too late to save the fetus.

Frequently, it is the nurse who first recognizes a breech presentation. On palpation, the hard vertex is felt in the fundus, and ballottement of the head can be done independently of the fetal body. FHTs are usually heard above

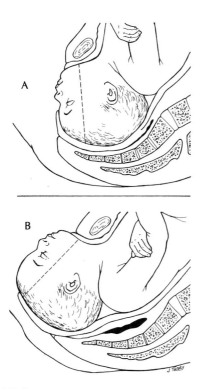

Figure 17-4 ▬▬▬▬▬
Mechanism of birth in mentoanterior position. **A,** The submentobregmatic diameter at the outlet. **B,** The fetal head is born by movement of flexion.

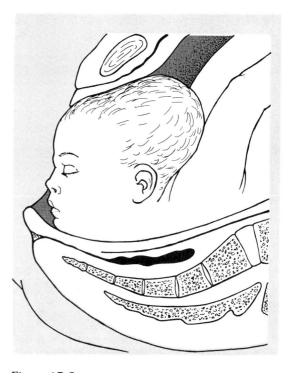

Figure 17-5 ▬▬▬▬▬
Mechanism of birth in mentoposterior position. Fetal head is unable to extend farther. The face becomes impacted.

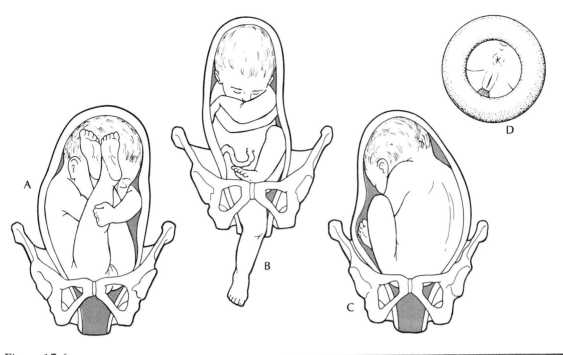

Figure 17-6

Breech presentation. **A**, Frank breech. **B**, Incomplete (footling) breech. **C**, Complete breech in LSA position. **D**, On vaginal examination, the nurse may feel the anal sphincter. The tissue of the fetal buttocks feels soft.

the maternal umbilicus. Passage of meconium from compression of the fetal intestinal tract during labor and descent through the birth canal is common.

Maternal implications

• Cesarean delivery may be done.

Fetal-neonatal implications

• Higher perinatal mortality rate (five times greater for breech infants than for cephalic infants)

• Increased risk of prolapsed cord, especially in incomplete breeches, because space is available between the cervix and presenting part

• Increased risk of cervical cord injuries due to hyperextension of the fetal head during vaginal delivery

• Increased risk of birth trauma, including intracranial hemorrhage, spinal cord injuries, brachial plexus palsy, and fracture of the upper extremities (Collea, 1984)

Interventions   Some clinicians may do an external version between the thirty-seventh week of pregnancy and the time that labor begins. If the version is successful and the fetus remains in cephalic presentation, a vaginal delivery is anticipated.

The fetus in breech presentation during labor requires careful assessment because of the increased risk of prolapsed cord. FHR is assessed frequently. The method of delivery is most usually cesarean, although some vaginal deliveries still occur. If the delivery is vaginal and proper flexion or descent of the head is delayed, the use of forceps, most commonly Piper forceps, on the aftercoming head may be necessary.

Transverse lie (shoulder presentation)   A transverse lie occurs in approximately 1 in 300–400 deliveries (Danforth, 1982). Maternal conditions associated with a transverse lie are grandmultiparity with relaxed uterine muscles, placenta previa, hydramnios, and preterm labor (Figure 17-7).

The long axis of the fetus lies across the woman's abdomen. On palpation, no fetal part is felt in the fundal portion of the uterus or above the symphysis. The fetal head may be

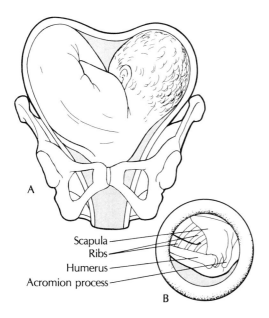

Scapula
Ribs
Humerus
Acromion process

Figure 17-7 ▰▰▰▰▰▰▰▰

Transverse lie. **A**, Shoulder presentation. **B**, On vaginal examination the nurse may feel the acromion process as the fetal presenting part.

palpated on one side and the breech on the other. FHTs are usually auscultated just below the midline of the umbilicus. During vaginal examination, the most commonly palpated presenting parts are the acromion process, the ridged thorax, or possibly an arm that is compressed against the fetal chest.

Maternal implications

• Dysfunctional labor
• Uterine rupture
• Cesarean delivery

Fetal-neonatal implications

• Increased risk of prolapsed cord

Interventions   As long as the fetus remains in a transverse lie, the only possible method of delivery is cesarean.

Compound presentation   A compound presentation is one in which there are two presenting parts such as occiput and fetal hand; occiput and fetal foot; or breech and fetal hand. Some compound presentations resolve themselves spontaneously, but others require additional manipulation at delivery.

Developmental Abnormalities

Macrosomia   Fetal **macrosomia** occurs when a neonate weighs more than 4000 g at birth. This condition is more common among offspring of large parents and diabetic women and in cases of grandmultiparity and postmaturity.

Maternal implications

• CPD
• Dysfunctional labor
• Soft tissue laceration during delivery
• Increased incidence of postpartal hemorrhage

Fetal-neonatal implications

• Cerebral trauma
• Excessive trauma to the fetal head
• Shoulder dystocia during delivery

Interventions   The maternal pelvis should be evaluated carefully if a large fetus is suspected. The labor is monitored closely for dysfunction, and the FHR is monitored continuously for signs of fetal distress.

After delivery, the neonate is assessed for skull fractures, cephalhematoma, fracture of the humerus and/or clavicle, and brachial plexus injury. The mother is assessed for uterine atony and postpartal hemorrhage.

Hydrocephalus   In hydrocephalus, 500–1000 mL of cerebrospinal fluid accumulates in the ventricles of the fetal brain. When this occurs before delivery, severe CPD results because of the enlarged cranium of the fetus.

With the use of ultrasound during pregnancy, diagnosis of this fetal abnormality is more likely. Once the woman is in labor, hydrocephalus should be suspected if labor contractions progress, yet the fetal head does not enter the birth canal. If a hydrocephalic fetus is in vertex presentation, the person doing a vaginal examination will feel wide suture lines and a globular cranium.

Maternal implications   Obstruction of labor can occur, with resulting uterine rupture.

Fetal-neonatal implications   The outlook for the fetus is questionable. If hydrocephalus is identified early in the gestation, intrauterine surgery may be performed to place a shunt, thereby preventing excessive accumulation of fluid in the fetal head. This surgery is not currently available to all mothers in all parts of the country.

If enlargement of the fetal head continues, the fetus-neonate is usually brain damaged and may die during delivery or shortly afterward. Frequently, other congenital malformations, such as myelomeningocele, accompany this condition.

Interventions Depending on the degree of hydrocephalus, the parents will be involved in some difficult decision making regarding the delivery method chosen. The nurse can help by providing information and answering questions. Cesarean delivery provides the least trauma to the fetal head. After delivery, skilled personnel need to be on hand to assess the newborn and provide supportive care as necessary.

Multiple Gestation

As discussed in Chapter 4, two fetuses that develop from one fertilized ovum are categorized as monozygotic (identical) twins. Dizygotic (fraternal) twins, the result of the fertilization of two separate ova, are not identical. If the twins are of the same sex, the placenta is examined in the pathology laboratory to determine whether the twins are monozygotic or dizygotic.

According to Pritchard, MacDonald, and Gant (1985), the incidence of monozygotic twins has no correlation with race, heredity, age, parity, and fertility therapy. However, these factors figure significantly in the incidence of dizygotic twins.

Identification of multiple gestation
During the prenatal period, any fetal growth, movement, or heart tone findings not in keeping with gestational age should lead the examiner to suspect a multiple gestation. Ultrasound examination can provide a positive diagnosis.

Maternal implications Early in the pregnancy, spontaneous abortions are more common, possibly because of genetic defects, poor placental development, or poor implantation. The woman may experience more physical discomfort during her pregnancy, such as shortness of breath, dyspnea on exertion, backaches,

and pedal edema. Other associated problems include increased incidence of PIH, maternal anemia, hydramnios, and placenta previa.

Complications during labor include abnormal fetal presentations; preterm labor; inadequate uterine contractions due to overstretching of the myometrium, abruptio placentae before labor begins, during labor with ROM, or after delivery of the first twin; and increased risk of postpartal hemorrhage due to decreased uterine tone.

Fetal-neonatal implications The perinatal mortality rate is four times greater for the first twin and five times greater for the second twin than for a singleton baby. Fetal problems include decreased intrauterine growth rate for each fetus, increased incidence of fetal anomalies, increased risk of preterm labor and the associated problems of a preterm baby, and abnormal presentations (Collea, 1984).

Interventions Antepartally, the woman may need counseling about diet and daily activities. The nurse can help her plan meals to meet her increased needs. An increase of 300 calories or more over the recommended daily dietary allowance established by the Food and Nutrition Board of the National Research Council is advised for uncomplicated pregnancy (see Table 8-1). The daily intake of protein should be increased as much as 1.5 g/kg of body weight. Daily iron supplements of 60–80 mg and an additional 1 mg of folic acid are recommended.

Counseling about daily activities may include encouraging the woman to plan frequent rest periods during the day. The rest period will have optimal effects if the woman rests in a side-lying position (which increases uteroplacental blood flow) and elevates the lower legs and the feet to reduce edema. Back discomfort may be relieved by pelvic rocking, maintaining good posture, and using good body mechanics when lifting objects or moving about.

With twins, any combination of presentations and positions can occur (Figure 17-8). An ultrasound test may be done just prior to labor or in early labor to determine the presentation and positions to make decisions about the method of delivery.

During labor, both fetuses are assessed by auscultation or electronic monitoring. Care is taken to identify the location of each twin's FHR

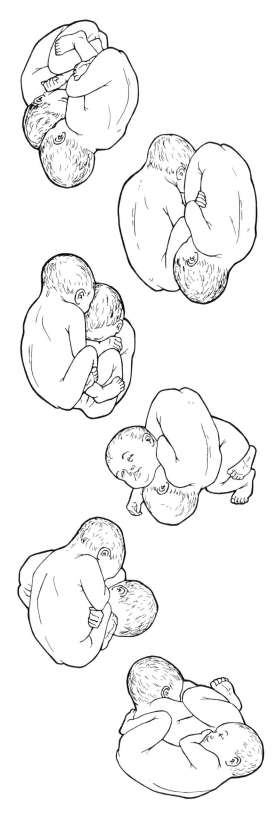

so that changes in rate can be evaluated. Signs of distress must be identified immediately. The woman's labor is assessed for dysfunctional patterns.

Vaginal delivery is facilitated when the larger fetus is in vertex presentation and is the first to be born. Uterine relaxation can be obtained with halothane if internal podalic version of the second twin is needed. However, if the first fetus is in a breech presentation, a cesarean delivery is recommended (Collea, 1984). Delivery of preterm twins is also by cesarean to minimize birth trauma.

Cesarean delivery is advocated in the presence of fetal distress, previous cesarean birth, CPD, placenta previa, and severe PIH. When the second twin is larger than the first and CPD exists, cesarean delivery should be performed (Pritchard, MacDonald, and Gant, 1985).

The nurse must prepare to receive two neonates instead of one. This means a duplication of everything, including resuscitation equipment, radiant warmers, and newborn identification papers and bracelets. Two staff members should be available for newborn resuscitation.

Fetal Distress

The most commonly observed initial signs of fetal distress include meconium-stained amniotic fluid (in a vertex presentation) and decelerations in FHR. Fetal scalp blood samples demonstrating a pH value of 7.20 or less provide a more sophisticated indication of fetal problems and are generally obtained when questions about fetal status arise. (For further discussion see p. 292.)

A variety of factors may contribute to fetal distress. The most common are related to cord compression, uteroplacental insufficiency, and preexisting maternal disease.

Maternal implications   Indications of fetal distress greatly increase the psychologic stress a laboring woman must face. The professional staff may become so involved in assessing fetal status and initiating corrective measures that they fail to give explanation and emotional support to the woman and her partner. It is imperative to provide full explanations of the problem and comfort to the couple. In many instances, if delivery is not imminent, the woman must

Figure 17-8
Types of twin presentations.

undergo cesarean delivery. This method of delivery may be a source of fear for the couple and of frustration, too, if they prepared for a shared vaginal delivery experience.

Fetal-neonatal implications   Prolonged fetal hypoxia may lead to mental retardation or cerebral palsy and ultimately to fetal death.

Interventions   When evidence of possible fetal distress develops, initial interventions include changing the maternal position and administering oxygen by mask at 6–7 L/min. If continuous electronic fetal monitoring has not been used prior to this time, it is usually instituted. Fetal scalp blood samples are also taken. Probable cause of the distress is ascertained, and further actions are based on a complete assessment of maternal-fetal status. The Nursing Care Plan on fetal distress (pp. 350–352) offers a guideline for dealing with fetal distress caused by various conditions.

Intrauterine Fetal Death

Fetal death, often referred to as *fetal demise*, accounts for one-half of the perinatal mortality after the 20th week of pregnancy. The first indication is usually cessation of fetal movement. Diagnosis of intrauterine fetal death (IUFD) is confirmed by ultrasound when no fetal heart action is visualized and there is evidence of overriding of the fetal cranial bones (Spalding's sign).

In 75% of these cases, spontaneous labor begins within 2 weeks of the fetal death (Quilligan, 1980). If labor does not occur within 2 weeks, oxytocin or prostaglandins may be administered to induce labor.

Prolonged retention of the fetus may lead to severe emotional stress for the woman and her partner. In addition, thromboplastin is released from the fetal tissues and may lead to DIC. (DIC is also referred to as *consumption coagulopathy*.)

The parents of a stillborn infant suffer a devastating experience, precipitating an intense emotional trauma. During the pregnancy, the couple has already begun the attachment process, which now must be terminated through the grieving process. Guidelines for nursing support of such parents are presented in Chapter 26.

Placental Problems

The most common types of placental problems are abruptio placentae, placenta previa, and abnormalities in placental formation and structure. Because the placenta is very vascular, problems are usually associated with maternal and possibly fetal hemorrhage. Abruptio placentae is a major emergency in labor and delivery and requires rapid, effective interventions. Although placenta previa is primarily an antepartal problem, it is presented here for the sake of comparison. Causes and sources of hemorrhage are highlighted in the box Essential Facts to Remember.

 ESSENTIAL FACTS TO REMEMBER

Causes and Sources of Hemorrhage

Causes and sources	Signs and symptoms
ANTEPARTAL PERIOD	
Abortion	Vaginal bleeding Intermittent uterine contractions Rupture of membranes
Placenta previa	Painless vaginal bleeding after seventh month
Abruptio placentae Marginal (partial)	Vaginal bleeding; no increase in uterine pain
Central (severe)	No vaginal bleeding Extreme tenderness of abdominal area Rigid, boardlike abdomen Increase in size of abdomen
INTRAPARTAL PERIOD	
Placenta previa	Bright red vaginal bleeding
Abruptio placentae	Same signs and symptoms as listed for the types of abruptio placentae
Uterine atony in stage III	Bright red vaginal bleeding, ineffectual contractility
POSTPARTAL PERIOD	
Uterine atony	Boggy uterus Dark vaginal bleeding Presence of clots
Retained placental fragments	Boggy uterus Dark vaginal bleeding Presence of clots
Lacerations of cervix or vagina	Firm uterus Bright red vaginal bleeding

Abruptio placentae Abruptio placentae is the separation of the placenta from the site of implantation on the uterine wall prior to delivery of the infant. The incidence is about 1% (Danforth, 1982). Women with a parity of five or more, older than 30, and having PIH are at increased risk of abruptio placentae.

Clinical manifestations Abruptio placentae is subdivided into three types (Figure 17-9).

- *Central.* In this situation, the placenta separates centrally, and the blood is trapped between the placenta and the uterine wall. Entrapment of the blood results in concealed bleeding.
- *Marginal.* In this case, the blood passes between the fetal membranes and the uterine wall and escapes vaginally (also called Marginal sinus rupture).
- *Complete.* Massive vaginal bleeding is seen in the presence of total separation.

The signs and symptoms of these three types of placental abruption are given in the Essential Facts to Remember—Differential Signs and Symptoms of Abruptio Placentae and Placenta Previa. In severe cases of central abruptio placentae, the blood invades the myometrial tissues between the muscle fibers. This occurrence accounts for the uterine irritability that is a significant sign of abruptio placentae. If hemorrhage continues, eventually the uterus turns entirely blue. After delivery of the neonate, the uterus contracts poorly. This condition is known as *Couvelaire uterus* and frequently necessitates hysterectomy.

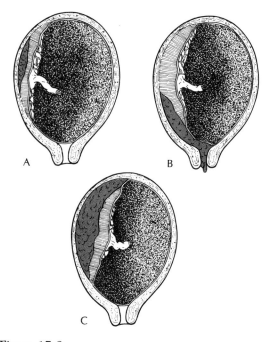

Figure 17-9
Abruptio placentae. **A**, Central abruption with concealed hemorrhage. **B**, Marginal abruption with external hemorrhage. **C**, Complete abruption. (Reprinted with permission of Ross Laboratories, Columbus, OH 43216. From Clinical Educational Aid no. 12.)

✺ ESSENTIAL FACTS TO REMEMBER

Differential Signs and Symptoms of Abruptio Placentae and Placenta Previa

Abruptio Placentae			Placenta Previa
CENTRAL	MARGINAL	COMPLETE	
No overt bleeding from vagina	Dark red vaginal bleeding	Massive vaginal bleeding	Bright red bleeding
Rigid abdomen	Nonrigid abdomen	Rigid abdomen	Nonrigid abdomen
Acute pain in abdominal area	Tenderness over uterus	Acute pain in abdominal area	No pain
Decreased blood pressure	Decreased blood pressure	Profound shock	Effect on blood pressure and pulse depends on amount of bleeding

As a result of the damage to the uterine wall and the retroplacental clotting with central abruption, large amounts of thromboplastin are released into the maternal blood supply. This in turn triggers the development of DIC and resultant hypofibrinogenemia. Fibrinogen levels, which are ordinarily elevated in pregnancy, may drop in minutes to the point at which blood will no longer coagulate due to the separation of the placenta.

Maternal implications   Maternal mortality is approximately 6%. Problems following delivery depend in large part on the severity of the intrapartal bleeding, coagulation defects (DIC), hypofibrinogenemia, and time between separation and delivery. Moderate to severe hemorrhage results in hemorrhagic shock, which may prove fatal to the mother if it is not reversed. In the postpartal period, mothers who have suffered this disorder are at risk for hemorrhage and renal failure due to shock, vascular spasm, intravascular clotting, or a combination of the three.

Fetal-neonatal implications   Perinatal mortality associated with premature separation of the placenta is about 15%. In severe cases, in which most of the placenta has separated, infant mortality is 100%. In less severe separation, fetal outcome depends on the level of maturity. The most serious complications in the neonate arise from preterm labor, anemia, and hypoxia. If fetal hypoxia progresses unchecked, irreversible brain damage or fetal demise may result. With thorough assessment and prompt action on the part of the health team, fetal and maternal outcomes can be improved.

Interventions   The nursing assessment begins when the woman is admitted. Any sudden change, such as an aching pain in the abdomen, may signal the separation of the placenta during labor. Other important signs that should be noted include irritability of the uterus, faint or absent FHTs, fetal hyperactivity, meconium-stained amniotic fluid, increase in fundal height, any increase in bleeding, and symptoms of shock. Frequently, shock symptoms appear disproportionate to blood loss. See Nursing Care Plan—Hemorrhage.

The psychologic needs of this woman cannot be overestimated. Maternal apprehension increases as the clinical picture changes. Factual reassurance and an explanation of the procedures and events are essential for the emotional well-being of the expectant couple. The nurse can reinforce positive aspects of the woman's condition, such as normal FHTs, normal vital signs, and decreased evidence of bleeding.

If the separation is mild and gestation is near term, labor may be induced and the fetus delivered vaginally. If ROM and oxytocin infusion by pump do not induce labor within 8 hours, a cesarean delivery is usually done. A longer delay increases the risk of increased hemorrhage, with resulting hypofibrinogenemia. Supportive treatment to decrease the risk of DIC includes typing and cross-matching for blood transfusions (at least three units), clotting mechanism evaluation, and intravenous fluids.

In cases of moderate to severe placental separation, hypofibrinogenemia is treated before delivery by intravenous infusion of cryoprecipitate or plasma. Cesarean delivery is then performed.

Postpartally, the nurse continues to monitor the mother's fluid intake, fluid output, and vital signs closely. The uterus is palpated frequently for atony. In addition, the nurse must be alert for signs of postpartal hemorrhage.

Placenta previa   In **placenta previa**, the placenta is implanted in the lower uterine segment instead of in the upper portion of the uterus. This implantation may be on a portion of the lower segment or over the internal cervical os. As the lower uterine segment contracts and dilates in the later weeks of pregnancy, the placental villi are torn from the uterine wall, thus exposing the uterine sinuses at the placental site. Bleeding begins, but because its amount depends on the number of sinuses exposed, initially it may be either scanty or profuse.

The cause of placenta previa is unknown. Statistically it occurs in about 1 in every 167 deliveries, with 20% being complete, and is more common in multiparas (Pritchard, MacDonald, and Gant, 1985). Women with a previous history of placenta previa as well as those who have undergone a low cervical cesarean delivery appear to be at greater risk.

Text continued on p. 372.

NURSING CARE PLAN
Hemorrhage

PATIENT ASSESSMENT

History

Identify factors predisposing to hemorrhage:
1. Presence of preeclampsia-eclampsia (PIH)
2. Overdistention of the uterus
   a. Multiple pregnancy
   b. Hydramnios
3. Grandmultiparity
4. Advanced age
5. Uterine contractile problems
   a. Hypotonicity
   b. Hypertonicity
6. Painless vaginal bleeding after seventh month
7. Presence of hypertension
8. Presence of diabetes
9. History of previous hemorrhage or bleeding problems, blood coagulation defects, abortions
10. Retained placental fragments
11. Cervical and/or vaginal lacerations

Determine religious preference to establish whether client will permit a blood transfusion

Physical Examination

Severe abdominal pain (central abruptio placentae)
External or concealed bleeding (see Essential Facts to Remember, p. 366)
Painless vaginal hemorrhage (placenta previa)
Shock symptoms (decreased blood pressure, increased pulse, pallor)
Uterine tetany or uterine atony
Portwine amniotic fluid with abruptio placentae
Degree of hemorrhage
Changes in FHR

Laboratory Evaluation

Hemoglobin and hematocrit
Type and cross-match
Fibrinogen levels

PLAN OF CARE

Nursing Priorities

1. If IV is not present, start one in large vein with large-bore plastic cannula
2. Evaluate blood loss (if possible, measure or weigh blood-soaked pads to facilitate adequate replacement)
3. Monitor vital signs, particularly pulse and BP
4. Measure urine output
5. Administer oxygen as necessary
6. Evaluate fetal status
7. Maintain fetal life-support mechanisms
8. Do not perform vaginal or rectal exam until placenta previa has been ruled out

Client/Family Educational Focus

1. Provide information regarding the cause of the hemorrhage
2. Discuss the assessment techniques and treatment associated with the hemorrhage
3. Provide opportunities for questions and individual concerns of the client and her family

Problem	Nursing interventions and actions	Rationale
Blood loss	Observe, record, and report blood loss	Monitoring the amount of blood loss aids in determining appropriate interventions
	Assess patient experiencing decrease in blood volume using following paremeters:	
	1. Monitor rate and quality of respirations continuously	Initially respiratory rate increases as a result of sympathoadrenal stimulation, resulting in increased metabolic rate; pain and anxiety may cause hyperventilation
	2. Measure pulse rate	Increased pulse rate is an effect of increased epinephrine
	3. Assess pulse quality by direct palpation	Reflects circulatory status
	Determine pulse deficit by comparing apical-radial rates	Thready pulse indicates vasoconstriction and reflects decreased cardiac output; peripheral pulses may be absent if vasoconstriction is intense
		Bounding pulse may indicate overload

NURSING CARE PLAN (continued)
Hemorrhage

Problem	Nursing interventions and actions	Rationale
	4. Compare present BP with patient's baseline BP; note pulse pressure	Hypotension indicates loss of large amount of circulatory fluid or lack of compensation in circulatory system As cardiac output decreases, there is usually a fall in pulse pressure Peripheral vasoconstriction may make accurate readings difficult
	5. Monitor urine output (decrease to less than 30 mL/hr is sign of shock): a. Insert Foley catheter b. Measure output hourly c. Measure specific gravity to determine concentration of urine	Vasoconstrictor effect of norepinephrine decreases blood flow to kidneys, which decreases glomerular filtration rate and the output of urine Inability to concentrate urine may indicate renal damage from vasoconstriction and decreased blood perfusion
	6. Assess skin for presence of following: a. Pallor and cyanosis: *Pallor* in brown-skinned persons appears yellowish-brown; black-skinned individuals appear ashen gray; generally pallor may be observed in mucous membranes, lips, and nail beds *Cyanosis* is assessed by inspecting lips, nail beds, conjunctiva, palms, and soles of feet at regular intervals; evaluate capillary refilling by pressing on nail bed and observing return of color; compare by testing your own nail bed b. Coldness c. Clamminess	Skin reflects amount of vasoconstriction Pallor is determined by intensity of vasoconstriction Cyanosis occurs when the amount of unoxygenated hemoglobin in the blood is ≤5 g/dL blood Produced by slow blood flow
	Assess state of consciousness frequently Measure CVP: normal CVP is 5–10 cm H_2O	Caused by sympathetic stimulation of sweat glands Diminished cerebral blood flow causes restlessness and anxiety; as shock progresses, state of consciousness decreases Provides estimation of volume of blood returning to heart and ability of both chambers in right heart to propel blood Low CVP indicates a decrease in the circulating volume of blood (hypovolemia)
	Assess amount of blood loss: 1. Count pads 2. Weigh pads and chux (1 g = 1 mL blood approximately) 3. Record amount in a specific amount of time (for example, 50 mL bright red blood on pad in 20 min)	In obstetric patients, blood is replaced according to estimates of actual blood loss, rather than using parameters of increased and decreased BP

NURSING CARE PLAN (continued)
Hemorrhage

Problem	Nursing interventions and actions	Rationale
Reduction of hemoglobin	Position patient in supine position with right hip elevated	Position keeps more blood volume available to vital centers Avoids pressure on vena cava
	Avoid Trendelenburg position	Trendelenburg position shifts heavy uterus against diaphragm and may compromise respiratory function
	Administer whole blood Administer O$_2$ by face mask at 4–7 L/min	Corrects reduced oxygen-carrying capacity Woman in labor is mouth breather; using face mask assures better oxygen delivery
Hypovolemia	Relieve decreased blood pressure by administration of whole blood While waiting for whole blood to be available, infuse isotonic fluids, plasma, plasma expanders, or serum albumin	Hypotension results from decreased blood volume Degree of hypovolemia may be assessed by CVP, hemoglobin, and hematocrit
Fluctuations in blood perfusion to vital organs	Monitor urine output hourly: 1. 50 mL/hr or more indicates safe renal perfusion 2. Less than 25 mL/hr indicates inadequate renal perfusion (tubular ischemia and necrosis can result) Monitor adequacy of fluid volume by evaluating CVP	Provides excellent measure of kidney perfusion
Marginal abruptio placentae	If abruptio placentae is diagnosed, nurse and physician will: 1. Evaluate blood loss. 2. Assess uterine contractile pattern and tenderness 3. Monitor maternal vital signs 4. Assess fetal status 5. Assess cervical dilatation and effacement 6. Rule out placenta previa 7. Perform amniotomy and begin oxytocin infusion if labor does not start immediately or is ineffective	Bleeding often stops as shock develops but resumes as circulation is restored. Provides information on type of abruption and maternal and fetal status.
Central abruptio placentae with severe blood loss	1. Perform same assessments as for marginal abruptio placentae 2. Monitor CVP 3. Replace blood loss 4. Effect immediate delivery 5. Observe for signs and symptoms of disseminated intravascular coagulation (DIC)	
Uterine atony immediately after delivery	1. Assess contractility of uterus and amount of vaginal bleeding. 2. Postpartally, massage uterus until firm and administer oxytocics per protocol or physician order	Muscle fibers that have been overstretched or overused do not contract well; contraction of muscle fibers over open placental site is essential; slight relaxation of uterus muscle fibers leads to continuous oozing of blood

NURSING CARE PLAN (continued)
Hemorrhage

Problem	Nursing interventions and actions	Rationale
Cervical and/or vaginal lacerations	1. Assess blood loss 2. Assess uterine contractility	
Fetal distress	Assess and monitor fetal heart rate (normal range 120–160 beats/min)	Hemorrhage from woman disrupts blood flow pattern to fetus, possibly compromising fetal status
	Observe for meconium in amniotic fluid	Hypoxia causes increased motility of fetal intestines and relaxation of abdominal muscles, with release of meconium into amniotic fluid
	Assist in obtaining fetal blood sample (pH <7.2 indicates severe jeopardy)	
Fear	Inform patient about procedures	Fear and anxiety affect release of catecholamines
	Remain calm Provide support	Increases patient's confidence
Depletion of fibrinogen	Evaluate blood levels; at term, normal fibrinogen level is 375–700 mg/dL; critical level required to clot blood is 100 mg/dL Observe for signs and symptoms of DIC	Fibrinogen and fibrin are lost because of their accumulation in a retroplacental clot; further fibrinogen loss and additional coagulation failure may result from intravascular clotting and fibrinolysis
DIC	Monitor the administration of blood components as necessary (whole blood, platelets, cryoprecipitate, plasma) Presence of hemorrhage— note previous interventions and rationale Minimize anxiety with an empathetic approach and explanations	Maintain the hematocrit value at 30% and above; elevate the platelet count and the fibrinogen levels Increase client's feelings of security

NURSING CARE EVALUATION

Blood loss is corrected
Vital signs remain within normal range
FHTs are present and within normal range

NURSING DIAGNOSIS*	SUPPORTING DATA	NURSING ORDERS
Decreased cardiac output related to hypovolemia and decreased venous return	Excessive bleeding or concealed bleeding Decreased blood pressure and/or changes in pulse pressure Pallor, cyanosis Decreased hematocrit values Decreased fibrinogen levels Decreased urine output Anxiety and/or restlessness Decreased central venous pressure	Assess patient status Correctly assess blood loss Monitor vital signs Monitor urine output Assist woman in maintaining side-lying position or supine position with a towel rolled under the right hip to displace the uterus to the left Monitor lab studies
Fear related to hemorrhage	Anxiety Expressed concerns and questions	Explain what is happening and each treatment Give correct, honest information Answer questions honestly

*These are a few examples of nursing diagnoses that may be appropriate for a woman with this condition. It is not an inclusive list and must be individualized for each woman.

The types of placenta previa are as follows (Figure 17-10):

- *Complete or total placenta previa.* The placenta totally covers the internal os.
- *Partial placenta previa.* A small portion of the placenta covers the internal os.
- *Low-lying or marginal placenta previa.* The placental edge is attached very close to but does not cover the internal os.

Clinical manifestations   Painless, bright red vaginal bleeding is the best diagnostic sign of placenta previa. If this sign should develop during the last 3 months of a pregnancy, placenta previa should always be considered until ruled out by examination. Generally, the first bleeding episode is scanty. If no rectal or vaginal examinations are performed, it often subsides spontaneously. However, each subsequent hemorrhage is more profuse.

The uterus remains soft, and if labor begins, it relaxes fully between contractions. The FHR usually remains stable unless profuse hemorrhage and maternal shock occur. As a result of the placement of the placenta, the fetal presenting part is often unengaged, and transverse lie is common.

Diagnosis   Ultrasound may be used to visualize the position of the placenta. If a woman is admitted at or near term with profuse vaginal bleeding or a history of painless vaginal bleeding and ultrasound is not available, a double set-up procedure may be done to permit the physician to perform a vaginal examination safely. A complete placenta previa can be felt over the internal cervical os. A double set-up involves examining the woman in the delivery room; if delivery is imminent, a vaginal delivery is done. If the examination triggers profuse vaginal bleeding, a cesarean delivery is done quickly. (See Figure 17-11.)

The presence of placenta previa increases maternal risks in the postpartal period. Hemorrhage, which may occur when the placental site is located in the lower uterine segment, is a primary danger. This is the passive section of the uterus, and the contractility of this section of muscle fiber is poor. Uterine rupture could occur as a result of the weakening of the uterine musculature by the ingrowth of the placenta and the presence of its blood sinuses. Uterine infection from prolonged rupture of membranes, retained placental fragments, and possible anemia are also risks.

Fetal-neonatal implications   The prognosis for the fetus depends on the extent of placenta previa. Changes in the FHR and meconium staining of the amniotic fluid may be apparent. In a profuse bleeding episode, the fetus is compromised and does suffer some hypoxia. FHR monitoring is imperative when the woman is admitted, particularly if a vaginal delivery is anticipated. This is important because the presenting part of the fetus may obstruct the flow of blood from the placenta or umbilical cord. If fetal distress occurs, delivery is by cesarean birth.

After delivery, blood sampling should be done to determine whether the intrauterine bleeding episodes of the woman have caused anemia in the newborn.

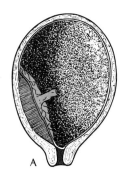
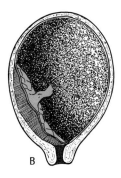
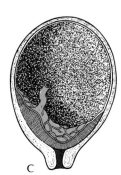

Figure 17-10

Placenta previa. **A**, Low placental implantation. **B**, Partial placenta previa. **C**, Total placenta previa. (Reprinted with permission of Ross Laboratories, Columbus, OH 43216. From Clinical Educational Aid no. 12.)

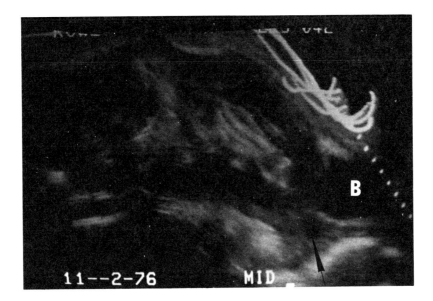

Figure 17-11

Ultrasound of placenta previa.

Interventions   Care of the woman with painless late gestational bleeding depends on (a) the week of gestation during which the first bleeding episode occurs and (b) the amount of bleeding. If the gestation is less than 37 weeks and if bleeding is scanty or has stopped, the placenta should be localized by ultrasound. If placenta previa is ruled out, a vaginal examination may be performed with a speculum to assess the cause of bleeding (such as cervical lesions). If placenta previa is diagnosed, then *expectant management* is used to delay delivery until about 37 weeks' gestation to allow the fetus to mature. Expectant management involves stringent regulation of nursing care as follows:

1. Bed rest with only bathroom privileges as long as the woman is not bleeding

2. No rectal or vaginal exams

3. Assessment of blood loss, pain, and uterine contractility

4. Assessment of FHTs with external fetal monitor

5. Monitoring of vital signs

6. Complete laboratory evaluation: hemoglobin, hematocrit, Rh factor, and urinalysis

7. Intravenous fluid (Ringer's lactate) during bleeding episodes

8. Two units of cross-matched blood available for transfusion

9. Communication with patient and family about what is happening and encouragement of their questions

If frequent, recurrent, or profuse bleeding persists, a cesarean delivery is performed.

At 37 weeks, delivery is performed either by the vaginal route or by cesarean birth. This decision is based on knowledge of the degree of previa and of the feasibility of inducing labor. If the placenta does not cover the os, membranes are ruptured and a vaginal delivery is anticipated. If bleeding becomes profuse, a cesarean delivery is done.

Other placental problems   Other problems of the placenta are presented in Table 17-1 and in Figure 17-12.

Problems Associated with Umbilical Cord

Prolapsed umbilical cord   A prolapsed umbilical cord results when the umbilical cord precedes the fetal presenting part. When this occurs, pressure is placed on the umbilical cord, as it is trapped between the presenting part and the maternal pelvis. Consequently, the vessels carrying blood to and from the fetus are compressed (see Figure 17-13).

Prolapse of the cord may occur with rupture of the membranes if the presenting part is not well engaged in the pelvis.

Table 17-1
Placental and Umbilical Cord Variations

Placental variation	Maternal implication	Fetal-neonatal implications
Succenturiate Placenta One or more accessory lobes of fetal villi develop on the placenta.	Postpartal hemorrhage from retained lobe	
Circumvallate Placenta A double fold of chorion and amnion form a ring around the umbilical cord on the fetal side of the placenta.	Increased incidence of late abortion, antepartal hemorrhage, and preterm labor	Fetal death
Battledore Placenta The umbilical cord is inserted at or near the placental margin.	Increased incidence of preterm labor and bleeding	Prematurity, fetal distress
Velamentous insertion of the umbilical cord The vessels of the umbilical cord divide some distance from the placenta in the placental membranes.	Hemorrhage if one of vessels is torn	Fetal distress, hemorrhage

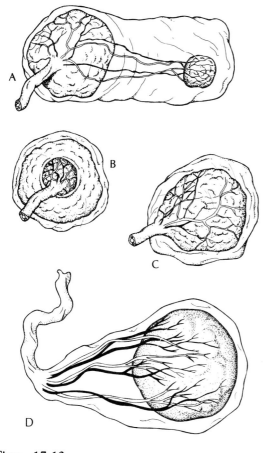

Figure 17-12
Placental variations. **A**, Succenturiate placenta. **B**, Circumvallate placenta. **C**, Battledore placenta. **D**, Placenta with a velamentous umbilical cord insertion.

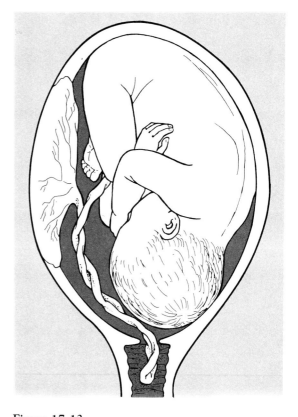

Figure 17-13
Prolapse of the umbilical cord.

Maternal implications   Although a prolapsed cord does not directly precipitate physical alterations in the woman, her immediate concern for the baby creates enormous stress. The woman may need to deal with some unusual interventions, a cesarean delivery, and in some circumstances, death of the baby.

Fetal-neonatal implications   Compression of the cord results in decreased blood flow and leads to fetal distress. If labor is occurring, the cord is compressed further with each contraction. If the pressure on the cord is not relieved, the fetus will die.

Interventions   Because there are few outward signs of cord prolapse, each pregnant woman is advised to call her physician or nurse-midwife when the membranes rupture and to go to the office, clinic, or birthing facility. A sterile vaginal examination determines if there is danger of cord prolapse. If the presenting part is well engaged, the risk of cord prolapse is minimal, and ambulation may be encouraged. If the presenting part is not well engaged, bed rest is recommended to prevent cord prolapse.

Because cord prolapse can be associated with fetal death, some physicians and nurse-midwives may insist that bedrest be maintained regardless of fetal engagement. This can lead to conflict if the laboring woman and her partner do not hold the same opinions. The nurse can ease this situation by helping communication between the physician or nurse-midwife and the couple.

When the woman is in labor, ROM (whether spontaneous or with amniotomy) signals the need for immediate auscultation of the FHR for 1 full minute. During labor, any alteration of FHR or presence of meconium in the amniotic fluid indicates the need to assess for the presence of cord prolapse.

If a prolapsed cord is found on vaginal examination, the examiner keeps his or her gloved fingers in the vagina and applies gentle pressure against the presenting part to relieve pressure on the cord. The woman is directed to turn to a side-lying or knee-chest position. The physician or nurse-midwife is notified immediately. Vaginal delivery is possible if:

- The cervix is completely dilated.

- Pelvic measurements are adequate.

If these conditions are not present, cesarean delivery is the method of choice. The woman is taken to the delivery room while the examiner continues to relieve the pressure on the cord until the infant has been delivered.

Problems Associated with Amniotic Fluid

Amniotic fluid embolism   **Amniotic fluid embolism** can occur after a labor with very intense, frequent contractions or from oxytocin induction with hypertonic uterine contractions. In the presence of a small tear in the amnion or chorion high in the uterus, the fluid may leak into the chorionic plate and enter the maternal circulation. The fluid can also enter at areas of placental separation or cervical tears. Under pressure from the contracting uterus, the fluid is driven into the maternal system. The more debris in the amniotic fluid (such as meconium), the greater the maternal problems.

Maternal implications   This condition frequently occurs during or after the delivery when the woman has had a difficult, rapid labor. Suddenly she experiences respiratory distress, circulatory collapse, acute hemorrhage, and cor pulmonale as the embolism blocks the vessels of the lungs. The woman exhibits a sudden onset of dyspnea, cyanosis, cardiovascular collapse, shock, and coma. If she survives for more than 1 hour, she has a 50% chance of developing DIC caused by thromboplastin-like material in the amniotic fluid. This results in massive hemorrhage.

Maternal mortality is approximately 85% (Duff, 1984). In suspected cases in which women survive, it is difficult to determine whether an amniotic fluid embolism actually occurred since specific tests are not available.

Fetal-neonatal implications   Delivery must be facilitated immediately to obtain a live birth. In many cases, the delivery has already occurred, or the fetus can be delivered vaginally with forceps. If labor has been tumultuous (very strong, frequent contractions), the fetus may suffer problems associated with dysfunctional labor.

Interventions Any woman exhibiting chest pain, dyspnea, cyanosis, frothy pink sputum, tachycardia, hypotension, and massive hemorrhage needs the cooperation and skills of every member of the health team if her life is to be saved. Medical and nursing interventions are supportive.

Every delivery room should be equipped with a working oxygen unit. In the absence of the physician, the nurse administers oxygen under positive pressure until medical help arrives. An intravenous line is quickly established. If respiratory and cardiac arrest occurs, cardiopulmonary resuscitation (CPR) is initiated immediately.

The nurse readies the equipment necessary for blood transfusion and for the insertion of the CVP line. As the blood volume is replaced, using fresh whole blood to provide clotting factors, the central venous pressure (CVP) is monitored frequently. In the presence of cor pulmonale, fluid overload could easily occur.

Hydramnios **Hydramnios** occurs when over 2000 mL of amniotic fluid is in utero. The exact cause of hydramnios is unknown. In some instances, hydramnios is associated with fetal malformations that affect the fetal swallowing mechanism and neurologic disorders such as spina bifida or myelomeningocele. This condition is also associated with anencephaly; the fetus is thought to urinate excessively due to overstimulation of the cerebrospinal centers.

Maternal implications When the amount of amniotic fluid is over 3000 mL, the woman experiences shortness of breath and edema in the lower extremities from compression of the vena cava. Milder forms of hydramnios occur more frequently and are associated with minimal symptoms. Hydramnios is associated with such maternal disorders as diabetes and Rh sensitization and with multiple gestations.

Antepartally, if the amniotic fluid is removed rapidly, abruptio placentae can result from too sudden a change in the size of the uterus. Because of overdistention of uterine muscles, uterine dysfunction can occur intrapartally, and the incidence of postpartal hemorrhage increases.

Fetal-neonatal implications Fetal malformations and premature delivery are common with hydramnios; thus perinatal mortality is high. Prolapsed cord can occur when the membranes rupture, a further complication for the fetus. The incidence of malpresentations is also increased.

Interventions Hydramnios should be suspected when the fundal height increases out of proportion to the gestational age. As the amount of fluid increases, the nurse may have difficulty palpating the fetus and auscultating the FHTs. In more severe cases, the maternal abdomen appears extremely tense and tight on inspection. Sonography reveals large spaces between the fetus and the uterine wall. Also at this time, an anencephalic infant or a dilated fetal stomach resulting from esophageal atresia may be identified, and multiple gestation may be confirmed.

If the accumulation of amniotic fluid has become severe enough to cause maternal dyspnea, hospitalization and removal of the excessive fluid are required. This can be done by amniocentesis. The amniocentesis is performed with the aid of sonography to prevent inadvertent damage to the fetus and placenta, and the fluid is removed slowly to prevent abruption.

For nursing measures during amniocentesis, see Chapter 11.

Oligohydramnios **Oligohydramnios**, a severe reduction and concentration of the amniotic fluid, is a rare maternal finding. The exact cause of this condition is unknown. It is found in cases of postmaturity, with IUGR secondary to placental insufficiency, and in fetal conditions associated with renal and urinary malfunction (Pritchard, MacDonald, and Gant, 1985).

Maternal implications Labor can by dysfunctional, and progress is slow.

Fetal-neonatal implications Fetal hypoxia may occur due to umbilical cord compression.

Complications Involving the Passage

The passage includes the maternal bony pelvis, beginning at the pelvic inlet and ending at the pelvic outlet, and the maternal soft tissues within these anatomic areas. A contracture (narrowed diameter) in any of the described areas can result in CPD if the fetus is larger than the pelvic diameters. Abnormal fetal presentations and positions occur in CPD as the fetus attempts to accommodate to its passage.

The gynecoid and anthropoid pelvic types usually are adequate for vertex delivery, but the android and platypelloid types predispose to CPD. Certain combinations of types also can result in pelvic diameters inadequate for vertex delivery. (See Chapter 12 for a description of pelvis types and their implications for childbirth.)

Contractures of the Inlet

Contracture of the pelvic inlet is indicated by a diagonal conjugate less than 11.5 cm. The primary risk is that the narrowed diameter will not permit engagement of the fetal presenting part. If engagement does occur, the fetus may assume a malpresentation, such as face or shoulder.

The management of inlet contractures begins with assessment of the pelvic configuration, the size and presentation of the fetus, uterine activity, cervical dilatation, and any problems during previous labors and deliveries. These findings influence the decision to proceed with a trial labor or to do a cesarean delivery.

Contractures of the Midpelvis

Contractures of the midpelvis are more common than inlet contractures. Although a satisfactory method of measuring the midpelvis manually does not exist, prominent spines, converging pelvic walls, or a narrow sacrosciatic notch can be ascertained on vaginal examination. Midpelvis contractures cause transverse arrest of the head, leading to potentially difficult midforceps delivery.

The treatment goal is to allow the natural forces of labor to push the biparietal diameter of the fetal head beyond the potential interspinous obstruction.

A bulging perineum and crowning indicate that the obstruction has been passed.

Contractures of the Outlet

Contractures of the outlet and midpelvis almost always occur simultaneously (Mengert and Steer, 1984). A diameter of less than 8 cm between the inner surface of the ischial tuberosities constitutes an outlet contracture. Whether vaginal delivery can occur depends on the woman's measurements and fetal size.

Implications of Pelvic Contractures

Maternal implications   Labor is prolonged in the presence of CPD. ROM can result from the force of the unequally distributed contractions being exerted on the fetal membranes. In obstructed labor, where the fetus cannot descend, uterine rupture can occur. With delayed descent, necrosis of maternal soft tissues can result from pressure exerted by the fetal head. Eventually, necrosis can cause fistulas from the vagina to other nearby structures. Difficult forceps deliveries can also result in damage to maternal soft tissue.

Fetal-neonatal implications   If the membranes rupture and the fetal head has not entered the inlet, there is a danger of cord prolapse. Excessive molding and/or overriding of the sutures may occur. A large caput succedaneum (see Chapter 20) may form. If the labor and delivery are particularly difficult, skull fracture and/or intracranial hemorrhage may occur.

Interventions   The adequacy of the maternal pelvis for a vaginal delivery should be assessed intrapartally as well as antepartally. During the intrapartal assessment, the size of the fetus and its presentation, position, and lie must also be considered. (See Chapter 13 for intrapartal assessment techniques.)

The nurse should suspect CPD when labor is prolonged, cervical dilatation and effacement are slow, and engagement of the presenting part is delayed. Contractions should be monitored continuously, and the labor progress should be charted on the Friedman graph. The fetus should also be monitored continuously.

If the physician is uncertain whether the infant will be delivered vaginally, a trial of labor may be given. The woman is allowed to labor to determine if the forces of the uterine contractions can overcome the actual or suspected disproportion. No fetal descent, ineffective contractions, and lack of progressive dilatation and effacement of the cervix are evidence of the failure of the trial of labor, and cesarean delivery is done.

The couple may need support in coping with the stresses of this complicated labor. The nurse should keep the couple informed of what is happening and explain the procedures that are being used. This knowledge reassures the couple that measures are being taken to resolve the problem.

Complications of Third and Fourth Stages

Postpartal Hemorrhage

Postpartal hemorrhage is a loss of blood in excess of 500 mL in the first 24 hours following delivery. Immediate postpartal hemorrhage is most commonly caused by uterine atony and lacerations of the vagina and cervix.

Retained placenta   The placenta should be delivered within 30 minutes following the birth of the infant. If it does not, or if hemorrhage occurs after the delivery of the newborn but before delivery of the placenta, the cause is frequently a retained placenta. In this instance, the physician observes the firmness of the fundus and administers fundal massage if needed. When the placenta is ready to separate, fundal massage helps to express (deliver) the placenta. If signs of placental separation have not occurred, the physician manually removes the placenta by inserting a gloved hand into the uterus and placing the fingers at the placental margin. Then the placenta is gently separated from the uterine wall. During this procedure, the other hand remains on the uterine fundus, externally.

After delivery of the placenta, the consistency of the fundus is assessed. If it is boggy and bleeding continues, vigorous massage is instituted. Oxytocics (Pitocin, Methergine, or Ergotrate) may be given. If the bleeding persists, the physician undertakes bimanual uterine compression. If intravenous infusion is not already occurring, a line is established, and oxytocin is added at a rapid rate. Blood transfusions may be ordered. Oxygen at 4–7 L/min is given by face mask. The physician manually checks the uterine cavity for retained placental fragments and also inspects the cervix and vagina for lacerations. The combination of bimanual compression, oxytocics, and blood transfusion is usually effective in treating uterine atony. The fundus should be assessed frequently for the next few hours to see that it remains contracted.

Placenta accreta   *Placenta accreta*, a type of retained placenta, is very serious because the chorionic villi attach directly to the myometrium of the uterus. Placenta accreta cannot be manually removed from the uterus as described above. An abdominal hysterectomy is usually required to control bleeding.

Uterine atony   Relaxation of the uterus (or insufficient contractions) following delivery can frequently be anticipated in the presence of the following:

- Overdistention of the uterus due to multiple fetuses, macrosomic fetus, or hydramnios
- Dysfunctional labor that has already indicated the uterus is contracting in an other-than-normal pattern
- Oxytocin stimulation or augmentation during labor
- Use of anesthetics that produces uterine relaxation

Hemorrhage from uterine atony may be slow and steady rather than sudden and massive. The blood may escape from the vagina or collect in the uterus. Because of the increased blood volume associated with pregnancy, changes in maternal blood pressure and pulse may not occur until blood loss has been significant.

After delivery of the placenta, the fundus should be palpated to assure that it is firm and well contracted. If it is not firm, vigorous massage should be instituted. Oxytocics may be given.

Retained placental fragments   Hemorrhage from retained placental fragments is not usually a cause of immediate postpartal hemorrhage but tends to be a major cause of later postpartal bleeding. To prevent this type of hemorrhage, the placenta should be inspected after delivery for evidence of missing pieces or cotyledons. The membranes should be inspected for absent sections or for vessels that traverse from the edge of the placenta outward along the membranes, which may indicate placenta succenturiate and a retained lobe. The uterine cavity may be checked for retained placental fragments or membranes.

Lacerations   Lacerations of the cervix or vagina may be indicated when bright red vaginal bleeding persists in the presence of a well-contracted uterus. Shock that is out of proportion to blood loss may result from uterine laceration. Upper vaginal lacerations are most frequently in the posterior fornix. The physician inspects the lower aspects of the uterus, cervix, and vagina. If lacerations are found, they are sutured.

Inversion of uterus   Uterine inversion occurs when the uterus turns inside out during the third stage of labor. This rare occurrence can be caused by a lax uterine wall coupled with undue tension on an umbilical cord when the placenta has not separated. Forceful pressure on the fundus with a dilated cervix and sudden emptying of the uterine contents may be contributing factors. Maternal bleeding with shock is rapid and profound.

Interventions   The physician manually replaces the uterus by grasping the vaginal mass, spreading the cervical ring with the fingers and thumb, and steadily forcing the fundus upward. The patient is often placed under deep anesthesia. Occasionally tocolytic agents are given (Oxorn, 1980).

Nursing interventions should be directed at management of shock. Volume replacement should be a priority. The nurse starts an intravenous infusion and sees that a blood sample is collected for type and cross-matching. The nurse monitors blood pressure and pulse rate every 5 minutes until the anesthesiologist arrives and is ready to assume this duty.

Careful monitoring of the intake and output is vital. An indwelling catheter is usually inserted into the bladder after the uterus is replaced. The uterus should be assessed frequently to ensure it remains contracted.

Genital Tract Trauma

Hematoma   The most common site of a genital tract hematoma is the lateral vaginal wall in the area of the ischial spines. If the hematoma is 3 cm or less and does not enlarge, it does not require therapy. A hematoma that continues to enlarge may allow enough blood loss to cause shock, sensations of intense internal pressure, and severe pain. In this instance, the hematoma should be drained, and the bleeding point located and ligated (Work, 1982).

Nursing measures are directed first toward further assessment when the patient complains of intense pressure and pain in the perineal or rectal area. The perineum should be inspected for bruising or areas of swelling. Maternal blood pressure and pulse are assessed.

Signs and symptoms of shock in the presence of a well-contracted uterus and no visible vaginal blood loss should alert the nurse to the possibility of hematoma. The hematoma may be palpated by gentle rectal exam, although this procedure may be quite uncomfortable for the woman. After alerting the physician, the nurse continues to monitor vital signs and may initiate intravenous fluids if hypovolemic shock is developing.

Perineal lacerations   A laceration of the perineal tissues may occur when the perineal tissues have been stretched too much or the episiotomy has been extended. Lacerations of the vagina and perineum are classified as first, second, third, or fourth degree (Pritchard, MacDonald, and Gant, 1985).

- First-degree lacerations involve the perineal skin and vaginal mucosa.
- Second-degree lacerations include underlying fascia and muscle in addition to the skin and vaginal mucosa.
- Third-degree lacerations include all of the above and extend to the anal sphincter.
- Fourth-degree lacerations include all of the above and tear through the anal sphincter extending up the rectal wall.

Lacerations are repaired by suturing. Nursing measures begin with careful assessment of the perineum for swelling and bruising. Cold packs may be applied to increase comfort. In the postpartum period, additional comfort measures include sitz baths, use of a perineal light and topical anesthetic spray to the perineum.

Complicated Childbirth: Effects on the Family

A complicated pregnancy and difficult labor and delivery are crisis situations that can test the coping mechanisms of every individual involved. In Chapter 26, the responses of families suffering complications during pregnancy and birth are discussed at length.

Summary

Childbirth is traditionally viewed as normal and happy, and usually it is. However, many complications may develop that represent a hazard to the woman and her unborn child. It is essential to assess a laboring woman carefully and provide her with appropriate care to prevent or treat problems.

References

Andrews CM, Andrews EC: Nursing, maternal postures, and fetal position. *Nurs Res* 1983; 32:336.

Bishop EH: Acceleration of fetal pulmonary maturity. *Obstet Gynecol* (Suppl) 1981; 58:48.

Boehm FH, Acker D: Prevention and treatment of premature labor. In: *Gynecology and Obstetrics.* Sciarri JJ (editor). Philadelphia: Harper & Row, 1984.

Collea JV: Choosing a method for breech delivery. *Contemp Ob/Gyn* April 1984; 23:27.

Creasy RK: When preterm labor threatens. *Contemp Ob/Gyn* January 1984; 23:26.

Danforth D: *Obstetrics and Gynecology*, 4th ed. Philadelphia: Harper & Row, 1982.

Duff P: Defusing the dangers of amniotic fluid embolism. *Contemp Ob/Gyn* August 1984; 24:127.

Flood B, Naeye RL: Factors that predispose to premature rupture of the fetal membranes. *J Obstet Gynecol* March/April 1984; 13:119.

Foster SD: Ritrodrine for arrest of premature labor. *MCN* 1981; 6:204.

Genest M: Preparation for childbirth evidence for efficacy, a review. *J Obstet Gynecol Neonat Nurs* 1981; 10:82.

Giacoia GP, Yaffe S: Perinatal pharmacology, chap 100. In: *Gynecology and Obstetrics.* Vol 3. Sciarri JJ (editor). Philadelphia: Harper & Row, 1982.

Katz M, Benedetti TJ, Yonezawa R: Minimizing side effects from β-adrenergic tocolytics. *Contemp Ob/Gyn* October 1983; 22:169.

Lipshitz J: Beta-adrenergic agonists. *Semin Perinatol* July 1981; 5:252.

Lipshitz J, Schneider JM: Inhibition of labor, chap 87. In: *Gynecology and Obstetrics.* Vol 3. Sciarri JJ (editor). Philadelphia: Harper & Row, 1980.

Mengert WF, Steer CM: Pelvic capacity, chap 53. In: *Gynecology and Obstetrics.* Vol 2. Sciarri JJ (editor). Philadelphia: Harper & Row, 1984.

Oxorn H: *Human birth and delivery*, 4th ed. New York: Appleton-Century-Crofts, 1980.

Philipsen T, Eriksen PS, Lynggard F: Pulmonary edema following ritrodine-saline infusion in premature labor. *Obstet Gynecol* September 1981; 58(3):304.

Pritchard JA, MacDonald PC, Gant NF: *Williams Obstetrics*, 17th ed. New York: Appleton-Century-Crofts, 1985.

Quilligan EJ: *Current Therapy in Obstetrics and Gynecology*. Philadelphia: Saunders, 1980.

Sasmor JL, Grossman E: Childbirth education in 1980. *J Obstet Gynecol Neonat Nurs* May/June 1981; 10(3):155.

Work BA: Caring for genital tract birth trauma. *Contemp Obstet Gynecol* November 1982; 20:82.

Zacharias JF: Childbirth education classes: Effects on attitudes toward childbirth in high-risk indigent women. *J Obstet Gynecol Neonat Nurs* 1981; 10:265.

Additional Readings

Benedetti TS: Coping with shoulder dystocia. *Contemp Ob/Gyn* June 1984; 23(6):29.

Cefalo RC: Abnormalities of labor. *Clin Obstet Gynecol* March 1982; 25(1):103.

Chez RA, Bowes WA: Meconium: When and how to suction. *Contemp Ob/Gyn* April 1984; 23(4):61.

Gimovsky ML, Petrie RH: Strategy for choosing the best delivery route for the breech baby. *Contemp Ob/Gyn* April 1983; 21(4):201.

Marshall CL: Coping with an unsuspected second twin. *Contemp Ob/Gyn* August 1984; 24(2):165.

Meissner JE: Predicting a patient's anxiety level during labor: A two part assessment tool. *Nurs 80* 1980; 10:50.

O'Brien W, Cefalo RC: Evaluation of x-ray pelvimetry and abnormal labor. *Clin Obstet Gynecol* March 1982; 25(1):157.

Rayburn WF et al: Umbilical cord length and intrapartum complications. *Obstet Gynecol* 1981; 57(4):450.

18
Elective Obstetric Procedures

Chapter Contents

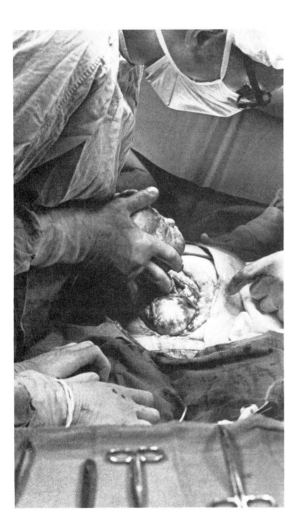

Objectives

- Describe the various methods of version and the nursing interventions for each method.

- Discuss the use of amniotomy in current maternity care.

- Compare methods for inducing labor, explaining their advantages and disadvantages.

- Describe the types of episiotomies performed, the rationale for each, and the associated nursing interventions.

- Describe the indications for forceps delivery and types of forceps that may be used.

- Discuss the use of vacuum extraction including indications, procedure, complications, and related nursing interventions.

- Explain the indications for cesarean birth, impact on the family unit, preparation and teaching needs, and associated nursing interventions.

Key Terms ▬▬▬▬▬

amniotomy	induction of labor
episiotomy	version

The use of operative and other obstetric procedures has increased in recent years. More childbearing women are being identified as high risk, and these births need to be assisted to reduce the possible dangers to the woman and infant. In addition, certain obstetric procedures are performed to accommodate the wishes of the expectant family or the physician.

Obstetric procedures discussed in this chapter are versions, amniotomy, induction of labor, episiotomy, forceps delivery, vacuum extraction, and cesarean birth.

Version _____

Version is the alteration of fetal position by abdominal or intrauterine manipulation to achieve a more favorable fetal position for delivery.

External or Cephalic Version

The infant can be rotated from a breech or transverse position to cephalic position by external abdominal manipulation. This version may be done before term and is more successful in multiparous women with relaxed abdominal walls.

The prerequisites for cephalic version are as follows (Pritchard, MacDonald, and Gant, 1985; VanDorsten et al., 1981):

1. The presenting part must not be engaged.

2. The abdominal wall must be thin enough to permit accurate palpation.

3. The uterine wall must not be irritable.

4. There must be a sufficient quantity of amniotic fluid in the uterus, and the membranes must be intact.

Contraindications include the following:

1. CPD disproportion that would prevent a vaginal delivery

2. Third-trimester bleeding

3. Low implantation of the placenta

4. Previous uterine surgery

Before an external or cephalic version, the woman receives ritodrine intravenously to relax the uterus. Under continuous fetal monitoring, the fetus is turned from breech to vertex presentation (Figure 18-1).

Nursing interventions   Nursing care during an external version includes assessment of maternal blood pressure every 5 minutes and continuous monitoring of the fetus. These assessments should continue for 30 minutes after the version.

Internal or Podalic Version

Internal or podalic version is used to rotate a fetus in a vertex or transverse position to a breech position. The only indication for this is for the delivery of the second twin (Pritchard, MacDonald, and Gant, 1985). In this procedure, after the first twin is delivered, the physician reaches into the uterine cavity, grasps one or both feet of the second twin and draws them through the cervix.

Amniotomy _____

Amniotomy, the artificial rupturing of membranes, is probably the most common operative procedure in obstetrics. Amniotomy

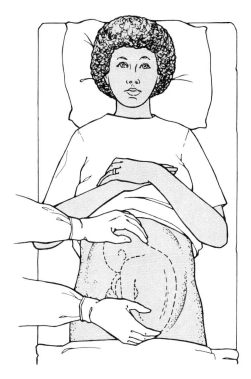

Figure 18-1

External version of fetus. A new technique for version involves pressure on the fetal head and buttocks so that the fetus completes a "backward flip" or "forward roll."

is often performed after active labor begins. The procedure is thought to shorten labor because when the hard fetal head comes in better contact with the cervix during contractions, dilatation occurs more quickly.

Possible problems associated with amniotomy are:

1. Maternal intrauterine infection and fetal infection due to introduction of bacteria or prolonged ROM
2. Increased incidence of early decelerations during labor because of the increased pressure on the fetal head
3. Prolapsed umbilical cord, which may occur when the amniotic fluid escapes from the uterus and when the presenting part is not well engaged

Nursing interventions   The procedure, expected effects, and possible problems are

explained to the childbearing couple. The fetal presentation, position, and station are assessed because amniotomy is usually delayed until engagement has occurred. The woman is positioned in a semireclining position and draped to provide privacy. The FHR is assessed just prior to and immediately after the amniotomy, and the two FHR assessments are compared. If there are marked changes, the nurse should check for prolapse of the cord. The amniotic fluid is inspected for amount, color, odor, and the presence of meconium or blood. The perineal area is cleansed and dried after the procedure. The chux should be changed frequently to maintain comfort. Because there is now an open pathway for organisms to ascend into the uterus, strict sterile technique must be observed during vaginal examinations. In addition, the number of vaginal examinations must be kept to a minimum, and the woman's temperature should be monitored every 2 hours.

Induction of Labor

The American College of Obstetricians and Gynecologists defines **induction of labor** as the deliberate initiation of uterine contractions prior to their spontaneous onset (Hughes, 1972). The procedure may be either elective or medically indicated because of the presence of a maternal and/or fetal problem.

Elective induction is defined by the Food and Drug Administration as "the initiation of labor for the convenience of an individual with a term pregnancy who is free of medical indications." The advisability of elective induction is questionable because of the associated maternal risks and the possibility of delivering a preterm infant.

Medically indicated induction may be considered in the presence of diabetes mellitus, renal disease, severe PIH, abruptio placentae, premature ROM, postterm pregnancy, severe fetal hemolytic disease, and intrauterine fetal death (Cibils, 1981).

Contraindications

All contraindications to spontaneous labor and vaginal delivery are contraindications to induction (Cibils, 1981).

The major maternal contraindications are:

- Previous uterine incision
- CPD
- Presence of herpesvirus hominis type 2
- Placenta previa centrally located
- Overdistention of the uterus (hydramnios, multiple gestation)

The major fetal contraindications are:

- Severe fetal distress or positive CST
- Preterm fetus
- Breech or transverse presentation

Before an induction is attempted, assessment must indicate that both the woman and unborn child are ready for labor. This assessment includes evaluation of fetal maturity and cervical readiness.

Labor Readiness

Fetal maturity Gestational age of the fetus can be determined throughout the gestational period by ultrasound examination. Amniotic fluid studies also provide important information on fetal maturity. (See Chapter 11 for a discussion of methods to assess fetal maturity.)

Cervical readiness The findings of vaginal examinations help determine whether cervical changes favorable to induction have occurred. Bishop (1964) developed a prelabor scoring system that has proved helpful in predicting the inducibility of women (Table 18-1). Components evaluated are cervical dilatation, effacement, consistency, and position as well as the station of the fetal presenting part. A score of 0, 1, 2, or 3 is given to each assessed characteristic. The higher the total score for all the criteria, the more likely it is that labor will ensue. The lower the total score, the higher the failure rate. A favorable cervix is the most important criterion for a successful induction.

The presence of a cervix that is anterior, soft, more than 50% effaced, and dilated at least 3 cm, with the fetal head at +1 station or lower is favorable for a successful induction (Danforth, 1982).

Methods

The most frequently used methods of induction are amniotomy, intravenous oxytocin infusion, or both.

Amniotomy The mechanism by which amniotomy stimulates labor is unknown. However, under favorable conditions, which include cervical readiness and position of the fetal head against the lower segment and dipping into the pelvis, about 80% of women at term go into active labor within 24 hours after amniotomy (Cibils, 1981).

The advantages of amniotomy as a method of labor induction are as follows:

1. The contractions elicited are similar to those of spontaneous labor.
2. There is usually no risk of hypertonus or rupture of the uterus.
3. The woman does not require as close surveillance as in oxytocin infusion.
4. Fetal monitoring is facilitated because amniotomy does not interfere with the following:
   a. Scalp blood sampling for pH determinations
   b. Scalp electrode application
   c. Intrauterine catheter placement

Table 18-1
Prelabor Status Evaluation Scoring System*

Factor	Assigned value			
	0	**1**	**2**	**3**
Cervical dilatation	Closed	1-2 cm	3-4 cm	5 cm or more
Cervical effacement	0%-30%	40%-50%	60%-70%	80% or more
Fetal station	−3	−2	−1, 0	+1, or lower
Cervical consistency	Firm	Moderate	Soft	
Cervical position	Posterior	Midposition	Anterior	

*Modified from Bishop, E. H. Reprinted with permission from the American College of Obstetricians and Gynecologists. *Obstetrics and Gynecology.* Vol. 24, 1964.

5. The color and composition of amniotic fluid can be evaluated.

The following are the disadvantages of amniotomy:

1. During the procedure there is a risk of compression of the umbilical cord (McKay and Mahan, 1983).

2. Once an amniotomy is done, delivery must occur regardless of subsequent findings that suggest delaying birth.

3. The danger of a prolapsed cord is increased.

4. There is a risk of infection from ascending organisms.

5. Compression and molding of the fetal head are increased.

6. Labor may not be successfully induced, resulting in cesarean delivery.

See discussion of nursing care after amniotomy on p. 383.

Prostaglandin administration In some centers, prostaglandin gel PGE_2 is being used to ripen the cervix and induce labor. The gel is placed in a diaphragm, which is inserted into the vagina and placed against the cervix. The gel may be removed if side-effects, such as hypertonus or hyperactivity of the uterus, nausea, and vomiting, develop. Prostaglandin gel may also be administered in suppository form. The suppository is placed in the posterior vaginal fornix (Macer et al., 1984). Research is currently being conducted to determine if the administration of prostaglandins is safe and effective.

Oxytocin infusion Intravenous administration of oxytocin is an effective method of initiating uterine contractions (inducing labor). It may also be used to augment labor or to stimulate or enhance contractions that are ineffective. Ten units of oxytocin (Pitocin) are added to 1 L of intravenous fluid (usually 5% dextrose in balanced salt solution—for example, 5% dextrose in lactated Ringer's). The resulting mixture will contain 10 mU of oxytocin per milliliter, and the prescribed dose can be easily calculated. A second bottle of intravenous fluid is prepared and used to start and maintain the infusion. This avoids infusing a large dose of oxytocin as the line is begun and provides additional fluids while the oxytocin solution is being kept at a low infusion rate. After the infusion is started, the oxytocin solution is piggy-backed to the primary tubing and the infusion is delivered with an infusion pump to ensure accuracy. The FDA (1978) recommends an initial dosage of 1–2 mU/min and further states the dosage "may be gradually increased in increments of no more than 1–2 mU/min until the patient experiences a contraction pattern similar to normal labor."

During administration, the goal is to achieve contractions every 2–3 minutes of good intensity, each of which lasts 40–50 seconds. The uterus should relax to normal baseline tone between contractions.

Oxytocin induction is not without some risks. Rapid progression of infusion rates or continuance of a particular rate without adequate assessment of the uterine contractions may lead to hyperstimulation of the uterus, fetal distress due to decreased placental perfusion, a rapid labor and delivery with the danger of cervical or perineal lacerations, or uterine rupture. Water intoxication may occur if large doses are given in electrolyte-free solution over a prolonged period of time (Cibils, 1981).

Nursing interventions Constant observation and accurate assessments are mandatory to provide safe, optimal care for both woman and fetus. Baseline data (maternal temperature, pulse, respiration, blood pressure, and FHR) should be obtained before beginning the infusion. A fetal monitor is used to provide continuous data. Many institutions recommend obtaining a 15-minute recording before the infusion is started to obtain baseline data on uterine contractions and FHR. Before each advancement of the infusion rate, assessments of the following should be made:

• Maternal blood pressure and pulse

• Rate and reactivity of the FHR tracing (any bradycardia or decelerations are noted)

• Contraction status, frequency, intensity, duration, and resting tone between contractions

During the induction, urinary output is assessed to identify any problems with retention, fluid deficit, and possibility of the development of water intoxication. As contractions are established, vaginal examinations are done to evaluate cervical dilatation, effacement, and station. The frequency of vaginal examinations primarily depends on the number of pregnancies and on characteristics of the contractions. For example, a nullipara who has contractions every 5–7 minutes, each lasting 30 seconds, and who does not perceive her contractions does not usually require a vaginal examination. When her contractions are every 2–3 minutes, lasting 50–60 seconds with good intensity, a vaginal examination will be needed to evaluate her progress.

For additional information on nursing interventions, see Drug Guide—Oxytocin, and Nursing Care Plan—Induction of Labor.

Oxytocin may be given intravenously for augmentation of labor; see Drug Guide—Oxytocin for further discussion.

Episiotomy

An **episiotomy** is a surgical incision of the perineal body extending downward from the vaginal opening (Carter and Wolber, 1981). The purposes of an episiotomy are to prevent lacerations, to minimize stretching of the perineal tissues, and to decrease trauma to the fetal head during descent and delivery.

The routine use of episiotomies is becoming an increasingly controversial issue. Various authors have found no evidence to support the reasons for episiotomies just listed (Cogan and Edmunds, 1977; Banta and Thacker, 1982). However, most medical textbooks still advocate the prophylactic use of this procedure.

A regional or local block is given in preparation for the episiotomy. The episiotomy is performed just before delivery, when the presenting part is beginning to crown but before there is excessive stretching of the perineal tissues. The incision begins at the midline and may be extended down the midline through the perineal body, or it may extend at a 45° angle in a mediolateral direction to the right or left (Figure 18-2). A midline episiotomy is preferred if the perineum is of adequate length and no difficulty during delivery is anticipated because blood loss is less, the incision is easy to repair, and the incision heals with less discomfort. The

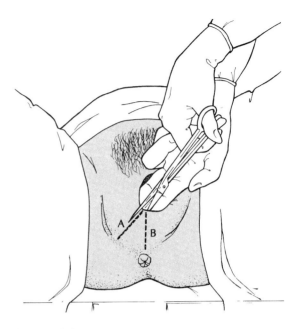

Figure 18-2

The two most common types of episiotomies are mediolateral (**A**) and midline (**B**).

major disadvantage is that the midline incision may extend through the anal sphincter and rectum. In the presence of a short perineum or an anticipated difficult delivery, a mediolateral episiotomy provides more room for delivery and decreases the possibility of a traumatic extension into the rectum. The mediolateral episiotomy may be complicated by greater blood loss, a longer healing period, and more discomfort postpartally.

Nursing interventions   During repair of the episiotomy (*episiorrhaphy*), the woman needs nursing support because she may have sensations of pressure. Placing a hand on her shoulder and talking with her can comfort her and distract her from the repair process.

The application of ice packs during the first eight hours after repair helps to alleviate pain and swelling. The episiotomy site should be inspected every 15 minutes during the first hour after delivery and thereafter daily for redness, swelling, tenderness, and hematomas. (See Chapter 25 for additional discussion of relief measures.)

Text continued on p. 392.

DRUG GUIDE
Oxytocin (Pitocin)

OVERVIEW OF OBSTETRIC ACTION

Oxytocin (Pitocin) exerts a selective stimulatory effect on the smooth muscle of the uterus and of the blood vessels. Oxytocin affects the myometrial cells of the uterus by increasing the excitability of the muscle cell, increasing the strength of the muscle contraction, and supporting propagation of the contraction (movement of the contraction from one myometrial cell to the next). Its effect on the uterine contraction depends on the dosage used and on the excitability of the myometrial cells. During the first half of gestation, little excitability of the myometrium occurs and the uterus is fairly resistant to the effects of oxytocin. However, from midgestation on, the uterus responds increasingly to exogenous intravenous oxytocin. When at term, cautious use of diluted oxytocin, administered intravenously, results in a slow rise of uterine activity. Depending on the rate of infusion, the maximum effect is achieved in 20–60 minutes. The half-life of exogenous circulating oxytocin is 3 minutes; half-life of uterine response is about 15 minutes (Cibils, 1981).

Oxytocin is used to induce labor at term and to augment uterine contractions in the first and second stages of labor. Oxytocin also may be used immediately after delivery to stimulate uterine contraction and thereby control uterine atony.

Oxytocin is not thought to cross the placenta because of its molecular weight and the presence of oxytocinase in the placenta (Giacoia and Yaffe, 1982). Oxytocin has an antidiuretic effect.

Route, dosage, frequency

For induction of labor: Add 10 units oxytocin (1 mL) to 1000 mL of intravenous solution. (The resulting concentration is 10 mU oxytocin per 1 mL of intravenous fluid.) Using an infusion pump, administer IV, starting at 0.5 mU/min and increasing the rate stepwise every 20 minutes until good contractions (every 2–3 minutes, each lasting 40–60 seconds) are achieved or to a maximum rate of 20 mU/minute (Cibils, 1981).

0.5 mU/min =	3 mL/hr	8	mU/min =	48 mL/hr
1.0 mU/min =	6 mL/hr	10	mU/min =	60 mL/hr
1.5 mU/min =	9 mL/hr	12	mU/min =	72 mL/hr
2 mU/min =	12 mL/hr	15	mU/min =	90 mL/hr
4 mU/min =	24 mL/hr	18	mU/min =	108 mL/hr
6 mU/min =	36 mL/hr	20	mU/min =	120 mL/hr

For augmentation of labor: Prepare and administer IV oxytocin as for labor induction. Increase rate until labor contractions are of good quality.

For administration after delivery of placenta: One dose of 10 units oxytocin (1 mL) is given intramuscularly or by slow intravenous push.

Maternal contraindications

Severe preeclampsia-eclampsia

Predisposition to uterine rupture (in nullipara over 35 years of age, paragravida 4 or more, overdistention of the uterus, previous major surgery of the cervix or uterus)

Cephalopelvic disproportion

Malpresentation or malposition of the fetus, cord prolapse

Preterm infant

Rigid, unripe cervix; total placenta previa

Presence of fetal distress

Maternal side effects

Hyperstimulation of the uterus results in hypercontractility, which in turn may cause the following:

Abruptio placentae

Impaired uterine blood flow → fetal hypoxia

Rapid labor → cervical lacerations

Rapid labor and delivery → lacerations of cervix, vagina, perineum, uterine atony, fetal trauma

Uterine rupture

Water intoxication (nausea, vomiting, hypotension, tachycardia, cardiac arrhythmia) if oxytocin is given in electrolyte-free solution

Hypotension with rapid IV administration postpartum

Effect on fetus/neonate

Fetal effects are primarily associated with the presence of hypercontractility of the maternal uterus. Hypercontractility causes a decrease in the oxygen supply to the fetus, which is reflected by irregularities and/or decrease in FHR. Hyperbilirubinemia.

NURSING CONSIDERATIONS

Explain induction or augmentation procedure to client

Apply fetal monitor and obtain 15-minute tracing to assess FHR before starting IV oxytocin

For induction or augmentation of labor, start with primary IV and piggy-back secondary IV with oxytocin

Assure continuous fetal and uterine contraction monitoring

Assess FHR, maternal blood pressure, pulse, and uterine contraction frequency, duration, and resting tone before each increase in oxytocin infusion rate

Record all assessments and IV rate on monitor strip and on client's chart

Record all client activities (such as change of position, vomiting) and procedures done (amniotomy, sterile vaginal examination) and administration of analgesics on monitor strip to allow for interpretation and evaluation of tracing

Assess cervical dilatation as needed

Utilize nursing comfort measures

Discontinue IV oxytocin infusion and infuse primary solution when (a) fetal distress is noted (bradycardia, late or variable decelerations, meconium staining); (b) uterine contractions are more frequent than every 2 minutes; (c) sustained uterine contractions are seen; or (d) insufficient relaxation of the uterus between contraction or a steady increase in resting tone are noted; in addition to discontinuing IV oxytocin infusion, turn client to side, and if fetal distress is present, administer oxygen by tight face mask at 4–7 L/min; notify physician

NURSING CARE PLAN
Induction of Labor

CLIENT ASSESSMENT

History

Previous pregnancies
Present pregnancy course
Childbirth preparation
Estimated gestational age

Physical Examination

1. Examination of pregnant uterus (Leopold's maneuvers to determine fetal size and position)
2. Vaginal examination to evaluate cervical readiness
   a. Ripe cervix: feels soft to the examining finger, is located in a medial to anterior position, is more than 50% effaced, and is dilated at least 3 cm
   b. Unripe cervix: feels firm to the examining finger, is long and thick, perhaps in a posterior position, with little or no dilatation
3. Presence of contractions
4. Membranes intact or ruptured
5. Fetal size (Leopold's maneuvers, ultrasonography)
6. Fetal readiness
7. CPD evaluation
8. Maternal vital signs and FHR before beginning induction

Laboratory Evaluation

Fetal maturity tests (L/S ratio, creatinine concentrations, ultrasonography)

Maternal blood studies (CBC, hemoglobin, hematocrit, blood type, Rh factor)
Urinalysis

PLAN OF CARE

Nursing Priorities

1. Monitor and evaluate status of mother and fetus continuously throughout the induction
2. Provide continuous physical and emotional support
3. Evaluate and monitor uterine response to induction
4. Evaluate and monitor fetal response to induction
5. Continuously evaluate client for complications associated with induction (abruptio placentae, fetal distress, any rise or decrease in maternal BP, hemorrhage, shock, uterine rupture, tetanic contractions)

Client/Family Educational Focus

1. Provide information regarding the induction procedure including action and side effects of medications, and expected action
2. Provide information regarding the fetal monitor, how it works, and the information that can be obtained from it
3. Provide opportunities for questions and individual concerns of the client and family

Problem	Nursing interventions and actions	Rationale
Client preparation	Assess client's feelings regarding induction Client may ask, "Will this work?" "How long will it take?" "Will it hurt more?" Assess client's knowledge base regarding the induction process Provide needed information (for example, when the cervix is ripe, contractions should begin in 30–60 minutes); length of labor depends on a number of factors	Client may be apprehensive about what will happen or feel a sense of failure that she cannot "go into labor by herself" After assessing knowledge base, appropriate information can be given to allay apprehension
	Assess knowledge of breathing techniques; if client does not have a method to use, teach breathing techniques before starting oxytocin infusion	Use of breathing techniques during contractions will help relaxation; although client may be apprehensive about induction, teaching a new breathing method will be easier before contractions are present
Changing client status Maternal vital signs	Assess maternal BP and pulse before beginning induction and then before each increase in infusion rate; do not advance infusion rate in presence of maternal hypertension or hypotension or radical changes in pulse rate	To establish baseline data and to assess client response to induction; client status may change rapidly

NURSING CARE PLAN (continued)
Induction of Labor

Problem	Nursing interventions and actions	Rationale
Cervical dilatation	Evaluate cervical dilatation by vaginal examination with each oxytocin dosage; increase after labor is established	When cervix responds by stretching or pulling, *do not* increase oxytocin dosage; overdosage may occur, causing rapid labor with possible cervical lacerations and fetal damage; when there is no change in the cervix, additional oxytocin is needed
Fetal status	Assess FHR by continuous electronic fetal monitoring. Obtain 15-minute tracing prior to beginning induction to evaluate fetal status; *do not* start infusion or advance rate (if induction has already begun) if FHR is not in range of 120–160 beats/min, if decelerations are present, or if variability decreases	Will provide continuous data regarding fetal response to induction
Contraction status	Apply monitor to obtain 15 minutes of tracing prior to starting induction	Establishes baseline data
	Assess contraction frequency, duration, and intensity prior to each increase in infusion rate	Evaluates uterine response to induction
	Do not increase rate of infusion if contractions are every 2–3 minutes, lasting 40–60 seconds, with moderate intensity	Desired effect has been obtained
	Discontinue oxytocin infusion if: 1. Contractions are more frequent than every 2 minutes 2. Contraction duration exceeds 75–90 seconds 3. Uterus does not relax between contractions	Uterus is being overstimulated and serious complications may develop for woman and fetus
Discomfort from contractions	Provide support to client as she uses breathing techniques	Contractions may build up more quickly with oxytocin induction
	Encourage use of effleurage, back rub, and other supportive measures	Techniques help maintain relaxation and thereby decrease pain sensation
	Assess need for analgesia, obtain order and administer (as long as maternal BP, pulse, respiration and FHR are within normal range)	After labor is well established, analgesia may be given without delaying process
Inadequate labor response	Increase oxytocin IV infusion rate every 20 minutes until adequate contractions are achieved; do *not* exceed an infusion rate of 20 mU/min	Uterine response to oxytocin may be individualized
	Check infusion pump to assure oxytocin is infusing; check whether pump is on (chamber refills and empties, level of fluid in IV bottle becomes lower), if problem is found, correct it and restart infusion at beginning dose	Oxytocin may not be infusing due to pump, mechanical, or human error
	Check piggy-back connection to primary tubing to assure solution is not leaking	

NURSING CARE PLAN (continued)
Induction of Labor

Problem	Nursing interventions and actions	Rationale
Failed induction	Explain reasons, if known Provide support Discontinue oxytocin induction, continue to monitor maternal and fetal status until effects of oxytocin have subsided	Cervix may not have been "ready" (ripe) for induction; even though labor was not established, significant changes in the cervix may have occurred; oxytocin may have been improperly administered Failure of induction may increase client's feelings of failure or increase apprehension if delivery must be effected because of maternal or fetal problems
Hypotension	Position client on her side; encourage her to avoid supine position Monitor maternal BP and pulse and FHR every 15–20 minutes If client becomes hypotensive: 1. Keep her on her side, may change to other side 2. Discontinue oxytocin infusion 3. Increase rate of primary IV 4. Monitor FHR 5. Notify physician 6. Assess for cause of hypotension	To maintain optimal blood flow to uterus and placenta Woman is frequently on her back at beginning of induction while monitors are attached and IV is started; vena cava is obstructed, causing maternal hypotension, which may lead to fetal bradycardia; initial hypotension is secondary to peripheral vasodilation induced by oxytocin, which causes diminished blood supply to placenta and resultant decrease in O_2 supply to fetus Actions are directed toward improving blood flow and oxygenation of tissues
Infection	Use aseptic technique for starting and maintaining the IV Maintain sterile technique when doing vaginal exams Assess client's temperature every 4 hours if membranes are intact, and every 2 hours if membranes are ruptured Assess IV site for redness, swelling when membranes are ruptured; assess amniotic fluid for odor and discoloration	Asepsis reduces incidence of infection Organisms may be introduced during vaginal examinations Elevated temperature may signal infection May indicate local infection May be associated with chorioamnionitis
Water intoxication	Administer oxytocin in electrolyte solution Assess and record fluid intake and output Monitor for nausea, vomiting, hypotension, tachycardia, cardiac arrhythmias	Oxytocin has slight antidiuretic effect, especially when administered in electrolyte-free solutions Provides information on hydration status These are signs and symptoms of water intoxication; they must be differentiated from other problems
Delivery of preterm infant	Correlate tests done to establish gestational age; calculate gestational age Notify pediatrician and nursery personnel if infant is preterm and induction must continue for medical reasons	Prematurity can occur due to incorrect evaluation of fetal age; specialized care may be needed
Tetanic contractions	Observe contraction frequency and duration. In presence of contractions lasting over 90 seconds:	Contractions lasting over 90 seconds with decreased resting tone may result in fetal hypoxia

NURSING CARE PLAN (continued)
Induction of Labor

Problem	Nursing interventions and actions	Rationale
	1. Discontinue oxytocin infusion 2. Assess maternal status 3. Assess fetal status	Ruptured uterus or abruptio placentae can result from drug-induced tumultuous labor
Fetal hypoxia–asphyxia	Monitor FHR continuously (normal range is 120–160/min) In episodes of bradycardia (<120 beats/min) lasting for more than 30 sec, administer O_2 by face mask at 4–7 L/min Stop oxytocin infusion Position woman on left side if quick recovery of FHR does not occur Carefully evaluate fetal tachycardia (>160/min) Sustained tachycardia may necessitate discontinuation of oxytocin infusion Assess for presence of meconium staining	O_2 deficiency may occur over a long period of time; in cases of placental insufficiency or cord compression, compensated tachycardia may occur Persistent fetal tachycardia causes more prominent O_2 deficiency (hypoxia) and CO_2 increase in fetal blood; vasoconstriction occurs, with increased fetal blood flow through coronary arteries, brain, and placenta; this increased demand on myocardial performance leads to cardiac decompensation if oxygen exchange is impaired and hypoxia continues Fetal hypoxia may also cause central vasomotor center to release adrenal catecholamines; at term, this enhances depolarization of cardiac pacemaker cells, which will result in direct bradycardia Bradycardia or subsequent reflex tachycardia temporarily remedies the O_2 deficiency
Rapid delivery	Assist with rapid delivery; observe for: 1. Laceration of cervix and tissues in the birth canal 2. Fetal distress Evaluate postpartally: 1. Check mother for lacerations and contractility of fundus 2. Check neonate for birth injuries	Overstimulation or overdosage of oxytocin may occur as additional endogenous oxytocin is produced by maternal system Rapid delivery increases risk of cervical and soft tissue lacerations in birth canal Rapid labor and delivery may lead to uterine atony Pressure within fetal head changes rapidly with precipitous, rapid delivery; infant is prone to cerebral edema and hemorrhage

NURSING CARE EVALUATION
Normal sterile vaginal delivery is accomplished without complications (lacerations, precipitous delivery)
Postpartally the maternal fundus is firm; blood flow is moderate; blood pressure, pulse, and respirations are stable and within normal limits
Neonate's respirations, color, and temperature are within normal limits
Family bonding is begun by allowing interactions among mother, baby, and father in delivery room

NURSING CARE PLAN (continued)
Induction of Labor

NURSING DIAGNOSIS	SUPPORTING DATA	NURSING ORDERS
Knowledge deficit related to induction procedure	Client unable to verbalize the purpose and procedure Expresses questions and concerns regarding the induction	Explain the induction procedure including possible side-effects and associated problems Acquaint the couple with the fetal monitor and explain findings
Alteration in uterine blood flow related to hypertonic uterine contractions	Contraction frequency of less than every 2 minutes and duration exceeding 60–90 seconds Marked changes in FHR variability and rate Late decelerations	Carefully assess contraction pattern prior to any increase of infusion rate Carefully assess fetal status prior to any increase in infusion rate Follow protocols for induction Continuously monitor contraction and fetal status with electronic monitoring Decrease or discontinue infusion if contraction pattern is excessive or fetal distress is apparent

Forceps Deliveries

Forceps may be used to provide traction, to rotate the fetus, or both. There are two types of forceps deliveries. The delivery is termed *outlet forceps delivery* when the fetal head is visible on the perineum without spreading the labia. When the fetal head is higher than the level of the ischial spines, delivery is termed a *midforceps delivery*. Before a midforceps delivery can be performed, the lower part of the fetal head must be at the level of the ischial spines, and the biparietal diameter must have entered the inlet (engagement). Most midforceps deliveries involve rotation of the fetus from an occiput-posterior or occiput-transverse position to an occiput-anterior position. *High forceps deliveries* (application of forceps before engagement of the fetal head) are no longer done because they are extremely dangerous for the woman and the fetus.

Indications

Forceps may be used electively to shorten the second stage of labor by sparing the woman the pushing effort, or when regional or general anesthesia has affected the woman's motor innervation and she cannot push effectively. They are also advocated in preterm infant deliv-ery (Pritchard, MacDonald, and Gant, 1985), as discussed in Chapter 17.

Complications

Maternal complications may include lacer-ations of the birth canal and perineum and increased bleeding. Fetal complications usually arise as a result of pressure on the tissues of the fetal head, which may cause edema or bruis-ing. Incorrect placement of the forceps may also result in bruising, edema, and temporary paral-ysis of an area of the newborn's face. A difficult forceps delivery may result in cerebral edema or brachial plexus palsy in the newborn.

Prerequisites for Forceps Application

Use of forceps requires complete dilatation of the cervix and knowledge of the exact posi-tion and station of the fetal head. The mem-branes must be ruptured to allow a firm grasp on the fetal head. The presentation must be ver-tex or face with the chin anterior, and the head must be engaged, preferably on the perineum. *Under no circumstances should there be any CPD*.

Nursing interventions The nurse can explain the procedure briefly to the woman if she is awake. With adequate regional anesthesia, she should feel some pressure but no pain. The woman is encouraged to maintain breathing techniques to prevent her from pushing during application of the forceps (Figure 18-3). The nurse monitors contractions and with each contraction the physician will provide traction as the woman pushes. The nurse should monitor the FHR continuously until the delivery. It is not uncommon to observe bradycardia as traction is being applied to the forceps. Bradycardia results from head compression and is transient in nature.

The newborn is inspected for bruising and edema to the tissues of the face and head. Assessments for cerebral trauma and brachial plexus palsy are particularly important if there was a difficult forceps delivery.

Vacuum Extraction

In vacuum extraction, suction is used to help deliver the fetal head. The vacuum extractor is composed of a soft silicone cup attached by tubes to a suction bottle (pump). The suction cup, which comes in various sizes, is placed against the fetal occiput. The pump is used to create negative pressure (suction) inside the cup. Traction is applied in coordination with uterine contractions and the fetal head is delivered.

The most common indication for use of the vacuum extractor is a prolonged first stage of labor. Other indications include: (a) fetal distress; (b) malpositions such as OP or OT; and (c) maternal complications such as cardiopul-

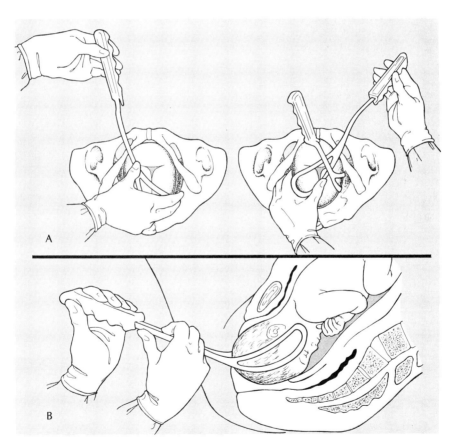

Figure 18-3

Application of forceps in occiput anterior (OA) position. **A,** The left blade is inserted along the left side wall of the pelvis over the parietal bone. **B,** The right blade is inserted along the right side wall of the pelvis over the parietal bone. **C,** With correct placement of the blades, the handles lock easily. During contractions, traction is applied to the forceps in a downward and outward direction to follow the birth canal.

monary disease, shock, PIH, and abruptio placentae (Greis et al., 1981).

Nursing interventions   During the procedure, the woman is informed about what is happening. If adequate regional anesthesia has been administered, the woman feels only pressure during the procedure. The FHR should be auscultated every 5 minutes or more frequently. The nurse should be ready to release the suction quickly in the event that the cup accidentally slips off during traction ("pull off") to prevent damage to the maternal tissues. Parents need to be informed that the caput on the baby's head will disappear in a few hours.

Assessment of the newborn should include inspection and continued observation for cerebral trauma and soft tissue necrosis.

Cesarean Birth

Cesarean birth is the delivery of the infant through an abdominal and uterine incision. Technologic and medical advancements have altered the attitude toward cesarean birth from a "procedure of last resort" to an "alternative birth method." In the United States the incidence of cesarean birth has increased from 5.5% in 1970 to approximately 15%–20% in 1984 (NIH, 1980; Pritchard, MacDonald, and Gant, 1985).

Indications for Cesarean Delivery

Cesarean births are performed in cases of breech presentation, fetal distress, dysfunctional labor, and uteroplacental insufficiency from maternal disease conditions. The most commonly occurring indication for cesarean delivery is dystocia caused by CPD. Other indications for this procedure include breech presentation, prolapsed cord, placenta previa, abruptio placentae, IUGR, prolonged ROM, genital herpes, prematurity, fetal distress and occasionally tumors blocking the vagina.

Maternal Mortality and Morbidity

Maternal mortality is two to four times greater in cesarean deliveries than vaginal deliveries (NIH, 1980; Amirikia, 1981). Mortality, although low (less than 0.02%), is most often due to anesthesia accidents and/or underlying medical conditions such as cardiac disease, renal disease, diabetes, or severe PIH.

Major complications resulting from cesarean birth include hemorrhage, injury to the bladder or intestines, trauma to the ovaries, endometritis, infection of the incision, and urinary tract infection. Elevated temperature occurs in 29%–85% of women after cesarean birth (Elliott, 1984). The risk to the fetus of a traumatic vaginal delivery must be weighed against the risk of maternal morbidity.

Types of Cesarean Deliveries

The type of cesarean is defined by the type of uterine incision that is made. The various uterine incisions include low-segment transverse, classic, and low classic (Figure 18-4). The type of uterine incision usually depends on the indication for the cesarean delivery. The choice of incision affects the woman's opportunity to have a subsequent vaginal delivery, as well as the risk of rupture at the site of the uterine scar during a subsequent labor.

Low-segment transverse incision   The low-transverse incision is the most common and preferred for the following reasons:

1. The lower segment is the thinnest portion of the uterus. Therefore, an incision in this area results in a minimal blood loss.

2. The concentration of the contractile proteins actin and myosin is least in the lower uterine segment. Thus the chance of uterine rupture during subsequent labor is less.

The limitations of the low-transverse incision are the following:

1. It takes longer to make and repair.

2. It is limited in size because of the presence of major blood vessels on either side of the uterus.

Classic cesarean incision   The classic incision is a vertical incision in the body of the uterus. It is used when there are adhesions from previous cesarean births, when the fetal position is the transverse lie, or when the placenta is implanted anteriorly. Because large blood vessels in the body of the uterus are cut, more blood is lost with this incision than with others,

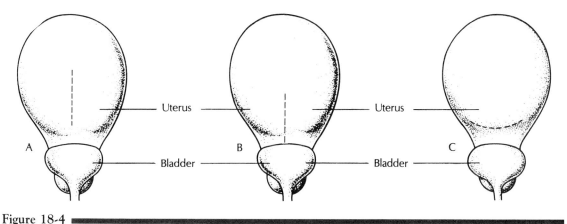

Figure 18-4 ▬▬▬▬▬▬▬▬▬▬▬▬▬▬▬▬▬▬
Types of uterine incisions for cesarean delivery. **A**, Classic. **B**, Low classic. **C**, Low-segment transverse.

and the risk of rupture of the uterine scar in subsequent labors is slightly increased.

Low classic incision   The low classic (low flap vertical) uterine incision is made into the lower uterine segment. Considered to be a compromise between the classic and transverse, the low classic incision is as safe as a transverse, yet can be extended into a classic if necessary.

Vaginal Birth After Cesarean Delivery

In North America, elective repeat cesarean births are common following a primary cesarean, and in 1984 one in 18 babies was delivered by repeat cesarean (Porreco and Meier, 1984). However, vaginal birth after cesarean (VBAC) is gaining acceptance in cases of nonrecurring indications (for example, cord accident, placenta previa, fetal distress). This trend had been influenced by consumer demand and a growing body of evidence suggesting that a properly conducted vaginal delivery after a cesarean poses less risk for maternal and neonatal mortality and morbidity than does a repeat cesarean (Porreco and Meier, 1984).

VBAC can be considered when:

1. Contraindications for vaginal delivery (such as CPD, placenta previa, and abruptio placentae) are ruled out.

2. Previous records with complete information about the previous cesarean birth, course of delivery, and postoperative recovery are available.

3. The woman and fetus can be monitored during labor.

4. A positive atmosphere can be maintained to facilitate the woman's comfort and decrease her anxiety (frequently, the medical and nursing staff are more concerned than current statistics indicate they need to be).

5. The uterus is explored after delivery to ascertain whether the uterine scar is intact.

Anesthesia for Cesarean Delivery

There is no perfect anesthetic for cesarean delivery. Each has its advantages, disadvantages, possible risks, and side-effects. Goals for anesthesia administration include safety, comfort, and emotional satisfaction for the client. There are two classifications of anesthesia for cesarean delivery: general and conduction (spinal and epidural). See Chapter 16 for further discussion.

Cesarean Birth—Nursing Interventions for the Family

Preparation for cesarean birth   Cesarean birth is an alternative method of delivery. Since one out of every five or six deliveries is a cesarean, preparation for this possibility should be an integral part of every childbirth education curriculum. (See the discussion in Chapter 9.) Ideally, all couples should be encouraged to discuss the possibility of a cesarean birth with their physician or nurse-midwife. They can also

Text continued on p. 400.

NURSING CARE PLAN
Cesarean Birth

CLIENT ASSESSMENT

History

Previous pregnancies
Course of recovery from previous cesarean births
Present pregnancy course
Estimated gestational age
Childbirth preparation
Sensitivity to medications and anesthetic agents
Past bleeding problems

Physical Examination

1. Fetal size, fetal status (FHR), and fetal maturity
2. Lung and cardiac status
3. Complete physical examination prior to
   administration of anesthetic

Laboratory Evaluation

CBC
Hemoglobin and hematocrit
Type and cross-match for two units whole blood
Rh
Prothrombin time
VDRL
Urinalysis

PLAN OF CARE

Nursing Priorities

1. Provide couple with factual information and support
   in preparation for their cesarean birth to enable them
   to make choices, feel in control, and minimize
   feelings of anxiety, loss, guilt, and helplessness
2. Support the couple's desires to participate in their
   birth experience within the constraints or options of
   the situation
3. Encourage couple to participate in making decisions
   about the cesarean birth and about care during the
   preparatory, recovery, and postpartal periods

Client/Family Educational Focus

1. Maintain "birth-oriented" approach
2. Explain preparatory procedures and postoperative
   care measures
3. Provide opportunity for questions and concerns of the
   client and family

Problem	Nursing interventions and actions	Rationale
Preparation for cesarean birth	Integrate cesarean birth information into childbirth preparation classes	Couples may deny the possibility of an unplanned cesarean birth Preparatory needs are basically the same for all couples anticipating childbirth Provides knowledge base that allows for adaptive coping responses should they deliver in either manner
	Emphasize the similarities between vaginal and cesarean delivery Minimize perceptions of "normal" versus "abnormal" birth Provide factual information	Enables couples to make choices and participate in their birth experiences
	Encourage couple to discuss with obstetrician the approach and birth preferences in the event of a vaginal or cesarean birth	Gives opportunity to discuss needs and desires; minimizes unrealistic expectations, disappointment, and/or feelings of loss Promotes understanding of options, beliefs of birth attendant, and hospital policies Allows couple to do anticipatory problem solving and develop effective coping behaviors
Anticipated or repeat cesarean birth	Encourage expression of feelings	Enables couple to work through fears, ambivalent or unresolved feelings and grief associated with inability to deliver vaginally

NURSING CARE PLAN (continued)
Cesarean Birth

Problem	Nursing interventions and actions	Rationale
	Assess reaction to and interpretation of past cesarean birth experiences	Identifies need for information and gives opportunity to work through fears or unresolved feelings
	Encourage the development of mutual support by couples sharing their experiences and common concerns	Decreases sense of being "different" or "alone" by realizing that their fears and concerns are not unique and feelings of anger or guilt are normal
Previous negative cesarean birth experiences	Create a safe, nonthreatening environment for couples to work through unresolved negative feelings	Negative feelings may contribute to distortion of information, impede learning, and affect expectations of upcoming birth experience
	Encourage couples to identify events that would make this birth experience more positive	Allows for anticipatory problem solving, and enhances ability to meet goals and expectations for birth event
Independence and sense of confidence	Maximize the couple's opportunities to have choices and make decisions	Increases sense of control over one's body and experiences
Preparation for emergency cesarean	Avoid "last-minute" approach	Avoids or minimizes reactions of anger, shock, resentment, panic, or crisis
	Keep couple informed as developments occur allowing for mutual decision making between the family and birth attendant	Gives couple control; helps them perceive their birth experience positively
	Informing them of the facts, alternatives, and consequences of nonintervention	
Effective communication	Cover important points of what to anticipate: 1. What is going to happen to the woman's body and how it will feel 2. What and why specific procedures will be done 3. How to handle discomfort associated with procedures	Increases coping capability because couple knows what to expect
	Provide couple with brief period of privacy	Gives opportunity for them to pool their coping strengths to deal with the anxiety of the situation
	Inquire if couple has any questions about the decision	Gives opportunity for further clarification
	Prepare couple in increments, giving information and rationale for each procedure	Crisis alters couple's ability to grasp information which they may hear or misinterpret
	Avoid silence	Often interpreted by the couple as frightening and/or negative
	Employ eye contact and therapeutic touch	Conveys a feeling of caring and reality orientation
Postpartal visit by nurse attending birth	Describe the birth events, minute-by-minute, event-by-event	Fills in the "missing pieces" of the birth experience
	Encourage parents to tell story as many times as needed	Enables parents to psychologically integrate the birth experience and resolve negative feelings
Inclusion of father (or significant other) in birth	Support the presence of the father during intrapartal and postpartal periods if desired	Promotes family bonding, minimizes "missing pieces"; calms the mother; makes for a shared experience

NURSING CARE PLAN (continued)
Cesarean Birth

Problem	Nursing interventions and actions	Rationale
	Provide accurate, current information as developments occur	Reduces feelings of confusion, helplessness, and anxiety
	Serve as a support system for the father	
	Initiate father-infant contact immediately after delivery if infant stable	Promotes family bonding
	Allow parents and baby to be together in recovery room	
Recovery from surgery	Assess vital signs every 5 min until stable, then every 15 min for an hour, then every 30 min until stable	Vital signs may vary in response to medications or anesthetic
Fluids and nutrition	Maintain intravenous infusion flow rate Check patency and inspect IV site for redness or swelling	IV fluids are maintained for 24–48 hours, or until bowel sounds are present; oxytocic agent is usually added to the IV infusion for a few hours after surgery to enhance contraction of uterine muscles
	Administer ice chips for first 24 hours, then advance diet as bowel sounds return	
Bladder drainage	Connect indwelling bladder catheter to dependent drainage. Catheter is usually removed 1–2 hours after IV fluids are discontinued	Enhances bladder emptying
	Measure urine output on first two voidings and check bladder for distention	Measuring urine provides information regarding adequate output and indicates whether the bladder is being emptied
Blood loss	Check hemoglobin and hematocrit a few hours after surgery and on first postoperative day	Identifies existence of anemia related to blood loss
Nausea and vomiting	Administer antiemetic as needed; check vital signs before administering	Establishes baseline vital signs; some antiemetics lower blood pressure
Pain	Administer pain medication as needed; assess vital signs before administering	Controls or alleviates pain at incision site and gas pains; establishes baseline vital signs, necessary because pain medications may lower blood pressure
	Monitor maternal use if she is nursing	Many drugs taken by the mother are passed into the breast milk
	Place woman in comfortable position and splint incision when she deep breathes or coughs	Provides support and relief of pain
Healing of incision	Inspect incision for redness, swelling, drainage, bruising, and separation of tissues	Healing of incision is facilitated when infection is absent; if signs of infection are present, antibiotic therapy is indicated
Bowel function	Auscultate bowel sounds	Bowel sounds are absent for 24–36 hours as a result of anesthetic and pain medication
	Progressive ambulation after 24 hours Discuss rationale for early ambulation and assist in the ambulation process Offer positive reinforcement for all attempts and steps in ambulation process	Ambulation enhances return of bowel function

NURSING CARE PLAN (continued)
Cesarean Birth

Problem	Nursing interventions and actions	Rationale
Pulmonary status	Turn woman and have her cough and deep breathe every 2 hours for 24 hours Splint incision while she is coughing or deep breathing	Provides aeration of lungs and assists in preventing pulmonary complications Promotes comfort
Hemorrhage	Evaluate firmness and position of fundus Palpate fundus after pain medication is administered to promote patient comfort	Monitor involution Palpation of fundus causes discomfort to the woman and is frequently neglected and therefore becomes increasingly important
	Fundus may be palpated from side of abdomen to avoid discomfort Evaluate lochia	Tenderness at incision site Lochia progresses from rubra to serosa to alba Increase in flow indicates inefficient contraction of uterus and/or subinvolution
Bonding	Enhance bonding by maintaining maternal comfort Provide information about the baby as soon as possible (such as sex, condition, and normalcy) Provide early opportunities for parent-infant interaction Discuss her feelings about the cesarean birth and her self-image as a mother	Interaction may be delayed because of recovery from anesthesia and discomfort in first few hours after delivery Feelings of failure associated with birthing experience can be generalized to ability to assume mothering role

NURSING CARE EVALUATION

No sign of infection
Involution proceeds normally
Client is discharged in good physical state
Education is provided for self-care and infant care

NURSING DIAGNOSIS	SUPPORTING DATA	NURSING ORDERS
Potential ineffective airway clearance	Reluctance to do deep breathing and coughing due to discomfort Rales, rhonchi Elevated temperature Productive cough	Assist with expelling secretions 1. Help woman turn, deep breathe and cough every 2 hours 2. Auscultate lungs 3. Splint abdomen while coughing 4. Provide fluids as soon as possible
Knowledge deficit about postoperative course	Expresses concerns or questions about specific aspects of recovery from cesarean delivery	Provide education 1. Assess present knowledge base and informational needs 2. Provide teaching about present care needs and home care

discuss their specific needs and desires. These might include participating in the choice of anesthetic and having the father present during the cesarean birth, for example.

Preparation for emergency cesarean delivery In reality, a couple is frequently ill prepared for the possibility of a cesarean delivery. Childbirth attendants sometimes wait until the last minute to inform the woman of the need for a cesarean delivery under the guise of "sparing the couple undue anxiety." Ironically, the woman's reaction to this delayed approach is not only excessive anxiety but also anger, shock, and resentment resulting in a state of crisis or panic (Affonso and Stichler, 1980). By contrast, the mutual decision approach between the birth attendants and the woman keeps the family fully informed as developments occur. The clinician presents all the facts, suggests alternatives, and describes likely outcomes of nonintervention, allowing the expectant parents to participate in the decision making. The opportunity to make choices and have control over their birthing experience is the major factor influencing a couple's positive perception of the event (Affonso and Stichler, 1980).

The period preceding surgery must be used to its greatest advantage. The couple needs some time and privacy to assimilate the information given to them and to pull together their strength to face this new crisis. It is imperative that caregivers utilize their most effective communication skills. The woman often interprets silence as indicating danger for her and her fetus, or she may think that the clinician is angry at her "failure" to perform (Affonso, 1981). The woman may experience panic or fear. She may be confused and numb to instructions. The attendant must address the salient points regarding what the couple may anticipate during the next few hours. Asking "What questions do you have about the decision?" gives the couple an opportunity for further clarification. The woman is best prepared in increments; she is given her information and the rationale for each procedure before it is begun. Before a procedure, the woman should be told (a) what the nurse or clinician is going to do; (b) why it is being done; and (c) what sensations she may experience. This allows the woman to give informed consent to the procedure. The woman experiences a sense of control, and therefore less helplessness and powerlessness.

Often the phenomenon of memory lapse is more pronounced during crisis or panic states. "Missing pieces" are unremembered events or segments of time. Although not unique to cesarean birth, this phenomenon contributes to a sense of loss or missing out for the woman. Her inability to remember may contribute to feelings of depression or anger. It is important for the delivery nurse to visit the woman during the postpartal period to fill in the "missing pieces."

Preparation of the woman for surgery involves more than the procedures of establishing intravenous lines and urinary catheter or doing an abdominal prep. As discussed previously, good communication skills are useful in helping the woman stay in control. Therapeutic touch and eye contact do much to maintain reality orientation and control. These measures reduce anxiety for the woman during the stressful preparatory period. The nurse should continually assess how the woman is perceiving the event and coping with her apprehension (Leach and Sproule, 1984; Lipson, 1984).

Before the surgery, the woman is given nothing by mouth, an abdominal and perineal prep is done (from below breasts to the pubic region), and an indwelling catheter to dependent drainage is inserted to prevent bladder distention and obstructed delivery. The woman must sign a consent form for surgery. At least two units of whole blood are readied for administration. An intravenous line is started, with an adequate size needle to permit blood administration, and preoperative medication is ordered. The pediatrician should be notified, and adequate preparation made to receive the infant. The nurse should make sure that the infant warmer is functional and that appropriate resuscitation equipment is available. The nurse assists in positioning the woman on the operating table. The FHR should be ascertained before surgery and during preparation, since fetal hypoxia can result from supine maternal hypotension. The operating table may be adjusted so it slants slightly to one side. This helps relieve the pressure of the gravid uterus on the vena cava and lessens the incidence of supine maternal hypotension. The suction should be in working order, and the urine collection bag should be positioned under the operating table to ensure proper drainage of urine.

Delivery   There are conflicting opinions and policies about fathers in the delivery room during a cesarean birth. It is interesting that the reasons for excluding them are similar to those once given for excluding fathers from attending vaginal birth. Examples of these opinions, which have since been proven to be invalid, include concerns about the father fainting, emotional trauma, increased risk of law suits or infection, and so on. The NIH Task Force on Cesarean Birth (1980), after considering this issue, concluded that "in spite of the widespread fears of adverse effects . . . there is no evidence of harm from fathers' participation." The position statement by the American College of Obstetrics and Gynecology states that they "cannot perceive strong medical indications or contraindications to the presence of fathers in the operating suite" (Affonso, 1981). In fact, the father's presence during the cesarean procedure leads to a more positive evaluation of the birth experience later by both the mother and father (Affonso, 1981). In addition, when the father is present for the delivery, the mother requires less postpartal medication for pain, experiences less loneliness, and is less anxious about the baby's health.

When the father attends the cesarean birth, he must scrub and wear the surgical gown and mask as do others in the operating suite. A stool can be placed at the bedside near the woman's head. The father can sit nearby to provide physical touch, visual contact, and verbal reassurance to his partner.

Other measures can be taken to promote the participation of the father who is not allowed or chooses not to be in the delivery room. They are:

1. Allowing the father to be near the delivery room where he can hear the newborn's first cry
2. Encouraging the father to carry or accompany the infant to the nursery for the initial assessment
3. Involving the father in postpartal care in the recovery room

In addition to meeting the emotional and informational needs of the expectant parents, other nursing functions are carried out to assure physiologic support and safety of the woman and neonate.

After delivery, the nurse assists the pediatrician with physiologic support of the neonate. After the infant's condition is stable, he or she should be shown to the woman if she is awake. The circulating nurse helps apply the dressing to the incision and, with the aid of other staff, transfers the woman to the recovery room.

Immediate postpartal recovery period. The postpartal recovery room must be equipped with suction and oxygen to ensure a patent airway and to protect from respiratory obstruction due to secretions. The recovery room nurse should check the woman's vital signs every 5 minutes until they are stable, then every 15 minutes for an hour, then every 30 minutes until she is discharged to the postpartal floor. The nurse should remain with the woman until she is stable.

The dressing and perineal pad must be checked every 15 minutes for at least an hour, and the fundus should be gently palpated to determine whether it is remaining firm. The fundus may be palpated from the side while the incision is supported with the other hand. Oxytocin is usually administered intravenously to promote the contractility of the uterine muscles. If the woman has been under general anesthesia, she should be positioned on her side to facilitate drainage of secretions, turned, and assisted with coughing and deep breathing every 2 hours for at least 24 hours. If she has received a spinal anesthetic, the level of anesthesia should be checked every 15 minutes until sensation has fully returned. The nurse monitors intake and output and observes the urine for bloody tinge, which could mean surgical trauma to the bladder. The physician prescribes medication, which should be administered as needed, to relieve the mother's pain and nausea. Facilitation of parent–infant interaction following birth and postpartal care is discussed in Chapter 24.

Summary ─────────────────

Elective and operative procedures are widely utilized in obstetrics. Amniotomy, the most common operative procedure, is performed to shorten labor. Labor can be induced when the fetus is mature and the cervix is ripe. Episiotomies reduce tearing of perineal tissues and promote their healing. Forceps were developed to assist in difficult delivery situations. Other procedures used in some deliveries include external and internal version and cesarean birth. Operative obstetrics provides a means for health care practitioners to promote the safety, health, and comfort of the laboring woman and her fetus.

Resource Groups

Cesarean/Support Education and Concern (C/Sec, Inc.) (66 Christopher Rd., Waltham, MA 02154)
Cesarean Association for Research, Education, Support, and Satisfaction (CARESS) (Burbank, Calif., 91510.)
Cesarean Birth Council (San Jose, Calif., 95101.)

References

Affonso DD: *Impact of Cesarean Childbirth*. Philadelphia: Davis, 1981.

Affonso DD, Stichler JF: Cesarean birth: Women's reactions. *Am J Nurs* March 1980; 80:468.

Amirikia H et al: Cesarean section: A 15-year review of changing incidence, indications, and risks. *Am J Obstet Gynecol* May 1981; 140:81.

Banta D, Thacker SB: The risks and benefits of episiotomy: A review. *Birth* Spring 1982; 9:25.

Bishop EH: Pelvic scoring for elective inductions. *Obstet Gynecol* 1964; 24:266.

Carter FB, Wolber PG: Episiotomy, chap 67. In: *Gynecology and Obstetrics*. Vol. 2. Sciarri JJ (editor). Hagerstown, Md.: Harper & Row, 1981.

Cibils LA: *Electronic Fetal-Maternal Monitoring*. Boston: PSG Publishing Co, 1981.

Cogan R, Edmunds EP: The unkindest cut. *Contemp Ob/Gyn* 1977; 9:55.

Danforth DN (editor): *Obstetrics and Gynecology*, 4th ed. Philadelphia: Harper & Row, 1982.

Elliott JP: Lavage to prevent postcesarean infection. *Contemp Ob/Gyn* May 1984; 23(5):43.

Giacoia GP, Yaffe S: Perinatal pharmacology, chap 100. In: *Gynecology and Obsterics*. Vol. 3. Sciarri JJ (editor). Philadelphia: Harper & Row, 1982.

Greis JB et al: Comparison of maternal and fetal effects of vacuum extraction with forceps or cesarean deliveries. *Obstet Gynecol* May 1981; 57:571.

Hughes EC (editor): *Obstetrics Gynecology Terminology*. Philadelphia: Davis, 1972.

Leach L, Sproule V: Meeting the challenge of cesarean births. *J Obstet Gynecol Neonatal Nurs* May/June 1984; 13(3):191.

Lipson JG: Repeat cesarean births: Social and psychological issues. *J Obstet Gynecol Neonatal Nurs* May/June 1984; 13(3):157.

Macer J, Buchanan D, Yonekura ML: Induction of labor with prostaglandin E_2 vaginal suppositories. *Obstet Gynecol* May 1984; 63(5):644.

McKay S, Mahan CS: How worthwhile are membrane stripping and amniotomy? *Contemp Ob/Gyn* December 1983; 22(6):173.

NIH Cesarean Birth Task Force. National Institute of Child Development statement on cesarean childbirth. US Department of Health and Human Services, Building HHH, Rm 447F8, Washington, DC 20201, 1980.

Orhue AA, Unuigbe JA, Ezimokhai M, Ojo VA: Outcome of induced labor in 931 term pregnancies. *Obstet Gynecol* 1984; 64(1):108.

Porreco RP, Meier PR: Repeat cesarean—Mostly unnecessary. *Contemp Ob/Gyn* September 1984; 24(3):55.

Pritchard JA, MacDonald PC, Gant, NF: *Williams Obstetrics*, 17th ed. New York: Appleton-Century-Crofts, 1985.

US Department of Health, Education, and Welfare. New restrictions on oxytocin use. *Food and Drug Administration Bulletin*. Vol 8, October/November 1978.

VanDorsten JP et al: Randomized control trial of external cephalic version with tocolysis in late pregnancy. *Am J Obstet Gynecol* October 1981; 141:417.

Additional Readings

Cain RL, Pedersen FA, Zaslow M et al: Effects of the father's presence or absence during a cesarean delivery. *Birth* Spring 1984; 11(1):10.

Crowell DH et al: Effects of induction of labor on the neurophysiologic functioning of newborn infants. *Am J Obstet Gynecol* January 1980; 136:48.

Datta S: Avoiding anesthetic complications in cesarean deliveries. *Contemp Ob/Gyn* May 1983; 21(5):151.

Luther FR et al: The effect of estrogen priming on induction of labor with prostaglandins. *Am J Obstet Gynecol* June 1980; 137:351.

O'Driscoll K, Geoghegan F: Haemorrhage in first born infants and delivery with obstetric forceps. *Br J Obstet Gynaecol* April 1981; 88:577.

Quilligan EJ: Making inroads against the C-section rate. *Contemp Ob/Gyn* January 1983; 21(1):221.

Sellers SM et al: Release of prostaglandins past amniotomy is not mediated by oxytocin. *Br J Obstet Gynaecol* January 1980; 87:43.

Shearer EC: Education for vaginal birth after cesarean. *Birth* Spring 1982; 9(1):31.

Wilf RT, Franklin JB: Six years' experience with vaginal births after cesareans at Booth Maternity Center in Philadelphia. *Birth* Spring 1984; 11(1):5.

She was a beautiful baby. She blew shining bubbles of sound. She loved motion, loved light, loved color and music and textures. . . . She was a miracle to me. . .

TILLE OLSEN

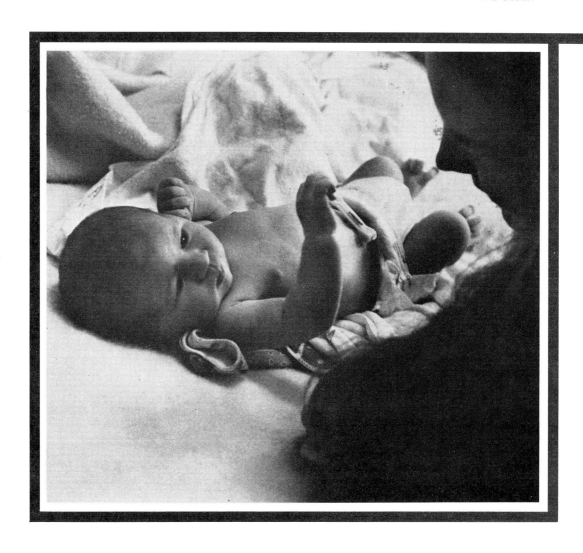

IV
The Newborn

19
Physiologic Responses of the Newborn to Birth

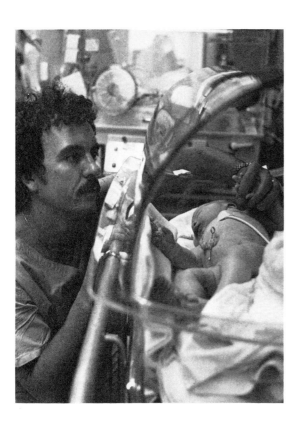

Chapter Contents

Respiratory Adaptations
Initiation of Breathing
Neonatal Pulmonary Physiology
Oxygen Transport
Characteristics of Neonatal Respiration

Cardiovascular Adaptations
Fetal-Neonatal Transition Circulation
Characteristics

Hematopoietic System
Neonatal Hematology

Temperature Regulation
Heat Loss
Heat Production

Hepatic Adaptation
Iron Storage and Red Blood Cell Production
Carbohydrate Metabolism
Physiologic Jaundice—Icterus Neonatorum
Coagulation

Gastrointestinal Adaptation

Renal Adaptation

Immunologic Adaptations

Neurologic and Sensory/Perceptual Functioning
Neurologic Adaptations
Motor Activity
States of the Newborn
Sensory Capacities of the Newborn

Objectives

• Describe the physiologic changes of the transition from intrauterine to extrauterine life.

- Outline the cardiovascular and respiratory changes necessary to maintain neonatal ventilation and perfusion.
- Compare fetal and neonatal hematopoietic systems.
- Describe nonshivering thermogenesis.
- Discuss the changing roles of the liver and gastrointestinal tract in the neonate.
- Determine the significance of the kidney in fluid and electrolyte balance in the neonate.
- Describe the immunologic response of the neonate.
- Describe the sensory/perceptual functioning of the newborn.

Key Terms

active acquired immunity	passive acquired immunity
brown adipose tissue (BAT)	periodic breathing
cardiopulmonary adaptation	physiologic anemia of infancy
conduction	physiologic jaundice
convection	radiation
evaporation	surfactant
meconium	thermal neutral zone (TNZ)

The neonatal period includes the time from birth through the twenty-eighth day of life. During this period, the newborn adjusts from intrauterine to extrauterine life. The nurse must be knowledgeable about a newborn's normal biopsychosocial adaptations to recognize deviations from it.

To begin life as an independent being, the neonate must immediately establish pulmonary ventilation in conjunction with marked circulatory changes. These radical and rapid changes are crucial to the maintenance of life. In contrast, all other neonatal body systems can change their functions or establish themselves over a prolonged period of time.

Respiratory Adaptations _____

The respiratory system is in a continuous state of development from fetal life to early childhood.

During the first 20 weeks of gestation, growth of the primitive lung is limited to the differentiation of pulmonary, vascular, and lymphatic structures.

At 20–24 weeks of fetal life, alveolar ducts begin to appear, followed by primitive alveoli at 24–28 weeks. During this time, the alveolar epithelial cells begin to differentiate into type I cells (structures necessary for gas exchange) and type II cells (structures that provide for the synthesis and storage of *surfactant*). **Surfactant** is composed of a group of surface-active phospholipids, of which one component, lecithin, is the most critical for alveolar stability.

At 28–32 weeks of gestation, the number of type II cells increases further, and surfactant is produced by a choline pathway within the type II cells. Surfactant production by this pathway peaks about 35 weeks of gestation, and remains high until term, paralleling late fetal lung development. At this time, the lungs are structurally developed enough to permit maintenance of good lung expansion and adequate exchange of gases (Avery, 1981).

Clinically, the peak production of surfactant by the choline pathway corresponds closely with the marked decrease in incidence of idiopathic respiratory distress syndrome after 35 weeks of gestation. Production of sphingomyelin remains constant throughout gestation. The neonate delivered before the L/S ratio is 2:1 will have varying degrees of respiratory distress. (See discussion of L/S ratio in Chapter 11.)

Initiation of Breathing

The ability of the neonate to breathe air immediately upon exposure to extrauterine life appears to be the consequence of weeks of intrauterine practice. Fetal breathing movements (FBMs) occur as early as 11 weeks' gestation. Goldstein and Reid (1980) propose that FBMs are essential for development of chest wall muscles (including the diaphragm) and to a lesser extent for regulating lung fluid volume and therefore lung growth.

That vital first breath is initiated by several chemical, thermal, sensory, physical, and mechanical stimuli. These are described next.

Chemical stimuli An important chemical stimulator that contributes to the onset of breathing is transitory asphyxia of the fetus and newborn. The elevation in P_{CO_2} and the decrease in pH and P_{O_2} are the natural outcome of normal vaginal delivery with cessation of placental gas exchange and umbilical cord pulsation and cutting. Although brief periods of asphyxia are a significant stimulator, prolonged asphyxia is abnormal.

Thermal stimuli   The significant decrease in environmental temperature after delivery (from 98.6F to 70–75F or 37C to 21–23.9C) is a major stimulus for initiation of breathing. As nerve endings in the skin are stimulated, the newborn responds with rhythmic respirations. Excessive cooling may result in profound depression and evidence of cold stress (see Chapter 22).

Sensory and physical stimuli   As the fetus is delivered from a quiet environment to one of sensory abundance, a number of physical and sensory influences help respiration begin. They include the numerous tactile, auditory, and visual stimuli of birth. Historically, vigorous stimulation was provided by slapping the buttocks or heels of the newborn, but today greater emphasis is placed on gentle physical contact. Thoroughly drying the infant, for example, provides stimulation in a far more comforting way and decreases heat loss.

Mechanical events   Fetal lungs continuously produce fluid during the latter half of intrauterine development. This secretion fills the lungs almost completely, expanding air spaces. Some of the fluid drains out of the lungs into the amniotic fluid and is swallowed by the fetus. The respiratory passages of a normal term fetus contain approximately 80–110 mL of fluid, which must be removed at the time of delivery to permit adequate movement of air. Approximately one-third of the fluid is squeezed out of the lungs as the fetal chest is compressed by the birth canal during a vaginal delivery. The subsequent recoil of the chest wall after the birth of the newborn's trunk is thought to produce a small passive inspiration of air to replace the fluid that was squeezed out. The remaining lung fluid is drawn back farther into the lung with each breath and is later absorbed into the bloodstream through the pulmonary capillaries and lymphatics. At the same time, air is also forced into the proximal airways. An air-liquid interface (the surface boundary between these two components) is established in the smaller airways and alveoli. It is not known how quickly the remaining alveolar fluid is reab-

sorbed, but under normal circumstances it is reabsorbed after a few breaths or within the first hour after birth (Korones, 1981). Figure 19-1 summarizes the initiation of respiration.

The initial expiration should clear the airways of accumulated fluid and permit inspiration. However, it is wise to suction mucus and fluid from the newborn's mouth with a suction device (such as a DeLee mucus trap or bulb syringe) as the head and shoulders are delivered and as the infant stabilizes (see Procedure 14-1 and Chapter 14).

Problems associated with lung clearance and/or initiation of respiratory activity may be precipitated by a variety of factors such as (a) underdeveloped lymphatics, which decrease the rate at which the fluid is absorbed from the lungs, or (b) complications antenatally or during labor and delivery that interfere with adequate lung expansion and result in increased pulmonary vascular resistance and decreased blood flow. These complications include inadequate compression of the chest wall in a very small neonate, the absence of chest wall compression in the neonate delivered by cesarean birth, or severe asphyxia at birth.

Neonatal Pulmonary Physiology

The first breath of life—the gasp in response to tactile, thermal, mechanical, and chemical changes associated with birth—initiates the serial opening of the alveoli. Thus begins the transition from a fluid-filled environment to an air-breathing existence, and from a dependent intrauterine existence to an independent extrauterine life.

To maintain life, the lungs must function immediately after birth. Two radical changes must take place for the lungs to function. First, pulmonary ventilation must be established through continued lung expansion following birth. Second, a marked increase in the pulmonary circulation must occur.

The ability of the lung to maintain oxygen (oxygenation) and carbon dioxide exchange (ventilation) is influenced by such factors as lung compliance and airway resistance. Lung compliance (the ability of the lung to fill with air easily) is influenced by the elastic recoil of the lung tissue and by anatomic variation.

The infant's relatively large heart and mediastinal structures reduce available lung space. The large abdomen further encroaches on the high

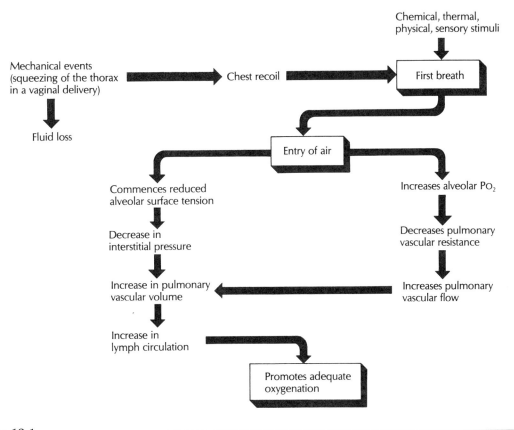

Figure 19-1
Initiation of respiration in the neonate.

diaphragm to decrease lung space. Anatomically, the neonatal chest has weak intercostal muscles, a rigid rib cage with horizontal ribs, and a high diaphragm that inhibits available space for lung expansion.

Ventilation is also impeded by airway resistance. A reduction in the size of the airway or continued retention of secretions within the airway greatly increase resistance to the flow of air in and out of the lungs.

Surface forces (such as the changing radii of the alveoli during respiration) further affect lung compliance because pressure must be used to overcome the surface-tension forces within the alveoli.

Because of surface tension within the alveoli, they would collapse upon expiration if it were not for surfactant. Surfactant reduces the surface tension during expiration (less pressure is required to hold the alveolus open) and maintains alveolar stability.

The surfactant system develops systematically as gestation progresses. Examination of amniotic fluid for other phospholipids and L/S ratio is an accepted way to evaluate fetal lung maturity (see Chapter 11). Although the L/S ratio continues to be used extensively to determine fetal lung maturity, phosphatidyglycerol (PG) is a more mature component of the surfactant complex. Its presence in the amniotic fluid appears to ensure fetal lung maturity and reduces the incidence of false-positive L/S ratio readings, a common occurrence in the pregnant diabetic client, for example.

Oxygen Transport

The transportation of oxygen to the peripheral tissues depends on the type of hemoglobin in the red blood cell. In the fetus and neonate, a variety of hemoglobins exist, the most significant being fetal hemoglobin (Hb F) and adult hemoglobin (Hb A). Approximately 70%–90% of hemoglobin in the fetus and neonate is of the fetal variety. The greatest difference between Hb F and Hb A is related to the transport of oxygen.

In the newborn, the greater affinity of Hb F for oxygen causes the shift to the left in the oxygen dissociation curve. More oxygen is bound to Hb F, which makes oxygen saturation in the newborn relatively greater than in the adult, but less oxygen is available to the tissues at any partial pressure. This is beneficial for the fetus, who must maintain adequate oxygen uptake in the presence of very low oxygen tension (umbilical venous Po_2 cannot exceed the uterine venous Po_2). Because of this phenomenon, hypoxia in the neonate is particularly difficult to recognize because of the high concentration of oxygen in the blood. Clinical manifestations of cyanosis are lacking until low blood levels of oxygen are present. Shifts to the left in the curve also may be caused by alkalosis (increased pH) and hypothermia. Acidosis, hypercarbia, and hyperthermia may cause the oxygen dissociation curve to shift to the right.

Characteristics of Neonatal Respiration

Normal neonatal respiration rate is 30–50 breaths/min. Initial respirations may be largely diaphragmatic, with shallow and irregular depth and rhythm. Additionally, they are primarily abdominal and synchronous with the chest movement. Short periods of apnea are to be expected. When the breathing pattern is characterized by apnea lasting 5–15 seconds, **periodic breathing** is occurring. Periodic respiration is rarely associated with differences in skin color or heart rate changes, nor does it have prognostic significance. Tactile or other sensory stimulation increases the inspired oxygen and converts periodic breathing patterns to normal breathing patterns. Neonatal sleep states particularly influence respiratory patterns. With deep sleep, the pattern is reasonably regular. Periodic breathing occurs with rapid-eye-movement (REM) sleep, and grossly irregular breathing is evident with motor activity, sucking, and crying.

The neonate is an obligatory nose breather, and any obstruction will cause respiratory distress, so it is important to keep the throat and nose clear. If respirations drop below 30 or exceed 60 per minute when the infant is at rest, or if dyspnea or cyanosis occurs, the physician should be notified. (Some initial dyspnea or cyanosis may be

normal.) Any increased use of the intercostal muscles (retracting) may also indicate respiratory distress.

Cardiovascular Adaptations

With the onset of respiration, the functions of the cardiovascular and respiratory systems become interrelated; hence the term **cardiopulmonary adaptation**. When air enters the lungs, the rise in alveolar Po_2 stimulates the relaxation of the pulmonary arteries, which in turn decreases the pulmonary vascular resistance. Simultaneously, lowered surface tension decreases interstitial pressure. Immediately, the vascular flow in the lung increases by 20%, followed by subsequent increases of 85% at 7 hours of life and 100% at 24 hours of life (Smith and Nelson, 1976). The greater blood volume contributes to the conversion from fetal circulation to neonatal circulation. After the establishment of pulmonary circulation, blood is well distributed throughout the lung, although the alveoli may or may not be fully ventilated.

Increased shunting is common in the early neonatal period, largely through fetal circulation channels, the bronchial circulation, and collapsed alveoli. The bidirectional flow, or right-to-left shunting through the ductus arteriosus, may divert a significant amount of blood away from the lungs depending on the pressure changes of respiration, crying, and the cardiac cycle. For adequate oxygenation to occur, the heart must deliver sufficient blood to the lungs.

Fetal-Neonatal Transition Circulation

During fetal life, blood with higher oxygen content is diverted to the heart and brain. Blood in the descending aorta is less oxygenated and supplies the kidney and intestinal tract. Limited amounts of blood, pumped from the right ventricle toward the lungs, enter the pulmonary vessels. In the fetus, increased pulmonary resistance forces most of the blood through the ductus arteriosus into the descending aorta (see Figure 4-7). Expansion of the lungs with the first breath decreases the pulmonary vascular resistance, as the clamping of the cord raises systemic vascular resistance and left atrial pressure. This physiologic mechanism marks the beginning of neonatal circulation and the integration of the cardiovascular and respiratory systems (Figure 19-2). Five major areas of change occur in cardiopulmonary adaptation.

1. *Increased aortic pressure and decreased venous pressure.* When the cord is cut, the placental vascular bed is eliminated and the intravascular space is reduced. Consequently, aortic (systemic) blood pressure is increased. At the same time, when the newborn is separated from the placenta, blood return via the inferior vena cava is decreased, resulting in a small decrease in pressure within the venous circulation.

2. *Increased systemic pressure and decreased pulmonary artery pressure.* Pressure increases in the systemic circulation because severing the placenta produces greater systemic resistance. At the same time, adequate lung expansion produces increased pulmonary blood flow, while the increased blood Po_2 associated with initiation of respirations produces vasodilatation. The combination of increased pulmonary blood flow and vasodilatation results in decreased pulmonary artery resistance. As a result, the systemic vascular pressure decreases, causing perfusion of the other body systems.

3. *Closure of the foramen ovale.* Closure of the foramen ovale is a function of atrial pressures. In utero, pressure is greater in the right atrium, and the foramen ovale is open. Decreased pulmonary resistance and increased pulmonary blood flow result in increased pulmonary venous return into the left atrium, thereby increasing left atrial pressure slightly. The decreased pulmonary vascular resistance also causes a decrease in right atrial pressure. The pressure gradients are now reversed, left atrial pressure is greater, and the foramen ovale is functionally closed. Although the foramen ovale closes 1–2 hours after birth, a slight right-to-left shunting may occur in the early neonatal period. Any increase in pulmonary resistance may result in reopening of the foramen ovale, causing a right-to-left shunt. Permanent closure occurs within several months.

4. *Closure of the ductus arteriosus.* Initial elevation of the systemic vascular pressure above the pulmonary vascular pressure increases pulmonary blood flow by causing a reversal of the flow through the ductus arteriosus. Blood now flows from the aorta into the pulmonary artery. Furthermore, although the presence of oxygen causes the pulmonary arterioles to dilate, an

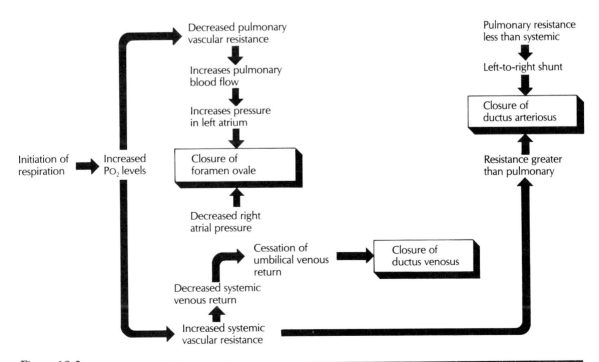

Figure 19-2
Transitional circulation—conversion from fetal to neonatal circulation.

increase in blood Po_2 triggers the opposite response in the ductus arteriosus—it constricts. If the lungs fail to expand or if Po_2 levels drop, the ductus remains patent. Fibrosis of the ductus occurs within 3 weeks, but functional closure is accomplished within 15 hours after birth.

5. *Closure of the ductus venosus.* Although the mechanism of initiating closure of the ductus venosus is not known, it appears to be related to mechanical pressure changes after severing of the cord, redistribution of blood, and cardiac output. Closure of the bypass forces perfusion of the liver. Anatomic fibrosis occurs within 3–7 days (Korones, 1981) (Figure 19-3).

Characteristics

Heart rate   Shortly after the first cry and the advent of cardiopulmonary circulation, the newborn heart rate accelerates to 175–180 beats/min. Thereafter, the rate follows a fairly uniform course, slowing to 115 beats/min at 4–6 hours of life, then rising and plateauing to approximately 120 beats/min at 12–24 hours of life (Smith and Nelson, 1976). The range of the heart rate in the full-term neonate is 100 beats/min while asleep and 120–150 while awake; it may be as high as 180 while crying.

Heart murmurs   Murmurs are usually produced by turbulent blood flow. Murmurs may be heard when blood flows across an abnormal valve or across a stenosed valve, when there is an atrial septal or ventricular septal defect, or when there is increased flow across a normal valve. A transient murmur is often heard in newborns before the ductus arteriosus closes completely.

Blood pressure   During the newborn period, the blood pressure tends to be the highest immediately after birth, and then descends to its lowest level about 3 hours after. By days 4–6 of life, the blood pressure rises to a level approximately the same as the initial level (Smith and Nelson, 1976). Blood pressure is particularly sensitive to the changes in blood volume that occur in the transition to neonatal circulation (Figure 19-4).

Blood pressure values during the first 12 hours of life vary with the birth weight. In the full-term resting neonate, the average blood pres-

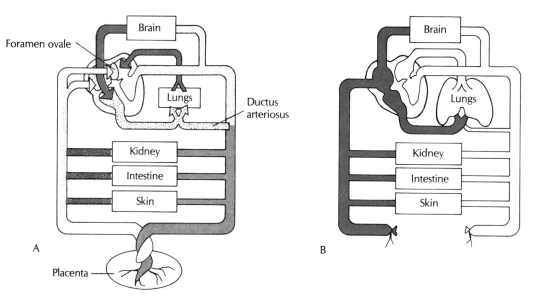

Figure 19-3

A, Schematic representation of fetal circulation. Oxygenated blood leaves the placenta by way of the umbilical vein (vessel without stippling). It flows into the portal sinus in the liver (not shown), and a variable portion of it perfuses the liver. **B,** Schematic representation of circulation in the normal newborn. After expansion of the lungs and ligation of the umbilical cord, pulmonary blood flow increases and left atrial and systemic arterial pressures rise while pulmonary arterial and right heart pressures fall. (From Avery GB: *Neonatology: Pathophysiology and Management of the Newborn.* Philadelphia: Lippincott, 1981, pp, 184–185.)

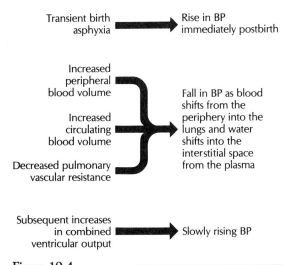

Figure 19-4
Response of blood pressure to neonatal changes in blood volume.

sure is 74/47 mm Hg; in the preterm newborn, it averages 64/39 mm Hg. Crying may cause an elevation of 20 mm Hg in both the systolic and diastolic blood pressure, thus accurate measurement is more likely in the quiet newborn.

Hematopoietic System

Fetal erythrocytes are larger than those present at birth but fewer in number. After birth, the red blood cell (RBC) count gradually increases as cell size decreases. Neonatal RBCs have a life span of 80–100 days, approximately two-thirds the life span of an adult's RBC. In neonatal red blood cells, about 5% of the RBCs retain their nucleus.

Hematologic values in the newborn are modified by several factors, which include (Smith and Nelson, 1976):

1. *Delayed cord clamping and the normal shift of plasma to the extravascular spaces.* Placental vessels contain about 100 mL of blood at term, the majority of which can be transfused into the newborn by positioning the neonate below the level of the placenta and by late clamping of the cord. If the neonate receives this transfusion of blood, it is reflected by a rise in hemoglobin level and an increase in the hematocrit to 65% about 48 hours after birth (compared with 48% when the cord is clamped immediately).

2. *Gestational age.* Increasing gestational age

is associated with more RBCs and greater hemoglobin concentration.

3. *Prenatal and/or perinatal hemorrhage.* Significant prenatal or perinatal bleeding decreases the hematocrit level and causes hypovolemia.

4. *The site of the blood sample.* Blood samples taken from veins are more accurate than those taken from capillaries. The concentration of RBCs is increased in capillary blood because peripheral blood flow is sluggish.

Neonatal Hematology

In the first days of life, hematocrit may rise by 1–2 g/dL above fetal levels as a result of placental transfusion, low oral fluid intake, and diminished extracellular fluid volume. By 1 week postnatally, peripheral hemoglobin is comparable to fetal blood counts. The hemoglobin level declines progressively thereafter (Hatch and Sumner, 1981), creating a phenomenon known as **physiologic anemia of infancy**.

Leukocytosis is a normal finding because the trauma of birth stimulates increased production of neutrophils during the first week of life. Neutrophils then decrease to 35% of the total leukocyte count by 2 weeks of age. Eventually, lymphocytes become the predominant type of leukocyte and the total white blood count falls.

Blood volume of the term infant is estimated to be 80–85 mL/kg of body weight. The true blood volume varies with the amount of blood received during placental transfusion.

The concentration of serum electrolytes in the blood indicates the fluid and electrolyte status of the newborn. These values as well as normal blood values for the term infant are as follows:

Laboratory data	Normal range
Hemoglobin	15–20 g/dL
Hematocrit	43%–61%
WBC	10,000–30,000/mm³
Neutrophils	40%–80%
Immature WBC	3%–10%
Platelets	100,000–280,000/mm³
Sodium mmol/L	124–156
Potassium mmol/L	5.3–7.3
Chloride mmol/L	90–111
Calcium mg/dL	7.3–9.2
Glucose mg/dL	40–97

Temperature Regulation

Temperature regulation is the maintenance of thermal balance by the dissipation of heat to the environment (heat loss) at a rate equal to the production of heat. Newborns are *homeothermic*; they attempt to stabilize their internal body temperatures within a narrow range in spite of significant temperature variations in their environment.

Thermoregulation in the newborn is closely related to the rate of metabolism and oxygen consumption. Within a specific environmental temperature range, called the **thermal neutral zone (TNZ)**, the rates of oxygen consumption and metabolism are minimal and internal body temperature is maintained because of thermal balance. For an unclothed full-term neonate, the range of the TNZ is an ambient temperature of 32–34C (89.6–93.2F). The limits for an adult are 26–28C (78.8–82.4F). Thus, the normal newborn requires higher environmental temperatures to maintain a thermal neutral environment.

Several neonatal characteristics affect the establishment of a TNZ. One of these is the decreased subcutaneous fat and thin epidermis of the newborn. Blood vessels are closer to the skin than those of an adult. Therefore, the circulating blood is influenced by changes in environmental temperature, and in turn influences the hypothalamic temperature-regulating center.

The flexed posture of the term infant decreases the surface area exposed to the environment, thereby reducing heat loss. Other neonatal characteristics such as size and age may also affect the establishing of a TNZ. Preterm SGA neonates require higher environmental temperatures to achieve a thermal neutral environment while a larger, well-insulated newborn may be able to cope with lower environmental temperature. If the environmental temperature falls below the lower limits of the TNZ, the neonate responds with increased oxygen consumption and metabolism, which results in greater heat production. Prolonged exposure to the cold may result in depleted glycogen stores and acidosis. Oxygen consumption can also increase when the environmental temperature is above the TNZ.

Heat Loss

A newborn is at a distinct disadvantage in maintaining a normal temperature. With a larger body surface in relation to mass and a limited amount of insulating subcutaneous fat, the newborn loses about four times the heat of an adult (Danforth, 1982). Because of the risk of hypothermia, minimizing heat loss in the newborn after delivery is imperative (see Chapters 14 and 21 for nursing measures).

Two major routes of heat loss are from the internal core of the body to the body surface and from the external surface to the environment. Usually the core temperature is 0.5C higher than the skin temperature, resulting in continuous transfer of heat to the surface. The greater the difference in temperatures between core and skin, the more rapid the transfer. Heat loss from the body surface to the environment takes place in four ways—convection, radiation, evaporation, and conduction.

- **Convection** is the loss of heat from the warm body surface to the cooler air currents. Air-conditioned rooms, oxygen by mask, and removal from an incubator for procedures done without an overhead warmer increase convective heat loss of the neonate.

- **Radiation** losses occur when heat transfers from the heated body surface to cooler surfaces and objects not in direct contact with the body. The walls of a room or of an incubator are potential causes of heat loss by radiation, even if the ambient temperature of the isolette is within the thermal neutral range for that infant.

- **Evaporation** is the loss of heat incurred when water is converted to a vapor. The newborn is particularly prone to lose heat by evaporation immediately after delivery when the infant is wet with amniotic fluid and during baths.

- **Conduction** is the loss of heat to a cooler surface by direct skin contact. Chilled hands, cool scales, cold examination tables, and cold stethoscopes can cause loss of heat by conduction.

After birth, the highest losses of heat are generally due to radiation, convection, and thermal conduction. The neonate initially can respond to the cooler environmental temperature with adequate peripheral vasoconstriction, but this mechanism becomes less effective because of the minimal amount of fat insulation, large body surface, and ongoing thermal conduction.

Heat Production

When exposed to a cool environment, the newborn requires additional heat. The neonate has several physiologic mechanisms that increase heat production, or *thermogenesis*. These include increased basal metabolic rate, muscular activity, and chemical thermogenesis (also called *nonshivering thermogenesis*).

Nonshivering thermogenesis (NST), an important mechanism of heat production unique to the newborn, uses the infant's stores of **brown adipose tissue** (also called *brown fat*). Brown adipose tissue **(BAT)** is the primary source of heat in the cold-stressed neonate. It first appears in the fetus at about 26–30 weeks of gestation and continues to increase until 2–5 weeks after the birth of a full-term infant, unless the fat is depleted by cold stress. BAT is deposited in the midscapular area, around the neck, and in the axillas, with deeper placement around the trachea, esophagus, abdominal aorta, kidneys, and adrenal glands (Figure 19-5). BAT constitutes 2%–6% of the newborn's total body weight. Brown fat receives its name from its dark color, which is due to its enriched blood supply, dense cellular content, and abundant nerve endings.

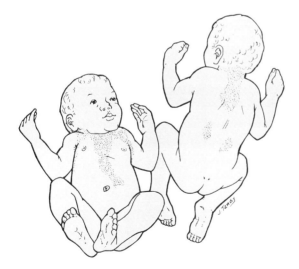

Figure 19-5 ▬▬▬▬
The distribution of brown adipose tissue (BAT) in the neonate. (From Davis V: Structure and function of brown adipose tissue in the neonate. *J Obstet Gynecol Neonat Nurs* November/December 1980; 9:364.)

Nonshivering thermogenesis occurs when skin receptors perceive a drop in the environmental temperature and in response transmit sensations to the central nervous system, which in turn stimulates the sympathetic nervous system. Norepinephrine, released by the adrenal gland and at local nerve endings in the brown fat, causes the metabolism of triglycerides to fatty acids, thereby releasing heat, which is distributed to the body.

Shivering, muscular activity common in the cold adult, is rarely seen in the newborn, although it has been observed at ambient temperatures of 15C (59F) or less. If an infant shivers, his or her metabolic rate has already doubled. The extra muscular activity does little to produce needed heat.

After being exposed to cold, an infant with a depleted supply of brown fat will have limited or no metabolic response. Increased basal metabolism due to hypothermia results in increased oxygen consumption. A decrease in the environmental temperature of 2C is a drop sufficient to double the oxygen consumption of a term neonate (Avery and Taeusch, 1984).

The normal term neonate is usually able to cope with the increase in basal metabolism, but the preterm neonate may be unable to increase ventilation to the necessary level of oxygen consumption. As a consequence, maintaining an optimal thermal environment is an absolute necessity to prevent neonatal cold stress and the resulting metabolic physiologic responses. (See Chapter 22 for discussion of cold stress.)

Hypoxia and the effect of certain drugs (such as meperidine) may also prevent metabolism of brown fat. Meperidine given to the laboring woman leads to a greater fall in the newborn's body temperature during the neonatal period. It is important to remember that neonatal hypothermia prolongs and increases the effects of many analgesic and anesthetic drugs in the neonate.

Hepatic Adaptation ▬▬▬▬▬▬

The newborn's liver is relatively large, occupying about 40% of the abdominal cavity. The liver's role in iron storage, carbohydrate metabolism, conjugation of bilirubin, and coagulation is discussed next.

Iron Storage and Red Blood Cell Production

Neonatal iron stores are determined by total body hemoglobin content and length of gestation. If the mother's iron intake during pregnancy has been adequate, the infant will have stored enough iron to last until the fifth month of neonatal life. At this time, foods containing iron or iron supplements must be given to prevent anemia in the infant.

Carbohydrate Metabolism

Neonatal carbohydrate reserves are relatively low. One-third of this reserve is in the form of liver glycogen. Glucose, stored as glycogen in the fetal liver starting during weeks 9–10 of gestation (Korones, 1981), is the major source of energy for the fetus. At term, neonatal glycogen stores are twice those of an adult.

Glucose is the main source of energy in the first few hours (4–6) after delivery. The blood glucose level falls rapidly and then stabilizes at values of 50–60 mg/dL for several days; by the third postnatal day, values increase to 60–70 mg/dL. Blood glucose levels are influenced by a balance between liver glucose output and peripheral uptake and by body temperature, insulin concentration, and muscular activity.

If the fetus or neonate experiences hypoxia, the glycogen stores are used and may be depleted to meet metabolic requirements. As stores of liver and muscle glycogen and blood glucose decrease, the neonate compensates by changing from a predominantly carbohydrate metabolism to fat metabolism. Energy is derived from fat and protein as well as from carbohydrates. The amount and availability of these fuel sources depend on constraints imposed by immature metabolic pathways (lack of specific enzymes or hormones) in the first few days of life.

Physiologic Jaundice—Icterus Neonatorum

The fetal liver begins to metabolize bilirubin at 12 weeks of gestation, but this ability disappears by 36 weeks. The fetus does not conjugate bilirubin because unconjugated bilirubin can cross the placenta to be excreted. *Conjugation* of bilirubin is the conversion of this yellow lipid-soluble pigment into a water-soluble pigment. **Physiologic jaundice** is caused by accelerated destruction of fetal RBCs, impaired conjugation of bilirubin, and increased bilirubin reabsorption from the intestinal tract. This condition does not have a pathologic basis, but rather is a normal biologic response of the newborn.

Five interacting factors give rise to physiologic jaundice (Avery and Taeusch, 1984).

1. *Increased amounts of bilirubin delivered to the liver.* The increased blood volume due to delayed cord clamping combined with accelerated RBC destruction leads to an increased bilirubin level in the blood. The erythrocyte (RBC) life span is 80–100 days instead of 120, as in the adult. A proportionately larger amount of non-erythrocyte bilirubin is formed in the neonate. Therefore, newborns have two to three times greater production or breakdown of bilirubin.

2. *Defective uptake of bilirubin from the blood.* Inadequate formation of hepatic binding proteins results in higher bilirubin levels.

3. *Defective conjugation of the bilirubin.* Decreased glucuronyl-transferase activity results in greater bilirubin values. (An expanded discussion of the conjugation of bilirubin is found in Chapter 22.) An enzyme found in breast milk is thought to further impede the conjugation of bilirubin.

4. *Defect in bilirubin excretion.* A congenital infection may cause impaired excretion. Delay in introduction of bacterial flora and decreased intestinal mobility can also delay excretion.

5. *Increased reabsorption of bilirubin.* Bilirubin is increased with reduced bowel motility, which enhances the reabsorption of bilirubin from the intestine via the enterohepatic pathway.

About 50% of full-term neonates and 80% of preterm neonates exhibit physiologic jaundice on about the second or third day after birth. The characteristic yellow color results from increased levels of unconjugated bilirubin, which are a normal product of RBC breakdown and reflect a temporary inability of the body to eliminate bilirubin. The signs of physiologic jaundice appear *after* the first 24 hours postnatally. This differentiates physiologic jaundice from pathologic jaundice (Chapter 22), which is clinically seen at birth or within the first 24 hours of postnatal life. Serum levels of bilirubin are usually about 4–6 mg/dL before yellow coloration of the skin and sclera appears.

During the first week, unconjugated bilirubin levels in physiologic jaundice should not exceed 12 mg/dL in the full-term or preterm newborn (Avery, 1981). Peak bilirubin levels are reached between days 3 and 5 in the full-term infant and between days 5 and 6 in the preterm infant. These values are established for European and American newborns. Chinese, Japanese, Korean, and American Indian neonates have considerably higher bilirubin levels that persist for longer periods with no apparent ill effects (Gartner and Lee, 1977).

The nursery environment may hinder the early detection of the degree and type of jaundice. Pink walls and artificial lights mask the beginning of jaundice in newborns. Observations in daylight assist in early recognition by eliminating distortions caused by artificial lights. Some nursery procedures are designed to decrease the probability of high bilirubin levels. These actions are as follows:

- The infant's body temperature is maintained at 97.6F (36.4C) or above. Chilling results in acidosis, which in turn decreases available serum albumin-binding sites and causes elevated unconjugated bilirubin levels.

- Stool is evaluated for amount and type. Bilirubin is eliminated in the feces; inadequate defecation may result in reabsorption and recycling of bilirubin.

- Early feedings are encouraged to promote fecal elimination and bacterial colonization and to provide caloric intake necessary for formation of hepatic binding proteins.

If jaundice is suspected, the nurse can quickly assess the neonate's coloring by pressing his or her skin with a finger. As the blanching occurs, the nurse can observe the yellow coloring. If jaundice becomes apparent, nursing care is directed toward keeping the neonate well hydrated and promoting intestinal elimination. For specific nursing management and therapies, see p. 537.

Physiologic jaundice may be very upsetting to parents; they require emotional support and thorough explanation of the condition. Hospitalization of the newborn for a few additional days may be upsetting to parents. They are encouraged to provide for the emotional needs of their newborn by continuing to feed, hold, and caress the infant. If the mother is discharged, the parents should be encouraged to return for feedings and feel free to telephone or visit whenever possible. In many instances, the mother, especially if she is breast-feeding, may decide to remain hospitalized with her infant; this decision should be supported. As an alternative to extended hospitalization, some infants are able to utilize home phototherapy programs (*American Journal of Nursing*, 1984).

Breast-feeding jaundice Breast-feeding is implicated in prolonged jaundice in some newborns. The breast milk of some women is thought to contain an enzyme that inhibits glucuronyl transferase or to contain several times the normal breast milk concentration of certain free fatty acids, which may inhibit the conjugation of bilirubin. The newborn's bilirubin level begins to rise about the fourth day after the mother's mature milk has come in. The level peaks at 2–3 weeks of age and may reach 15–20 mg/dL. Interruption of nursing may be advised if bilirubin reaches 16–17 mg/dL (Avery, 1981). Within 48 hours after discontinuing breast-feeding, the neonate's serum bilirubin levels begin to fall and return to normal levels by 4–8 days. (See Essential Facts to Remember—Jaundice.)

 ESSENTIAL FACTS TO REMEMBER

Jaundice

Physiologic jaundice:

- Physiologic jaundice occurs *after* the first 24 hours of life.

- During first week of life, bilirubin should not exceed 12 mg/dL.

- Bilirubin levels peak at 3–5 days in term infants.

Breast-milk jaundice:

- Bilirubin levels begin to rise about the fourth day after mature breast milk comes in.

- Peak of 15–20 mg/dL is reached at 2–3 weeks of age.

- It may be necessary to interrupt nursing for a short period when bilirubin reaches 16–17 mg/dL.

Many physicians believe that breast-feeding may be resumed once other causes of jaundice have been ruled out. The bilirubin concentrations may rise (Avery, 1981) but should not reach previous high levels. Nursing mothers need encouragement and support in their desire to nurse their infants, assistance and instruction regarding pumping and expressing milk during the interrupted nursing period, and reassurance that nothing is wrong with their milk or mothering abilities.

Coagulation

The liver plays an important part in blood coagulation during fetal life and continues this function to some degree during the first few months following birth. Coagulation factors II, VII, IX, and X (synthesized in the liver) are activated under the influence of vitamin K and therefore are considered vitamin K–dependent. The absence of normal flora needed to synthesize vitamin K in the newborn gut results in low levels of vitamin K and creates a transient blood coagulation deficiency between the second and fifth day of life. From a low point at about 2–3 days after birth, these coagulation factors rise slowly, but do not approach normal adult levels until 9 months of age or later. Increasing levels of these vitamin K–dependent factors indicate a response to dietary intake and bacterial colonization of the intestines. Although usually no clinical consequences arise, an injection of vitamin K (Aqua-MEPHYTON) is given prophylactically on the day of birth to combat the deficiency. (Hemorrhagic disease of the newborn is discussed in more depth in Chapter 22.) Other coagulation factors having low cord blood levels are XI, XII, and XIII. Fibrinogen and factors V and VIII are near adult ranges (Buchanan, 1978).

Platelet counts at birth are in the same range as for adults, but neonates may manifest mild transient platelet-functioning defect.

Prenatal maternal therapy with diphenylhydantoin sodium (Dilantin) or phenobarbital (Luminal) causes abnormal clotting factors studies and neonatal bleeding in the first 24 hours after birth. Infants born to mothers receiving coumadin (Warfarin) compounds may bleed because these agents cross the placenta and accentuate existing vitamin K–dependent clotting factor deficiencies.

Gastrointestinal Adaptation

By 36–38 weeks of fetal life, the gastrointestinal system is fully mature, with enzymatic activity and the ability to transport nutrients. The term neonate has adequate intestinal and pancreatic enzymes to digest most simple carbohydrates, proteins, and fats.

The carbohydrates requiring digestion in the newborn are usually disaccharides (lactose, maltose, and sucrose). Lactose is the primary carbohydrate in the breast-feeding newborn and is generally easily digested and well absorbed. The only enzyme lacking is pancreatic amylase, which remains relatively deficient during the first few months of life. Therefore, newborns have trouble digesting starches (changing more complex carbohydrates into maltose).

Although proteins require more digestion than carbohydrates, they are well digested and absorbed from the neonatal intestine.

The neonate digests and absorbs fats less efficiently because of the minimal activity of the pancreatic enzyme lipase. The neonate excretes about 10%–20% of the dietary fat intake, compared with 10% for the adult. The newborn absorbs the fat in breast milk more completely than the fat in cow's milk because it consists of more medium-chain triglycerides and breast milk contains lipase. (See Chapter 21 for further discussion of infant nutrition.) In utero, swallowing is accompanied by gastric emptying and peristalsis of the fetal intestinal tract. By the end of gestation, in preparation for extrauterine life, peristalsis becomes much more pronounced.

Air enters the stomach immediately after birth. The small intestine is filled within 2–12 hours and the large bowel within 24 hours. The salivary glands are immature at birth, and the infant produces little saliva until about age 3 months. The newborn's stomach has a capacity of about 50–60 mL. It empties intermittently, starting within a few minutes of the beginning of a feeding. Two to 4 hours after feeding, the stomach is completely empty. The newborn's gastric pH is equal to an adult's, but stomach contents become less acidic in about a week and remain less acid than those of adults for 2–3 months.

The cardiac sphincter is immature, as is nervous control of the stomach, so some regurgitation may be noted in the neonatal period. Regurgitation of the first few feedings during the first day or two of life can usually be lessened by avoiding overfeeding and by burping the newborn well during and after the feeding.

When no other signs and symptoms are evident, vomiting is often self-limiting and ceases within the first few days of life. However, vomiting or continuous regurgitation should be observed closely. If the neonate has swallowed bloody or purulent amniotic fluid, lavage may be indicated to relieve the problem.

Adequate digestion and absorption are essential for neonatal growth and development. If optimal nutritional support is available, postnatal growth ideally should parallel intrauterine growth; that is, after 30 weeks of gestation, the fetus gains 30 g per day and adds 1.2 cm to body length daily. To gain weight at the intrauterine rate, the term neonate requires 120 calories per kilogram per day. Following birth, caloric intake is often insufficient for weight gain until the neonate is 5–10 days old. During this time, there may be a weight loss of 5%–15%. Failure to lose weight when caloric intake is inadequate may indicate fluid retention. Shift of intracellular water to extracellular space and insensible water loss account for the 5%–15% weight loss.

Normal term neonates pass meconium within 12 hours of life or at least within 48 hours (Avery and Tauesch, 1984). **Meconium** is formed in utero from the amniotic fluid and its constituents, with intestinal secretions and shed mucosal cells. It is recognized by its thick, tarry, dark green appearance. Transitional (thin brown to green) stools consisting of part meconium and part fecal material are passed for the next day or two, after which the stools become entirely fecal. Generally, the stools of a breast-fed newborn are pale yellow (but may be pasty green); they are more liquid and more frequent than those of formula-fed neonates, whose stools are paler. Frequency of bowel movement varies, but range from one every 2–3 days to as many as ten daily. (See Essential Facts to Remember—Physiologic Adaptations to Extrauterine Life.)

Renal Adaptation

The newborn's kidneys are relatively large and may extend below the iliac crests; they are most easily palpable through the abdominal wall soon after birth. Because the infant pelvis is too small to contain it, the bladder is also an abdominal organ.

The physiologic features of the neonatal kidney include the following:

1. The kidney has its full number of functioning nephrons.

2. The newborn kidneys are unable to dispose of water and solutes easily because of decreased glomerular filtration ability.

3. The nephron has the ability to reabsorb sodium (Na^+) and hydrogen ion (H^+), and concentrate urine.

4. The kidney has limited tubular reabsorption, which leads to inappropriate loss of substances such as amino acids and bicarbonate. With increased loss of bicarbonate and buffering capacity, there is a predisposition to acidosis and electrolyte imbalances.

By 4 months of gestation, urine is found in the fetal bladder, and amniotic fluid analysis indicates that the fetus voids in utero. About 17% of newborns void at delivery, 92% by 24 hours, and 99% within 48 hours. A neonate who has not voided after 24 hours should be assessed for adequacy of fluid intake, bladder distention, restlessness, and symptoms of pain. The physician should be notified.

ESSENTIAL FACTS TO REMEMBER

Physiologic Adaptations to Extrauterine Life

- Periodic breathing may be present

- Desired skin temperature 36–36.5C, stabilizes 4–6 hours after birth

- Desired blood glucose level reaches 60–70 mg/dL by third postnatal day

- Stools: Meconium (thick, tarry, dark green)
  Transitional stools (thin, brown to green)
  Breast-fed infants (yellow gold, soft, or mushy)
  Bottle-fed infants (pale yellow, formed, and pasty)

Unless edema is present, normal urinary output is often limited, and the voidings are scanty until fluid intake increases. (The fluid of edema is eliminated by the kidneys, so infants with edema have a much higher urinary output.) The first 2 days postnatally, the newborn voids 2 to 6 times daily; with a urine output of 30–60 mL per day. Subsequently, the neonate voids 5 to 25 times every 24 hours, with a volume of 30–50 mL/kg/24 hr. The initial bladder volume is 6–44 mL of urine.

Full-term neonates are not able to concentrate urine to the same extent as the adult. The maximum concentrating ability of the newborn is a specific gravity of 1.025. Feeding practices may affect the osmolarity of the urine. The inability of the neonate to further concentrate urine is due to the limited excretion of solutes in the growing newborn. The ability to concentrate urine fully is reached by about 3 months of age.

After the first voiding, the newborn's urine frequently appears cloudy (due to presence of mucus) and has a high specific gravity, which decreases as fluid intake increases. Occasionally pink stains ("brick dust spots") appear on the diaper. These are caused by urates and are harmless. Blood may occasionally be observed on the diapers of female infants. This *pseudomenstruation* is related to the withdrawal of maternal hormones. Males may have bloody spotting from a circumcision. In the absence of apparent causes for bleeding, the physician should be notified. Normal urine during early infancy is straw-colored and almost odorless, although certain drugs or the presence of infection give the urine an odor.

The normal values of a urinalysis for a neonate include the following:

Protein < 5–10 mg/dL

WBC < 2–3

RBC 0

Casts 0

Bacteria 0

Immunologic Adaptations

The newborn possesses varying degrees of nonspecific and specific immunity. The nonspecific mechanism is *opsonization*, the coating of invasive bacteria to ready them for ingestion by phagocytes. Specific immunity is provided by *immunoglobulins*, a type of antibody secreted by lymphocytes and plasma cells into the body fluids.

The cells that constitute the immune system appear early in fetal life, but usually are not fully activated until sometime after birth. Opsonization, for example, is impaired at birth. Albumin and globulin, however, are present throughout the last trimester of gestation.

Of the three major types of immunoglobulins primarily involved in immunity—IgG, IgA, and IgM—only IgG crosses the placenta. The pregnant woman forms antibodies in response to illness or immunization. This process is called **active acquired immunity**. When IgG antibodies are transferred to the fetus in utero, **passive acquired immunity** results, since the fetus does not produce the antibodies itself. IgG is very active against bacterial toxins.

Because the maternal immunoglobin is transferred primarily during the third trimester, preterm infants (especially those born prior to 34 weeks) may be more susceptible to infection. In general, newborns have immunity to tetanus, diphtheria, smallpox, measles, mumps, poliomyelitis, and a variety of other bacterial and viral diseases. The period of resistance varies: Immunity against common viral infections such as measles may last 4–8 months, whereas immunity to certain bacteria may disappear within 4–8 weeks.

The normal newborn does produce antibodies in response to an antigen, but not as effectively as an older child would. It is customary to begin immunization at 2 months of age, and then the infant can develop active acquired immunity.

IgM immunoglobulins are produced in response to blood group antigens, gram-negative enteric organisms, and some viruses in the expectant mother. Because IgM does not normally cross the placenta, most or all is produced by the fetus beginning at 10–15 weeks' gestation. Elevated levels of IgM at birth may indicate placental leaks or, more commonly, antigenic stimulation in utero. Consequently, elevations suggest that the infant was exposed to an intrauterine infection such as syphilis or a TORCH infection. The lack of available maternal IgM in the newborn also accounts for the infant's susceptibility to Gram-negative enteric organisms such as *E. coli*.

The functions of IgA immunoglobulins are not fully understood. IgA appears to provide protection mainly on secreting surfaces such as the respiratory tract, gastrointestinal tract, and eyes. Serum IgA does not cross the placenta and is not normally produced by the fetus in utero. Unlike the other immunoglobulins, IgA is not affected by gastric action. Colostrum, the forerunner of breast milk, is very high in secretory form of IgA. Consequently, it may be of significance in providing some passive immunity to the infant of a breast-feeding mother (Charles and Larsen, 1984).

Limited information is available on the remaining two immunoglobulins, IgE and IgD. IgE, which does not cross the placenta, contains skin-sensitizing antibodies. IgD has no known distinctive antibody function or activity and is found in minimal amounts in the cord blood.

Neurologic and Sensory/ Perceptual Functioning

Neurologic Adaptations

The formation and maturation of the nervous system is influenced minimally, if at all, by the actual birth process. Because many complex biochemical and histologic changes have yet to occur in the neonatal brain, the postnatal period is considered a time of risk in regard to the development of the brain and nervous system. For neurologic development, including intellectual development, to proceed, the brain and associated nervous system must mature in an orderly, unhampered fashion.

The neonate responds to and interacts with the environment from the moment of birth in a predictable pattern of behavior that is influenced by the intrauterine experience. Brazelton (1975) found a positive association between newborn behavior and the nutritional status of the pregnant woman. Neonates with higher birth weight responded more to visual and auditory cues and exhibited more mature motor activity than low-birth-weight newborns.

Maternal behavior and experiences, such as smoking and emotional shocks, may also affect the fetus.

The fetus is exposed to a variety of external and internal stimuli that might influence neonatal behavior. For example, neonates exposed to intense noise during fetal life are markedly less reactive to loud sounds postnatally. The ability of the newborn to cope with stressors is manifested in behavioral responses ranging from dealing quietly with the stimulation, to becoming overreactive and tense, to displaying a combination of the two reactions.

Motor Activity

The organization and the quality of the newborn's motor activity are influenced by a number of factors including the following (Brazelton, 1984):

- Sleep-alert states
- Presence of environmental stimuli, such as heat, light, cold, and noise
- Conditions causing a chemical imbalance, such as hypoglycemia
- Hydration status
- State of health
- Recovery from the stress of labor and delivery

The performance of complex behavioral patterns may be reflective of neonatal integrity. Neonates who can bring a hand to their mouth may be demonstrating motor coordination as well as a self-quieting technique, thus increasing the complexity of the behavioral response. Neonates also possess complex, organized defensive motor patterns as exhibited by the ability to remove an obstruction, such as a cloth across the face.

States of the Newborn

The state of consciousness of the neonate can be divided into two categories, the sleep state and the alert state (Brazelton, 1984). Subcategories are identified under each major category.

Sleep states   The sleep states are as follows:

1. *Deep or quiet sleep.* Deep sleep is characterized by closed eyes with no eye movements, regular, even breathing, and jerky motions or startles at regular intervals. Behavioral reponses to external stimuli are likely to be delayed. Startles are rapidly suppressed, and changes in state are not likely to occur.

2. *Active REM.* Irregular respirations, eyes closed with REM, irregular sucking motions, minimal activity, and irregular but smooth movement of the extremities can be observed in active REM sleep. Environmental and internal stimuli initiate a startle reaction and a change of state.

Sleep cycles in the neonate have been recognized and defined according to duration. The length of the cycle depends on the age of the neonate. At term, REM active sleep and quiet sleep occur in intervals of 45–50 minutes. About 45%–50% of the total sleep of the neonate is active sleep, 35%–45% is quiet (deep) sleep, and 10% of sleep is transitional between these two periods. It is hypothesized that REM sleep stimulates the growth of the neural system. Over a period of time, the neonate's sleep-wake patterns become diurnal; that is, the infant sleeps at night and stays awake during the day. (See Chapter 21 for a short discussion of assessment of neonatal states.)

Alert states The following are subcategories of the alert state (Brazelton, 1984):

1. *Drowsy or semidozing.* The behaviors common to the drowsy state are open or closed eyes, fluttering eyelids, semidozing appearance, and slow, regular movements of the extremities. Mild startles may be noted from time to time. Although the reaction to a sensory stimulus is delayed, a change of state often results.

2. *Wide awake (quiet alert).* In the wide-awake state, the neonate is alert and follows and fixates on attractive objects, faces, or auditory stimuli. Motor activity is minimal, and the response to external stimuli is delayed.

3. *Active awake.* The eyes are open and motor activity is quite intense with thrusting movements of the extremities in the active-awake state. Environmental stimuli cause increase in startles or motor activity, but individual reactions are difficult to distinguish because of generalized high activity level.

4. *Crying.* Intense crying is accompanied by jerky motor movements. Crying serves several purposes for the newborn. It may be a distraction from disturbing stimuli such as hunger and pain. Fussiness often allows the neonate to discharge energy and reorganize behavior. Most important,

crying elicits an appropriate response of help from the parents.

Waking states that last for varying amounts of time are influenced by fatigue, hunger, and needs of the newborn. In the first 30–60 minutes after birth, many neonates display an alert state, characteristic of the first period of reactivity. (Periods of reactivity are discussed in Chapter 21.) About 12–18 hours after birth, the infant is again alert when the second period of reactivity occurs. These alert states tend to be short the first 2 days of life to allow the newborn to recover from the birth. Subsequently, alert states are of choice or of necessity (Brazelton, 1984). Increasing choice of wakefulness by the neonate indicates a maturing capacity to achieve and maintain consciousness. Heat, cold, and hunger are but a few of the stimuli that can cause wakefulness by necessity. Once the disturbing stimuli are removed, sleep tends to recur.

Sensory Capacities of the Newborn

The newborn is able to process and respond to complex visual stimulation. For example, when a bright light is flashed into the neonate's eyes, the initial response is blinking, constriction of the pupil, and perhaps a slight startle reaction. However, with repeated stimulation, the newborn's response repertoire gradually diminishes and disappears; this is known as *habituation.* The capacity to ignore repetitious disturbing stimuli is a neonatal defense mechanism readily apparent in the noisy well-lighted nursery.

In addition to being able to disregard specific stimuli, the newborn has the ability to be alert to, to follow, and to fixate on complex visual stimuli that are appealing and attractive. The newborn prefers the human face and eyes and bright shiny objects. As the face or object comes into the line of vision, the neonate responds with bright, wide eyes, still limbs, and fixed staring. This intense visual involvement may last several minutes, during which time the neonate is able to follow the stimulus from side to side. Figure 19-6 illustrates this response. The newborn uses this sensory capacity to become familiar with family, friends, and surroundings (Figure 19-7).

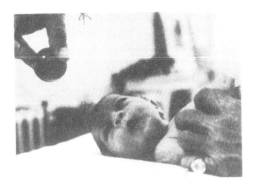

Figure 19-6 ▬▬▬▬▬▬▬▬
Head turning to follow. (From Avery ME, Taeusch HW, *Schaeffer's Diseases of the Newborn*. Philadelphia: W. B. Saunders, 1984, p. 71. Reprinted by permission.)

Auditory capacity   The newborn responds to auditory stimulation with a definite, organized behavior repertoire. The stimulus used to assess auditory response should be selected to match the state of the newborn. A rattle is appropriate for light sleep, a voice for an awake state, and a clap for deep sleep. As the neonate hears the sound, the cardiac rate rises, and a minimal startle reflex may be observed. If the sound is appealing, the newborn will become alert and search for the site of the auditory stimulus.

Olfactory capacity   Neonates are able to distinguish their mother's breast pads from those of other mothers by 1 week postnatally (Brazelton, 1984). Apparently this phenomenon is related to the neonate's ability to select by smell.

Taste and sucking   The newborn responds differently to varying tastes. Sugar, for example, increases sucking. Sucking pattern variations also exist in newborns fed cow's milk or human breast milk (Brazelton, 1984). When breast-feeding, the neonate sucks in bursts with frequent regular pauses. The bottle-fed newborn tends to suck at a regular rate with infrequent pauses.

When awake and hungry, the neonate displays rapid searching motions in response to the rooting reflex. Once feeding begins, the newborn establishes a sucking pattern according to the method of feeding. Finger sucking is not only present postnatally, but in utero. The neonate frequently uses sucking as a self-quieting activity, which assists in the development of self-regulation.

Tactile capacity   The neonate is very sensitive to being touched, cuddled, and held. Often a mother's first response to an upset or crying newborn is touching or holding. Swaddling, placing a hand on the infant's abdomen, or holding the arms to prevent a startle reflex are other methods of soothing the newborn. The settled neonate is then able to attend to and interact with the environment.

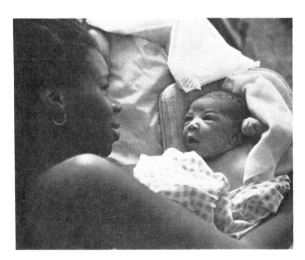

Figure 19-7 ▬▬▬▬▬▬▬▬
Newborn's visual involvement and attentiveness to his mother. (Photo by Suzanne Arms.)

Summary ▬▬▬▬▬▬▬▬▬▬▬

Birth propels the infant from a warm, weightless, fluid environment into a cold, dry, pressurized environment within a short time. After separation from the placenta, the infant must maintain all major body functions independently. Immediate initiation of respiration and changes in the circulatory patterns are essential for extrauterine life. Within 24 hours after birth, the newborn's renal, gastrointestinal, hematologic, metabolic, and neurologic systems must function sufficiently to maintain extrauterine life.

A basic understanding of these physiologic and neuro-behavioral changes helps the nurse effectively assess (Chapter 20) and intervene (Chapter 21) to meet the health needs of the newborn and his or her family.

References

American Journal of Nursing. Jaundiced babies bloom with home phototherapy. *Am J Nurs* 1984; 84(7):871.

Avery GB: *Neonatology: Pathophysiology and Management of the Newborn*. Philadelphia: Lippincott, 1981.

Avery ME, Taeusch HW. *Schaeffer's Diseases of the Newborn*, 5th ed. Philadelphia: Saunders, 1984.

Brazelton TB: Neonatal behavior and its significance. In: *Schaeffer's Diseases of the Newborn*, 5th ed. Avery ME, Taeusch HW (editors). Philadelphia: Saunders, 1984.

Brazelton TB et al: Biomedical variables and neonatal performance of Guatemalan infants. Paper presented to American Academy of Cerebral Palsy, 1975, New Orleans, La.

Buchanan GR: Neonatal coagulation: Normal physiology and pathophysiology. *Clin Haematol* 1978; 7:85.

Charles D, Larsen B. How colostrum and milk protect the newborn. *Contemp Obstet Gynecol* 1984; 24(1):143.

Danforth DH (editor): *Obstetrics and Gynecology*, 4th ed. Philadelphia: Harper & Row, 1982.

Gartner LM, Lee KS: Jaundice and liver disease. In: *Neonatal Perinatal Medicine*, Behrman RE (editor). St. Louis: Mosby, 1977.

Goldstein JD, Reid LM: Pulmonary hypoplasia resulting from phrenic nerve agenesis and diaphragmatic amyoplasia. *J Pediatr* 1980; 97:282.

Hatch DJ, Sumner E: *Neonatal Anaesthesia*. Chicago: Year Book Medical Publishers, 1981.

Korones SB: *High-Risk Newborn Infants: The Basis for Intensive Care Nursing*, 3rd ed. St. Louis: Mosby, 1981.

Smith CA, Nelson NM: *The Physiology of the Newborn Infant*, 4th ed. Springfield, Ill.: Thomas, 1976.

Additional Readings

Avery ME, Fletcher BD, Williams RG: *The Lung and Its Disorders in the Newborn Infant*, 4th ed. Philadelphia: Saunders, 1981.

Brazelton TB: Behavioral competence of the newborn infant. *Sem Perinatol* 1979; 3:35.

Bryan A: Control of respiration in the newborn. *Clin Perinatol* 1978; 5:293.

Gartner LM, Lee KS: Effect of starvation and milk feeding on intestinal bilirubin absorption. (Abstract.) *Gastroenterology* 1979; 77:A13.

Gorski PA et al: Stages of behavioral organization in the high risk neonate: Theoretical and clinical considerations. *Sem Perinatol* 1979; 3:61.

Hill ST et al: The effect of early parent-infant contact on newborn body temperature. *J Obstet Gynecol Neonat Nurs* 1979; 8:287.

Hutton NJ et al: Urine collection in the neonate: Effect of different methods on volume, specific gravity, and glucose. *J Obstet Gynecol Neonat Nurs* 1980; 9:165.

Oehler JM: *Family-Centered Neonatal Nursing Care*. Philadelphia: Lippincott, 1981.

Parker S, Brazelton TB: Newborn behavioral assessment: Research prediction, and clinical uses . . . . the Brazelton neonatal behavioral assessment scale. *Child Today* 1981; 10(4):2.

Porth CM et al: Temperature regulation in the newborn. *Am J Nurs* 1978; 78:1691.

20
Nursing Assessment of the Newborn

Chapter Contents

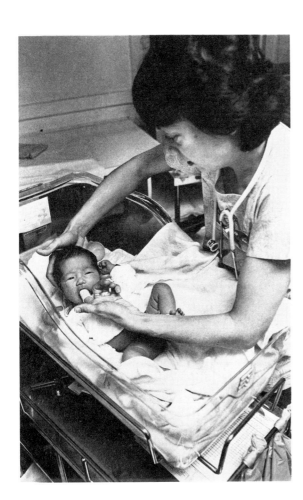

Objectives

- Describe the normal physical characteristics of the newborn.

- Identify the various methods of determining gestational age.

- Describe the neurologic and/or neuromuscular characteristics of the newborn and the reflexes that may be present at birth.

- Describe the function of the neonatal behavioral assessment.

Key Terms

acrocyanosis
Brazelton's neonatal
　behavioral
　assessment
caput succedaneum
cephalhematoma
Erb-Duchenne
　paralysis
Epstein's pearls
erythema toxicum
gestational age
　assessment tools

milia
molding
Mongolian spots
Moro reflex
pseudomenstruation
rooting reflex
scarf sign
telangiectatic nevi
　(stork bites)
tonic neck reflex

Unlike the adult, the newborn communicates needs primarily by behavior. Because the nurse is the most consistent observer of the newborn, he or she must be able to interpret this behavior into information about the neonate's condition and to respond with appropriate nursing interventions. This chapter focuses on the assessment of the neonate and on interpretation of the findings.

Assessment of the newborn is a continuous process designed to evaluate development and adjustments to extrauterine life. In the delivery room, the Apgar scoring procedure and careful observation of the neonate form the basis of assessment and are correlated with information such as:

- Maternal history
- Duration of labor
- Maternal analgesia and anesthesia
- Complications of labor or delivery
- Treatment instituted in the delivery room, in conjunction with determination of clinical gestational age
- Consideration of the classification of newborns by weight and gestational age and by neonatal mortality risk
- Physical examination of the newborn

An initial physical assessment of the newborn is done in the delivery room (Chapter 14). When the newborn is transferred to the nursery, the nurse performs a brief physical examination, estimates gestational age, and completes the admitting procedures (see Chapter 21). A more complete physical examination is performed by the physician or nurse practitioner within 24 hours after birth. This chapter describes the correct procedure for estimating gestational age and performing the newborn physical examination.

Estimation of Gestational Age

Traditionally, the gestational age of a neonate was determined from the date of the pregnant woman's last menstrual period. This method was accurate only 75%–85% of the time. Because of the problems that develop with the infant who is preterm or whose weight is inappropriate for gestational age, a more accurate system was developed to evaluate each newborn. Once learned, this evaluation can be made in a few minutes.

Clinical **gestational age assessment tools** have two components: external physical characteristics and neurologic and/or neuromuscular development evaluations. Physical characteristics generally include sole creases, amount of breast tissue, amount of lanugo, cartilagenous development of the ear, testicular descent, and scrotal rugae or labial development. These objective clinical criteria are not influenced by labor and delivery.

During the first 24 hours of life, the newborn's nervous system is unstable; thus, neurologic evaluation findings based on reflexes or assessments dependent on the higher brain centers may not be reliable. If the neurologic findings drastically deviate from the gestational age derived by evaluation of the external characteristics, a second assessment is done in 24 hours.

Of the current gestational assessment aids, Dubowitz and Dubowitz's tool is the most thoroughly documented and validated way to assess intrauterine growth alterations and preterm neonates (Robertson, 1979). This assessment tool lists physical characteristics and neuromuscular tone components to be assessed upon admission to the nursery.

Ballard's *estimation of gestational age* by maturity rating is a simplified version of the Dubowitz tool. The Ballard tool omits some of the neuromuscular tone assessments such as head lag, ventral suspension (which is difficult

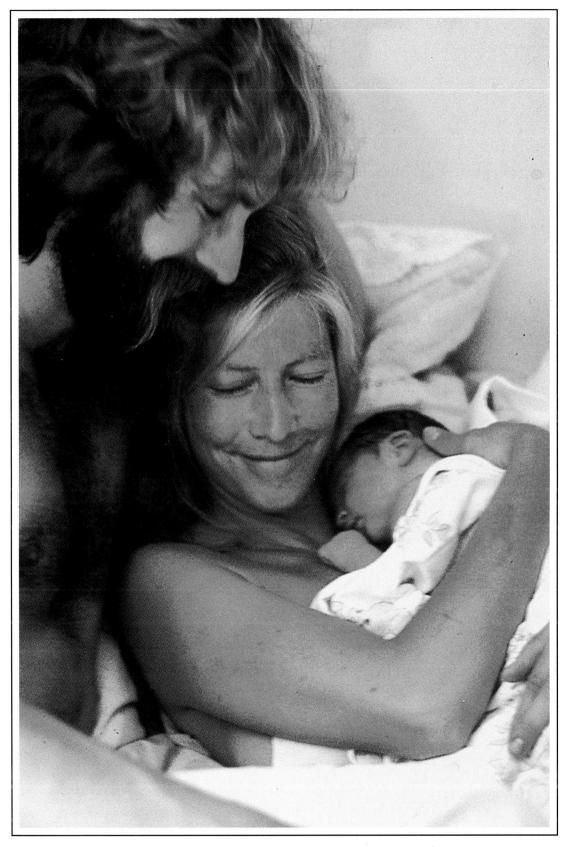

Plate I Beginnings…

Plate II   Linea nigra

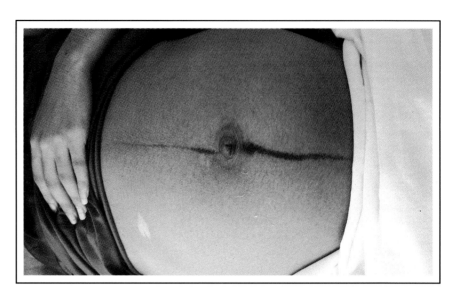

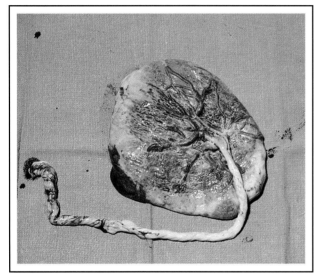

Plate III   Fetal side of placenta

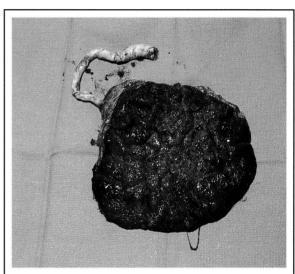

Plate IV   Maternal side of placenta

Plate V   Acrocyanosis

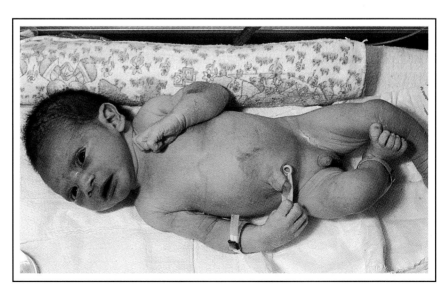

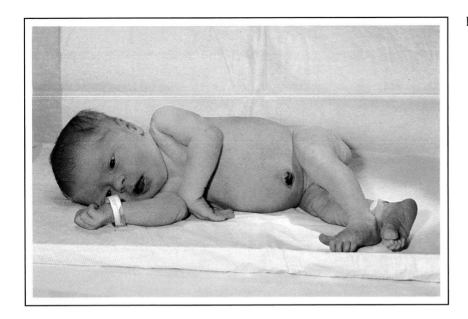

Plate VI Normal newborn

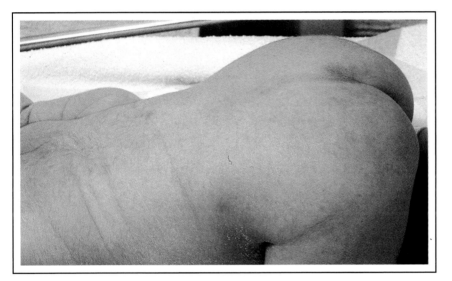

Plate VII Mongolian spots

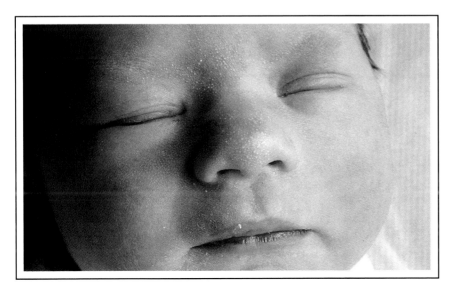

Plate VIII Facial milia

Plate IX   Stork bites

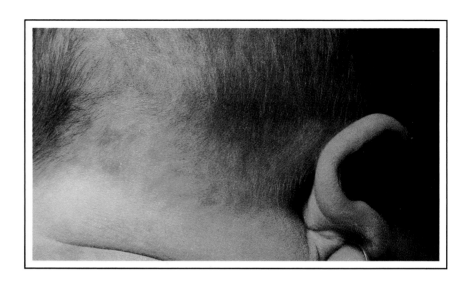

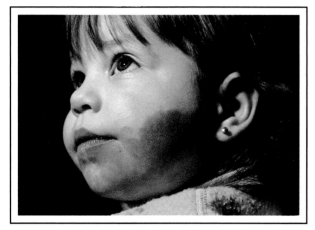

Plate X   Portwine stain

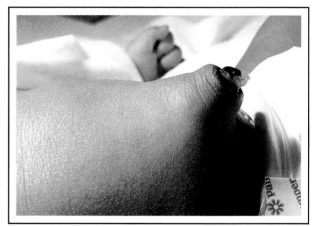

Plate XI   Umbilical hernia

Plate XII   Erythema toxicum

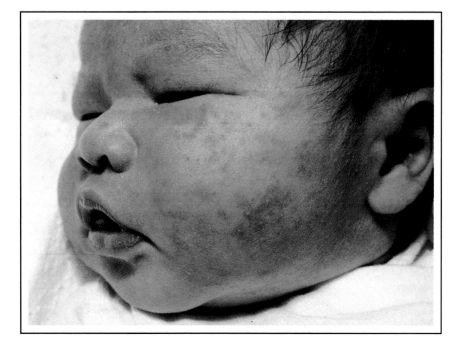

to assess in the very ill neonate), and leg recoil. The scoring method of Ballard's tool is much like that of the Dubowitz tool; each physical and neuromuscular finding is given a value, and the total score is matched to a gestational age (Figure 20-1). The maximum score on the Ballard's tool is 50, which corresponds to a gestational age of 44 weeks.

Estimation of Gestational Age
by Maturity Rating
Symbols: X=First exam   O=Second exam

Neuromuscular Maturity

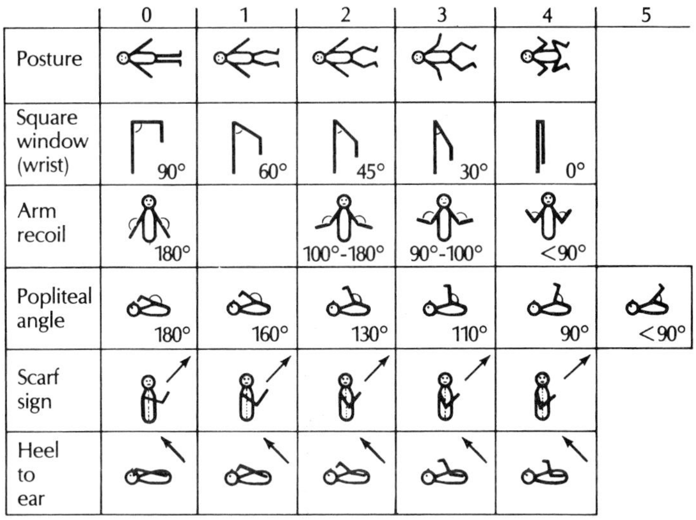

Gestation by dates _____ wks.

Birth date _____ Hour _____ am/pm

APGAR _____ 1 min _____ 5 min

Score	Wks
5	26
10	28
15	30
20	32
25	34
30	36
35	38
40	40
45	42
50	44

Physical Maturity

	0	1	2	3	4	5
Skin	gelatinous red, transparent	smooth pink, visible veins	superficial peeling and/or rash, few veins	cracking pale area, rare veins,	parchment, deep cracking, no vessels	leathery, cracked, wrinkled
Lanugo	none	abundant	thinning	bald areas	mostly bald	
Plantar creases	no crease	faint red marks	anterior transverse crease only	creases anter. 2/3	creases cover entire sole	
Breast	barely percept.	flat areola, no bud	stippled areola, 1-2 mm bud	raised areola, 3-4 mm bud	full areola, 5-10 mm bud	
Ear	binna flat, stays folded	sl. curved pinna, soft with slow recoil	well-curv. pinna, soft but ready recoil	formed and firm with instant recoil	thick cartilage, ear stiff	
Genitals (male)	scrotum empty, no rugae		testes decending, few rugae	testes down, good rugae	testes pendulous, deep rugae	
Genitals (female)	prominent clitoris and labia minora		majora and minora equally prominent	majora large, minora small	clitoris and minora completely covered	

Figure 20-1

Newborn maturity rating and classification. (From Ballard JL et al: A simplified assessment of gestational age. *Pediatr Res* 1977; 11:374. Figure adapted from "Classification of the low-birth-weight infant" by A. Y. Sweet in *Care of the High-Risk Infant* by M. H. Klaus and A. A. Fanaroff, W. B. Saunders Co., Philadelphia, 1977, p. 47.)

For example, upon completing a gestational assessment of a 1-hour-old newborn, the nurse gives a score of 3 to all the physical characteristics, for a total of 18, and gives a score of 3 to all the neuromuscular assessments, for a total neurologic score of 18. The physical characteristics score of 18 is added to the neurologic score of 18 for a total score of 36, which correlates with 38+ weeks' gestation. Since all infants vary slightly in the development of physical characteristics and maturation of neurologic function, there will be greater variance in each of these scores instead of all being 3, as in the example.

Both these tools lose accuracy when neonates of less than 28 weeks' or over 43 weeks' gestation are assessed. An additional tool is Brazie and Lubchenco's "Estimation of Gestational Age Chart" (Appendix D). Some nurseries use the physical characteristics component of this tool as an initial assessment for all neonates admitted to the nursery.

In carrying out gestational age assessments, the nurse should keep in mind that some maternal conditions such as PIH and diabetes may affect certain gestational assessment components and warrant further study. Maternal diabetes, although it appears to accelerate fetal growth, seems to retard maturation. Maternal hypertensive states, which retard growth, seem to speed maturation.

Assessment of Physical Characteristics

The nurse first evaluates observable characteristics without disturbing the infant. Selected physical characteristics common to both gestational assessment tools are presented here in the order in which they might be evaluated most effectively:

1. *Resting posture*, although a neuromuscular component, should be assessed as the infant lies undisturbed on a flat surface (Figure 20-2).

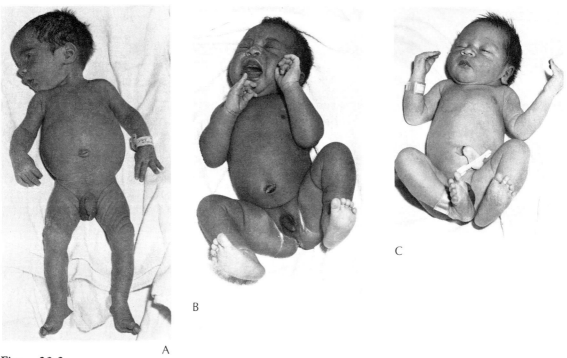

Figure 20-2

Resting posture. **A**, Infant exhibits beginning of flexion of the thigh. The gestational age is approximately 31 weeks. Note the extension of the upper extremities. **B**, Infant exhibits stronger flexion of the arms, hips, and thighs. The gestational age is approximately 35 weeks. **C**, The full-term infant exhibits hypertonic flexion of all extremities. (From Dubowitz L, Dubowitz V: *Gestational Age of the Newborn*. Menlo Park, Calif.: Addison-Wesley, 1977.)

2. *Skin* in the preterm neonate appears thin and transparent, with veins prominent over the abdomen early in gestation. As term approaches, the skin appears opaque because of increased subcutaneous tissue. Disappearance of the protective vernix caseosa promotes skin desquamation.

3. *Lanugo*, a fine hair covering, decreases as gestational age increases. The amount of lanugo is greatest at 28–30 weeks and then disappears, first from the face, then from the trunk and extremities.

4. *Sole (plantar) creases* are reliable indicators of gestational age in the first 12 hours of life. After this, the skin of the foot begins drying, and creases appear. Development of sole creases begins at the top portion of the sole and, as gestation progresses, proceeds to the heel (Figure 20-3). Plantar creases vary with race. Black infants' sole creases are less developed at term (Damoulaki-Sfakianaki et al., 1972).

5. *Breast tissue and areola* are palpated by application of the forefinger and middle finger

to the breast area. Although Figure 20-4 shows the thumb and forefinger being applied so that the reader can see the areola, during actual assessment the nipple should not be grasped with thumb and forefinger because skin and subcutaneous tissue will prevent accurate estimation of size. The nurse can cause trauma to the breast tissue if this procedure is not done gently. As gestation progresses, the breast tissue mass and areola enlarge. However, a large breast tissue mass can occur as a result of conditions other than advanced gestational age. The infant of a diabetic mother tends to be large for gestational age (LGA) and the accelerated development of breast tissue is a reflection of subcutaneous fat deposits. Small for gestational age (SGA) term or postterm newborns may have utilized subcutaneous fat (which would have been deposited as breast tissue) to survive in utero; as a result, their lack of breast tissue may indicate a gestational age of 34–35 weeks, even though other factors indicate a *term* or *postterm* neonate.

6. *Ear form and cartilage distribution* develop with gestational age. The cartilage gives

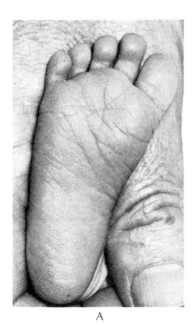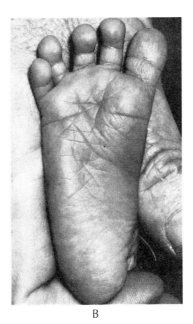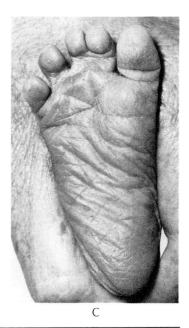

| A | B | C |

Figure 20-3

Sole creases. **A,** Infant has a few sole creases on the anterior portion of the foot. Note the slick heel. The gestational age is approximately 35 weeks. **B,** Infant has a deeper network of sole creases on the anterior two-thirds of the sole. Note the slick heel. The ges-

tational age is approximately 37 weeks. **C,** The full-term infant has deep sole creases down to and including the heel. (From Dubowitz L, Dubowitz, V: *Gestational Age of the Newborn.* Menlo Park, Calif.: Addison-Wesley, 1977.)

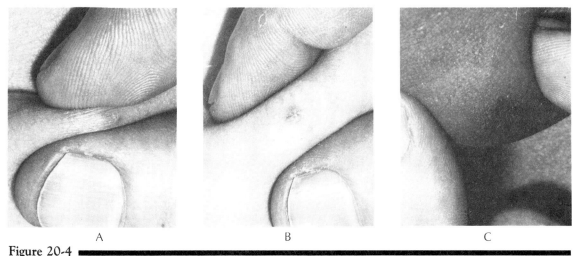

A   B   C

Figure 20-4

Breast tissue. **A,** Infant has a barely visible areola and nipple. No tissue is palpable. The gestational age is less than 33 weeks. **B,** Infant has a visible raised area. On palpation the area is 4 mm. The gestational age is 38 weeks. **C,** Infant has a 10 mm breast tissue area. The gestational age is 40–44 weeks. The thumb and forefinger are used here so that the reader can visualize the areola; during actual assessment only the forefinger and middle finger should be used for palpation. (From Dubowitz L, Dubowitz V: *Gestational Age of the Newborn*. Menlo Park, Calif.: Addison-Wesley, 1977.)

the ear its shape and substance (Figure 20-5). An infant of less than 34 weeks' gestation has little cartilage, so the ear folds over on itself and remains folded. By contrast, the term neonate's pinna is firm, stands away from the head, and springs back quickly from folding.

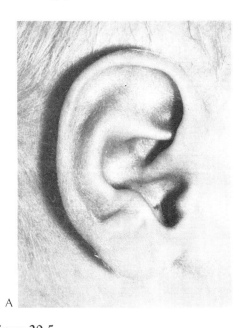

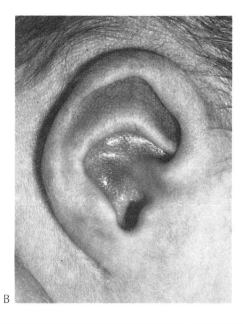

A   B

Figure 20-5

Ear form and cartilage. **A,** The ear of the infant at approximately 36 weeks' gestation shows incurving of the upper two-thirds of the pinna. **B,** Infant at term shows well-defined incurving of the entire pinna. (From Dubowitz L, Dubowitz V: *Gestational Age of the Newborn*. Menlo Park, Calif.: Addison-Wesley, 1977).

7. *Male genitals* are evaluated for size of the scrotal sac, the presence of rugae, and descent of the testes (Figure 20-6). Prior to 36 weeks, the small scrotum has few rugae, and the testes are palpable in the inguinal canal. By 36–38 weeks, the testes are in the upper scrotum, and rugae have developed over the anterior portion of the scrotum. By term, the testes are generally in the lower scrotum, which is pendulous and covered with rugae.

The appearance of the *female genitals* depends in part on subcutaneous fat deposition and therefore relates to fetal nutritional status (Figure 20-7). The clitoris varies in size and occasionally is so large that it is difficult to identify the sex of the infant. This may be caused by adrenogenital syndrome, which causes the adrenals to secrete excessive amounts of androgen and other hormones.

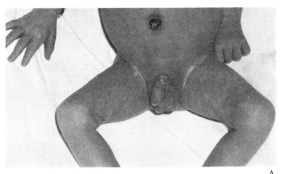
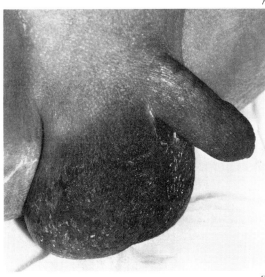

Figure 20-6
Male genitals. **A**, A preterm infant's testes are not within the scrotum. The scrotal surface has few rugae. **B**, Term infant's testes are generally fully descended. The entire surface of the scrotum is covered by rugae. (From Dubowitz L, Dubowitz V: *Gestational Age of the Newborn*. Menlo Park, Calif.: Addison-Wesley, 1977.)

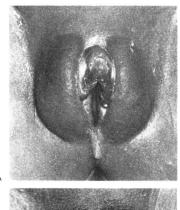

A

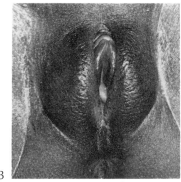

B

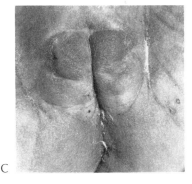

C

Figure 20-7
Female genitals. **A**, Infant has a prominent clitoris. The labia majora are widely separated, and the labia minora, viewed laterally, would protrude beyond the labia majora. The gestational age is 30–36 weeks. **B**, The clitoris is still visible; the labia minora are now covered by the larger labia majora. The gestational age is 36–40 weeks. **C**, The term infant has well-developed, large labia majora that cover both the clitoris and labia minora. (From Dubowitz L, Dubowitz V: *Gestational Age of the Newborn*. Menlo Park, Calif.: Addison-Wesley, 1977.)

Other physical characteristics assessed by some gestational age scoring tools include the following:

1. *Vernix* covers the preterm infant. The postterm infant has no vernix. After noting vernix distribution, the delivery room nurse dries the newborn to prevent evaporative heat loss, thus disturbing the vernix. The delivery room nurse must communicate to the neonatal nurse the amount of vernix and the areas of vernix coverage.

2. *Hair* of the preterm infant has the consistency of matted wool or fur and lies in bunches rather than in the silky, single strands of the term infant's hair.

3. *Skull firmness* increases as the infant matures. In a term neonate the bones are hard, and the sutures are not easily displaced. The clinician should not attempt to displace the sutures forceably.

4. *Nails* appear and cover the nail bed at about 20 weeks' gestation. Nails extending beyond the fingertips may be indicative of post-term neonate.

Assessment of Neurologic Status

The central nervous system of the human fetus matures at a fairly constant rate. Specific neurologic parameters correlated to gestational age have been established. Tests have been designed to evaluate neurologic status as manifested by neuromuscular tone development. In the fetus, neuromuscular tone develops from the lower to the upper extremities. The neurologic evaluation requires more manipulation and disturbances than the physical evaluation of the neonate. These assessments are difficult to carry out if the newborn is ill and requires supportive therapies that tend to immobilize the infant.

The neuromuscular evaluation (see Figure 20-1) is best performed when the infant has stabilized. The following characteristics are evaluated:

1. *Ankle dorsiflexion* is determined by flexing the ankle on the shin. The examiner uses a thumb to push on the sole of the neonate's foot while the fingers support the back of the neonate's leg. Then the angle formed between the foot and the interior leg is measured (Figure 20-8). This sign can be influenced by intrauterine position and congenital deformities.

2. The *square window sign* is elicited by flexing the neonate's hand toward the ventral forearm. The angle formed at the wrist is measured (Figure 20-9).

3. *Recoil* is a test of flexion development. Because flexion first develops in the lower extremities, recoil is first tested in the legs. The neonate is placed on his or her back on a flat surface. With a hand on the neonate's knees and while manipulating the hip joint, the nurse places the neonate's legs in flexion, then extends them parallel to each other and flat on the surface. The response to this maneuver is recoil of the neonate's legs. According to gestational age, they may not move or they may return slowly or quickly to the flexed position.

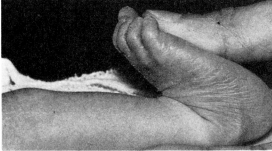

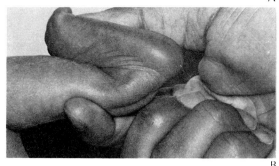

Figure 20-8 ▬▬▬
Ankle dorsiflexion. **A,** A 45° angle is indicative of 32–36 weeks' gestation. A 20° angle is indicative of 36–40 weeks' gestation. **B,** An angle of 0° is common at gestational age of 40 weeks or more. (From Dubowitz L, Dubowitz V: *Gestational Age of the Newborn*. Menlo Park, Calif.: Addison-Wesley, 1977.)

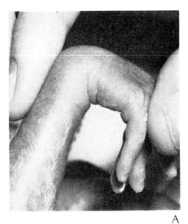
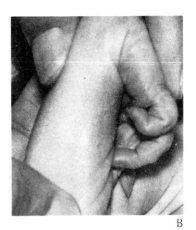
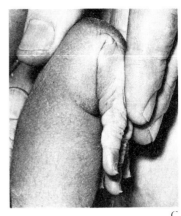

A   B   C

Figure 20-9

Square window sign. **A,** This angle is 90° and suggests an immature newborn of 28–32 weeks' gestation. **B,** A 30° angle is commonly found from 38–40 weeks' gestation. **C,** A 0° angle occurs from 40–42 weeks. (From Dubowitz L, Dubowitz V: *Gestational Age of the Newborn.* Menlo Park, Calif.: Addison-Wesley, 1977.)

Recoil in the upper extremities is tested by flexion at the elbow and extension of the arms at the neonate's side.

4. The *popliteal angle* is determined with the infant supine and flat. The thigh is flexed on the chest, and the examiner places an index finger behind the infant's ankle to extend the lower leg. The angle formed is then measured. Results vary from no resistance in the very immature infant to an 80° angle in the term infant.

5. The *heel-to-ear maneuver* is performed by placing the infant in a supine position and then gently drawing the foot toward the ear on the same side until resistance is felt. Both the popliteal angle and the proximity of foot to ear are assessed. In a very immature infant, the leg will remain straight and the foot will go to the ear or beyond. Maneuvers involving the lower extremities of newborns who had frank breech presentation should be delayed to allow for resolution of leg positioning (Ballard et al., 1979).

6. The **scarf sign** is elicited by placing the neonate supine and drawing an arm across the chest toward the infant's opposite shoulder until resistance is met. The location of the elbow is then noted (Figure 20-10).

7. Head lag (*neck flexors*) is measured by pulling the neonate to a sitting position and noting the degree of head lag. Total lag is common in infants up to 34 weeks' gestation, whereas postmature infants (42 weeks) will hold their head in front of their body line.

8. Ventral suspension (*horizontal position*) is evaluated by holding the infant prone on the examiner's hand. The position of head and back and degree of flexion in the arms and legs are then noted. Some flexion of arms and legs indicates 36–38 weeks' gestation; fully flexed extremities, with head and back even, are characteristic of a term neonate.

9. *Major reflexes* such as sucking, rooting, grasping, Moro, tonic neck, and others are evaluated and scored.

Determination of gestational age and correlation with birth weight (Figure 22-1) enables the nurse to assess the infant more accurately and to anticipate possible physiologic problems. This information is then used in conjunction with a complete physical examination to determine priorities and to establish a plan of care appropriate to the individual infant.

Physical Examination

After the initial determination of gestational age and related potential problems, a more extensive physical assessment is done. The nursing student is expected to be able to do most of the assessments, although she or he may not be required to know all the alterations and possible causes. The nurse should choose a warm,

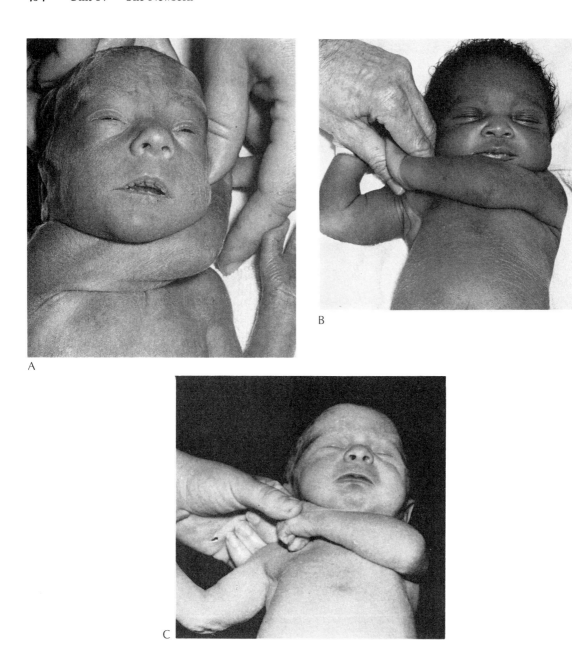

Figure 20-10

Scarf sign. **A**, No resistance is noted until after 30 weeks' gestation. The elbow can be readily moved past the midline. **B**, The elbow is at midline at 36–40 weeks' gestation. **C**, Beyond 40 weeks' gestation, the elbow will not reach the midline. (From Dubowitz L, Dubowitz V: *Gestational Age of the Newborn*. Menlo Park, Calif.: Addison-Wesley, 1977.)

well-lighted area that is free of drafts. Completing the physical assessment in the presence of the parents provides an opportunity to acquaint them with their unique newborn. The examination should be performed in a systematic manner and all findings recorded. When assessing the physical and neurologic status of the newborn, the nurse should first consider general appearance and then proceed to specific areas.

General Appearance

The newborn's head is disproportionately large for the body. The center of the baby's body is the umbilicus rather than the symphysis pubis, as in the adult. The body appears long and the extremities short. The flexed position that the neonate maintains contributes to the apparent shortness of the extremities. The hands are tightly clenched. The neck looks short because the chin rests on the chest. Newborns have a prominent abdomen, sloping shoulders, narrow hips, and rounded chests. They tend to stay in a flexed position similar to the one maintained in utero and will offer resistance when the extremities are straightened. After a breech delivery, the feet are usually dorsiflexed, and it may take several weeks for the newborn to assume typical newborn posture.

Weight and Measurements

The normal full-term Caucasian newborn has an average birth weight of 3405 g (7 lb, 8 oz), whereas Black, Oriental, and American Indian newborns are usually somewhat smaller. Other factors that influence weight are age and size of parents, health of mother, and the interval between pregnancies. After the first week and for the first 6 months, the neonate's weight will increase about 198 g (7 oz) weekly.

Approximately 70%–75% of the neonate's body weight is water. During the initial newborn period (the first 3 or 4 days), there is a physiologic weight loss of about 5%–10% for term infants because of fluid shifts. This weight loss may reach 15% for preterm infants. Large babies may also tend to lose more weight because of greater fluid loss in proportion to birth weight. If weight loss is greater than expected, clinical reappraisal is indicated. Factors contributing to weight loss include small fluid intake resulting from delayed breast-feeding or a slow adjustment to the formula, increased volume of meconium excreted, and urination. Weight loss may be marked in the presence of temperature elevation because of associated dehydration.

The length of the normal newborn is difficult to measure because the legs are flexed and tensed. To measure length, the nurse should place infants flat on their backs with legs extended as much as possible (Figure 20-11). The average length is 49.4 cm (19.5 in), with the range being 45.8–52.3 cm (18–20.5 in). The newborn will grow approximately an inch a

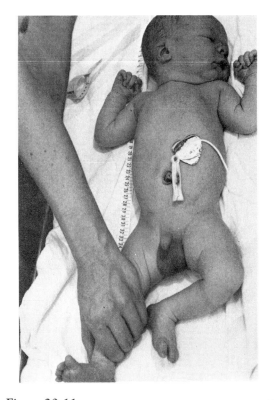

Figure 20-11
Measuring the length of a newborn. From Swearingen PL: *Photo-Atlas of Nursing.* Menlo Park, Calif.: Addison-Wesley, 1984.)

month for the next 6 months. This is the period of most rapid growth.

At birth, the newborn's head is one-third the size of an adult's head. The circumference of the newborn's head is 33–35 cm (13–14 in). For accurate measurement, the tape is placed over the most prominent part of the occiput and brought to just above the eyebrows (Figure 20–12A). The circumference of the newborn's head is approximately 2 cm greater than the circumference of the newborn's chest at birth and will remain in this proportion for the next few months. (Factors that alter this measurement are discussed on p. 439.)

The average circumference of the chest at birth is 32 cm (12.5 in). Chest measurements should be taken with the tape measure at the lower edge of the scapulas and brought around anteriorly directly over the nipple line (Figure 20-12B). The abdominal circumference or girth may also be measured at this time by placing

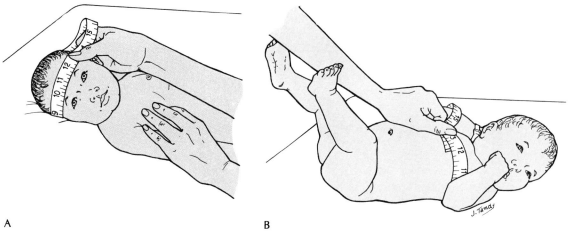

A   B

Figure 20-12

A, Measuring the head circumference of the newborn. **B**, Measuring the chest circumference of the newborn.

the tape around the newborn's abdomen at the level of the umbilicus, with the bottom edge of the tape at the top edge of the umbilicus. (See Essential Facts to Remember—Measurements.)

 ESSENTIAL FACTS TO REMEMBER

Measurements

Weight:

Average: 3405 g (7 lb, 8 oz)

Range: 2950–3515 g (6 lb, 8 oz–7 lb, 12 oz)

Weight depends on racial origin and maternal age and size

Physiologic weight loss: 5%–10% for term infants, up to 15% for preterm infants

Growth: 7 oz (198 g) per week for first 6 months

Length:

Average: 49.4 cm (19.5 in)

Range: 45.8–52.3 cm (18–20.5 in)

Growth: 1 inch (2.5 cm) per month for first 6 months.

Head circumference:

33–35 cm (13–14 in)

Approximately 2 cm larger than chest circumference

Temperature

Initial assessment of the newborn's temperature is critical. In utero, the temperature of the fetus is about the same as or slightly higher than the expectant mother's. When the infant enters the outside world, his or her temperature can suddenly drop as a result of exposure to cold drafts and the skin's heat-loss mechanisms. Upon arrival in the nursery, a newborn's skin temperature may be as low as 36C (96.8F) if the newborn was not dried and placed under a radiant warmer in the delivery room (Korones, 1981). The temperature should stabilize within 8–12 hours. Temperature should be monitored at least every hour until stable, then every 4 hours for 24 hours (Standards and Recommendations for Hospital Care of Newborn Infants, 1977). Many institutions use a continuous probe, or measurements are obtained every 15–30 minutes for the first hour, then each hour for 4 hours. (See Chapter 19 for a discussion of the physiology of temperature regulation.)

The temperature may be taken either by axilla or rectally (Figure 20-13). In some agencies the initial temperature is taken rectally; other agencies rely exclusively on axillary methods. The rectal route is not recommended as a routine method as it may predispose to rectal mucosal irritation and increase chances of perforation (Avery, 1981). If the temperature is taken rectally, the nurse holds the thermometer in the rectum for 5 minutes. Care must be taken

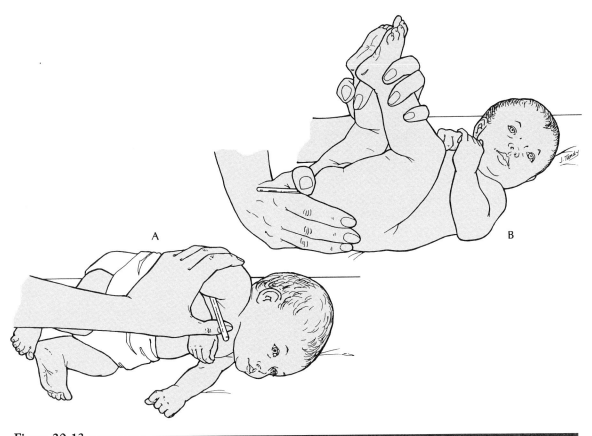

Figure 20-13
The axillary temperature should be taken for 3 minutes. The newborn's arm should be tightly but gently pressed against the thermometer and the newborn's side as illustrated. The rectal thermometer must be held in place for 5 minutes and the legs supported.

to avoid inserting the thermometer too far. It is not unusual for an imperforate anus to be diagnosed initially when the nurse is unable to take the temperature rectally.

Axillary temperature reflects skin temperature and the body's compensatory response to changes in the thermal environment. Some clinicians question the accuracy of axillary temperature in the first 24 hours of life because peripheral circulation is poor in newborns. Skin temperature assessment allows time for initiation of interventions prior to a more serious fall in the core temperature as assessed by rectal temperatures. If the axillary method is used, the thermometer must remain in place at least 3 minutes (Standards and Recommendations for Hospital Care of Newborn Infants, 1977) unless an electronic thermometer is used. Axillary temperatures can be misleading because of friction caused by apposition of inner arm skin and upper chest wall and nearness of brown fat to the probe. The best measure of skin temperature is by means of continuous skin probe rather than axillary temperature, especially for small neonates.

Temperature instability, a deviation of more than 1C (2F) from one reading to the next, or a subnormal temperature may indicate an infection. In contrast with an elevated temperature in older children, an increased temperature in a newborn may indicate reactions to too much covering, too hot a room, or dehydration. Dehydration, which tends to increase body temperature, occurs in newborns whose feedings have been delayed for any reason. Newborns respond to overheating (temperature greater than 37.5C or 99.5F) by increased restlessness and eventually by perspiration. The perspiration is initially seen on the head and face, then on the chest.

Skin

The skin of the newborn should be pink-tinged or ruddy in color and warm to the touch. The ruddy color results from increased concentration of red blood cells in the blood vessels and from limited subcutaneous fat deposits.

Acrocyanosis   **Acrocyanosis** (bluish discoloration of the hands and feet) may be present in the first 2–6 hours after birth. This condition is due to poor peripheral circulation, which results in vasomotor instability and capillary stasis, especially when the newborn is exposed to cold. If the central circulation is adequate, the blood supply should return quickly when the skin is blanched with a finger.

Harlequin Sign   *Harlequin* (clown) color change is occasionally noted: A deep red color develops over one side of the infant's body while the other side remains pale, so that the skin resembles a clown's suit. This color change results from a vasomotor disturbance in which blood vessels on one side dilate while the vessels on the other side constrict. It usually lasts from 1–20 minutes. Affected neonates may have single or multiple episodes.

Jaundice   *Jaundice* is evaluated by blanching the tip of the nose or the gum line. This procedure must be carried out in appropriate lighting. If jaundice is present, the area will appear yellowish immediately after blanching. Evaluation and determination of the cause of jaundice must be initiated immediately to prevent possibly serious sequelae. The jaundice may be related to breast-feeding (small incidence), hematomas, or immature liver function, or it may be caused by blood incompatibility or severe hemolytic process.

Erythema neonatorum toxicum   **Erythema toxicum** is a perifollicular eruption of lesions that are firm, vary in size from 1–3 mm, and consist of a white or pale yellow papule or pustule with an erythematous base. The rash may appear suddenly, usually over the trunk and diaper area, and is frequently widespread. The lesions do not appear on the palms of the hands or the soles of the feet. The peak incidence is at 24–48 hours of life. Diagnosis may be confirmed by obtaining a smear of aspirated pustule, which after staining shows numerous eosinophils and no bacteria are cultured. The cause is unknown and no treatment is necessary. The lesions disappear in a few hours or days.

Skin turgor   *Skin turgor* is assessed to determine hydration status, the need to initiate early feedings, and the presence of any infectious processes.

Vernix caseosa   *Vernix caseosa*, a whitish cheeselike substance, covers the fetus while in utero and lubricates the skin of the newborn. The skin of the term or postterm infant has less vernix and is frequently dry, and peeling is common, especially on the hands and feet. **Milia**, which are plugged sebaceous glands, appear as raised white spots on the face, especially across the nose.

Mongolian spots   **Mongolian spots** are macular areas of bluish-black pigmentation found on the lumbar dorsal area and the buttocks. They are common in Oriental and Black infants and newborns of other dark-skinned races. They gradually fade during the first or second year of life.

Forceps marks   Forceps marks may be present after a difficult forceps delivery. The newborn may have reddened areas over the cheeks and jaws. It is important to reassure the parents that these will disappear, usually within 1 or 2 days. Transient facial paralysis resulting from the forceps pressure is a rare complication.

Telangiectatic nevi   **Telangiectatic nevi, or "stork bites,"** appear as pale pink or red spots and are frequently found on the eyelids, nose, lower occipital bone, and nape of the neck. These lesions are common in light-complexioned neonates and are more noticeable during periods of crying. These areas blanch easily, have no clinical significance, and usually fade by the second birthday.

Nevus flammeus   *Nevus flammeus*, or port-wine stain, is a capillary angioma directly below the epidermis. It is a nonelevated, sharply demarcated, red to purple birthmark. The size and shape is variable but it commonly appears on the face. It does not grow in size, does not fade with time, and does not blanch. In the Black infant, the nevus flammeus appears jet black in color. The birthmark may be concealed by using an opaque cosmetic cream such as "covermark."

Nevus vasculosus *Nevus vasculosus*, or "strawberry mark," is a capillary hemangioma. It consists of newly formed and enlarged capillaries in the dermal and subdermal layers. It is a raised, clearly delineated, dark red, rough-surfaced birthmark commonly found in the head region. Such marks usually grow (often rapidly) for several months and become fixed in size by 8 months. They then begin to shrink, and, except in rare cases, are completely gone by the time the child is 7 years old.

Birthmarks are frequently a cause of concern for the parents. The mother may be especially anxious, fearing that she is to blame ("Is my baby 'marked' because of something I did?"). Guilt feelings are common in the presence of misconceptions about the cause. Birthmarks should be identified and explained to the parents. By providing appropriate information about the cause and course of birthmarks, the nurse frequently relieves the fears and anxieties of the family.

Head

General appearance   The newborn's head is large (approximately one-fourth of the body size), with soft, pliable skull bones. The head may appear asymmetrical in the newborn of a vertex delivery. This asymmetry, called **molding**, is caused by overriding of the cranial bones during labor and delivery. Within a few days after delivery, the overriding usually diminishes and the suture lines become palpable. Because head measurements are affected by molding, a second measurement is indicated a few days after delivery. The heads of breech-born newborns and those delivered by cesarean birth are characteristically round and well shaped since pressure was not exerted on them during birth. Any extreme differences in head size may indicate microcephaly or hydrocephalus. Variations in the shape, size, or appearance of the head measurements may be due to *craniostenosis* (premature closure of the cranial sutures) and *plagiocephaly* (asymmetry caused by pressure on the fetal head during gestation).

Two *fontanelles* ("soft spots") may be palpated on the infant's head. Fontanelles, which are openings at the juncture of the cranial bones, can be measured with the fingers. Accurate measurement necessitates that the examiner's finger be measured in centimeters. The diamond-shaped *anterior fontanelle* is approximately 3–4 cm long by 2–3 cm wide. It is located at the juncture of the frontal and parietal bones. The *posterior fontanelle*, smaller and triangular, is formed by the parietal bones and the occipital bone. The fontanelles will be smaller immediately after birth than several days later because of molding. The anterior fontanelle closes within 18 months, whereas the posterior fontanelle closes within 8–12 weeks.

The fontanelles are a useful indicator of the newborn's condition. The anterior fontanelle may swell when the newborn cries or may pulsate with the heartbeat, which is normal. A bulging fontanelle usually signifies increased intracranial pressure, and a depressed fontanelle indicates dehydration. The sutures between the cranial bones should be palpated for amount of overlapping.

In addition to being inspected for degree of molding and size, the head should be evaluated for soft tissue edema and bruising.

Cephalhematoma   **Cephalhematoma** is a collection of blood resulting from ruptured blood vessels between the surface of a cranial bone and the periosteal membrane. The scalp in these areas feels loose and slightly edematous. These areas emerge as defined hematomas between the first and second day. Although external pressure may cause the mass to fluctuate, it does not increase in size when the infant cries. Cephalhematomas may be unilateral or bilateral and do not cross suture lines. They are relatively common in vertex deliveries and may disappear within 2–3 weeks or very slowly over subsequent months (Danforth, 1982). Figure 20-14 shows a cephalhematoma.

Caput succedaneum   **Caput succedaneum** is a localized, easily identifiable soft area of the scalp, generally resulting from a long and difficult labor or vacuum extraction. The sustained pressure of the presenting part against the cervix results in compression of local blood vessels, and venous return is slowed. This causes

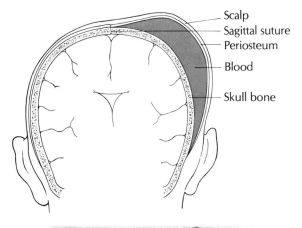

Scalp
Sagittal suture
Periosteum
Blood
Skull bone

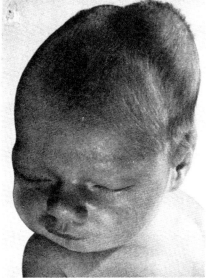

Figure 20-14

Cephalhematoma is a collection of blood between the surface of a cranial bone and the periosteal membrane. Cephalhematoma over left parietal bone. (Photo: Reproduced with permission from Potter, E. L. and Craig, J. M.: *Pathology of the Fetus and Infant*, 3rd ed. Copyright © 1975 by Year Book Medical Publisher, Inc. Chicago.)

an increase in tissue fluids, an edematous swelling, and occasional bleeding under the periosteum. The caput may vary from a small area to a severely elongated head. The fluid in the caput is reabsorbed within 12 hours or a few days after birth. Caputs resulting from vacuum extractors are sharply outlined, circular areas up to 2 cm thick. They disappear more slowly than naturally occurring edema. It is possible to distinguish between a cephalhematoma and a caput

because the caput overrides suture lines (Figure 20-15), whereas the cephalhematoma, because of its location, never crosses a suture line.

Face

The newborn's face is well designed to help the infant suckle. Sucking (fat) pads are located in the cheeks, and a labial tubercle is frequently found in the center of the upper lip. The chin is recessed, and the nose is flattened. The lips are sensitive to touch, and the sucking reflex is easily initiated.

Symmetry of the eyes, nose, and ears is evaluated. See the Neonatal Physical Assessment Guide, p. 451, for deviations in symmetry and variations in size, shape, and spacing of facial features. Facial movement symmetry should be assessed to determine presence of facial palsy.

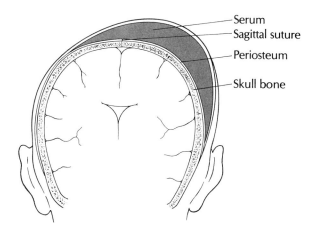

Serum
Sagittal suture
Periosteum
Skull bone

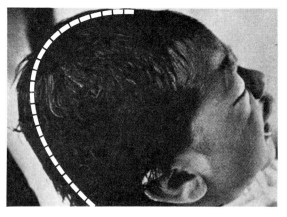

Figure 20-15

Caput succedaneum is a collection of fluid (serum) under the scalp. (Photo courtesy Mead Johnson and Company, Evansville, Ind.)

Facial paralysis appears when the neonate cries; the affected side is immobile and the palpebral (eyelid) fissure widens (Figure 20-16). Paralysis may result from forceps delivery or pressure on the facial nerve from the maternal pelvis during birth. Facial paralysis usually disappears within a few days to 3 weeks.

Eyes   The eyes of the Caucasian neonate are a blue or slate blue gray. Scleral color tends to be bluish because of its relative thinness. The infant's eye color usually is established at approximately 3 months, although it may change any time up to 1 year. Dark-skinned neonates tend to have dark eyes at birth.

The eyes should be checked for size, equality of pupil size, reaction of pupils to light, blink reflex to light, and edema and inflammation of the eyelids. The eyelids are usually edematous during the first few days of life because of the delivery and the instillation of silver nitrate drops in the newborn's eyes. Chemical conjunctivitis appears a few hours after the instillation of the silver nitrate drops but disappears without treatment in 1–2 days. If infectious conjunctivitis exists, the infant has the same purulent exudate as in chemical conjunctivitis, but it is caused by staphylococci or a variety of Gram-negative bacteria and requires treatment with ophthalmic antibiotics. Onset is usually after the second day.

Edema of the orbits or eyelids may persist for several days until the neonate's kidneys can evacuate the fluid.

Small subconjunctival hemorrhages appear in about 10% of newborns and are commonly found on the inner aspect of the sclera. These are caused by the changes in vascular tension during birth. They will remain for a few weeks and are of no pathologic significance. Parents need reassurance that the infant is not bleeding from within the eye and that vision will not be impaired.

The neonate may demonstrate transient strabismus caused by poor neuromuscular control of eye muscles (Figure 20-17). It gradually regresses in 3–4 months. The "doll's eye" phenomenon is also present for about 10 days after birth. As the newborn's head position is changed to the left and then to the right, the eyes move to the opposite direction. This results from underdeveloped integration of head-eye coordination.

The nurse should observe the neonate's pupils for opacities or whiteness. Congenital cataracts should be suspected in infants of mothers with a history of rubella, cytomegalic inclusion disease, or syphilis.

The cry of the neonate is commonly tearless because the lacrimal structures are immature at birth and are not usually fully functional until the second month of life. Some infants may produce tears during the neonatal period. Poor oculomotor coordination and absence of

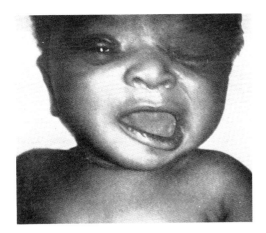

Figure 20-16
Facial paralysis. Paralysis of right side of face from injury to right facial nerve. (Courtesy of Dr. Ralph Platow. In Potter, E. L. and Craig, J. M.: *Pathology of the fetus and infant*, 3rd ed. Copyright © 1975 by Year Book Medical Publishers, Inc. Chicago.)

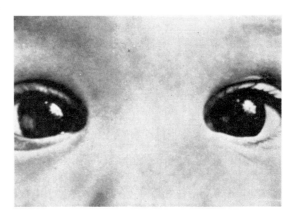

Figure 20-17
Transient strabismus may be present in the newborn due to poor neuromuscular control. (Courtesy Mead Johnson and Company, Evansville, Ind. 47721.)

accommodation limit visual abilities, but the newborn does have peripheral vision and can fixate on near objects (9–12 in) for short periods (Ludington-Hoe, 1983). The newborn can perceive faces, shapes, and colors and begins to show visual preferences early. The neonate blinks in response to bright lights, to a tap on the bridge of the nose (glabellar reflex), or to a light touch on the eyelids. Pupillary light reflex is also present. Examination of the eye is best accomplished by rocking the newborn from an upright position to the horizontal a few times or by other methods that will elicit an opened-eye response.

Nose   The neonate's nose is small and narrow. Infants are characteristically nose breathers for the first few months of life. The newborn generally removes obstructions by sneezing. Nasal patency is assured if the neonate breathes easily with mouth closed. If respiratory difficulty occurs, the nurse checks for choanal atresia.

The newborn has the ability to smell after the nasal passages are cleared of amniotic fluid and mucus. This ability is demonstrated by the search for milk. Infants will turn their heads toward the milk source, whether bottle or breast.

Mouth   The lips of the newborn should be pink, and a touch on the lips should produce sucking motions. Saliva is normally scant. The taste buds are developed prior to birth, and the newborn can easily discriminate between sweet and bitter.

The easiest way to completely examine the mouth is to gently stimulate infants to cry by depressing their tongue, thereby causing them to open the mouth fully. It is extremely important to observe the entire mouth to look for a cleft palate, which can be present even in the absence of a cleft lip. The examiner places a clean index finger along the hard and soft palate to feel for any openings.

Occasionally, an examination of the gums will reveal *precocious teeth* on the lower central incisor. If they appear loose, they should be removed to prevent aspiration. Gray-white lesions (*inclusion cysts*) on the gums may be confused with teeth. On the hard palate and gum margins, **Epstein's pearls**, small glistening white specks (keratin-containing cysts) that feel hard to the touch are often present. These

usually disappear in a few weeks and are of no significance. Thrush may appear as white patches that look like milk curds adhering to the mucous membranes and that cause bleeding when removed. Thrush is caused by *Candida albicans*, often acquired from an infected vaginal tract during birth, and is treated with a preparation of nystatin (Mycostatin).

A neonate who is *tongue-tied* has a ridge of frenulum tissue attached to the underside of the tongue at varying lengths from its base, causing a heart shape at the tip of the tongue. "Clipping the tongue," or cutting the ridge of tissue, is not recommended. This ridge does not affect speech or eating, but cutting does create an entry for infection.

Transient nerve paralysis resulting from birth trauma may be manifested by asymmetrical mouth movements when the neonate cries or by difficulty with sucking and feeding.

Ears   The ears of the newborn may be crumpled or flattened against the skull and should have well-formed cartilage (one appropriate for gestational age). In the normal newborn, the top of the ear should be parallel to the outer and inner canthus of the eye. The ears should be inspected for shape, size, and position. *Low-set ears* are characteristic of many syndromes and may indicate chromosomal abnormalities (especially trisomies 13 and 18), mental retardation, and/or internal organ abnormalities, especially bilateral renal agenesis as a result of embryologic developmental deviations (Figure 20-18). *Preauricular skin tags* may be present. They are ligated at the base and allowed to slough off.

Following the first cry, the newborn can hear. Hearing becomes acute as mucus from the middle ear is absorbed and the eustachian tube becomes aerated.

Downs and Silver (1972) have identified the following risk factors associated with potential hearing loss:

- The presence of hearing loss in any family member prior to the age of 50 years

- Serum bilirubin level greater than 20 mg/dL for the full-term newborn

- Suspected maternal rubella infection during pregnancy, resulting in congenital rubella syndrome

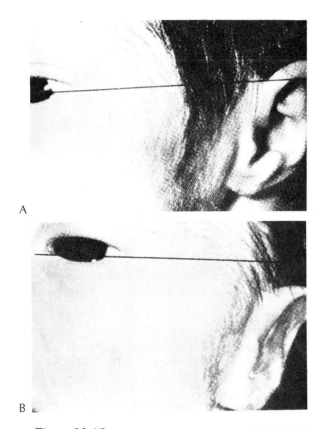

A

B

Figure 20-18 ▬▬▬▬▬
The position of the external ear may be assessed by drawing a line across the inner and outer canthus of the eye to the insertion of the ear. **A**, Normal position. **B**, True low-set. (Courtesy Mead Johnson and Company, Evansville, Ind. 47721.)

- Defects of the ear, nose, or throat
- Small neonatal size, particularly less than 1500 g at birth

The newborn's hearing is evaluated by response to loud or moderately loud noises unaccompanied by vibrations. The sleeping neonate should stir or awaken in response to the nearby sounds.

Neck

A short neck, creased with skin folds, is characteristic of the normal newborn. Because muscle tone is not well developed, the neck cannot support the full weight of the head, which rotates freely. The head lags considerably when the neonate is pulled from a supine to a sitting position, but the prone infant is able to raise the head slightly. The neck is palpated for masses and presence of lymph nodes and is inspected for webbing. Adequacy of range of motion and neck muscle function is determined by fully extending the head in all directions. Injury to the sternocleidomastoid muscle (congenital torticollis) must be considered in the presence of neck rigidity.

The clavicles are evaluated for evidence of fractures, which occasionally occur during difficult deliveries or in neonates with broad shoulders. The normal clavicle is straight. If fractured, a lump and a grating sensation during movements may be palpated along the course of the side of the break. The Moro reflex (p. 449) is also elicited to evaluate bilateral equal movement of the arms. If the clavicle is fractured, the response will be demonstrated only on the unaffected side.

Chest

The thorax is cylindrical at birth, and the ribs are flexible. The general appearance of the chest should be assessed. A protrusion at the lower end of the sternum, called the *xiphoid cartilage*, is frequently seen. It is under the skin and will become less apparent after several weeks as the infant accumulates adipose tissue.

Engorged breasts occur frequently in male and female newborns. This condition, which occurs by the third day, is a result of maternal hormonal influences and may last up to 2 weeks. The infant's breast should not be massaged or squeezed, because this practice may cause a breast abscess. Extra or *supernumerary nipples* are occasionally noted below and medial to the true nipples (Figure 20-19). These harmless pink spots vary in size and do not contain glandular tissue (Korones, 1981). Accessory nipples can be differentiated from a pigmented nevi (mole) by placing the fingertips alongside the accessory nipple and pulling the adjacent tissue laterally. The accessory nipple will appear dimpled.

Cry

The neonate's cry should be strong, lusty, and of medium pitch. A high-pitched, shrill cry is abnormal and may indicate neurologic disorders or hypoglycemia. Cries vary in length from 3–7 min after consoling measures are used. The neonate's cry is an important method of communication and alerts caretakers to changes in his or her condition and needs.

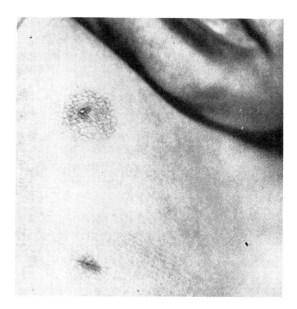

Figure 20-19

Extra or supernumerary nipples may appear below and medial to the true nipples. (Courtesy Mead Johnson and Company, Evansville, Indiana 47721)

Respiration

Normal breathing for a term newborn is predominantly diaphragmatic, with associated rising and falling of the abdomen during inspiration and expiration. Any signs of respiratory distress, nasal flaring, intercostal or xiphoid retraction, expiratory grunt or sigh, seesaw respirations, or tachypnea should be noted. Hyperextension (chest appears high) or hypoextension (chest appears low) of the anteroposterior diameter of the chest should also be noted. Both the anterior and posterior chest are auscultated. Some breath sounds are heard better when the neonate is crying, but localization and identification of breath sounds are difficult in the newborn. Because sounds may be transmitted from the unaffected lung to the affected lung, the absence of breath sounds cannot be diagnosed. Air entry may be noisy in the first couple of hours until lung fluid resolves, especially in cesarean births.

Heart

Heart rates are rapid (120–180 beats/min) in neonates but fluctuate a great deal. Auscultation provides the nurse with valuable assessment data. The heart is examined for rate and rhythm, position of apical impulse, and heart sound intensity.

The pulse rate is variable and follows the trend of respirations in the neonatal period. The pulse rate is influenced by physical activity, crying, state of wakefulness, and body temperature. Auscultation is performed over the entire precordia, below the left axilla, and below the scapula. Apical pulse rates are obtained by auscultation for a full minute preferably when the neonate is asleep.

The placement of the heart in the chest should be determined when the neonate is in a quiet state. The heart is relatively large at birth and is located high in the chest, with its apex somewhere between the fourth and fifth intercostal space.

A shift in the mediastinum to either side may indicate pneumothorax, dextrocardia (heart placement on the right side of the chest), or a diaphragmatic hernia. The experienced nurse can diagnose these and many other problems early with a stethoscope. Normally, the heart beat has a "toc tic" sound. A slur or slushing sound (usually after the first sound) may indicate a *murmur*. Although 90% of all murmurs are transient and are considered normal (Korones, 1981), they should be observed closely by a physician.

In infants, a low-pitched, musical murmur heard just to the right of the apex of the heart is fairly common. Occasionally, significant murmurs will be heard, including the murmur of a patent ductus arteriosus, aortic or pulmonary stenosis, or small ventricular septal defect. See Chapter 22 for a discussion of congenital heart defects.

Mottling (lacy pattern of dilated blood vessels under the skin) also occurs as a result of general circulation fluctuations. It may last several hours to several weeks or may come and go periodically.

Peripheral pulses (brachial, femoral, pedal) are also evaluated to detect any lags or unusual characteristics. Brachial pulses are palpated bilaterally for equality and compared with the femoral pulses. Femoral pulses are palpated by applying gentle pressure with the middle finger over the femoral canal. Decreased or absent femoral pulses indicate coarctation of the aorta and require additional investigation. A wide difference in blood pressure between the upper and lower extremities also indicates coarctation. The measurement of blood pressure is best accomplished by using the Doppler technique or a 1–2 inch cuff and a stethoscope over the brachial artery.

Blood pressures are not routinely measured on newborns unless they are having distress, are premature, or are suspected of some anomaly. For pertinent aspects of vital signs, see Essential Facts to Remember—Vital Signs.

Abdomen

Without disturbing the infant, the nurse can learn a great deal about the newborn's abdomen. It should be cylindrical and protrude slightly. A certain amount of laxness of the abdominal muscles is normal. A scaphoid appearance suggests the absence of abdominal contents. No cyanosis should be present, and few if any blood vessels should be apparent to the eye. There should be no gross distention or bulging. The more distended the abdomen, the tighter the skin becomes, with engorged vessels appearing. Distention is the first sign of many of the abnormalities found in the gastrointestinal tract.

ESSENTIAL FACTS TO REMEMBER

Vital Signs

Pulse:

120–150 beats/min

During sleep as low as 100 beats/min; if crying, up to 180 beats/min

Apical pulse is counted for one (1) full minute

Respirations:

30–50 respirations/min

Predominantly diaphragmatic but synchronous with abdominal movements

Blood Pressure:

80–60/45–40 mm Hg at birth

100/50 mm Hg at day 10

Temperature:

Axillary: 36.5–37C (97.7–98.6F)

Skin: 36–36.5C (96.8–97.7F)

Rectal: 36.6–37.2C (97.8–99F)

Abdominal palpation should be done systematically. The nurse palpates each of the four abdominal quadrants and moves in a clockwise direction until all four quadrants have been palpated for softness, tenderness, and the presence of masses.

Umbilical Cord

Initially the umbilical cord is white and gelatinous in appearance, with the two umbilical arteries and one umbilical vein readily apparent. Because a single umbilical artery is frequently associated with congenital anomalies, the vessels should be counted as part of the newborn assessment. The cord begins drying within 1 or 2 hours after delivery and is shriveled and blackened by the second or third day. Within 7–10 days, it sloughs off, although a granulating area may remain for a few days longer.

Cord bleeding is abnormal and may result because the cord was inadvertently pulled or because the cord clamp was loosened. Foul-smelling drainage is also abnormal and is generally caused by infection. Such infection requires immediate treatment to prevent the development of septicemia. If the neonate has a patent urachus (abnormal connection between the umbilicus and bladder), moistness or draining urine may be apparent at the base of the cord.

Genitals

Female infants The labia majora, labia minora, and clitoris are examined, and the nurse notes the size of each as appropriate for gestational age. A vaginal tag or hymenal tag is often evident and will usually disappear in a few weeks. During the first week of life, the neonate may have a vaginal discharge composed of thick whitish mucus. This discharge, which can become tinged with blood, is referred to as **pseudomenstruation** and is caused by the withdrawal of maternal hormones. Smegma, a white cheeselike substance, is often present under the labia.

Male infants The penis is inspected to determine whether the urinary orifice is correctly positioned. *Hypospadias* occurs when the urinary meatus is located on the ventral surface of the penis. It occurs most commonly in whites in the United States. *Phimosis* is a condition commonly occurring in newborn males in which the opening of the prepuce is narrowed and the foreskin cannot be retracted over the glans. This condition may interfere with urination, so the adequacy of the urinary stream should be evaluated.

The scrotum is inspected for size and symmetry and should be palpated to verify the presence of both testes. The testes are palpated separately between the thumb and forefinger, with the thumb and forefinger of the other hand placed together over the inguinal canal. Scrotal edema and discoloration are common in breech deliveries. Hydroceles are common in newborns and should be identified.

Anus

The anal area is inspected to verify that it is patent and has no fissure. Imperforate anus and rectal atresia may be ruled out by a digital examination. The passage of the first meconium stool is also noted. Atresia of the gastrointestinal tract or meconium ileus with resultant obstruction must be considered if the infant does not pass meconium in the first 24 hours of life.

Extremities

Extremities are examined for gross deformities, extra digits or webbing, clubfoot, and range of motion. The normal neonate's extremities appear short, are generally flexible, and move symmetrically.

Arms and hands Nails extend beyond the fingertips in term infants. Fingers and toes should be counted. *Polydactyly* is the presence of extra digits on either the hands or feet. Polydactyly is more common in Blacks. If the infant has polydactyly and the parents do not, a dominant genetic disorder can be ruled out. *Syndactyly* refers to fusion (webbing) of fingers or toes. Hands should be inspected for normal palmar creases. A single palmar crease, called *simian line* (see Figure 3-13) is frequently present in children with Down syndrome. (See Chapter 3 for further discussion.)

Brachial palsy, which is partial or complete paralysis of portions of the arm, results from trauma to the brachial plexus during a difficult delivery. It occurs most commonly when strong traction is exerted on the head of the neonate in an attempt to deliver a shoulder lodged behind the symphysis pubis in the presence of shoulder dystocia. Brachial palsy may also occur during a breech delivery if an arm becomes trapped over the head and traction is exerted.

The portion of the arm affected is determined by the nerves damaged. **Erb-Duchenne paralysis** involves damage to the upper arm (fifth and sixth cervical nerves) and is the most common type. Injury to the eighth cervical and first thoracic nerve roots and the lower portion of the plexus produces the relatively rare *lower arm injury*. The *whole arm type* results from damage to the entire plexus.

With Erb-Duchenne paralysis, the infant's arm lies limply at the side. The elbow is held in extension, with the forearm pronated. The infant is unable to elevate the arm, and the Moro reflex cannot be elicited on the affected side (Figure 20-20). When lower arm injury occurs, paralysis of the hand and wrist results; complete paralysis of the limb occurs with the whole arm type.

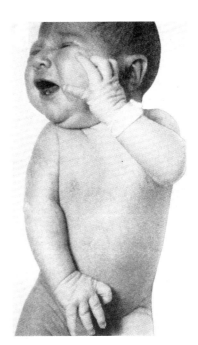

Figure 20-20 ▬▬▬▬
Erb's palsy resulting from injury to fifth and sixth cervical roots of brachial plexus. (Photo: Reproduced with permission from Potter, E. L. and Craig, J. M.: *Pathology of the Fetus and Infant*, 3rd ed. Copyright © 1975 by Year Book Medical Publishers, Inc. Chicago.)

Treatment involves passive range-of-motion exercises to prevent muscle contractures and to restore function. The nurse should carefully instruct the parents in the correct method of performing the exercises and provide for supervised practice sessions. In more severe cases, splinting of the arm is indicated until the edema decreases. The arm is held in a position of abduction and external rotation with the elbow flexed 90°. The "Statue of Liberty" splint is commonly used, although similar results are obtained by attaching a strip of muslin to the head of the crib and tying the other end around the wrist, thereby holding the arm up.

Prognosis is related to the degree of nerve damage resulting from trauma and hemorrhage within the nerve sheath. Complete recovery occurs within a few months with minimal trauma. Moderate trauma may result in some partial paralysis. Recovery is unlikely with severe trauma, and muscle wasting may develop.

Legs and feet   The legs of the newborn should be of equal length, with symmetrical skin folds. *Ortolani's maneuver* is performed to rule out the possibility of congenital hip dysplasia. With the neonate supine, the nurse places thumbs on the inner thighs and fingers on the outer aspect of the neonate's leg from the knee to the head of the femur. The legs are flexed, then abducted and pressed downward. If a click is felt under the index finger and there is resistance to abduction, a dislocation exists (Figure 20-21).

The feet are then examined for evidence of a talipes deformity (clubfoot). Intrauterine position frequently causes the feet to appear to turn inward (Figure 20-22). If the feet can easily be returned to the midline by manipulation, no treatment is indicated. Further investigation is indicated when the foot will not turn to a midline position or align readily.

Back

With the neonate prone, the nurse examines the back. The spine should appear straight and flat, since the lumbar and sacral curves do not develop until the infant begins to sit. The base of the spine is then examined for a dermal sinus. The nevus pilosus ("hairy nerve") is only occasionally found at the base of the spine in newborns, but it is significant because it is frequently associated with spina bifida.

Neurologic Status

The neurologic examination assesses the intactness of the neonatal nervous system. It should begin with a period of observation, noting the general physical characteristics and

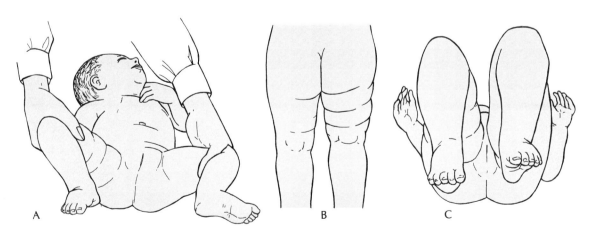

Figure 20-21

Early signs of congenital dislocation of the right hip. **A**, Limitation of abduction and click is felt. **B**, Asymmetry of skin folds and prominence of trochanter. **C**, Shortening of femur. (Reprinted with permission of Ross Laboratories, Columbus, Ohio 43216)

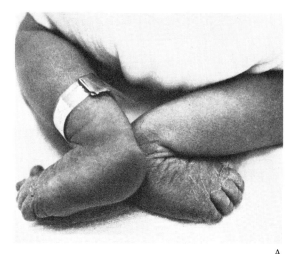

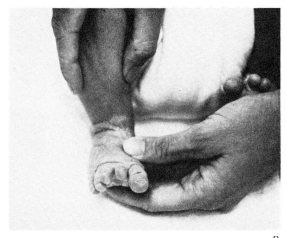

A

B

Figure 20-22

A, Bilateral talipes equinovarus seen with infant in supine position. **B**, To determine the presence of clubfoot, the nurse moves the foot to the midline. Resistance indicates true clubfoot.

behaviors of the newborn. Important behaviors to assess are the state of alertness, resting posture, cry, and quality of muscle tone and motor activity.

Partially flexed extremities with the legs abducted to the abdomen is the usual position of the neonate. When awake, the newborn may exhibit purposeless, uncoordinated bilateral movements of the extremities. If these movements are absent, minimal, or obviously asymmetrical, neurologic dysfunction should be suspected. Eye movements are observable during the first few days of life. An alert neonate is able to fixate on faces and brightly colored objects. If a bright light shines in the newborn's eyes, the blinking response is elicited. The cry of the newborn should be lusty and vigorous. High-pitched cries, weak cries, or no cries are all causes for concern.

Muscle tone is evaluated with the head of the neonate in a neutral position as various parts of the body are passively moved. The newborn is somewhat hypertonic; that is, resistance to extending the elbow and knee joints should be noted. Muscle tone should be symmetrical. Diminished muscle tone and flaccidity require further evaluation.

Neonatal tremors are common in the full-term infant and must be evaluated to differentiate them from a convulsion. A fine jumping of the muscle is likely to be a central nervous system disorder and requires further evaluation. Tremors may also be related to hypoglycemia or hypocalcemia. Neonatal seizures may consist of no more than chewing or swallowing movements, deviations of the eyes, rigidity, or flaccidity because of central nervous system immaturity.

Specific deep tendon reflexes can be elicited in the neonate but have limited value unless they are obviously asymmetrical. The knee jerk is brisk; a normal ankle clonus may involve three or four beats. Plantar flexion is present.

The central nervous system of the newborn is immature and characterized by a variety of reflexes. Because the newborn's movements are uncoordinated, methods of communication are limited, and control of bodily functions drastically limited, the reflexes serve a variety of purposes. Some are protective (blink, gag, sneeze), some aid in feeding (rooting, sucking), and some stimulate human interaction (grasping). Neonatal reflexes and general neurologic activity should be carefully assessed.

The most common reflexes found in the normal neonate are the following:

- *Tonic neck reflex.* The **tonic neck reflex** (*fencer position*) is elicited when the neonate is supine and the head is turned to one side. In response, the extremities on the same side straighten, whereas on the opposite side they flex (Figure 20-23). This reflex may not be seen during the early neonatal period, but once it appears it persists until about the third month.

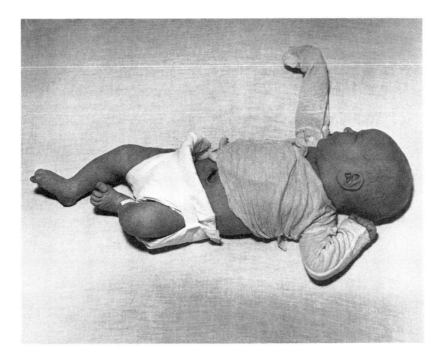

Figure 20-23
Tonic neck reflex.

- *Moro reflex.* The **Moro reflex** is elicited when the neonate is startled by a loud noise or is lifted slightly above the crib and then suddenly lowered. In response, the infant straightens arms and hands outward while the knees flex. Slowly the arms return to the chest, as in an embrace. The fingers spread, forming a C, and the infant may cry.

- *Grasp reflex.* If the palm is stimulated with a finger or object, the infant grasps and holds it firmly enough to be lifted momentarily from the crib.

- *Rooting reflex.* The **rooting reflex** is elicited when the side of the infant's mouth or cheek is touched. In response, the newborn turns toward that side and opens the lips to suck (Figure 20-24).

- *Sucking reflex.* When an object is placed in the neonate's mouth, a sucking motion begins.

- *Babinski reflex.* Hyperextension of all toes occurs when one side of the sole is stroked from the heel upward across the ball of the foot.

- *Trunk incurvation.* When the infant is prone, stroking the spine causes the pelvis to turn to the stimulated side.

In addition to these reflexes, the infant can blink, yawn, cough, sneeze, and draw back from pain (protective reflexes). Neonates can even move a little on their own. When placed on their

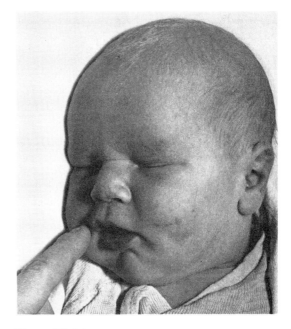

Figure 20-24
Rooting reflex.

stomachs, they push up and try to crawl (*prone crawl*). When he or she is held upright with one foot touching a flat surface, the neonate puts one foot in front of the other and walks (*stepping reflex*) (Figure 20-25). This reflex is more pronounced at birth and is lost in 1–2 months.

Brazelton (1984) recommends the following steps as a means of assessing central nervous system integration:

1. Insert a clean finger into the newborn's mouth to elicit a sucking reflex.
2. As soon as the neonate is sucking vigorously, assess hearing and vision responses by noting sucking changes in the presence of a light, rattle, and a voice.
3. The neonate should respond with a brief cessation of sucking followed by continuous sucking with repetitious stimulation.

This examination demonstrates auditory and visual integrity as well as the ability for complex behavioral interactions.

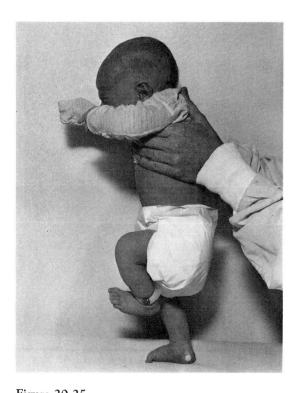

Figure 20-25
Stepping reflex disappears after about 1 month.

Neonatal Physical Assessment

Following is a guide for systematically assessing the newborn. Normal findings, alterations, and related causes are presented, in correlation with suggested nursing responses. The findings are typical for a full-term neonate.

Neonatal Behavioral Assessment

Two conflicting forces influence parents' perceptions of their infant. One is the parents' preconceptions, based on hopes and fears, of what their newborn will be like. The other is their initial reaction to the infant's temperament, behaviors, and physical appearance. Nurses can assist parents in identifying their infant's specific behaviors.

Brazelton (1973) developed a tool that has revolutionized our understanding and perception of the newborn's capabilities and responses, permitting us to recognize each infant's individuality. **Brazelton's neonatal behavioral assessment** tool provides valuable guidelines for assessing the newborn's state changes, temperament, and individual behavior patterns. It provides a means by which the health care provider, in conjunction with the parents (primary caregivers), can identify and understand the individual newborn's states. Parents learn which responses, interventions, or activities best meet the special needs of their infant, and this understanding fosters positive attachment experiences.

The assessment tool attempts to identify the infant's repertoire of behavioral responses to the environment and also documents the infant's neurologic adequacy. The examination usually takes 20 to 30 minutes and involves about 30 different tests and maneuvers. The scale includes 27 behavioral items, each scored on a 9-point scale, and 20 elicited reflexes, which are scored on a 3-point scale.

Some items are scored according to the infant's response to specific stimuli. Others, such as consolability and alertness, are scored

Text continued on p. 462.

NEONATAL PHYSICAL ASSESSMENT GUIDE

Assessment and normal findings	Alterations and possible causes*	Nursing responses to data base†
VITAL SIGNS **Blood pressure** At birth: 80–60/45–40 mm Hg Day 10: 100/50 mm Hg (may be unable to measure diastolic pressure with standard sphygmomanometer)	Low BP (hypovolemia, shock)	Monitor BP in all cases of distress, prematurity, or suspected anomaly Low BP; refer to physician immediately so measures to improve circulation are begun
Pulse: 120–150 beats/min (if asleep 100/min; if crying, up to 180/min)	Weak pulse (decreased cardiac output) Bradycardia (severe asphyxia) Tachycardia (over 160 beats/min at rest) (infection, CNS problems)	Assess skin perfusion by blanching (capillary refill test) Correlate finding with BP assessments; refer to physician Carry out neurologic and thermoregulation assessments
Respirations 30–50 breaths/min Synchronization of chest and abdominal movements Diaphragmatic and abdominal breathing	Tachypnea (pneumonia, RDS) Rapid, shallow breathing (hypermagnesemia due to large doses given to mothers with PIH)	Identify sleep-wake state; correlate with respiratory pattern Evaluate for all signs of respiratory distress; report findings to physician
Transient tachypnea	Expiratory grunting, subcostal and substernal retractions; flaring of nares (respiratory distress); apnea (cold stress, respiratory disorder) Respirations below 30 breaths/min (maternal anesthesia or analgesia)	
Crying Strong and lusty Moderate tone and pitch	High-pitched, shrill (neurologic disorder, hypoglycemia) Weak or absent (CNS disorder, laryngeal problem)	Discuss neonate's use of cry for communication Assess and record abnormal cries
Temperature Axilla 36.5–37C (97.7–98.6F) Rectal 36.6–37.2C (97.8–99F); 36.8C (98.8F) desired Heavier neonates tend to have higher body temperatures	Elevated temperature (room too warm, too much clothing or covers, dehydration, sepsis, brain damage) Subnormal temperature (brain stem involvement, cold) Swings of more than 2F from one reading to next or subnormal temperature (infection)	Notify physician of elevation or drop Counsel parents on possible causes of elevated or low temperatures, appropriate home care measures, when to call physician Teach parents how to take rectal and/or axillary temperature; assess parents' information regarding use of thermometer; provide teaching as needed
Weight 2950–3515 g (6.5–7.75 lb)	<2748 g (<6 lb) = SGA or preterm infant >4050 g (>9 lb) = LGA (infants of diabetic mothers)	Plot weight and gestational age to identify high-risk infants Ascertain body build of parents Counsel parents regarding appropriate caloric intake
Within first 3 to 4 days, normal weight loss of 5%–15% Large babies tend to lose more due to greater fluid loss in proportion to birth weight	Loss greater than 15% (small fluid intake, loss of meconium and urine, feeding difficulties)	Notify physician of net losses or gains Calculate fluid intake and losses from all sources (insensible water loss, radiant warmers, and phototherapy lights)

*Possible causes of alterations are placed in parentheses.
†This column provides guidelines for further assessment and initial nursing interventions.

NEONATAL PHYSICAL ASSESSMENT GUIDE (continued)

Assessment and normal findings	Alterations and possible causes*	Nursing responses to data base†
Length 45 cm (18 in) to 52.3 cm (20.5 in) Grows 10 cm (4 in) during first 3 months	Less than 45 cm (congenital dwarf) Short/long bones proximally (achondroplasia) Short/long bones distally (Ellis-Van Creveld syndrome)	Assess for other signs of dwarfism Determine other signs of skeletal system adequacy Plot progress at subsequent well-baby visits
POSTURE Body usually flexed, hands tightly clenched, neck appears short as chin rests on chest In breech deliveries, feet are usually dorsiflexed	Only extension noted, inability to move from midline (trauma, hypoxia, immaturity) Constant motion	Record spontaneity of motor activity and symmetry of movements If parents express concern about neonate's movement patterns, reassure and evaluate further if appropriate
SKIN Color Color consistent with racial background	Pallor of face, conjunctiva (anemia, hypothermia, anoxia)	Discuss with parents common skin color variations to allay fears
Pink-tinged or ruddy color over face, trunk, extremities	Beefy red (hypoglycemia, immature vasomotor reflexes, polycythemia)	Document extent and time of occurrence of color change
Common variations: acrocyanosis, circumoral cyanosis, or harlequin color change	Meconium staining (fetal distress) Icterus (hemolytic reaction from blood incompatibility, sepsis)	Obtain Hb and hematocrit values Assess for respiratory difficulty Differentiate between physiologic or pathologic jaundice
Mottled when undressed	Cyanosis (choanal atresia, CNS damage or trauma, respiratory or cardiac problem, cold stress)	Assess degree of (central or peripheral) cyanosis and possible causes; refer to physician
Minor bruising over buttocks in breech presentation and over eyes and forehead in facial presentations		Discuss with parents cause and course of minor bruising related to labor and delivery
Texture Smooth, soft, flexible; may have dry, peeling hands and feet	Generalized cracked or peeling skin (SGA or postterm; blood incompatibility; metabolic, kidney dysfunction)	Report to physician
	Seborrhea-dermatitis (cradle cap) Absence of vernix (postmature) Yellow vernix (bilirubin staining)	Instruct parents to shampoo the scalp and anterior fontanelle area daily with soap; rinse well; avoid use of oil
Elastic, returns to normal shape after pinching	Maintains tent shape (dehydration)	Assess for other signs and symptoms of dehydration
Pigmentation Clear; milia across bridge of nose or forehead will disappear within a few weeks		Advise parents not to pinch or prick these pimplelike areas
Café-au-lait spots (one or two)	Six or more (neurologic disorder such as Van Recklinghausen disease, cutaneous neurofibromatosis)	
Mongolian spots common in dark-skinned infants		Assure parents of normalcy of this pigmentation; it will fade in first year or two

*Possible causes of alterations are placed in parentheses.
†This column provides guidelines for further assessment and initial nursing interventions.

NEONATAL PHYSICAL ASSESSMENT GUIDE (continued)

Assessment and normal findings	Alterations and possible causes*	Nursing responses to data base†
Erythema toxicum	Impetigo (group A β-hemolytic streptococcus or *Staphylococcus aureus* infection)	If impetigo occurs, instruct parents about hand-washing and linen precautions during home care
Telangiectatic nevi birthmarks	Hemangiomas: Nevus flammeus (port-wine stain) Nevus vascularis (strawberry hemangioma) Cavernous hemangiomas	Collaborate with physician Counsel parents about birthmark's progression to allay misconceptions Record size and shape of hemangiomas Refer for follow-up at well-baby clinic
Rashes	Rashes (infection)	Assess location and type of rash (macular, papular, vesicular) Obtain history of onset, prenatal history, and related signs and symptoms
Petechiae of head or neck (breech presentation, cord around neck)	Generalized petechiae (clotting abnormalities)	Determine cause; advise parents if further health care is needed
HEAD		
General appearance, size, movement Round, symmetrical, and moves easily from left to right and up and down; soft and pliable	Asymmetrical, flattened occiput on either side of head (plagiocephaly) Head held at angle (torticollis) Unable to move head side-to-side (neurologic trauma)	Instruct parents to change infant's sleeping positions frequently Determine adequacy of all neurologic signs
Circumference: 33–35 cm (13–14 in); 2 cm greater than chest circumference	Extreme differences in size may be; microencephaly (Cornelia de Lange syndrome, CID, rubella, toxoplasmosis, chromosome abnormalities), hydrocephalus (meningomyelocele achondroplasia), anencephaly (neural tube defect) Head is 3 cm or more larger than chest circumference (preterm, hydrocephalus)	Measure circumference from occiput to frontal area using metal or paper tape Measure chest circumference using metal or paper tape and compare to head circumference Record measurements on growth chart Reevaluate at well-baby visits
Common variations: Molding Breech and cesarean newborns' heads are round and well shaped	Cephalhematoma (trauma during delivery) Caput succedaneum (long labor and delivery)	Reassure parents regarding common manifestations due to birth process and when they should disappear
Fontanelles Palpation of juncture of cranial bones Anterior fontanelle; 3–4 cm long by 2–3 cm wide, diamond-shaped	Overlapping of anterior fontanelle (malnourished or preterm infant)	Discuss normal closure times with parents and care of "soft spots" to allay misconceptions
Posterior fontanelle; 1–2 cm at birth, triangle-shaped	Premature closure of sutures (craniostenosis) Late closure (hydrocephalus)	Refer to physician Observe for signs and symptoms of hydrocephalus
Slight pulsation	Moderate to severe pulsation (vascular problems)	Refer to physician

*Possible causes of alterations are placed in parentheses.
†This column provides guidelines for further assessment and initial nursing interventions.

NEONATAL PHYSICAL ASSESSMENT GUIDE (continued)

Assessment and normal findings	Alterations and possible causes*	Nursing responses to data base†
Moderate bulging noted with crying or pulsations with heartbeat	Bulging (increased intracranial pressure, meningitis) Sunken (dehydration)	Evaluate hydration status
HAIR		
Texture		
Smooth with fine texture variations (Note: variations dependent on ethnic background)	Coarse, brittle, dry hair (hypothyroidism) White forelock (Waardenburg syndrome)	Instruct parents regarding routine care of hair and scalp
Distribution		
Scalp hair high over eyebrows (Spanish-Mexican hairline begins mid-forehead and extends down back of neck)	Low forehead and posterior hairlines may indicate chromosomal disorders	Assess for other signs of chromosomal aberations Refer to physician
FACE		
Symmetrical movement of all facial features, normal hairline, eyebrows and eyelashes present		Assess and record symmetry of all parts, shape, regularity of features, sameness or differences in features
Spacing of features		
Eyes at same level; nostrils equal size, cheeks full, and sucking pads present	Eyes wide apart—ocular hypertelorism (Apert syndrome, cri-du-chat, Turner syndrome)	Observe for other signs and symptoms indicative of disease states or chromosomal aberrations
Lips equal on both sides of midline	Abnormal face (Down syndrome, cretinism, gargoylism)	
Chin recedes when compared to other bones of face	Abnormally small jaw—micrognathia (Pierre Robin syndrome, Treacher Collins syndrome)	Maintain airway Initiate surgical consultation and referral
Movement		
Makes facial grimaces	Inability to suck, grimace, and close eyelids (cranial nerve injury)	Initiate neurologic assessment and consultation
Symmetrical when resting and crying	Asymmetry (paralysis of facial cranial nerve)	Assess and record symmetry of all parts, shape, regularity of features, sameness or differences in features)
EYES		
General placement and appearance		
Bright and clear; even placement; slight nystagmus	Gross nystagmus (damage to third, fourth, and sixth cranial nerves)	
Concomitant strabismus	Constant and fixed strabismus	Reassure parents that strabismus is considered normal up to 6 months
Move in all directions		
Blue or slate blue gray	Lack of pigmentation (albinism) Brushfield spots (may indicate Down syndrome)	Discuss with parents any necessary eye precautions Assess for other signs of Down syndrome
Brown color at birth in dark-skinned infants		Discuss with parents that permanent eye color is usually established by 3 months of age.
Eyelids		
Position: above pupils but within iris, no drooping	Elevation or retraction of upper lid (hyperthyroidism)	Assess for signs of hydrocephalus and hyperthyroidism

*Possible causes of alterations are placed in parentheses.
†This column provides guidelines for further assessment and initial nursing interventions.

NEONATAL PHYSICAL ASSESSMENT GUIDE (continued)

Assessment and normal findings	Alterations and possible causes*	Nursing responses to data base†
	"Setting sun" (hydrocephalus), ptosis (congenital or paralysis of oculomotor muscle)	Evaluate interference with vision in subsequent well-baby visits
Eyes on parallel plane Epicanthal folds in Oriental and 20% of Caucasian newborns	Upward slant in non-Orientals (Down syndrome) Epicanthal folds (Down syndrome, cri-du-chat syndrome)	Assess for other signs of Down syndrome
Movement Blink reflex in response to light stimulus		
Inspection Edematous for first few days of life, resulting from delivery and instillation of silver nitrate (chemical conjunctivitis); no lumps or redness	Purulent drainage (infection); infectious conjunctivitis (staphylococcus or Gram-negative organisms) Marginal blepharitis (lid edges red, crusted, scaly)	Initiate good hand-washing Refer to physician Evaluate infant for seborrheic dermatitis; scales can be removed easily
Cornea Clear Corneal reflex present	Ulceration (herpes infection); large cornea or corneas of unequal size (congenital glaucoma) Clouding, opacity of lens (cataract)	Refer to ophthalmologist Assess for other manifestations of congenital herpes; institute nursing care measures
Sclera May appear bluish in newborn, then white; slightly brownish color frequent in Blacks	True blue sclera (osteogenesis imperfecta)	Refer to physician
Pupils Pupils are equal in size, round, and react to light by accommodation	Anisocoria—unequal pupils (CNS damage) Dilatation or constriction (intracranial damage, retinoblastoma, glaucoma) Pupils nonreactive to light or accommodation (brain injury)	Refer for neurologic examination
Slight nystagmus in infant who has not learned to focus Pupil light reflex demonstrated at birth or by 3 weeks of age	Nystagmus (labyrinthine disturbance, CNS disorder)	
Conjunctiva Chemical conjunctivitis Subconjunctival hemorrhage	Pale color (anemia)	Obtain hematocrit and hemoglobin Reassure parents that chemical conjunctivitis will subside in 1–2 days and subconjunctival hemorrhage disappears in a few weeks
Palpebral conjunctiva (red but not hyperemic)	Inflammation or edema (infection, blocked tear duct)	
Vision 20/150 Tracks moving object to midline Fixed focus on objects at a distance of about 7 in; may be difficult to evaluate in newborn Prefers faces, geometric designs, and black and white to colors	Cataracts (congenital infection)	Record any questions about visual acuity and initiate follow-up evaluation at first well-baby checkup

*Possible causes of alterations are placed in parentheses.
†This column provides guidelines for further assessment and initial nursing interventions.

NEONATAL PHYSICAL ASSESSMENT GUIDE (continued)

Assessment and normal findings	Alterations and possible causes*	Nursing responses to data base†
Lashes and lacrimal glands		
Presence of lashes (lashes may be absent in preterm infants)	No lashes on inner two-thirds of lid (Treacher Collins syndrome); bushy lashes (Hurler syndrome); long lashes (Cornelia de Lange syndrome)	
Cry commonly tearless	Excessive tearing (plugged lacrimal duct, natal narcotic abstinence syndrome)	Demonstrate to parents how to milk blocked tear duct Refer to ophthalmologist if tearing is excessive before third month of life
NOSE		
Appearance		
External nasal aspects		
May appear flattened as a result of delivery process	Continued flat or broad bridge of nose (Down syndrome)	Arrange consultation with specialist
Small and narrow in midline; even placement in relationship to eyes and mouth	Low bridge of nose; beaklike nose (Apert syndrome, Treacher Collins syndrome) Upturned (Cornelia de Lange syndrome)	Initiate evaluation of chromosomal abnormalities
Patent nares bilaterally (nose breathers)	Blockage of nares (mucus and/or secretions)	Inspect for obstruction of nares
Sneezing common to clear nasal passages	Flaring nares (respiratory distress) Choanal atresia	
MOUTH		
Function of facial, hypoglossal, glossopharyngeal, and vagus nerves		
Symmetry of movement and strength	Mouth draws to one side (transient seventh cranial nerve paralysis due to pressure in utero or trauma during delivery, congenital paralysis)	Initiate neurologic consultation Administer eye care if eye on affected side is unable to close
	Fishlike shape (Treacher Collins syndrome)	
Presence of gag, swallowing, and sucking reflexes Adequate salivation	Suppressed or absent reflexes	Evaluate other neurologic functions of these nerves
Palate (soft and hard)		
Hard palate dome-shaped Uvula midline with symmetrical movement of soft palate	High-steepled palate (Treacher Collins syndrome)	
Palate intact, sucks well when stimulated Epithelial (Epstein's) pearls appear on mucosa	Clefts in either hard or soft palate (polygenic disorder)	Initiate a surgical consultation referral Assure parents that these are normal in newborn and will disappear at 2 or 3 months of age
Esophagus patent; some drooling common in newborn	Excessive drooling or bubbling (esophageal atresia)	Test for patency of esophagus
Tongue		
Free-moving in all directions, midline	Lack of movement or asymmetrical movement Tongue-tied	Further assess neurologic functions· Test reflex elevation of tongue when depressed with tongue blade

*Possible causes of alterations are placed in parentheses.
†This column provides guidelines for further assessment and initial nursing interventions.

NEONATAL PHYSICAL ASSESSMENT GUIDE (continued)

Assessment and normal findings	Alterations and possible causes*	Nursing responses to data base†
	Deviations from midline (cranial nerve damage)	Check for signs of weakness or deviation
Pink color, smooth to rough texture, noncoated	White cheesy coating (thrush) Tongue has deep ridges	Differentiate between thrush and milk curds Reassure parents that tongue pattern may change from day to day
Tongue proportional to mouth	Large tongue with short frenulum (cretinism, Down and other syndromes)	Evaluate in well-baby clinic to assess development delays Initiate referrals
EARS		
External ear		
Without lesions, cysts, or nodules	Nodules, cysts, or sinus tracts in front of ear Adherent earlobes Preauricular skin tags	Evaluate characteristics of lesions Counsel parents to clean external ear with washcloth only; discourage use of cotton-tip applicators Refer to physician for ligation
Hearing		
With first cry, eustachian tubes are cleared		
Absence of all risk factors	Presence of one or more risk factors	Assess history of risk factors for hearing loss
Attends to sounds; sudden or loud noise elicits Moro reflex	No response to sound stimuli (deafness)	Test for Moro reflex
NECK		
Appearance		
Short, straight, creased with skin folds	Abnormally short neck (Turner syndrome) Arching or inability to flex neck (meningitis, congenital anomaly)	Report findings to physician
Posterior neck lacks loose extra folds of skin	Webbing of neck (Turner syndrome, Down syndrome, trisomy 18)	Assess for other signs of the syndromes
Clavicles		
Straight and intact	Knot or lump on clavicle (fracture during difficult delivery)	Obtain detailed labor and delivery history; apply figure-8 bandage
Moro reflex elicitable	Unilateral Moro reflex response on unaffected side (fracture of clavicle, brachial palsy, Erb-Duchenne paralysis)	Collaborate with physician
Symmetrical shoulders	Hypoplasia	
CHEST		
Appearance and size		
Circumference: 32.5 cm, 1–2 cm less than head Wider than it is long		Measure at level of nipples after exhalation
Normal shape without depressed or prominent sternum Lower end of sternum (xiphoid cartilage) may be protruding; is less apparent after several weeks Sternum 8 cm long	Funnel chest (congenital or associated with Marfan syndrome) Continued protrusion of xiphoid cartilage (Marfan syndrome, "pigeon chest") Barrel chest	Determine adequacy of other respiratory and circulatory signs Assess for other signs and symptoms of various syndromes

*Possible causes of alterations are placed in parentheses.
†This column provides guidelines for further assessment and initial nursing interventions.

NEONATAL PHYSICAL ASSESSMENT GUIDE (continued)

Assessment and normal findings	Alterations and possible causes*	Nursing responses to data base†
Expansion and retraction		
Bilateral expansion	Unequal chest expansion (pneumonia, pneumothorax respiratory distress)	Assess respiratory effort regularity, flaring of nares, difficulty on both inspiration and expiration
No intercostal, subcostal, or supracostal retractions	Retractions (respiratory distress)	Record and consult physician
Auscultation		
Breath sounds are louder in infants	Decreased breath sounds (decreased respiratory activity, atelectasis, pneumothorax)	Perform assessment and report to physician any positive findings
Chest and axilla clear on crying	Increased breath sounds (resolving pneumonia or in cesarean births)	
Bronchial breath sounds (heard where trachea and bronchi closest to chest wall, above sternum and between scapulae)		
Bronchial sounds bilaterally	Adventitious or abnormal sounds (respiratory disease or distress)	
Air entry clear		
Rales may indicate normal newborn atelectasis		
Cough reflex absent at birth appears in 2 or more days		
Breasts		
Flat with symmetrical nipples	Lack of breast tissue (preterm or SGA)	
Breast tissue diameter 5 cm or more at term		
Distance between nipples 8 cm		
Breast engorgement occurs on third day of life; liquid discharge may be expressed in term infants	Breast abscesses	Reassure parents of normalcy of breast engorgement
Nipples	Supernumerary nipples Dark-colored nipples	
HEART		
Auscultation		
Location: lies horizontally, with left border extending to left of midclavicle		
Regular rhythm and rate	Arrhythmia (anoxia), tachycardia, bradycardia	All arrhythmia and gallop rhythms should be referred
Determination of point of maximal impulse (PMI)	Malpositioning (enlargement, abnormal placement, pneumothorax, dextrocardia, diaphragmatic hernia)	Initiate cardiac evaluation
Usually lateral to midclavicular line at third or fourth intercostal space		
Functional murmurs	Location of murmurs (possible congenital cardiac anomaly)	Evaluate murmur: location, timing, and duration; observe for accompanying cardiac pathology symptoms; ascertain family history
No thrills		

*Possible causes of alterations are placed in parentheses.
†This column provides guidelines for further assessment and initial nursing interventions.

NEONATAL PHYSICAL ASSESSMENT GUIDE (continued)

Assessment and normal findings	Alterations and possible causes*	Nursing responses to data base†
Horizontal groove at diaphragm shows flaring of rib cage to mild degree	Marked rib flaring (vitamin D deficiency) Inadequacy of respiratory movement	Initiate cardiopulmonary evaluation; assess pulses and blood pressures in all four extremities for equality and quality

ABDOMEN
Appearance
  Cylindrical with some protrusion; appears large in relation to pelvis; some laxness of abdominal muscles
  No cyanosis, few vessels seen
  Diastasis recti—common in Black infants
	Distention, shiny abdomen with engorged vessels (gastrointestinal abnormalities, infection, congenital megacolon)
	Scaphoid abdominal appearance (diaphragmatic hernia)
	Increased or decreased peristalsis (duodenal stenosis, small bowel obstruction)
	Localized flank bulging (enlarged kidneys, ascites, or absent abdominal muscles)
		Examine abdomen thoroughly for mass or organomegaly
		Measure abdominal girth
		Report deviations of abdominal size
		Assess other signs and symptoms of obstruction
		
		Refer to physician

Umbilicus
  No protrusion of umbilicus
  Protrusion of umbilicus common in Black infants
  Bluish white color
  Cutis navel (umbilical cord projects); granulation tissue in navel
	Umbilical hernia
	Patent urachus (congenital malformation)
	Omphalocele
	Gastroschisis
	Redness or exudate around cord (infection)
	Yellow discoloration (hemolytic disease, meconium staining)
		Measure umbilical hernia by palpating the opening and record; it should close by 1 year of age; if not, refer to physician
		Instruct parents on cord care and hygiene

Two arteries and one vein apparent Begins drying 1–2 hours after birth No bleeding	Single umbilical artery (congenital anomalies)	
Auscultation and percussion Soft bowel sounds heard shortly after birth; heard every 10–30 sec	Bowel sounds in chest (diaphragmatic hernia) Absence of bowel sounds Hyperperistalsis (intestinal obstruction)	Collaborate with physician Assess for other signs of dehydration and/or infection
Femoral pulses Palpable, equal, bilateral	Absent or diminished femoral pulses (coarctation of aorta)	Monitor blood pressure in upper and lower extremities

Inguinal area
  No bulges along inguinal area
  No inguinal lymph nodes felt
	Inguinal hernia	Initiate referral
		Continue follow-up in well-baby clinic

Bladder
  Percusses 1–4 cm above symphysis
  Emptied about 3 hours after birth; if not, at time of birth
  Urine—inoffensive, mild odor
	Failure to void within 24 hours after birth
	Exposure of bladder mucosa (exstrophy of bladder)
	Foul odor (infection)	

*Possible causes of alterations are placed in parentheses.
†This column provides guidelines for further assessment and initial nursing interventions.

NEONATAL PHYSICAL ASSESSMENT GUIDE (continued)

Assessment and normal findings	Alterations and possible causes*	Nursing responses to data base†
GENITALS		
Gender clearly delineated	Ambiguous genitals	Refer for genetic consultation
Male		
Penis		
Slender in appearance, 2.5 cm long, 1 cm wide at birth	Micropenis (congenital anomaly) Meatal atresia	Observe and record first voiding
Normal urinary orifice, urethral meatus at tip of penis	Hypospadias, epispadias	Collaborate with physician in presence of abnormality
Noninflamed urethral opening	Urethritis (infection)	Palpate for enlarged inguinal lymph nodes and record painful urination
Foreskin adheres to glans; prepuce can be retracted beyond urethral opening	Ulceration of meatal opening (infection, inflammation)	Evaluate whether ulcer is due to diaper rash; counsel regarding care
Uncircumcised foreskin tight for 2–3 months	Phimosis—if still tight after 3 months	Instruct parents to retract foreskin gently for cleaning at monthly intervals after 4 months of age
Circumcised Erectile tissue present		Teach parents how to care for circumcision
Scrotum		
Skin loose and hanging or tight and small; extensive rugae and normal size	Large scrotum containing fluid (hydrocele)	Shine a light through scrotum (transilluminate) to verify diagnosis
Normal skin color	Red, shiny scrotal skin (orchitis)	
Scrotal discoloration common in breech		
Testes		
Descended by birth; not consistently found in scrotum	Undescended testes (cryptorchidism)	If testes cannot be felt in scrotum, gently palpate femoral, inguinal, perineal, and abdominal areas for presence
Testes size 1.5–2 cm at birth	Enlarged testes (tumor) Small testes (Klinefelter syndrome or adrenal hyperplasia)	Refer and collaborate with physician for further diagnostic studies
Female		
Mons		
Normal skin color; area pigmented in dark-skinned infants		
Labia majora cover labia minora; symmetrical size appropriate for gestational age	Hematoma, lesions	Evaluate for recent trauma
Clitoris		
Normally large in newborn Edema and bruising in breech delivery	Hypertrophy (hermaphroditism)	
Vagina		
Urinary meatus and vaginal orifice visible (0.5 cm circumference)	Inflammation; erythema and discharge (urethritis)	Collect urine specimen for laboratory examination
Vaginal tag or hymenal tag disappears in a few weeks	Congenital absence of vagina	Refer to physician
Discharge; smegma under labia	Foul-smelling discharge (infection)	Collect data and further evaluate reason for discharge

*Possible causes of alterations are placed in parentheses.
†This column provides guidelines for further assessment and initial nursing interventions.

NEONATAL PHYSICAL ASSESSMENT GUIDE (continued)

Assessment and normal findings	Alterations and possible causes*	Nursing responses to data base†
Bloody or mucoid discharge	Excessive vaginal bleeding (blood coagulation defect)	
BUTTOCKS AND ANUS		
Buttocks symmetrical	Pilonidal dimple	Examine for possible sinus Instruct parents about cleansing this area
Anus patent and passage of meconium within 24–48 hours after birth	Imperforate anus, rectal atresia (congenital gastrointestinal defect)	Evaluate extent of problems Initiate surgical consultation Perform digital examination to ascertain patency
No fissures, tears, or skin tags	Fissures	
EXTREMITIES AND TRUNK		
Short and generally flexed; extremities move symmetrically through range of motion but lack full extension	Unilateral or absence of movement (spinal cord involvement) Fetal position continued or limp (anoxia, CNS problems, hypoglycemia)	
All joints move spontaneously; good muscle tone, of flexor type, birth to 2 months	Spasticity when infant begins using extensors (cerebral palsy, lack of muscle tone, "floppy baby" syndrome)	Collaborate with physician
Arms		
Equal in length	Brachial palsy (difficult delivery)	
Bilateral movement	Erb-Duchenne paralysis	
Flexed when quiet	Muscle weakness, fractured clavicle Absence of limb or change of size (phocomelia, amelia)	
Hands		
Normal number of fingers	Polydactyly (Ellis-Van Creveld syndrome) Syndactyly—one limb (developmental anomaly) Syndactyly—both limbs (genetic component)	Report to physician
Normal palmar crease	Simian line on palm (Down syndrome)	
Normal size hands	Short fingers and broad hand (Hurler syndrome)	
Nails present and extend beyond fingertips in term infant	Cyanosis and clubbing (cardiac anomalies) Nails long (postterm)	
Spine		
C-shaped spine Flat and straight when prone Slight lumbar lordosis Easily flexed and intact when palpated At least half of back devoid of lanugo Full-term infant in ventral suspension should hold head at 45° angle, back straight	Spina bifida occulta (nevus pilosus) Dermal sinus Myelomeningocele Head lag, limp, floppy trunk (neurologic problems)	Evaluate extent of neurologic damage; initiate care of spinal opening

*Possible causes of alterations are placed in parentheses.
†This column provides guidelines for further assessment and initial nursing interventions.

NEONATAL PHYSICAL ASSESSMENT GUIDE (continued)

Assessment and normal findings	Alterations and possible causes*	Nursing responses to data base†
Hips		
No sign of instability	Sensation of abnormal movement, jerk, or snap of hip dislocation	Examine all newborn infants for dislocated hip prior to discharge from hospital
Hips abduct to more than 60°		If this is suspected, refer to orthopedist for further evaluation Reassess at well-baby visits
Inguinal and buttock skin creases		
Symmetrical inguinal and buttock creases	Asymmetry (dislocated hips)	Refer to orthopedist for evaluation, counsel parents regarding symptoms of concern and therapy
Legs		
Legs equal in length	Shortened leg (dislocated hips)	Refer to orthopedist for evaluation
Legs shorter than arms at birth	Lack of leg movement (fractures, spinal defects)	Counsel parents regarding symptoms of concern and discuss therapy
Feet		
Foot is in straight line	Talipes equinovarus (true clubfoot)	Discuss differences between positional and true clubfoot with parents
Positional clubfoot—based on position in utero		
Fat pads and creases on soles of feet		Teach parents passive manipulation of foot Refer to orthopedist if not corrected by 3 months of age
Talipes planus (flat feet) normal under 3 years of age		Reassure parents that flat feet are normal in infant
NEUROMUSCULAR		
Motor function		
Symmetrical movement and strength in all extremities	Limp, flaccid, or hypertonic (CNS disorders, infection, dehydration fracture)	Appraise newborn's posture and motor functions by observing activities and motor characteristics
May be jerky or have brief twitchings	Tremors (hypoglycemia, hypocalcemia, infection, neurologic damage)	Evaluate electrolyte imbalance and neurologic functioning
Head lag not over 45°	Delayed or abnormal development (preterm, neurologic involvement)	
Neck control adequate to maintain head erect briefly	Asymmetry of tone or strength	

*Possible causes of alterations are placed in parentheses.
†This column provides guidelines for further assessment and initial nursing interventions.

as a result of continuous behavioral observations throughout the assessment. (For a complete discussion of all test items and maneuvers, the student is referred to Brazelton, 1973.)

The nurse should observe the newborn's sleep-wake patterns as discussed in Chapter 21, the rapidity with which the infant moves from one state to another, the ability to be consoled, and the ability to diminish the impact of disturbing stimuli. The scale items and maneuvers and the *sleep-alert states* in which they are assessed are categorized as follows:

Habituation The infant's ability to diminish or shut down innate responses to specific repeated stimuli, such as a rattle, bell, light, or pinprick to heel, is assessed.

Orientation to inanimate and animate visual and auditory assessment stimuli How often and where the newborn attends to auditory and visual stimuli are observed. The infant's orientation to the environment is determined by an ability to respond to clues given by others and by a natural ability to fix on and to follow a visual object horizontally and vertically. This capacity and parental appreciation of it are important for positive communication between infant and parents; the parents' visual (*en face*) and auditory (soft, continuous voice) presence stimulates their infant to orient to them. Inability or lack of response may indicate visual or auditory problems. It is important for parents to know that their infant can turn to voices by 3 days of age and can become alert at different times with a varying degree of intensity in response to sounds.

Motor activity   Several components are evaluated. Motor tone of the newborn is assessed in the most characteristic state of responsiveness. This summary assessment includes overall use of tone as the neonate responds to being handled—whether during spontaneous activity, prone placement, or horizontal holding—and overall assessment of body tone as the neonate reacts to all stimuli.

Variations   Frequency of alert states, state changes, color changes (throughout all states as examination progresses), activity, and peaks of excitement are assessed.

Self-quieting activity   Assessment is based on how often, how quickly, and how effectively newborns can use their resources to quiet and console themselves when upset or distressed. Considered in this assessment are such self-consolatory activities as putting hand to mouth, sucking on a fist or the tongue, and attuning to an object or sound. The infant's need for outside consolation must also be considered, for example, seeing a face; being rocked, held, or dressed; using a pacifier; and having extremities restrained.

Cuddliness or social behaviors   This area encompasses the infant's need for and response to being held. Also considered is how often the newborn smiles. These behaviors influence the parents' self-esteem and feelings of acceptance or rejection. Schaeffer and Emerson's (1964) study indicated that cuddling also appears to be an indicator of personality. Cuddlers appear to enjoy, accept, and seek physical contact; are easier to placate; sleep more; and form earlier and more intense attachments. Noncuddlers are active, restless, have accelerated motor devel-

opment, and are intolerant of physical restraint. Smiling, even as a grimace reflex, greatly influences parent-infant feedback. Parents identify this response as positive.

Summary

The various neonatal assessments and the data obtained from them are only as effective as the degree to which the findings are shared with the parents and incorporated into the interaction between parents and infant. Parents must be included in the assessment process from the moment of their child's birth. The Apgar score and its meaning should be explained immediately to the parents. As soon as possible, the parents should be a part of the physical and behavioral assessments. The examiner should emphasize the uniqueness of their infant.

The nurse can encourage the parents to identify the unique behavioral characteristics of their infant and to learn nurturing activities. Attachment is aided when parents are allowed to explore their infant in private, identifying individual physical and behavioral characteristics. The nurse's supportive responses to the parents' questions and observations are essential throughout the assessment process. With the nurse's help, attachment and the beginning of interactions between family members are established.

References

Avery, GB (editor): *Neonatology*, 2nd ed. Philadelphia: Lippincott, 1981.

Ballard JL et al: A simplified score for assessment of fetal maturation of newly born infants. *J Pediatr* November 1979; 95:5:769.

Brazelton T: *The Neonatal Behavioral Assessment Scale*. Philadelphia: Lippincott, 1973.

Brazelton T: Neonatal behavior and its significance. In: *Schaeffer's Diseases of the Newborn*, Avery ME, Taeusch HW (editors). Philadelphia: Saunders, 1984.

Damoulaki-Sfakianaki E et al: Skin creases on the foot and the physical index of maturity. Comparison between Caucasian and Negro infants. *Pediatrics* 1972; 50:483.

Danforth DN (editor): *Obstetrics and Gynecology*, 4th ed. Philadelphia: Harper & Row, 1982.

Downs MP, Silver HK: The A, B, C, D's to H.E.A.R. Early identification in nursery, office and clinic of the infant who is deaf. *Clin Pediatr* October 1972; 11:563.

Korones SB: *High-Risk Newborn Infants*, 3rd ed. St. Louis: Mosby, 1981.

Ludington-Hoe SM: What can newborns really see? *Am J Nurs* 1983; 83:1286.

Robertson A: Commentary: Gestational age. *J Pediatr* November 1979; 95:5:732.

Schaeffer H, Emerson P: Patterns of response to physical contact in early human development. *J Child Psychol Psychiatry* 1964; 5:1.

Standards and Recommendations for Hospital Care of Newborn Infants, 6th ed. Evanston, Ill.: American Academy of Pediatrics, 1977.

Additional Readings

Affonso D: The newborn's potential for interaction. *J Obstet Gynecol Neonat Nurs* November/December 1976; 5:9.

Clark AL, Affonso D: Infant behavior and maternal attachment: Two sides to the coin. *MCN* 1976; 1:94.

Lubchenco LO: Assessment of gestational age and development at birth. *Pediatr Clin North Am* 1970; 17:125.

Powell ML: *Assessment and Management of Developmental Changes and Problems in Children*, 2nd ed. St. Louis: Mosby, 1982.

Scanlon JW et al: *A System of Newborn Physical Examination*. Baltimore: University Park Press, 1979.

Sullivan R et al: Determining a newborn's gestational age. *MCN* January/February 1979; 4:38.

White PL et al: Comparative accuracy of recent abbreviated methods of gestational age determination. *Clin Pediatr* 1980; 19(5):319.

21

The Normal Newborn: Needs and Care

Chapter Contents

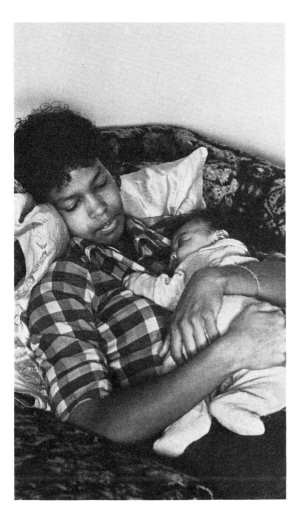

Objectives

- Discuss periods of reactivity after birth.

- Discuss the immediate and subsequent nursing care of the newborn.

- Compare various feeding preparations and the nutritional needs of the newborn.

- Identify common parental concerns regarding newborns.

- Describe the important information to be included in parent teaching.

Key Terms ▬▬▬▬▬▬▬▬▬

circumcision
newborn screening tests

Nursing assessments of the general characteristics, variations, and responses of each newborn reveal how extrauterine adaptation is proceeding. Based on their findings, nurses can individualize their care to meet the needs of each newborn.

Birth also marks the beginning of the expansion of the family unit. Thus, the nurse should be knowledgeable about family adjustments that need to be made, as well as the health care needs of the newborn. With such a background, the nurse can provide comprehensive care and promote the establishment of a well-functioning family unit. It is important that new parents return home with a positive feeling that they have the support, information, and skills to care for their child. Equally important is the need for the family to begin a unique relationship between family members and the new child. The cultural and social expectations of individual families and communities affect the way in which normal newborn care is carried out.

Nursing Observations and Care ▬▬▬▬▬▬▬▬▬

Nursing Management of the Newborn at Admission

In many hospitals the infant is placed in an observation nursery for several hours after birth. This procedure allows the nurse to assess the newborn carefully and to institute nursing care measures as needed. The observation nurs-ery is staffed at all times and must contain necessary emergency care equipment. Infants delivered in alternative birthing rooms or centers may be kept in the birthing room for observation rather than being taken to an observation nursery.

When the newborn is admitted to the observation nursery, identification is checked and confirmed. A concise verbal report of significant information is given to the nursery nurse. Essential data to be reported include the following:

1. *Condition of the newborn.* Essential information includes the newborn's Apgar scores at 1 and 5 minutes, resuscitative measures required in the delivery room, voidings, and passing of meconium. Complications to be noted are excessive mucus, delayed spontaneous respirations or responsiveness, abnormal number of cord vessels, and obvious physical abnormalities.

2. *Labor and delivery record.* A copy of the labor and delivery record should accompany the newborn to the nursery. The record has all significant data, for example, duration, course, and status of mother and fetus throughout labor and delivery. The labor and delivery nurse summarizes the data in a verbal report to the nursery nurse and takes particular care to note any variation or difficulties.

3. *Antepartal history.* Any maternal problems that may have compromised the fetus in utero are of immediate concern in the assessment of the newborn. Information about maternal age, EDC, previous pregnancies, and existing siblings is also included.

4. *Parent-infant interaction information.* Parental opportunities to hold their newborn and their desires regarding care, such as rooming-in and the type of feeding, are noted. Information about other children in the home, available support systems, and interactional patterns within each family unit assists in providing comprehensive care.

If no neonatal distress is apparent, the nurse proceeds with the admission nursery routine, taking the newborn's vital signs and performing actions to maintain body temperature and a clear airway. The initial temperature may be taken rectally to assess patency of the anus (care should be taken to avoid inserting the thermometer too far, which may perforate the intestines). Core temperature is then monitored either indirectly by obtaining an axillary temperature at intervals or by placing a skin probe on the abdomen of the newborn for continuous reading. Apical pulse and respirations are counted for a full minute and recorded. In some agencies, blood pressure is assessed by auscultation, palpation, or a Doppler instrument. The newborn is weighed in grams. This weight is converted to pounds for the parents' information (Figure 21-1). The scales are covered each

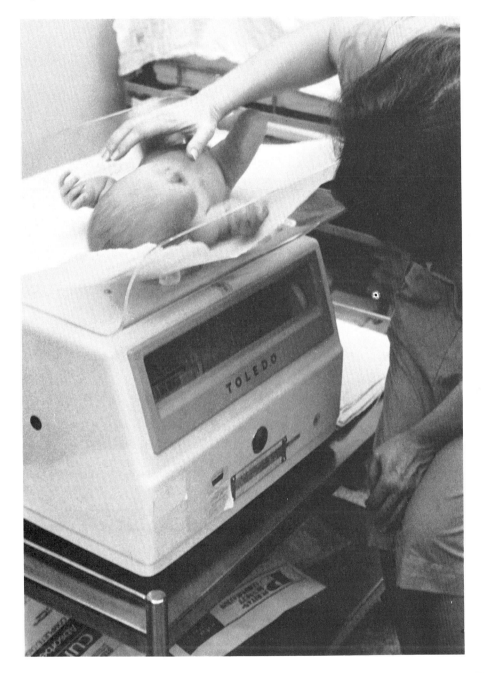

Figure 21-1

The scale is balanced before each weight, with the protective pad in place. The caretaker's hand is poised above the infant as a safety measure. (From Swearingen P: *The Addison-Wesley Photo-Atlas of Nursing Procedures*. Menlo Park, Ca.: Addison-Wesley, 1984.)

time an infant is weighed to prevent cross-infection and heat loss from conduction. The newborn is measured; the measurements are recorded in both centimeters and inches. Three routine measurements are (a) length, (b) circumference of the head, and (c) circumference of the chest. In some facilities, abdominal girth may also be determined. The nurse rapidly appraises the neonate's color, muscle tone, alertness, and general state. Basic assessments for estimating gestational age are done (for further discussion see Chapter 20).

A prophylactic injection of vitamin K is given intramuscularly in the lateral aspect of the thigh to prevent hemorrhagic problems (see the accompanying Drug Guide). The nurse is also responsible for giving the legally required prophylactic eye treatment for *Neisseria gonorrhoea*, which may have infected the neonate during the birth process. The traditional drug

of choice is 1% silver nitrate solution. To instill silver nitrate, the nurse punctures the wax container of 1% silver nitrate with a sterile needle, pulls down the infant's lower eyelid, and administers one or two drops into the lower conjunctival sac (Figure 21-2). After instillation, the eye is closed to spread the medication. The other eye is treated in the same manner. Controversy exists as to the value of flushing the eye with sterile water following the instillation of the silver nitrate.

Some practitioners now use an antibiotic ointment such as erythromycin (Ilotycin) instead of silver nitrate. Both of these medications may cause chemical conjunctivitis, which will cause the newborn some discomfort and may interfere with the neonate's ability to focus on the parents' faces (see the accompanying Drug Guide). The resulting edema and inflammation may cause undue concern if the parents

DRUG GUIDE
Erythromycin (Ilotycin)— Ophthalmic ointment

OVERVIEW OF NEONATAL ACTION

Erythromycin (Ilotycin) is utilized as prophylactic treatment of ophthalmia neonatorum, which is caused by the bacteria *Neisseria gonorrhoeae*. Preventive treatment of gonorrhea in the newborn is required by law. Erythromycin is also effective against ophthalmic chlamydial infections. It is either bacteriostatic or bactericidal depending on the organisms involved and the concentration of drug.

ROUTE, DOSAGE, FREQUENCY

Ophthalmic ointment is instilled as a narrow ribbon or strand, ¼-inch long, along the lower conjunctival surface of each eye, starting at the inner canthus. It is instilled only once in each eye. Administration may be done in the delivery room or later in the nursery so that eye contact is facilitated so that the bonding process is not interrupted.

NEONATAL SIDE EFFECTS

Sensitivity reaction; may interfere with ability to focus and may cause edema and inflammation. Side effects usually disappear in 24–48 hours.

NURSING CONSIDERATIONS

Wash hands immediately prior to instillation to prevent introduction of bacteria
Do not irrigate the eyes after instillation
Observe for hypersensitivity

DRUG GUIDE
Vitamin K₁ phytonadione (AquaMEPHYTON)

OVERVIEW OF NEONATAL ACTION

Phytonadione is used in prophylaxis and treatment of hemorrhagic disease of the newborn. It promotes liver formation of the clotting factors II, VII, IX, and X. At birth the neonate does not have the bacteria in the colon that is necessary for synthesizing fat-soluble vitamin K_1, therefore the newborn may have decreased levels of prothrombin during the first 5–8 days of life reflected by a prolongation of prothrombin time.

ROUTE, DOSAGE, FREQUENCY

Intramuscular injection is given in the lateral thigh muscle. A one-time only prophylactic dose of 0.5–1.0 mg is given in the delivery room or upon admission to the newborn nursery. May need to repeat 6–8 hours later especially if mother received anticoagulants during pregnancy.

NEONATAL SIDE EFFECTS

Pain and edema may occur at injection site. Possible allergic reactions such as rash and urticaria. Hyperbilirubinemia may occur in newborns or preterm infants given doses greater than 25 mg.

NURSING CONSIDERATIONS

Observe for bleeding (usually occurs on second or third day). Bleeding may be seen as generalized ecchymoses or bleeding from umbilical cord, circumcision site, nose, or gastrointestinal tract. Results of serial PT and PTT should be assessed.
Observe for jaundice and kernicterus especially in preterm infants.
Observe for signs of local inflammation.

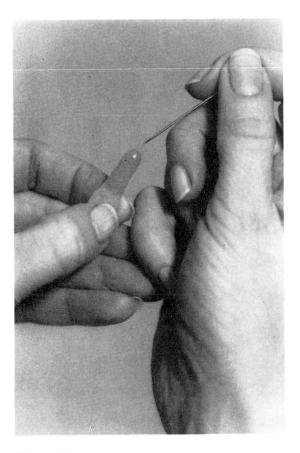
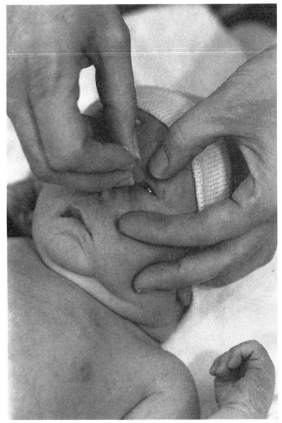

Figure 21-2

Silver nitrate instillation. **A**, Wax container is punctured with a needle. **B**, One or two drops of 1% silver nitrate solution are instilled in each lower conjunctival sac. (From Swearingen P: *The Addison-Wesley Photo-Atlas of Nursing Procedures*. Menlo Park, Ca.: Addison-Wesley, 1984.)

are not made aware of the need for the treatment. They should be told that the side effects will clear in 24–48 hours.

Eye-to-eye contact between the parents and child is of extreme emotional importance during the first hour after birth, and, as will be discussed later, the newborn is very alert during this time (Klaus and Kennell, 1982). To promote eye contact and attachment, prophylactic eye medication may be delayed to allow this important bonding opportunity.

A hematocrit and Dextrostix evaluation is routinely ordered for SGA and LGA infants in some institutions (see Procedure 22-4). Another routine but controversial practice in some institutions is removal of mucus from the stomach to help prevent possible aspiration. The practice can cause bradycardia and apnea in the unstabilized neonate.

The initial admission assessment serves as a basis for establishing nursing diagnoses regarding the infant and setting priorities for care and family education needs (Haun, Porter, and Chance, 1984). In many settings, the father accompanies the newborn to the nursery. This is an excellent opportunity for him to get to know his child as well as an excellent opportunity for the astute nurse to take note of the father's bonding process and comfort level with the newborn. The nurse must be aware that the father may be overwhelmed by the unfamiliar nursery setting. However, he will benefit from observing and interacting with the nurse who cares for his child.

Periods of Reactivity

The nurse must be able to assess accurately normal versus abnormal behavior. The neonate usually shows a predictable pattern of behavior during the first several hours after birth.

First period of reactivity   This phase lasts approximately 30 minutes after birth. During this phase the newborn is awake and active and may appear hungry and have a strong sucking reflex. This is a natural opportunity to initiate breast-feeding if this is the mother's choice. Bursts of random, diffuse movements alternating with relative immobility may occur. Respirations are rapid, as high as 80 breaths/min, and there may be retraction of the chest, transient flaring of the nares, and grunting. The heart rate is rapid and irregular. Bowel sounds are absent.

Sleep phase   The newborn's activity gradually diminishes, and the heart rate and respirations decrease as the infant enters the sleep phase. First sleep usually occurs an average of 3 hours after birth, and may last from a few minutes to 2–4 hours. During this period, the newborn will be difficult to awaken and will show no interest in sucking. Bowel sounds become audible, and cardiac and respiratory rates return to baseline values.

Second period of reactivity   The newborn is again awake and alert. This phase lasts 4–6 hours in the normal newborn. Physiologic responses are variable during this stage. The heart and respiratory rates increase; however, the nurse must be alert for apneic periods, which may cause a drop in the heart rate. The newborn must be stimulated to continue breathing during such times. The newborn may become mildly cyanotic or mottled during these fluctuations. Production of respiratory and gastric mucus increases, and the newborn responds by gagging, choking, and regurgitating.

Continued close observation is required to maintain a clear airway. Positioning on the side and nasal suctioning with a bulb syringe or a De Lee suction may also be necessary. The gastrointestinal tract becomes more active. The first meconium stool is frequently passed during this second active stage, and the initial voiding may also occur at this time. The newborn will indicate readiness for feeding by such behaviors as sucking, rooting, and swallowing. If feeding was not initiated in the first period of reactivity, it should be done at this time. See the section on feeding, p. 471, for further discussion of this first feeding.

Subsequent Nursing Management

After the initial admission assessment, the newborn's apical pulse and respirations are taken every 15–30 minutes for 1 hour, and then every 1–2 hours until stable.

Apical pulse is assessed while the neonate is at rest; heart rate, regularity, and murmurs should be noted.

The nurse must continue to assess the newborn's temperature closely and maintain body temperature in the range of 36.5–37.0C (97.7–98.6F). The axillary temperature should be monitored each hour for the first 4 hours and then once every 4 hours for the first 24 hours.

The newborn is placed in a warmer just after delivery to allow his or her temperature to return to normal (about 2–4 hours). When the newborn's temperature is normal and vital signs are stable, the infant may be bathed. However, this admission bath may be postponed for some hours if the condition dictates. Temperature is rechecked after the bath, and if the temperature is stable, the newborn is dressed, wrapped, placed in a crib, and given a trial period at room temperature. If the infant does not successfully maintain his or her temperature at 36.5C (97.7F), the newborn is returned to the warmer.

The nurse starts measures to prevent neonatal heat loss, such as using heat shields, keeping the infant dry and covered, and avoiding placement on cool surfaces or the use of cold instruments. The infant is also protected from drafts, open windows or doors, or air conditioners. Blankets and clothing are stored in a warm place. (See discussion on nonshivering thermogenesis and the mechanism of heat loss in Chapter 19.)

When the newborn's neurologic status is normal, vital signs are stabilized, and the first feeding has been tolerated (usually within 5–10 hours after birth), the infant is moved from the observation nursery area to the regular nursery. If rooming-in is desired, it may begin as soon as the newborn is transferred out of the observation nursery. However, some nurseries recommend that rooming-in be delayed for 24 hours. This recommendation is based on the knowledge that after 24 hours the amount of mucus in the newborn is decreased, the chance of choking is diminished, and the initial voiding and defecation have occurred and have been assessed.

During the first 24 hours of life, the nurse is constantly alert for signs of distress. If the newborn is with the parents during this period, extra care must be taken in their education so that they can appropriately maintain their newborn's temperature, recognize the hallmarks of physiologic distress, and know how to respond immediately to signs of respiratory problems. (See Essential Facts to Remember—Signs of Neonatal Distress.) The nurse also must be immediately available to support the family during the attachment process, which is taking place at this time.

A complete physical examination is done by the physician or nurse practitioner within the first 24 hours or prior to discharge. (See the Physical Assessment Guide in Chapter 20.)

Daily Nursery Observations and Care

Routine daily care varies for each nursery and even from one shift to the next. However, essential daily care of newborns should include the following:

- *Vital signs.* These are taken once a shift or more, depending on the newborn's status.
- *Weight.* The neonate should be weighed at the same time each day for accurate comparisons. A weight loss of up to 10% for term infants and 15% in preterm infants is expected during the first week of life. This is the result of limited intake and the loss of excess extracellular fluid. Parents should be told about the expected weight loss and the reason for it.
- *Overall color.* Changes in color may indicate the need for closer assessment of temperature or hematocrit and bilirubin levels.
- *Intake/Output.* Caloric and fluid intake are recorded as are voiding and stooling patterns.
- *Umbilical cord and circumcision.* Cord and circumcision care is provided, and records of that care are kept.
- *Newborn nutrition.* Caloric and fluid intake are recorded. The nurse is also responsible

 ESSENTIAL FACTS TO REMEMBER

Signs of Neonatal Distress

The most common signs of distress in the newborn are the following:

- Increased rate (more than 60/min) or difficult respirations
- Sternal retractions
- Excessive mucus
- Facial grimacing
- Cyanosis (generalized)
- Abdominal distention or mass
- Lack of meconium elimination within 24 hours after birth
- Inadequate urine elimination
- Vomiting of bile-stained material
- Unusual jaundice of the skin

for assisting the mother in breast-feeding or bottle-feeding her infant.

- *Parent education.* The nurse provides infant care classes for parents and encourages parents to participate in the care of their newborn.
- *Attachment.* Attachment is promoted by encouraging all family members to be involved with the new member of the family.

Newborn Feeding

Initial Feeding

It is the practice in most institutions to offer the newborn an initial feeding of plain sterile water approximately 1–4 hours after birth. Parents of breast-fed infants need to be informed of the rationale for it and of the fact that it will not hinder the newborn's intake of breast milk. If aspiration should occur, the water is readily absorbed by the lung tissue. Glucose water should not be used, since it will damage the newborn's lung tissue if aspirated (Avery, 1981). The sterile water provides an opportunity for the nurse to assess the effectiveness of the newborn's suck, swallow, and gag reflexes. A softer nipple made for preterm infants may be used if the newborn appears to tire easily. Extreme fatigue coupled with rapid respiration and circumoral cyanosis may indicate cardiovascular complications and should be assessed further. The initial feeding also provides an opportunity to assess the newborn for symptoms of tracheoesophageal fistula or esophageal atresia (see Chapter 22 for further discussion). In cases of esophageal atresia, the feeding is taken well initially, but as the esophageal pouch fills, the feeding is quickly regurgitated unchanged by stomach contents. If a fistula is present, the infant gags, chokes, regurgitates mucus, and may become cyanotic as fluid passes through the fistula into the lungs.

It is not unusual for the neonate to regurgitate some mucus and water following a feeding even though it was taken without difficulty. Consequently, the newborn is positioned on the side after a feeding to aid drainage and is observed carefully. To decrease this mucus, some nurseries routinely aspirate the stomach contents and do gastric lavage when the neonate is admitted from labor and delivery. Inability to pass the gastric tube suggests the possibility of atresia. The procedure should be stopped and the newborn assessed further.

Some mothers who plan to breast-feed will ask to nurse their newborns immediately following birth. This practice provides stimulation for milk production and aids in maternal-newborn attachment. If the newborn appears to have difficulty nursing, the sterile water feeding by the nurse allows an opportunity for assessment. If the water feeding is taken without difficulty and retained, the mother may resume breast-feeding. In formula-fed newborns, after a few successful swallows of sterile water, glucose water or formula may be substituted to give needed sugar and prevent hypoglycemia. The newborn may take 15–30 mL at this first feeding. The newborn's stomach will be filled within 3–5 minutes of sucking at the breast or bottle.

Feeding their newborn requires decisions by most new parents. The nurse provides information to assist them in the decision and can recommend an appropriate diet for the newborn. The information should include (a) an assessment of newborn nutritional needs, (b) adequate facts about the choice between breast- and bottle-feeding, and (c) suggestions about when to add supplemental foods.

Nutritional Needs of the Newborn

The newborn's diet must supply nutrients to meet the rapid rate of physical growth and development. A neonatal diet should include protein, carbohydrate, fat, water, vitamins, and minerals, and provide adequate calories. Recommendations shown in Table 21-1 are all based on limited research data but give generalizations about requirements for optimal nutrition for the first year of life.

The calories (110–120 cal/kg/day) in the newborn's diet are divided among protein, carbohydrate, and fat and should be adjusted according to the infant's weight. Protein is needed for rapid cellular growth and maintenance. The fat portion of the diet provides calories, regulates fluid and electrolyte balance, and develops the neonatal brain and neurologic system. Water requirements are high (140–160 mL/kg/day) in the newborn because of an inability to concentrate urine. Fluid needs are further increased in illness or hot weather. The iron intake of the infant will be affected by accu-

Table 21-1
Nutritional Needs of the Normal Newborn*

	At birth	At 1 year
Calories	120/kg	100/kg
Protein	1.9 g/100 kcal[†]	1.7 g/100 kcal[†]
Fat	30%–55% of total calories	30%–50% of total calories
Carbohydrate	35%–55% of total calories	35%–55% of total calories
Water	330 mL[‡]	700 mL
Calcium	388 mg	299 mg
Phosphate	132 mg	110 mg
Magnesium	16 mg	13.5 mg
Iron	7 mg	7 mg
Copper	Not established	Not established
Zinc	Not established	Not established
Vitamins		
A	100–200 IU[†]	100–200 IU[†]
D	0.4 mg/dL[†]	0.4 mg/dL[†]
E	0.4 mg/dL[†]	0.4 mg/dL[†]
K	75 mg/day[†]	75 mg/day[†]
C	10 mg/day[†]	10 mg/day[†]
Thiamine	0.2 mg/100 kcal[†]	0.2 mg/100 kcal[†]

*Adapted from information contained in Eckstein EF: *Food, People, and Nutrition.* Westport, Conn.: A V Publishing, 1980.
[†]Estimated to be approximately equivalent to levels in breast milk.
[‡]Approximately.

mulation of iron stores during the fetal life, and the mother's iron, and other food intake if she is breast-feeding. Ascorbic acid (usually in the form of fruit juices) and meat are known to enhance absorption of iron in the mother. Adequate minerals and vitamins are needed by the newborn to prevent deficiency states such as scurvy, cheilosis, and pellagra (Eckstein, 1980).

Breast milk: nutritional aspects The American Academy of Pediatrics (1980) recommends breast milk as the optimal food for the first 4–6 months of life. All factors being equal, breast milk is probably the best food for a newborn. The advantages are that breast milk contains antibodies to disease, is nonallergenic, and is not affected by unsafe water or insect-carried disease (Joseph, 1981). Breast milk and all its components are delivered to the infant in an unchanged form, and vitamins are not lost through processing and heating.

Breast milk is composed of lactose, lipids, polyunsaturated fatty acids, and amino acids, especially taurine. Larger amounts of lactose are present in breast milk than in formula milk. Some researchers feel the balance of amino acids in breast milk makes it the best food for neurologic development. Colostrum (the first milk) contains macrophages that appear to protect the newborn against respiratory infections, vomiting, allergy, and unexplained mortality (Palma and Adcock, 1981). Breast milk also contains an anti-infective organism called *Lactobacillus bifidus*, a natural protector against virulent disease strains in the gastrointestinal tract.

The American Academy of Pediatrics states that there is generally no need to give supplemental iron to breast-fed newborns before the age of 6 months. Supplemental iron may be detrimental to the ability of breast milk to protect the newborn by interfering with lactoferrin, an iron-binding protein that enhances the absorption of iron and has anti-infective properties.

If the breast-feeding mother is taking daily multivitamins, the newborn does not usually need extra vitamins. When the mother's diet or vitamin intake is inadequate or questionable, most pediatricians prescribe vitamins for the infant. Breast-fed newborns receive minerals in a more acceptable dose than do formula-fed infants (Riordan and Countryman, 1980).

One disadvantage of breast-feeding is that most drugs taken by the mother are transmitted through breast milk and may cause harm to the newborn (see Appendix E for specific drugs and their possible effect on the neonate). A mother's poor nutritional, physical, or mental health may be contraindications for breast-feeding. Difficulty in maintaining milk supply, sore nipples, and constant demand on her time may be other reasons not to breast-feed. Jaundice caused by breast milk may be yet another reason to not continue breast-feeding.

Formula: nutritional aspects Numerous types of commercially prepared lactose formulas meet the nutritional needs of the infant. These milk formulas contain different amounts of amino acids: tyrosine and phenylalanine are more prevalent in formula milk; the taurine present in breast milk is absent in cow's milk formula. Bottle-fed babies do gain weight a little faster than breast-fed babies because of the higher protein in commercially prepared formula than in human milk. Formula-fed infants generally double their weight within 3½–4 months, whereas nursing infants double their weight at about 5 months.

Formulas contain mostly saturated fatty acids, whereas breast milk is higher in unsaturated fatty acids. Calcium, sodium, and chloride occur in higher concentrations in some commercially made formulas, which may be detrimental to the newborn's kidneys. Their immature state may not be ready to handle such high loads of solutes. This high solute load may also lead to thirst in the formula-fed infant, causing overfeeding and possible obesity (Evans and Glass, 1979).

Another potential problem with formulas is an allergic reaction in the newborn. Before 6 months of age, the infant does not produce immunoglobulins to protect against allergic responses. Introduction of foreign-produced proteins in formula may cause an allergy.

Clinicians recommend iron-fortified formulas or supplements to those mothers who are bottle-feeding with non–iron fortified formulas as iron deficiency anemia is still very prevalent. Seven milligrams of iron per day is the recommended iron dosage. However, the nurse must be aware that too much iron in the form of the extra cereal or a too high formula iron content may interfere with the infant's natural ability to defend against disease (Picciano and Deering, 1980). Parents also need to be informed about the constipation that sometimes results from iron-enriched formula and about various methods of alleviating the constipation. Opinion varies about the use of vitamin supplements for newborns.

Many companies make an enriched formula that is similar to breast milk. These formulas all have sufficient levels of carbohydrate, protein, fat, vitamins, and minerals to meet the newborn's nutritional needs.

Whichever method of feeding is chosen, formula or breast milk, newborns should be given one of these feedings until 9 months to 1 year of age. Table 21-2 compares the components of breast milk, unmodified cow's milk, and a commercially standardized formula.

Neither unmodified cow's milk nor skim milk is an acceptable alternative for newborn feeding. The protein content in cow's milk is too high (50%–75% more than human milk), is poorly digested, and may cause bleeding of the gastrointestinal tract. Unmodified cow's milk is also inadequate in vitamins. Skim milk lacks adequate calories, fat content, and essential fatty acids necessary for proper development of the neonate's neurological system. It provides excessive protein and also causes problems as a result of altered osmolarity. Nutritionists advise against use of unmodified cow's milk or skim milk for children under 2 years of age.

Table 21-2

Composition of Mature Breast Milk, Unmodified Cow's Milk, and a Routine Infant Formula*

Composition/dL	Mature breast milk	Cow's milk	Routine formula (20 cal) with iron
Calories	75.0	69.0	67.0
Protein, g	1.1	3.5	1.5
Lactalbumin %	80	18	
Casein %	20	82	
Water, ml	87.1	87.3	
Fat, g	4.0	3.5	3.7
Carbohydrate, g	9.5	4.9	7.0
Ash, g	0.21	0.72	0.34
Minerals			
Na, mg	16.0	50.0	25.0
K, mg	51.0	144.0	74.0
Ca, mg	33.0	118.0	55.0
P, mg	14.0	93.0	43.0
Mg, mg	4.0	12.0	9.0
Fe, mg	0.1	Tr.	1.2
Zn, mg	0.15	0.1	0.42
Vitamins			
A, IU	240.0	140.0	158.6
C, mg	5.0	1.0	5.3
D, IU	2.2	1.4	42.3
E, IU	0.18	0.04	0.83
Thiamin, mg	0.01	0.03	0.04
Riboflavin, mg	0.04	0.17	0.06
Niacin, mg	0.2	0.1	0.7
Curd size	Soft	Firm	Mod. firm
	Flocculent	Large	Mod. large
pH	Alkaline	Acid	Acid
Anti-infective properties	+	±	–
Bacterial content	Sterile	Nonsterile	Sterile
Emptying time	More rapid		

*Avery GB: *Neonatology*, 2nd ed. Philadelphia: Lippincott, 1981, p. 1020.

Establishing a Feeding Pattern

Following the initial feeding, some hospitals establish artificial 4-hour time frames for feedings. This scheduling may present difficulties for the new mother trying to establish lactation. Breast milk is rapidly digested by the newborn, who may desire to nurse every 2–3 hours initially, with one or two feedings during the night.

Rooming-in permits the mother to feed the infant as needed. When rooming-in is not available, a supportive nursing staff and flexible nursery policies will allow the mother to feed on demand when the infant is hungry. Nothing is more frustrating to a new mother than attempting to nurse a newborn who is sound asleep because he or she is either not hungry or exhausted from crying. Once lactation is established and the family is home, a feeding pattern agreeable to both mother and child is usually established.

Formula-fed newborns may awaken for feedings every 2–5 hours but are frequently satisfied with feedings every 3–4 hours. Because formula is digested more slowly, the bottle-fed infant may go longer between feedings and may begin skipping the night feeding within about 6 weeks. This is very individualized depending on the size and development of the infant.

Both breast-fed and bottle-fed infants experience growth spurts at certain times and require increased feeding. The mother of a breast-fed infant may meet these increased demands by nursing more frequently to increase her milk supply. A slight increase in feedings will meet the needs of the formula-fed infant.

Providing nourishment for her newborn is a major concern of the new mother. Her feelings of success or failure may influence her self-concept as she assumes her maternal role. With proper instruction, support, and encouragement from professional persons, feeding becomes a source of pleasure and satisfaction to both parents and infant. (See Chapter 24 for a discussion of methods of assisting a mother to breast-feed or bottle-feed her newborn.)

Nutritional Assessment of the Infant

During the early months of life, the food offered to and consumed by infants will be instrumental in their proper growth and development. (See Essential Facts to Remember—Nutritional Needs of the Newborn.)

At each well-child visit the nurse assesses the nutritional status of the newborn. Assessment should include four components:

- Nutritional history from the parent
- Weight gain since the last visit
- Growth chart percentiles
- Physical examination

The nutritional history reports the type, amount, and frequency of milk and supplemental foods being given to the infant on a daily basis. The infant should gain 1 ounce per day for the first 6 months of life and 0.5 ounce per day for the second 6 months. Individual charts show the infant's growth with respect to height, weight, and head circumference. The important consideration is that infants continue to grow at their individual rates. The physical examination will assist in identifying any nutritional disorders. Edema, dermatitis, cheilosis, or bleeding gums may be caused by excess protein intake, or riboflavin, niacin, or vitamin C deficiency, respectively. Iron deficiency should be suspected in a pale, diaphoretic, irritable infant who is obese and consumes more than 35–40 ounces of formula per day (Driggers, 1980).

By calculating the nutritional needs of infants, the nurse can recommend a diet that supplies appropriate nutrition for infant growth and development. The assessment is especially helpful in counseling mothers of infants under 6 months of age in view of the tendency to add too many supplemental foods or offer too much formula to infants of this age. Usually this assessment will show that formula alone gives the infant enough calories so that introduction of solid foods can be delayed until later.

✺ ESSENTIAL FACTS TO REMEMBER

Nutritional Needs of the Newborn

- Caloric intake: 110–120 cal/kg/day
- Fluid requirements: 140–160 mL/kg/day
- Weight gain: First 6 months—1 oz/day
  Second 6 months—0.5 oz/day

Identification of appropriate nutritional intake can be done by comparing the infant's dietary intake with the desired caloric intake, weight, age, and the number of calories needed by the infant. Most commercial formulas prescribed for the normal healthy newborn contain 20 calories per ounce. If the infant is eating solids, the caloric value of those foods must be determined and included in the calculation of nutritional intake. With knowledge of the amount of calories needed by the infant according to weight and using Table 21-3, the nurse can counsel the parents about how many ounces per day the child needs to meet caloric requirements. The following case study shows the effectivenesss of these assessments (Markesberry, 1979).

——————— CASE STUDY* ———————

Ms. Leach brings Sue, age 1 month, to the clinic for a well-baby checkup. The baby measures 20½ inches and weighs 10 pounds. In relating the baby's dietary history, her mother says Sue was a healthy eater from day one. She drains her bottle in 5–12 minutes and by 2 weeks seemed hungry after the bottle. At that time she was already taking a full can of Similac (20 calories/ounce) concentrate (26 ounces diluted) a day, and feeding every 3 hours, so Ms. Leach added baby cereal to her nighttime feeding. Sue didn't accept cereal at first but took it readily when sugar was added. Now she's taking four tablespoons both morning and evening and has strained peaches or bananas once a day. Her daily calorie intake is as follows:

1 can Similac	520	calories
Cereal	88+	calories (formula or milk added to prepare cereal provides calories as does sugar)
Fruit	90	calories
Total Intake	698+	calories

A quick check of her caloric needs ... (Table 21-3) shows that at 10 pounds Sue should require 550 calories per day. This would be met by 27½ ounces of Similac alone. Her intake is well above suggested levels, a common finding in infants at this age.

*From Markesberry BA: Watching baby's diet: A professional and parent guide. *MCN* 1979; 4:177.

Table 21-3

Approximate Number of Ounces of 20 Calorie/Ounce Formula Needed to Meet Infant Caloric Needs*

Weight of infant	Caloric need (24 hr)	Ounces infant formula (24 hr)
Birth to 3 months		
6 lb	330	16.5
7 lb	385	19
8 lb	440	22
9 lb	495	25
10 lb	550	27.5
11 lb	605	30
12 lb	660	33
13 lb	715	36
14 lb	770	38.5
3-6 months		
10 lb	520	26
11 lb	572	28.5
12 lb	624	31
13 lb	676	34
14 lb	728	36.5
15 lb	780	39
16 lb	832	41.2
17 lb	884	44
18 lb	936	47
19 lb	988	49.5
20 lb	1040	52
21 lb	1092	54.5
22 lb	1144	57

*Reprinted with permission from Markesberry B: Watching baby's diet: A professional and parent guide. *Am J Nurs* 1979; 4:180.

Supplemental Foods

Opinions vary widely about when to add new foods and what kinds of supplemental foods to add to the infant's diet. Health care professionals need to help mothers plan their children's diet. If reasons are offered for why specific foods are given or withheld, more parental cooperation can be expected (Broussard, 1984).

The proper time to add foods to the infant's diet should be determined by the physiologic ability to accept other foods besides milk. Because breast milk or formula meets all the requirements of growth for the normal infant until 6 months of age, only after 6 months does the child need extra iron, water, carbohydrate, and vitamin C. Foods should be introduced one at a time to identify any food allergy, but the sequence of foods given is not critical.

Parents need to be advised that putting an infant to bed with a full bottle of formula or juice may foster tooth decay and ear infections. The infant needs extra water between meals when solid food is added because the solute load on the infant's kidneys will be increased. Mothers should be cautioned against adding extra salt or sugar to the infant's food; their long-term effects on the infant's future growth and blood pressure and the need for salt are currently under study. Some clinicians also advocate withholding cow's milk, eggs, and wheat until the infant is 6–9 months old. These are known to be allergenic substances for many persons.

Weaning

The decision to wean an infant from breast milk may be made because the child is 9–12 months old and can drink from a cup or because a separation of mother and child is imminent. Whatever the reason, the weaning process may cause emotional and physical trauma for the mother and the infant.

Weaning is a time of emotional separation for mother and baby: it may be difficult for them to give up the closeness of their nursing sessions. The nurse who is understanding about this possibility can help the mother to see that her infant is growing up and assist her to plan other activities to replace breast-feeding. A gradual approach is the easiest and most comforting way to wean the child from breast-feedings. Other activities can serve to enhance the parent–infant attachment process.

During weaning, the mother should substitute one cup-feeding or bottle-feeding for one breast-feeding session over several days so that her breasts gradually produce less milk. Over a period of several weeks she should substitute more cup-feedings or bottle-feedings for breast-feedings. Many mothers continue to nurse once a day in the early morning or late evening for several months until the milk supply is gone. The slow method of weaning will prevent breast engorgement and allows infants to alter their eating methods at their own rates.

Circumcision _____

Circumcision is a surgical procedure in which the prepuce of the penis is separated from the glans and a portion is excised. This permits exposure of the glans and easier retraction of the foreskin for cleaning purposes.

The parents make the decision about circumcision for their newborn male child. In most cases the choice is based on cultural, social, and family tradition. To guarantee informed consent, parents should be informed about possible long-term medical effects of circumcision and noncircumcision during the prenatal period. In the past, this procedure has been recommended for all newborn males. It is now recognized that in most cases this procedure is one of preference and not medically required (American Academy of Pediatrics, 1975).

Originally, circumcision was a rite of the Jewish religion. Proponents of the procedure cite studies that imply the incidence of cervical cancer is less in women married to circumcised men. The incidence of cancer of the penis is also lower in circumcised men. In addition, some believe circumcision allows for improved cleanliness and individual comfort. Opponents question the statistical data about cervical carcinoma and feel that neonatal circumcision predisposes to meatitis, which may eventually lead to meatal stenosis. Those opposed to circumcision maintain that continued retraction and good hygienic practices result in comparable cleanliness and comfort. Considerable controversy still exists regarding the pros and cons of circumcision.

To decrease the incidence of cold stress, the procedure is usually not done until the day prior to discharge, when the infant is well stabilized. Sometimes an infant is brought in after discharge for circumcision.

The nurse's responsibilities during a circumcision begin with checking to see that the circumcision permit is signed. Equipment is gathered, and then the infant is prepared by removing the diaper and placing him on a circumcision board or some other type of restraint (Figure 21-3).

A variety of techniques for circumcision is available (Figures 21-4, 21-5, 21-6), and all produce minimal bleeding. During the procedure, the nurse assesses the newborn's response. One consideration is pain experienced by the newborn. There is no question that he feels pain, but it is not known if he remembers the discomfort. Few physicians use anesthesia for this

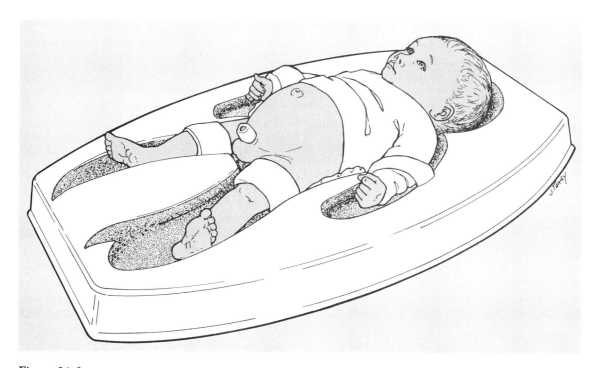

Figure 21-3
Proper positioning of the infant on a circumcision restraining board.

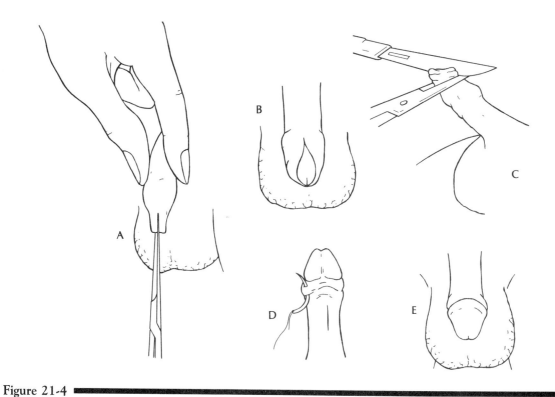

Figure 21-4
A and **B**, In this circumcision procedure, the prepuce is slit and retracted. **C**, Excess prepuce is then cut off.
D, The prepuce is sutured in place. **E**, Circumcised penis.

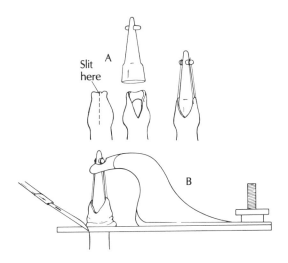

Figure 21-5
When the Yellen clamp is used for circumcision, the prepuce is drawn over the cone (**A**), and the clamp is applied (**B**). Pressure is maintained for 3–5 minutes, and then the excess prepuce is cut away.

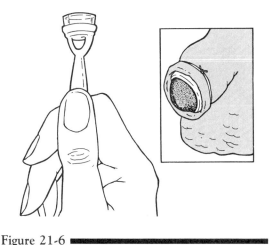

Figure 21-6
When the Plastibell is used for circumcision, the bell is fitted over the glans. Suture is tied around the bell's rim and the excess prepuce is cut away. The plastic rim remains in place for 3–4 days until healing takes place. The bell may be removed or allowed to fall off.

procedure. The nurse can provide comfort measures such as lightly stroking the baby's head and talking to him. Following the circumcision he should be held and comforted by his mother (Lubchenco, 1980).

After the circumcision a small petroleum jelly gauze strip may be applied to help control bleeding and to keep the diaper from adhering to the site. The petroleum jelly gauze is left in place for 1–2 days. It need not be changed unless it becomes contaminated with fecal material. The neonate's voiding should be assessed for amount, adequacy of stream, and presence of blood. If bleeding does occur, pressure is applied to the site with a sterile gauze, and the physician is notified. The neonate may be fussy for a few hours after the procedure or cry when he voids. He should be positioned on his side with the diaper fastened loosely to prevent undue pressure.

Before dismissal, the parents should be instructed to observe the penis for bleeding or possible signs of infection. A whitish yellow exudate around the glans is normal and not indicative of an infection. The exudate may be noted for about 2–3 days, and should not be removed, although the parents may be instructed to gently wash the penis and pat it dry. The diaper is loosely fastened for 2–3 days, because the glans remains tender for this length of time.

If a Plastibell is used, parents need to be informed that it will remain in place for about 3–4 days, then fall off (Figure 21-6).

Parent Education

Parents may be familiar with handling and caring for infants or this may be their first time to interact with a newborn. If they are new parents, the sensitive nurse gently teaches them by example and instructions geared to their needs and previous knowledge about the various aspects of newborn care.

The nurse observes how parents interact with their infant during feeding and caregiving activities. Rooming-in, even for a short time, offers opportunities for the nurse to provide information and evaluate whether the parents are comfortable with changing diapers, wrapping, handling, and feeding their newborn. Do both parents get involved in the infant's care? Is the mother depending on someone else to help her at home? Does the mother give excuses for not wanting to be involved in her baby's care? ("I am too tired," "My stitches hurt," or "I will learn later.") All these considerations need to be taken into account when evaluating the educational needs of the parents.

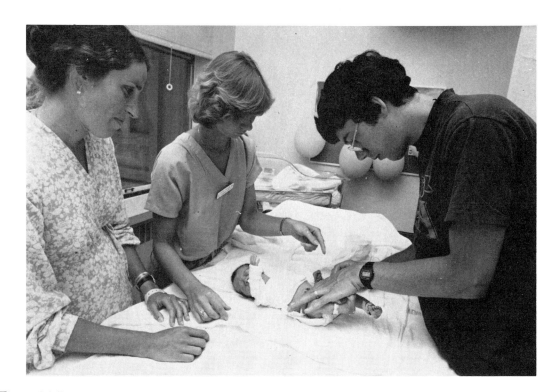

Figure 21-7
Individualizing parent education. Father returns demonstration of diapering his daughter.

Several methods may be used to teach parents about newborn care. Daily child care classes are a nonthreatening way to convey general information. Individual instruction is helpful to answer specific questions or to clarify an item that may have been confusing in class (Figure 21-7). Discharge planning is essential to verify the mother's knowledge when she leaves the hospital. Follow-up calls after discharge lend added support by providing another opportunity for mothers to have their questions answered. The essential areas to be covered by a nurse in educating parents before discharge are described in the following sections.

Positioning and Handling

Methods of positioning and handling the newborn are demonstrated to parents if needed. As the parents provide care, the nurse can instill parental confidence by giving them positive feedback. If the parents encounter problems, the nurse can suggest alternatives and serve as a role model.

How to pick up a newborn is one of the first concerns of anyone who has not handled many babies. When the infant is in the side-lying position, it is easily picked up by sliding one hand under the baby's neck and shoulders and the other hand under the buttocks or between the legs, then gently lifting the newborn from the crib. This technique provides security and support for the head (which the newborn is unable to support).

After the baby is out of the crib, one of the following holds may be used (Figure 21-8). The *cradle hold* is frequently used during feeding. It provides a sense of warmth and closeness, permits eye contact, frees one of the nurse's or parent's hands, and provides security because the cradling protects the infant's body. The *upright position* provides security and a sense of closeness and is ideal for burping the infant. One hand should support the neck and shoulders, while the other hand holds the buttocks or is placed between the newborn's legs. The *football hold* frees one of the caregiver's hands and permits eye contact. This hold is ideal for shampooing, carrying, or breast-feeding. It frees the mother to talk on the telephone or answer the door at home.

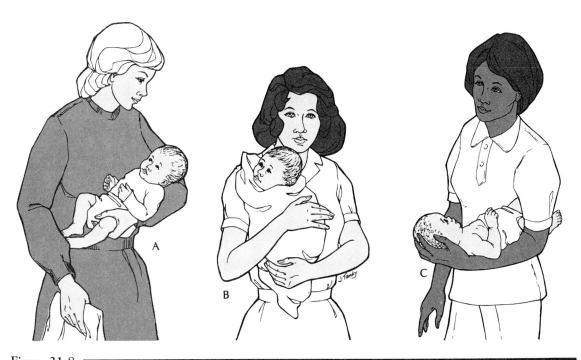

Figure 21-8
Various positions for holding an infant. **A**, Cradle hold. **B**, Upright position. **C**, Football hold.

The newborn infant is most frequently positioned on the side with a rolled blanket or diaper behind for support (Figure 21-9). This position aids drainage of mucus and allows air to circulate around the cord. It is also more comfortable for the newly circumcised male.

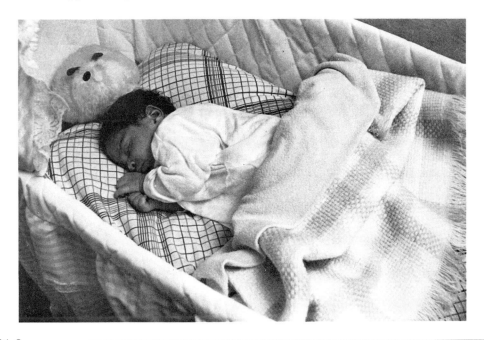

Figure 21-9
The most common sleeping position of the newborn is on the side. The little girl shown here does not need the additional support provided by a rolled blanket.

After feeding, the infant is placed on the right side to aid digestion and to prevent aspiration. Once the cord is healed, many infants prefer to lie prone. Newborns have enough head control to turn their heads side to side to prevent suffocation. The infant's position should be changed periodically during the early months of life, because neonatal skull bones are soft, and flattened areas may develop if the newborn consistently lies in one position.

Nasal and Oral Suctioning

Infants generally maintain air passage patency by coughing or sneezing. During the first few days of life, however, the newborn has increased mucus, and gentle suctioning with a bulb syringe may be indicated.

Parents have a great fear of their infant choking and may be relieved if they know what action to take. The nurse can demonstrate the use of the bulb syringe in the nose and mouth and have the parents do a return demonstration. The parents should repeat this demonstration before discharge so they will feel more confident and comfortable with the procedure. To suction the newborn, the bulb syringe is compressed, then the tip is placed in the nostril, and the bulb is permitted to reexpand slowly as the nurse or parent releases the compression on the bulb (Figure 21-10). The drainage is then compressed out of the bulb onto a tissue. The bulb syringe may also be used in the mouth if the newborn is spitting up and unable to handle the excess secretions. The bulb is compressed; the tip of the bulb syringe is placed about 1 inch in one side of the infant's mouth; and compression is released. This draws up the excess secretions. The procedure is repeated on the other side of the mouth. The center of the infant's mouth is avoided because suction in this area might stimulate the gag reflex. The bulb syringe should be washed in warm, soapy water and rinsed in warm water after each use. The bulb syringe should always be kept near the infant.

Bathing

An actual bath demonstration is the best way for the nurse to teach parents. Because excess bathing will dry out the baby's sensitive skin, bathing should be done every other day or twice

a week. Sponge baths are recommended for the first 2 weeks or until the umbilical cord completely falls off. The following information should be included in the demonstration. Supplies can be kept in a plastic bag or some type of container to prevent hunting for supplies each time. The supplies include two washcloths, two towels, two blankets, mild soap without much perfume (for example, Dial or Safeguard), shampoo, A and D or petroleum jelly (Vaseline) ointment, lotion, rubbing alcohol, cotton balls, two diapers, and clean clothes. The mother may want to use a small plastic tub for water, a clean kitchen or bathroom sink, or a large bowl. Expensive baby tubs are not necessary, but some parents may prefer to purchase them.

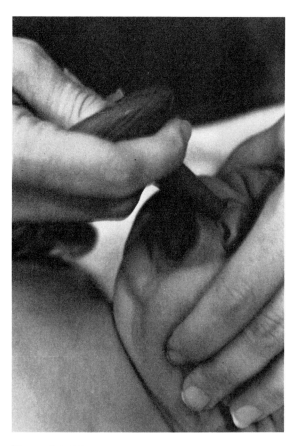

Figure 21-10 ▬▬▬▬▬
Nasal and pharyngeal suctioning. The bulb is compressed, then the tip is placed either in the nostril or mouth; the bulb is allowed to reexpand as the compression of the bulb is released. (From Swearingen P: *The Addison-Wesley Photo-Atlas of Nursing Procedures*. Menlo Park, Ca.: Addison-Wesley, 1984.)

Before starting, if no one else is at home, the parent may want to take the phone off the hook and put a sign on the door to prevent being disturbed. Having someone home during the first few baths will be helpful because that person can get items that were forgotten and provide moral support. The room should be warm and free of drafts.

Sponge bath After the supplies are gathered, the tub (or any of the containers mentioned above) is filled with water that is warm to the touch. The water temperature is tested with an albow or forearm. (Parents may also purchase a thermometer for bath water.) Soap should not be added to the water. The infant should be wrapped in a blanket, with a T-shirt and diaper on. This helps keep the newborn warm and secure.

To start the bath, a washcloth is wrapped around the index finger once. Each eye is gently wiped from inner to outer corner. This direction is the way eyes naturally drain and wiping in this direction prevents irritation of the eyes. A different spot on the washcloth is used for each eye to prevent cross-contamination. Some swelling and drainage may be common the first few days after birth. The ears are washed next by wrapping the washcloth once around an index finger and gently cleaning the external ear and behind the ear. Cotton swabs are never used in the ears because it is possible to put the swab too far into the ear and damage the ear drum. The remainder of the infant's face is then wiped with the soap-free washcloth. Many infants start to cry at this point. The face should be washed every day and the mouth and chin wiped off after each feeding.

The neck is washed carefully but thoroughly with the washcloth. Soap may now be used. Formula or breast milk and lint collect in the skin folds of the neck, so it may be helpful to sit the baby up, supporting the neck and shoulders with one hand while washing the neck with the other hand.

The baby's T-shirt is now removed and the blanket unwrapped. The chest, back, and arms are wet with the washcloth. The parent may then lather the hands with soap and wash the baby's chest, back, and arms. Care is taken to avoid wetting the cord. Soap is rinsed off with the wet washcloth, and the upper part of the body is dried with a towel or blanket. The baby's upper body is then wrapped with a dry clean blanket to prevent a chill.

Next the infant's legs are unwrapped, wet with the washcloth, lathered, rinsed, and well dried. If the infant has dry skin, a *small* amount of lotion or ointment (petroleum jelly or A and D ointment) may be used. Ointments are better than lotions for dry cracked feet and hands. Baby oil is not used, as it clogs skin pores. Powders aggravate dry skin and are also avoided.

The genital area is cleaned daily with soap and water and with water after each wet or dirty diaper. Girls are washed from the *front* of the genital area toward the rectum to avoid fecal contamination of the urethra and thus to the bladder. Newborn girls often have a thick, white mucus discharge or a slight bloody discharge from their vaginal area. This discharge is normal for the first 1–2 weeks of age and should be wiped off with a damp cloth at diaper changes.

Parents of uncircumcised baby boys should cleanse the penis daily. Daily retraction of the foreskin is controversial; consultation with the health care provider is desirable. Baby boys who have been circumcised need daily gentle cleansing. A very wet washcloth is rubbed over a bar of soap. The washcloth is squeezed above the baby's penis, letting the soapy water run over the circumcision site. The area is rinsed off with plain warm water and patted dry. A small amount of petroleum jelly or bactericidal ointment may be put on the circumcised area, but excessive amounts may block the meatus and should be avoided.

Baby powder (or cornstarch) is not recommended for diaper rash. Baby powder may cake with urine and irritate the infant's bottom. Corn starch may lead to a fungal infection. Both products may also be inhaled by the infant while being applied. If either powder or cornstarch is used, the parent should place a hand over the genital area during application. Ointments are more effective for diaper rash. If the ointment does not help the rash, parents using disposable diapers may try another brand of diaper. If cloth diapers are used, a different detergent or fabric softener may alleviate the problem. Persistent diaper rash should always be discussed with the clinician.

The umbilical cord should be kept clean and dry by cleansing it with alcohol-soaked cotton balls. The cord generally falls off in 7–14 days. Alcohol is used until the cord is completely gone. The diaper should be folded down to allow air to circulate around the cord. The physician should be consulted if bright red bleeding or puslike drainage occurs.

The last step in bathing is washing the infant's hair (some suggest doing this step first). The newborn is swaddled in a dry blanket, leaving only the head exposed and held in the football hold with the head tilted slightly downward to prevent water running in the eyes. Water should be brought to the head by a cupped hand. The hair is moistened and lathered with a small amount of shampoo. A *very* soft brush may be used to massage the shampoo over the entire head. The brush may be used over the soft spots. The hair is then rinsed and toweled dry. Oils or lotions are not used on the newborn's head. Brushing the infant's hair every day and washing the hair with a soft soapy brush during baths will prevent cradle cap.

Tub baths   The infant may be put in a tub after the cord has fallen off and the circumcision site is healed (approximately 2 weeks) (Figure 21-11). Infants usually enjoy a tub bath more than a sponge bath, although some newborns cry during either type. To prevent slipping, a washcloth is placed in the bottom of the tub or sink.

The parent places the newborn in the tub using the cradle hold and grasping the distal thigh. The neck is supported by the parent's elbow in the cradle position. Only 3 or 4 inches of water are needed in the tub. Because wet infants are slippery, some parents have found that pulling a cotton sock (with holes cut out for the fingers) over the arm will help prevent the baby from slipping. To wash the baby's back, the parent places his or her noncradling hand on the infant's chest with the thumb under the infant's arm closest to the parent. Gently tipping the baby forward onto the supporting hand frees the cradling arm to wash the back of the baby. After the bath the infant is lifted out of the tub in the cradle position, dried well, and wrapped in a dry blanket. The hair can then be washed in the same way as for a sponge bath.

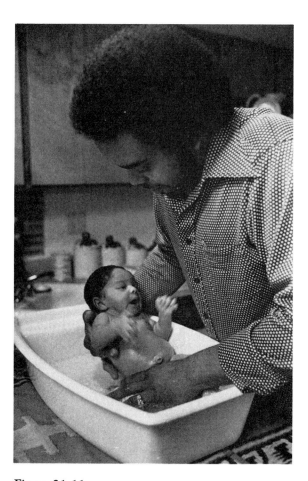

Figure 21-11
When bathing the infant, it is important to support the head. Note that the cord site has healed on this 2-week-old baby.

Nail Care

The nails of the newborn are seldom cut in the hospital. During the first days of life, the nails may adhere to the skin of the fingers, and cutting is contraindicated. Within a week the nails separate from the skin and frequently break off. If the nails are long or if infants are scratching themselves, the nails may be trimmed. This is most easily done while infants sleep. Nails should be cut straight across using adult cuticle scissors.

Wrapping the Newborn

Wrapping helps the newborn maintain body temperature and soothes him or her by providing a feeling of closeness and sense of security.

When wrapping, a blanket is placed on the crib (or secure surface) in the shape of a diamond. The baby's body is placed with the head at the upper corner of the diamond. The left corner of the blanket is wrapped around the infant and tucked under the right side (not too tightly—newborns need a little room to move). The bottom corner is then pulled up to the chest, and the right corner is wrapped around the baby's left side. This wrapping technique can be shared with a new mother so she will feel more skilled in handling her baby.

Dressing the Newborn

Newborns need to wear a T-shirt, diaper (plastic pants if using cloth diapers), and a sleeper. On a fairly cool day, they should also be wrapped in a light blanket while being fed. A good rule of thumb is for the parent to add one more light layer of clothing than the parent is wearing. Infants should wear hats outdoors to protect their sensitive ears from drafts. An infant may be covered with a blanket in air-conditioned stores. The blanket should be unwrapped or removed when inside a warm building.

At home the amount of clothing the infant wears is determined by the temperature. Families who maintain the home at 60–65F should dress the infant more warmly than those who maintain the temperature at 70–75F.

Diaper shapes vary and are subject to personal preference (Figure 21-12). Prefolded and disposable diapers are usually rectangular. Diapers may also be triangular or kite-folded. Extra material is placed in front for boys and toward the back for girls to aid in absorbency.

Infant clothing should be laundered separately using a mild soap or detergent. Diapers may be presoaked prior to washing. All clothing should be rinsed twice to remove soap and residue and to decrease the possibility of rash. Some infants may not tolerate the use of clothing treated with fabric softeners; in this case softeners should be avoided.

Temperature Assessment

The nurse must demonstrate how to take rectal and axillary temperatures for parents. A return demonstration is the only way to evaluate their understanding. The nurse shows them

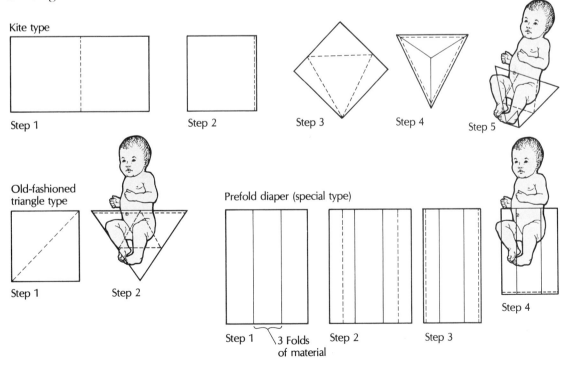

Figure 21-12
Three basic diaper shapes. Dotted lines indicate folds.

how to shake down a thermometer before inserting it.

When parents take a rectal temperature, the infant should be supine with the legs held up in one hand, exposing the rectum. The end of the rectal thermometer is lubricated with petroleum jelly and the thermometer is inserted just until the silver bulb is covered, approximately half an inch. The thermometer is held in place 5 minutes. A baby is never left alone with a thermometer in place. Normal rectal temperature is 36.6–37.2C (97.8–99F). Rectal temperatures are more accurate, and most pediatricians prefer that parents take temperatures this way.

To take an axillary temperature, the thermometer is placed under one of the infant's arms, making sure that the bulb of the thermometer is underneath the armpit. It is held in place 3–4 minutes (Figure 20-13). A parent only needs to take the newborn's temperature when any signs of illness are present. See Essential Facts to Remember—Signs of Illness in Newborns.

Parents are advised to call a physician immediately if any of these signs occur. Parents should also check with their physician for advice about over-the-counter medications they should have in the medicine cabinet. Flu, colds, teething, constipation, diarrhea, and other common ailments and their management should be discussed beforehand with the physician.

Stools and Urine

The appearance and frequency of newborn's stools can cause concern for parents. The nurse prepares parents by discussing and showing pictures of meconium stools, transitional stools, and the difference between breast-milk and formula stools. Although each baby develops his or her own stooling patterns, parents can be given an idea of what to expect. Parents should be told that breast-fed babies may have six to ten small, loose yellow stools per day, whereas formula-fed infants may have only one or two stools a day, which are more formed and brown. The parents may also be shown pictures of a constipated stool (small, pelletlike) and diarrhea (loose, green, or perhaps blood-tinged). Parents should understand that a green color is common in transitional stools so that

ESSENTIAL FACTS TO REMEMBER

Signs of Illness in Newborns

Parents should be alert to these signs of illness:

- Temperature above 38.4C (101F) or below 36.1C (97F)
- More than one episode of projectile vomiting
- Refusal of two feedings in a row
- Lethargy (listlessness)
- Cyanosis with or without a feeding
- Apnea

transitional stools are not confused with diarrhea the first week of a newborn's life.

Infants normally void (urinate) five to eight times per day. Less than five to eight wet diapers a day may indicate the newborn needs more fluids.

Sleep and Activity

Perhaps nothing is more individual to each neonate than the sleep-activity cycle. It is important for the nurse to recognize the individual variations of each newborn and to assist parents as they develop sensitivity to their infant's communication signals and rhythms of activity and sleep.

The newborn demonstrates several different sleep-wake states after the initial periods of reactivity described earlier. It is not uncommon for a neonate to sleep almost continuously for the first 2–3 days following birth, awakening only for feedings every 3–4 hours. Some newborns bypass this stage of deep sleep and may require only 12–16 hours of sleep. The parents need to know that this is normal.

Quiet sleep is characterized by regular breathing and no movement except for sudden body jerks. During this sleep state, normal household noise will not awaken the infant. In the *active sleep state*, the newborn has irregular breathing and fine muscular twitching. The newborn may cry out during sleep, but this does not mean he or she is uncomfortable or awake.

Unusual household noise may awaken the infant more easily in this state; however, the newborn will quickly go back to sleep.

Wide awake is a state in which newborns are quietly involved with the environment. They watch a moving mobile, smile, and, as they become older, discover and play with their hands and feet. When infants become uncomfortable due to wet diapers, hunger, or cold, they enter the *active awake and crying state*. In this state, the cause of the crying should be identified and eliminated. Sometimes parents are frustrated as they try to identify the external or internal stimuli that are causing the angry, hurt crying.

Crying   For the newborn, crying is the only means of vocally expressing needs. Parents and caregivers learn to distinguish different tones and qualities of the neonate's cry. The amount of crying is highly individual. Some will cry as little as 15–30 minutes in 24 hours or as long as 2 hours every 24 hours. When crying continues after causes such as discomfort or hunger are eliminated, the newborn may be comforted by swaddling or by rocking and other reassuring activity. Excessive crying should be noted and assessed, taking other factors into consideration. After the first 2–3 days, newborns settle into patterns that are individual to each infant and family.

Discharge Planning

The nurse can do much to help parents develop their competence in child care. By teaching parents how to meet their newborn's needs and ensure his or her safety, the nurse can get the new family off to a good start. The nurse also plays a vital role in fostering parent–infant attachment. See Chapter 23 for in-depth discussion of attachment process.

Safety Considerations

The nurse can be an excellent role model for parents in the area of safety. Newborns should always be positioned on the stomach or side with a blanket rolled up behind them. Correct use of the bulb syringe must be demonstrated. The baby should never be left alone anywhere but in the crib. The mother is reminded that while she and the newborn are together in the hospital, she should never leave the baby alone because newborns spit up frequently the first day or two after birth.

Accidents are the number one cause of death in children, with car accidents causing the most deaths, followed by poisonings. Half of the children killed or injured in automobile accidents could have been protected by the use of federally approved car seats. Newborns should go home from the hospital in a car seat (not infant carrier seat), and children should always ride in a car seat until 4 years of age (depending on size of the child), no matter how short the trip. In many states, the use of car seats for children up to the age of 4 years is mandatory.

All medications must be locked up. Newborns quickly grow into toddlers who can climb to medicine cabinets. Vitamins look like candy to a toddler. Whenever medication is given, children should be told they are taking medicine instead of calling it candy. Plants should be put above a toddler's reach; many are poisonous. All cleaning supplies must be moved to high, out-of-the-way cupboards. Parents are told to cover electrical outlets and keep electrical cords out of sight. Newborns do not need pillows or stuffed animals in the crib while they sleep; these items could cause suffocation.

Newborn Screening Program

Before the newborn and mother are discharged from the hospital, parents are informed about the normal screening tests for newborns and should be told when to return to the hospital or clinic to have the tests completed. **Newborn screening tests** detect disorders that cause mental retardation, physical handicaps, or death if left undiscovered. Inborn errors of metabolism usually can be detected within 1–2 weeks after birth and important treatment begun before any damage has occurred. The disorders that can be identified from a drop of blood obtained by a heel stick on the second or third day are galactosemia, homocystinuria, hypothyroidism, maple syrup urine disease, phenylketonuria (PKU), and sickle cell anemia. Parents should be instructed that a second blood specimen will be required from the newborn after 7–14 days when the newborn's metabolism is fully functioning. By this time the defects are clearly apparent and treatment initiated. Treatment of these conditions may be dietary or administration of the missing hormones. The inborn conditions cannot be cured but they can be treated. Although they are not contagious, they may be inherited (Chapter 3).

Discharge Care Needs

Each newborn will have variations in normal physiologic responses. Parents need to learn how to interpret these changes in their child. To assist parents in caring for their newborn at home, some physicians encourage pediatric prenatal visits so that this contact is established before the birth (Sprunger and Preece, 1981). Public health nurses have long been involved as guides in newborn care and parent education (Lauri, 1981). Hospitals are now expanding their primary care functions to the new family to include one home visit by the primary nurse who cared for the family in the hospital. The hospital nursery staff may also make themselves available as a 24-hour telephone resource for the new mother who needs additional support and consultation during the first few days at home with her newborn.

Routine well-baby visits should be scheduled with the clinic, pediatric nurse practitioner, or physician.

Parents should be taught all necessary caregiving methods before discharge. A checklist may be helpful to see if the teaching has been completed. The nurse needs to review all areas for understanding or questions with the mother, without rushing, taking time to answer all queries. The mother should have the physician's phone number, address, and any specific instructions. Having the nursery phone number is also reassuring to a new mother. The parents are encouraged to call with questions. The nurse may use this time to remind parents that normal weight loss is 5%–10% the first 3–5 days of age and that they can expect the baby to regain the birth weight by 10 days of age.

The newborn should have 5–8 wet diapers a day and progress from meconium stools through transitional stools to normal appearing formula or breast milk stools. The cord will usually fall off about 7–14 days after birth.

The final step of discharge planning is documentation. Any concerns of the parents or nurse are noted. The nurse records which demonstrations and/or classes the mother and/or father attended and their expressed understanding of the instructions given to them.

Parent education is a wonderful aspect of family-centered maternity care. The nurse who takes the time to get the family off to a good start can feel satisfied that the best care is being provided for all members of the family.

Summary

At the moment of birth, numerous adaptations must take place in the newborn's body systems. The nursing care of newborns is aimed at helping children adjust to the new environment and ensuring their well-being. In addition, the nurse uses his or her teaching skills to help the parents of the newborn adjust to their new role. Caretaking activities of the nurse and parents range from feeding and bathing the infant to providing sensory stimulation and emotional comfort.

References

American Academy of Pediatrics, Committee on Fetus and Newborn: Report of the Ad Hoc Task Force on Circumcision. *Pediatrics* October 1975, 56:610.

American Academy of Pediatrics, Committee on Nutrition: On the feeding of supplemental foods to infants. *Pediatrics* 1980; 65:1178.

Avery GB: *Neonatology*. Philadelphia: Lippincott, 1981.

Benitz WE, Tatro DS: *The Pediatric Drug Handbook*. Chicago: Year Book Medical Publishers, 1981.

Broussard AB: Anticipatory guidance—adding solids to the infant's diet. *J Obstet Gynecol Neonatal Nurs* July/August 1984; 13(4):239.

Driggers DA: Infant nutrition made simple. *Am Fam Physician* 1980; 22:113.

Eckstein EF: *Food, People and Nutrition*. Westport, Conn.: A. V. Publishing, 1980.

Evans HE, Glass L: Breastfeeding: Advantages and potential problems. *Pediatr Ann* 1979; 8:110.

Haun N, Porter E, Chance G: Care of the Normal Neonate. *The Canadian Nurse* October 1984; 80:37.

Joseph S: Anatomy of the infant formula controversy. *Am J Dis Child* 1981; 135:889.

Klaus MH, Kennell JH: *Parent-Infant Attachment*, 2nd ed. St. Louis: Mosby, 1982.

Lauri S: The public health nurse as a guide in infant child care and education. *J Adv Nurs* 1981; 6:297.

Lubchenco LO: Routine neonatal circumcision: A surgical anachronism. *Clin Obstet Gynecol* 1980; 23:1135.

Markesberry BA: Watching baby's diet: A professional and parent guide. *MCN* 1979; 4:177.

Palma PA, Adcock EW: Human milk and breast-feeding. *Am Fam Physician* 1981; 24:173.

Picciano MF, Deering RH: The influence of feeding regimens on iron status during infancy. *Am J Clin Nutr* 1980; 33:746.

Riordan JM, Countryman BA: Basics of breast-feeding. *J Obstet Gynecol Neonatal Nurs* 1980; 9(part 3):273.

Sprunger LW, Preece EW: Use of pediatric prenatal visits by family physicians. *J Fam Pract* 1981; 13:1007.

Additional Readings

Dallman PR: Inhibition of iron absorption by certain foods. *Am J Dis Child* 1980; 143:453.

Dunn DM, White DG: Interactions of mothers with their newborns in the first half-hour of life. *J Adv Nurs* 1981; 6:271.

Gilfoyle EM et al: *Children Adapt*. Thorofare, N.J.: Charles B. Slack, 1981.

Osborn LM et al: Hygiene care in uncircumcised infants. *Pediatrics* March 1981; 67:365.

Pelosi MA, Apuzzio J: Making circumcision safe and painless. *Contemp Ob/Gyn* 1984; 24:42.

Rong ML: *Manual of Newborn Care Plans*. Boston: Little, Brown, 1981.

22
Complications of the Neonate

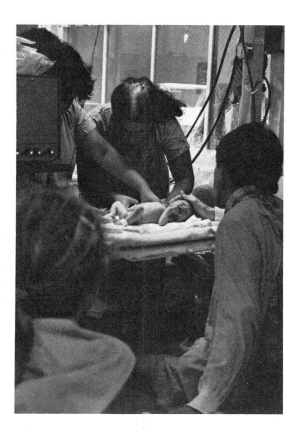

Chapter Contents

Cold Stress

Hypoglycemia

Hypocalcemia

Neonatal Jaundice
Mechanism of Bilirubin Conjugation
Hyperbilirubinemia
Nursing Management

Hemolytic Disease of the Newborn
Rh Incompatibility
ABO Incompatibility
Neonatal Assessment
Treatment of Hyperbilirubinemia and
Nursing Responsibilities
Support of the Family

Neonatal Anemia

Polycythemia

Hemorrhagic Disease

Necrotizing Enterocolitis

Infections
Sepsis Neonatorum
Group B Streptococcus
Syphilis
Gonorrhea
Herpesvirus Type 2
Monilial Infection (Thrush)

Infants with Congenital Heart Defects
Overview of Congenital Heart Defects
Clinical Signs and Symptoms in the Neonate
Nursing Assessment and Intervention

Other Congenital Anomalies

Objectives ■■■■■■■■■■■■■■■

- Compare the physiologic needs and complications of the preterm, small-for-gestational-age, and large-for-gestational-age infant and the underlying etiology of the various complications.

- Differentiate between postmaturity and placental insufficiency syndrome and explain why infants with these conditions sometimes require care similar to that for a preterm infant.

- Based on the labor record, Apgar score, and observable physiologic indicators, identify infants in need of resuscitation and the appropriate method of resuscitation.

- Based on clinical manifestations, differentiate the various types of respiratory distress (hyaline membrane disease, transient tachypnea of the newborn, and meconium aspiration syndrome) in the neonate.

- Identify the components of nursing care of an infant with respiratory distress syndrome.

- Differentiate between physiologic and pathologic jaundice based on onset, cause, possible sequelae, and specific management.

- Explain the set of circumstances that must be present for the development of erythroblastosis and ABO incompatibility and the nurse's role in the care of an infant with hemolytic disease.

- Identify the nursing responsibilities in phototherapy.

- Describe the assessment of clinical manifestations that would make the nurse suspect neonatal sepsis.

- Relate the dangers of untreated syphilis, gonorrhea, or herpesvirus type 2 to management of the infant in the neonatal period.

- Explain clinical and diagnostic manifestations and nursing care of necrotizing enterocolitis.

- Discuss selected metabolic abnormalities including cold stress, hypoglycemia, and hypocalcemia, and their effects on the neonate.

- Discuss selected hematologic variations and the nursing implications associated with each problem.

- Identify the nursing assessments that would make the nurse suspect a congenital cardiac defect during the early neonatal period.

- Discuss the nursing assessments of and initial interventions in selected congenital anomalies.

Key Terms ▰▰▰▰▰▰▰▰▰

bronchopulmonary
  dysplasia (BPD)
cold stress
drug-addicted infants
erythroblastosis
  fetalis
exchange transfusion
fetal alcohol syn-
  drome (FAS)
hydrops fetalis
hyperbilirubinemia
hypoglycemia

infant of diabetic
  mother (IDM)
kernicterus
large for gestational
  age (LGA)
phototherapy
polycythemia
postterm infant
preterm infant
respiratory distress
  syndrome (RDS)
small for gestational
  age (SGA)

Within the last 20 years, the field of neonatology has expanded greatly. In response to increasing knowledge about the neonate, many levels of nursery care have evolved: special care; transitional care; and low-, medium-, and high-risk care. The nurse is an important caregiver in all these nurseries. As a member of the multidisciplinary health care team, the nurse has contributed to the high level of perinatal care available today.

In addition to the availability of high-level neonatal care other factors influence the outcome for these at-risk infants. These factors include:

- Birth weight
- Gestational age
- Type and length of neonatal illness
- Environmental and maternal factors

Identification of High-Risk Infants _____

A high-risk infant is one who is susceptible to illness (morbidity) or even death (mortality) because of dysmaturity, immaturity, physical disorders, or complications of birth. In most cases, the infant is the product of a pregnancy involving one or more predictable risk factors, including the following:

- Low socioeconomic level of the mother
- Exposure to environmental dangers such as toxic chemicals
- Preexisting maternal conditions such as heart disease

- Obstetric factors such as age or parity
- Medical conditions related to pregnancy such as prenatal maternal infection
- Obstetric complications such as abruptio placentae

Various risk factors and their specific effects on the pregnancy outcome are listed in Table 6-1.

Because these factors and the perinatal risks associated with them are known, the birth of many high-risk neonates can often be anticipated and prepared for through adequate prenatal care. The pregnancy can be closely monitored, treatment can be instituted as necessary, and arrangements can be made for delivery to occur at a facility with appropriate equipment and personnel to care for both mother and child.

Identification of at-risk infants cannot always be made before labor, since the course of labor and delivery or how the infant will withstand the stress of labor is not known prior to the actual process. Thus during labor, fetal heart monitoring has played a significant role in detecting infants in distress.

Immediately after birth a valuable tool in identifying the high-risk neonate is the Apgar score. The lower the Apgar score at 5 minutes after birth, the higher the percentage of neurologic abnormalities (such as cerebral palsy) seen after 1 year. The percentage also increases significantly as birth weight decreases (Korones, 1981).

The newborn classification and neonatal mortality risk chart is another useful tool in identifying newborns at risk (Figure 22-1). Before this classification tool was developed, birth weight of less than 2500 g was the sole criterion for determination of immaturity. It was eventually recognized that an infant could weigh more than 2500 g but be immature. Conversely, an infant less than 2500 g might be functionally at term or beyond. Thus, birth weight and gestational age together became the criteria used to assess neonatal maturity and mortality risk.

According to the newborn classification and neonatal mortality risk chart, *gestation* is divided as follows:

- Preterm = 0–37 (completed) weeks
- Term = 38–41 (completed) weeks
- Postterm = 42+ weeks

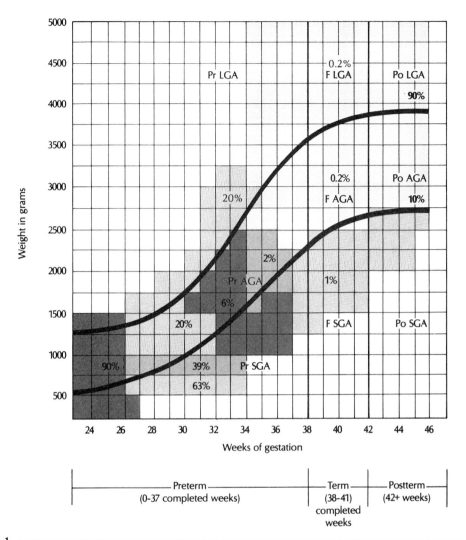

Figure 22-1

Newborn classification and neonatal mortality risk. (From Koops BL, Morgan LP, Battaglia FC: Neonatal mortality risk in relationship to birth weight and gestational age. *J Pediatr* 1982; 101(6):969.)

As shown in Figure 22-1, LGA infants are those above the curved line labeled ninetieth percentile. Appropriate-for-gestational-age (AGA) infants are those between the lines labeled 10th percentile and 90th percentile. SGA infants are those below the curved line labeled 10th percentile. A newborn is assigned to a category depending on birth weight and gestational age. For example, a newborn classified as Pr SGA is preterm and small for gestational age. The full-term newborn whose weight is appropriate for gestational age is classified F AGA.

Neonatal mortality risk is the chance of death within the neonatal period (see Chapter 1). As indicated in Figure 22-1, the neonatal mortality risk decreases as both gestational age and birth weight increase. Infants who are preterm and small for gestational age have the highest neonatal mortality risk. The mortality for LGA infants has decreased at most perinatal centers because of improved management of diabetes in pregnancy and increased recognition of potential problems with LGA infants.

Neonatal morbidity can be anticipated based on birth weight and gestational age. In Figure 22-2 the infant's birth weight is located in the vertical column, and the gestational age in weeks is found horizontally. The area where the two meet on the graph identifies commonly occurring problems. This tool assists in determining the needs of particular infants for special observation and care. For example, an infant of

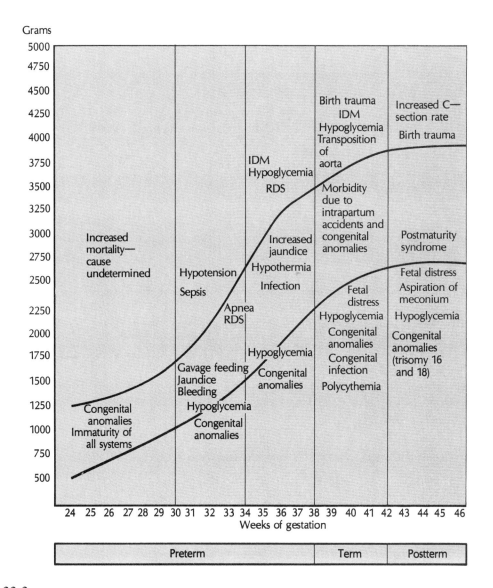

Figure 22-2

Neonatal morbidity by birth weight and gestational age. (From Lubchenco L: *The High-Risk Infant*. Philadelphia: Saunders, 1976, p. 122.)

2000 g at 40 weeks' gestation should be carefully assessed for evidence of fetal distress, hypoglycemia, congenital anomalies, congenital infection, and polycythemia.

Nursing Management of High-Risk Infants _____

Assessment of the at-risk newborn is an ongoing process. It begins with the history of the infant, which considers family and maternal history and other factors that may influence in utero development.

In the delivery room, the Apgar scores and careful observation are correlated with information about the duration of labor, maternal analgesia and anesthesia, and any complications of labor and delivery.

Assessment continues when the newborn is admitted to the nursery. All previous assessments, Apgar scores, and treatments instituted in the delivery room are evaluated in conjunction with the physical examination of the newborn. As discussed in Chapter 20, the physical examination includes all of the following:

- Complete head-to-toe assessment, observing for cardiorespiratory function, temperature, and congenital anomalies
- Clinical determination of gestational age
- Classification of the infant as AGA, SGA, or LGA and correlation with the morbidity risk for the specific classification (Figure 22-2)

When all the data are gathered and analyzed, the plan of care is developed. Nursing care of the at-risk infant depends on minute-to-minute observations of the changes in the neonate's physiologic status. It is essential to an infant's survival that the neonatal nurse understand the basic physiologic principles that guide nursing management of the at-risk neonate. The organization of nursing care must be directed toward:

- Decreasing physiologically stressful situations
- Constantly observing for subtle signs of change in clinical condition
- Interpreting laboratory data and coordinating interventions
- Conserving the infant's energy, especially in frail, debilitated preterm neonates

- Providing for developmental stimulation and sleep cycle
- Assisting the family in attachment behaviors

The success of the plan of care is confirmed by continuous assessments of the neonate's behavior, communication with family and health team members, and use of diagnostic measures.

The at-risk infant is the newest member of a family, and the parents should not be excluded from the plan of care. The importance of keeping them informed of their infant's progress, involving them in the care, and providing frequent opportunities for them to interact with their newborn and to voice their fears and concerns cannot be overemphasized.

Preterm (Premature) Infant

A **preterm infant** is any infant born before 38 weeks' gestation (Figure 22-3). The four categories of prematurity are:

1. *Less than 24 weeks' gestation*. These infants are very immature in their development and rarely survive.

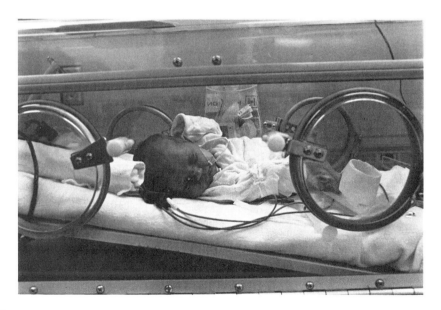

Figure 22-3
Preterm infant.

2. *24–30 weeks' gestation.* These infants may have alveolar development, but lack adequate surfactant, which results in severe RDS. However, with sophisticated supportive and therapeutic interventions, 27-to-30-week-old infants have a better chance for survival today.

3. *31–34 or 35 weeks' gestation.* Supportive measures may be necessary but are not as drastic. Survival chances are improved.

4. *36–37 weeks' gestation.* These infants are considered borderline or intermediate in their prematurity. They have characteristics of both term and preterm infants and may need minimal supportive therapy.

The preterm infant must travel the same complex pathway from intrauterine to extrauterine life as the term infant. Because of immaturity, the preterm neonate is unable to make this transition as smoothly. This section considers physiologic and nutritional factors associated with prematurity.

Respiratory and Cardiac Physiology and Considerations

The preterm infant's lungs are not fully mature and ready to take over the process of oxygen and carbon dioxide exchange without assistance until 37–38 weeks' gestation. Critical factors in the development of respiratory distress include:

1. The preterm infant's inability to produce adequate amounts of surfactant. (See Chapter 19 for discussion of respiratory adaptation and development.) When surfactant is decreased, compliance (ability of the lung to fill with air easily) is also lessened and the pressure needed to expand the lungs increases.

2. In the preterm infant, the muscular coat of pulmonary blood vessels is incompletely developed. Because of this, the pulmonary blood vessels do not constrict as well in response to decreased oxygen levels. This leads to left-to-right shunting of blood through the ductus arteriosus back into the lungs.

3. The ductus arteriosus usually responds to rising oxygen levels by vasoconstriction; in the preterm infant, who has higher susceptibility to hypoxia, the ductus may remain open. A patent ductus increases the blood volume to the lungs, causing pulmonary congestion, increased respiratory effort, and higher oxygen use.

Thermoregulation

Maintaining a normal body temperature in the preterm infant presents a nursing challenge. Heat loss is a major problem that the nurse can do much to prevent. Two limiting factors in heat production, however, are the availability of glycogen in the liver (glycogen stores are primarily laid down during the third trimester) and the amount of brown fat available for metabolism (the preterm infant does not have a full supply of brown fat). If the infant is chilled after birth, both glycogen and brown fat stores are metabolized rapidly for heat production, leaving the infant with no reserves in the event of future stress. Since the muscle mass is small in preterm infants, and muscular activity is diminished (they are unable to shiver), little heat is produced.

Heat loss occurs as a result of several physiologic and anatomic factors:

1. The preterm infant has a much larger ratio of body surface to body weight. This means that the infant's ability to produce heat (body weight) is much less than the potential for losing heat (surface area). The loss of heat in a preterm infant weighing 1500 g is five times greater per unit of body weight than in an adult (Korones, 1981).

2. The preterm infant has very little subcutaneous fat, which is the human body's insulation. Without adequate insulation, heat is easily conducted from the core of the body (warmer temperature) to the surface of the body (cooler temperature). Heat is lost from the body as the blood vessels, which lie close to the skin surface in the preterm infant, transport blood from the body core to the subcutaneous tissues.

3. The posture of the preterm infant is another important factor influencing heat loss. Flexion of the extremities decreases the amount of surface area exposed to the environment; extension increases the surface area exposed to the environment and thus increases heat loss. The gestational age of the infant influences the amount of flexion, from completely hypotonic and extended at 28 weeks to strong flexion displayed by 36 weeks (Figure 20-2).

In summary, the more preterm an infant the less able he or she is to maintain heat balance. Prevention of heat loss by providing a neutral thermal environment is one of the most important considerations in nursing management of the preterm infant (Noerr, 1984). (See Nursing Care Plan—Preterm Infants for Thermoregulation, p. 499.) Cold stress, with its accompanying severe complications, can be prevented (see p. 531).

Nutrition and Fluid Requirements

Providing adequate nutrition and fluids for the preterm infant is a major concern of the health care team. Early feedings are extremely valuable in maintaining normal metabolism and lowering the possibility of such complications as hypoglycemia, hyperbilirubinemia, and hyperkalemia. However, the preterm infant is at risk for complications that may develop because of immaturity of the digestive system.

Since the basic structure of the gastrointestinal (GI) tract is formed early in gestation, the preterm infant is able to take in suitable nourishment. However, although the GI structure is present, the ability to digest and absorb food efficiently develops later in gestation. As a result of GI immaturity, the preterm neonate has the digestive and absorption problems listed below:

- Limited ability exists to convert certain essential amino acids to nonessential amino acids. Certain amino acids, such as taurine and cysteine, are essential to the preterm infant but not to the term infant.

- Kidney immaturity causes an inability to handle the increased osmolarity of formula protein. The preterm infant requires a higher concentration of whey protein than casein.

- Difficulty absorbing saturated fats occurs because of decreased bile salts and pancreatic lipase.

- Lactose digestion may not be fully functional during the first few days of a preterm's life. The preterm neonate can digest and absorb most simple sugars.

- Deficiency of calcium and phosphorus may exist since two-thirds of these minerals are deposited in the last trimester. As a result the preterm infant is prone to rickets and significant bone demineralization.

Oral caloric intake necessary for growth in an uncompromised healthy preterm neonate is 120–150 kcal/kg/day. In addition to relatively high caloric needs, the preterm neonate requires more protein (3–4 g/kg/day) than the term neonate.

Formula for preterm neonates   The composition of the "best-suited formula" for the preterm infant is a subject of much discussion and research. Breast milk as the primary source of nutrition for the preterm infant has also been a topic of recent debate and research (McCormick, 1984).

It is now known that the quality as well as the quantity of protein ingested is important to the small preterm infant. To meet these needs, several higher-calorie, higher-protein formulas are available that meet the preterm infant's nutritional demands, yet do not overtax the concentration abilities of the immature kidneys.

Most preterm formulas contain protein with a whey/casein ratio of 60/40 (a similar proportion to that found in breast milk) and a caloric value of 24 calories per ounce. Similac Special Care and Enfamil Premature Formula are specially formulated for preterm neonates. Preterm formulas also need to contain MCT (medium chain triglycerides), and additional amino acids such as cysteine. The preterm neonate also needs calcium and vitamin D supplements to increase mineralization of bones. Multivitamins and vitamin E are required if the diet is high in MCT and if the infant is fed a formula with iron.

Breast milk is widely used to feed preterm infants. Besides its many benefits for the infant, it allows the mother to contribute to her infant's well-being (Figure 22-4). It is a nursing responsibility to inform mothers of their option to breast-feed if they choose to do so. The nurse should be aware of the advantages and possible disadvantages of breast-feeding, such as slower growth rate, hyponatremia, and lactose intolerance, if breast milk is the sole source of food.

Additional factors that influence the preterm neonate's nutrition are the immaturity of the renal system (inability to concentrate urine), immaturity of the respiratory system (weak or absent cough), and immaturity of the neurologic system (poor suck, gag, and swallow reflexes).

Text continued on p. 503.

NURSING CARE PLAN
Preterm Infants

PATIENT ASSESSMENT

History

1. Maternal history, including general, obstetric, and events of labor and delivery. Factors frequently associated with preterm delivery include:
   a. Age—very young mothers
   b. Closely spaced pregnancies
   c. Low socioeconomic group
   d. Previous history of preterm pregnancy
   e. Abnormalities of reproductive system: uterine malformations, incompetent cervix, infections (both urinary tract and systemic)
   f. Elective cesarean delivery
   g. Obstetric complications such as abruptio placentae, placenta previa, premature rupture of membranes, amnionitis
2. Fetal conditions associated with preterm delivery include:
   a. Blood incompatibility, with resultant erythroblastosis fetalis
   b. Multiple gestation
   c. Congenital infections

Physical Examination

1. Physical characteristics vary according to gestational age, but certain characteristics are frequently present:
   a. Skin—reddened, translucent, blood vessels readily apparent, lack of subcutaneous fat
   b. Nails—soft, short
   c. Lanugo—plentiful, widely distributed
   d. Small genitals (testes may not be descended)
   e. Head size—appears large in relation to body
   f. Ears—minimal cartilage, pliable, folded over
   g. Resting position—flaccid, froglike position
   h. Cry—weak, feeble
   i. Reflexes—poor sucking, swallowing, and gag
2. Gestational age determined by clinical assessment tools
3. Temperature fluctuates easily
4. Pulse taken apically—often rapid and irregular, normal range 120–160
5. Respirations—40–60 per minute, shallow, irregular, usually diaphragmatic with intermittent periodic breathing
6. Blood pressure—compare infant's BP with low-birth-weight newborn's BP normograms
7. Color usually pink or ruddy but may be acrocyanotic; observe for cyanosis, jaundice, pallor, or plethora
8. Activity—jerky, generalized movements (Note: seizure activity is abnormal)
9. Elimination—observe for patency of anus
10. Stool—first stool meconium; stool volume may be decreased because of hypomotility of intestine
11. Voiding—first voiding within 24 hours of birth; output scanty and infrequent for 1–3 days
12. Skull—bones pliable, fontanelle smooth and flat; presence of bulging may indicate CNS problem, depressed fontanelle suggests dehydration; observe for cephalhematoma or caput succedaneum
13. Evaluate for common preterm infant morbidities (see Figure 22-2)

Laboratory Examination

Chest x-ray (PA and left lateral)—clear with no infiltration

Complete blood count (CBC)

Rh determination if mother Rh negative and father Rh positive

Urinalysis on second voided specimen

Specific gravity every voiding—normal range 1.006–1.013

Hematest and reducing substance on all stools (if Hematest positive, consider necrotizing enterocolitis)

Dextrostix every 4–6 hours

Blood glucose level drawn if Dextrostix below 45 mg/mL

PLAN OF CARE

Nursing Priorities

1. Enhance respiratory efforts.
2. Promote homeostasis through provision of neutral thermal environment and through meeting nutrition and fluid needs.
3. Protect from infections.
4. Support psychologic well-being of parents and infant by facilitating positive parent-child bonding and sensory stimulation of infant.
5. Evaluate infant for possible complications and institute appropriate interventions.

Family Educational Focus

1. Discuss the implications of having a preterm infant in regard to respiratory immaturity, caloric and fluid requirements, and thermal instability.
2. Explain treatment modalities and their rationale.
3. Explore the long-term implications of such alteration on the achievement of developmental milestones for the first 2 years of life and evaluation of development based on chronological age
4. Provide opportunities to discuss questions and individual parental concerns regarding their preterm neonate.

NURSING CARE PLAN (continued)
Preterm Infants

Problem	Nursing interventions and actions	Rationale
Respiratory distress	Maintain airway patency through judicious suctioning. Position with head slightly elevated and neck slightly extended. Avoid increased oxygen consumption by maintaining adequate body temperature (97.7F ± 0.5F). Observe, record, and report signs of respiratory distress, including: 1. Cyanosis—serious sign when generalized 2. Tachypnea—sustained respiratory rate greater than 60/min after first 4 hr of life 3. Retractions 4. Expiratory grunting 5. Flaring nostrils 6. Apneic episodes 7. Presence of rales or ronchi on auscultation Implement treatment plan for respiratory distress, if indicated. Administer oxygen per physician order for relief of symptoms of respiratory distress.	Anatomic and physiologic characteristics predispose preterm infant to respiratory distress because: 1. Increased danger of obstruction results from small diameter of bronchi and trachea. 2. Newborn is nose breather and prone to nasal obstruction. 3. Chest wall musculature is weak and efficiency of cough reflex is decreased. 4. Cough and gag reflexes may be absent due to immaturity. 5. Lung surfactant necessary to maintain alveolar stability and prevent collapse is inadequate (Avery, 1981).
Heat losses	Increase environmental temperature to maintain thermal neutrality. Reflect principles of anatomy and physiology of temperature control and thermogenesis in planning of care. Minimize heat losses and prevent cold stress by: 1. Warming and humidifying oxygen without blowing over face in order to avoid increasing oxygen consumption 2. Maintaining skin in dry condition 3. Keeping isolettes, radiant warmers, and cribs away from windows and cold external walls and out of drafts; using heat shields with small infants 4. Using skin probe to monitor infant skin temperature at 36–37C 5. Avoiding placing infant on cold surfaces such as metal treatment tables, cold x-ray plates 6. Padding cold surfaces with diapers and using radiant warmers during procedures 7. Warming blood for exchange transfusions	A neutral thermal environment requires minimal oxygen consumption to maintain a normal core temperature. Body temperature fluctuates because: 1. Assuming a position of extension exposes a relatively large body surface in relation to body mass. 2. Infant lacks subcutaneous fat for adequate insulation. 3. Immature central nervous system provides poor temperature control. 4. Stores of brown fat for chemical thermogenesis are decreased; a small infant (less than 1200 g) can lose 80 cal/kg/day through radiation of body heat. Physical principles of heat loss include: 1. Evaporation—lungs and skin when cooling occurs as a result of water evaporation. 2. Convection—air currents. 3. Conduction—skin contact with cooler object. 4. Radiation—loss of warmth to cooler surrounding objects.

NURSING CARE PLAN (continued)
Preterm Infants

Problem	Nursing interventions and actions	Rationale
Caloric and fluid intake necessary for growth	Initiate feeding of sterile water at 2–4 hr of age in well preterm infant. Promote growth by providing caloric intake of 120–150 cal/kg/day in small amounts; increased slowly in small amounts (1–2 mL) given more frequently (every 2–3 hr). Supplement oral feedings with intravenous intake per physician orders. Feed specially formulated formulas such as Similac Special Care and Enfamil Premature formula. Utilize concentrated formulas that supply more calories in less volume, such as 24 calories/ounce. Feed with soft preemie nipple and burp frequently. Observe, record, and report signs of respiratory distress or fatigue occurring during feedings. Evaluate for signs of dehydration, including depressed fontanelle, poor skin turgor, decreased urine output, sunken eyeballs, and dry mucous membranes. Monitor daily weight, blood pH, normal urine output of 1–3 mL/kg/hour, specific gravity, Dipstix/Clinitest for evidence of glycosuria. Measure abdominal girth prior to each feeding. Utilize an orogastric or nasogastric tube or nasojejunal gavage feedings in small preterm infants not tolerating intermittent volumes of feeding per nipple. Facilitate continuous feedings and prevent vomiting by placing nasojejunal tube past pylorus. Initiate safety factors with gavage feedings (see Procedure 22-1): Determine presence of residual formula in stomach prior to initiating feeding by aspirating from gastric tube and replacing amount before remainder of feeding is given. Observe, record, and report complications of nasojejunal tube including misplacement, perforation, plugging, vomiting due to excessive volume, or sepsis.	Sterile water is desirable for first feedings because, in the presence of gastrointestinal tract abnormalities and/or aspiration of feeding, fewer pulmonary complications will result. Adequate nutritional and fluid intake promotes growth and prevents such complications as metabolic catabolism, hypoglycemia, and dehydration. Small, frequent feedings of high-calorie formula are used because of limited gastric capacity and decreased gastric emptying. Growth is evaluated by increase in weight, length, and body measurements. Early detection of abdominal distention aids in diagnosis of necrotizing enterocolitis. Suck, swallow, and gag reflexes are immature at birth in preterm infant. Nipple feeding, an active rather than passive intake of nutrition, requires energy expenditure and burning of calories by infant. Gavage feedings require less energy expenditure on the part of the preterm infant. Decrease in exertion is an important consideration in feeding an infant who is ill, has poorly developed suck reflex, or is less then 32 weeks' gestation. Presence of residual formula in stomach is indication of intolerance to amount of feeding or to increase in amount of feeding or is indicative of obstruction, paralytic ileus, or necrotizing enterocolitis.
Fatigue during feedings	Establish a nipple feeding program that is begun slowly and progresses slowly, such as nipple feed once per day, nipple feed once per shift, and then nipple feed every other feeding.	Residual feeding is calculated for example by: 1. Feeding order—24 mL every 2 hours. 2. Residual—3 mL.

NURSING CARE PLAN (continued)
Preterm Infants

Problem	Nursing interventions and actions	Rationale
	Monitor daily weight with anticipation of small amount of weight loss when nipple feedings start. Supplement gavage or nipple feedings with intravenous therapy per physician order until oral intake is sufficient to support growth.	3. Formula this feeding—21 mL plus 3 mL residual. Residual formula is readministered because digestive processes have already been begun. As infant matures, gavage feedings should be replaced with nipple feedings to assist in strengthening sucking reflexes and meeting psychologic needs.
	Develop a plan of care that involves parents in feeding of infant.	Involvement of parents in feeding of preterm infant is essential to development of attachment and expansion of parental knowledge and coping mechanisms.
	Observe, record, and report presence of complications such as hypoglycemia or hypocalcemia.	Preterm infant requires delicate balance for homeostasis and prevention of complications.
Susceptibility to infection	Initiate a plan of care to prevent exposure to infection such as hand washing, reverse isolation, and individual equipment. Implement treatment per physician orders in presence of infection (refer to section on sepsis neonatorum, p. 545, for review of nursing care).	Infection is common occurrence due to immaturity of immunologic system, increased use of invasive procedures and techniques, and more prolonged hospitalization.
Prolonged separation of infant and mother	Support emotionally the psychologic well-being of family, including positive maternal–child bonding and sensory stimulation of infant. Include parents in determining infant's plan of care and encourage their participation. Encourage parents to visit frequently. Provide opportunities for parents to touch, hold, talk to, and care for infant. Determine type and amount of sensory stimulation appropriate and implement sensory stimulation program. Prepare for discharge by instructing parent in such areas as feeding techniques, formula preparation (including bottle sterilization), and breast-feeding; bathing, diapering, and hygiene; temperature monitoring; administration of vitamins; sibling rivalry; care of complications and preventing exposure to infections; normal elimination patterns, normal reflexes and activity, and how to promote normal growth and development without being overprotective; returning for continued medical care; and availability of community resources if indicated.	Maternal bonding begins in first few hours or days following birth of an infant. Preterm infants experience prolonged periods of separation from their mothers, which necessitates intervention to ensure maternal–child bonding. Related to prolonged separation of preterm infants from their mothers following delivery is increased incidence of child neglect and child abuse. Parents should receive same postpartum teaching as any parent taking a new infant home. Mothers with preterm infants desiring to breast-feed will pump their breasts to keep milk flowing and in some situations to provide milk for their infant. This activity allows breast-feeding after discharge from hospital. Mothers need to understand the changes to expect in color of the infant's stool and number of bowel movements plus odor from bottle or breast-feeding in order to avoid unnecessary concern on mother's part. Preterm infants usually do not require referral to community agencies such as visiting nurse associations unless there is a specific

NURSING CARE PLAN (continued)
Preterm Infants

Problem	Nursing interventions and actions	Rationale
		problem requiring assistance. Infants with feeding problems or resolving complications or mothers unable to cope with sick infants are examples of conditions requiring referral to community resources.

Possible complications
  Apnea
  Pulmonary problems, including RDS, wet lung, atelectasis, pneumothorax
  Cold stress, hypocalcemia, hypoglycemia
  Sepsis neonatorum
  Retrolental fibroplasia
  Necrotizing enterocolitis
  Hyperbilirubinemia or kernicterus
  Anemia
		These additional possible complications are covered in the chapter.

NURSING CARE EVALUATION Respirations are 30–50 per minute, regular, with no episodes of apnea. Temperature is stable. Infant is gaining weight. Infant takes nipple feedings without developing fatigue. Complications are controlled or absent. Infant is active without jerky generalized movement.		Infant is free from infection or infection is controlled. Parent–child bonding is completed. Infant responds to sensory stimulation. Parents understand and can demonstrate knowledge of infant care, feeding, growth projections, prevention of exposure to infections, treatment of complications, and when to return for medical care.

NURSING DIAGNOSIS*	SUPPORTING DATA	NURSING ORDERS
Potential for injury related to impaired thermoregulatory mechanisms	Decreased temperature Lethargy Pallor Hypoglycemia	Provide stable environmental temperature 1. Monitor skin temperature continuously. 2. Correlate infant's skin temperature with environmental temperature setting. 3. Assess probe for proper placement, ensure that probe has good contact with infant's skin. 4. Maintain infant in warmed environment. 5. Use warmed blankets and equipment when working with infant.
Knowledge deficit related to care of infant in the home	Expressed concerns and questions regarding care of preterm infant in the home	Provide knowledge 1. Begin teaching about the infant when the infant is admitted. 2. Provide opportunities for parents to visit their infant in the nursery and to work with the infant. 3. Provide opportunities for return demonstrations.

*These are a few examples of nursing diagnoses that may be appropriate for a preterm infant. It is not an inclusive list and must be individualized for each newborn.

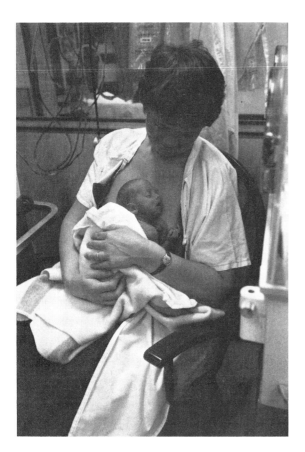

Figure 22-4

Mother visits intensive care unit to breast-feed her preterm infant. (Photo by Suzanne Arms.)

Nutritional intake is considered adequate when there is consistent weight gain of 20–30 g per day. Initially, no weight gain may be noted for several days, but total weight loss should not exceed 15% of the total birth weight or more than 1%–2% per day. Some institutions add the criteria of head circumference growth and increase in body length of 1 cm/week, once the neonate is stable.

Feeding regimens are established based on the weight and estimated stomach capacity of the neonate. In many instances it is necessary to supplement the oral feedings with parenteral fluids to maintain adequate hydration and caloric intake. See Nursing Care Plan for Preterm Infants for discussion of feeding regimens.

Calculation of fluid requirements must take into account both the weight of the neonate and postnatal age. In the preterm infant, more fluid is lost through the skin than in term infants because of decreased insulating fat and blood vessels close to the surface. In addition, higher environmental temperature, phototherapy, and radiant warmers may increase fluid loss an additional 50%.

Recommendations for fluid therapy in the preterm infant are approximately 80–100 mL/kg/day for day 1; 100–120 mL/kg/day for day 2; and 120–150 mL/kg/day by day 3 of life. These amounts may be increased up to 200 mL/kg/day if the infant is very small, receiving phototherapy, or under a radiant warmer. The infant may need less fluid if a heat shield is used, the environment is more humid, or humidified oxygen is being provided. (See Essential Facts to Remember—Nutrition of the Preterm Infant.)

Because of general immaturity, the preterm infant is susceptible to the following feeding problems:

1. Marked danger of aspiration and its associated complications because of the infant's poorly developed gag reflex, incompetent esophageal cardiac sphincter, and poor sucking and swallowing reflexes.

2. Small stomach capacity, which limits the amount of fluid that can be introduced to meet the infant's high caloric needs.

3. Decreased absorption of essential nutrients because of immaturity, malabsorption, and nutritional loss associated with vomiting and diarrhea.

4. Fatigue associated with sucking, which may lead to increased basal metabolic rate, increased oxygen requirements, and possible necrotizing enterocolitis (NEC).

 ESSENTIAL FACTS TO REMEMBER

Nutrition of the Preterm Infant

- Initially requires 80–100 ml/kg/day; may need more fluid if of lower birth weight
- Requires 120–150 cal/kg/day oral intake for growth
- Requires supplemental multivitamins, vitamin E, folic acid, and calcium
- Desired weight gain of 20–30 g/day
- Desired initial weight loss of only 1%–2%/day

5. Feeding intolerance and NEC due to diminished blood flow to the intestinal tract because of shock or prolonged hypoxia at birth.

Methods of feeding   The preterm infant is fed by various methods depending on the infant's gestational age, health and physical condition, and neurologic status. The two most common oral feeding methods are nipple and gavage feeding.

Nipple feeding   Preterm infants who have a coordinated suck and swallow reflex and those showing continued weight gain may be fed by nipple. To avoid excessive expenditure of energy a soft nipple is usually used.

Gavage feeding   Preterm infants who do not have coordinated swallow or suck reflexes require gavage feeding. Gavage feeding is also used when infants are losing weight because of the energy expenditure secondary to nippling. See Procedure 22-1.

PROCEDURE 22-1
Gavage Feeding

Objective	Nursing action	Rationale
Ensure smooth accomplishment of the procedure	Gather necessary equipment including: 1. No. 5 or No. 8 Fr. feeding tube 2. 10–30 mL syringe 3. ¼-in. paper tape 4. Stethoscope 5. Appropriate formula 6. Small cup of sterile water Explain procedure to parents	Considerations in choosing size of catheter include size of the infant, area of insertion (oral or nasal), and rate of flow desired. The very small infant (less than 1600 g) requires a 5 Fr. feeding tube; an infant greater than 1600 g may tolerate a larger tube. Orogastric insertion is preferred over nasogastric insertion as infants are obligatory nose breathers. If nasogastric insertion is used, a No. 5 catheter should be utilized to minimize airway obstruction. The size of the catheter will influence the rate of flow. The syringe is used to aspirate stomach contents prior to feeding, to inject air into the stomach for testing tube placement and for holding measured amount of formula during feeding. Tape is used to mark tube for insertion depth as well as for securing tube during feeding. Stethoscope is needed to auscultate rush of air into stomach when testing tube placement. Sterile water may be used to lubricate feeding tube when inserted nasally. With oral insertion, there are enough secretions in the mouth to lubricate the tube adequately. The cup of sterile water may also be used to test for placement by placing the end of the tube into the water to check for air bubbles from the lungs. However, this test may not be accurate as air may also be present in the stomach (Avery, 1981).
Insert tube accurately into stomach	Position infant on back or side with head of bed elevated. Take tube from package and measure the distance from the tip of the ear to the nose to the xiphoid process, and mark the point with a small piece of paper tape (Figure 22-5). If inserting tube nasally, lubricate tip in cup of sterile water. Shake excess drops to prevent aspiration.	This position allows easy passage of the tube. This measuring technique ensures enough tubing to enter stomach. Water should be used, as opposed to an oil-based lubricant, in the event tube is inadvertently passed into lung.

PROCEDURE 22-1 (continued)
Gavage Feeding

Objective	Nursing action	Rationale
	Stabilize infant's head with one hand, and pass the tube via the mouth (or nose) into the stomach, to the point previously marked. If the infant begins coughing or choking or becomes cyanotic or aphonic, remove the tube immediately.	Any signs of respiratory distress signal likelihood that tube has entered trachea. Orogastric insertion is less likely to result in passage into the trachea than nasogastric insertion.
	If no respiratory distress is apparent, lightly tape tube in position, draw up 0.5–1.0 mL of air in syringe, and connect it to tubing. Place stethoscope over the epigastrium and briskly inject the air (Figure 22-6).	Nurse should hear a sudden rush of air as it enters stomach.
	Aspirate stomach contents with syringe, and note amount, color, and consistency. Return residual to stomach unless otherwise ordered to discard it.	Residual formula should be evaluated as part of the assessment of infant's tolerance of gavage feedings. It is not discarded, unless particularly large in volume or mucoid in nature, because of the potential for causing an electrolyte imbalance.
	If only a clear fluid or mucus is found upon aspiration and if any question exists as to whether the tube is in the stomach, the aspirate can be tested for pH.	Stomach aspirate tests in the 1–3 range for pH.
Introduce formula into stomach without complication	Hold infant for feeding or position on right side if infant cannot be held.	Positioning on side decreases the risk of aspiration in case of emesis during feeding.
	Separate syringe from tube, remove plunger from barrel, reconnect barrel to tube, and pour formula into syringe.	Feeding should be allowed to flow in by gravity. It should not be pushed in under pressure with syringe.

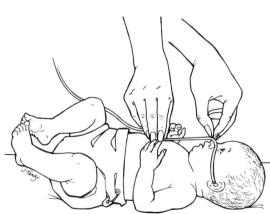

Figure 22-5
Measuring gavage tube length.

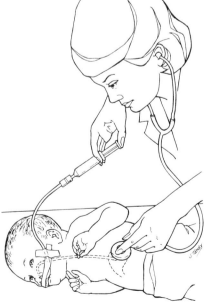

Figure 22-6
Auscultation for placement of gavage tube.

PROCEDURE 22-1 (continued)
Gavage Feeding

Objective	Nursing action	Rationale
	Elevate syringe 6–8 in. over infant's head. Allow formula to flow at slow, even rate.	Raising column of fluid increases force of gravity. Nurse may need to initiate flow of formula by inserting plunger of syringe into barrel just until formula is seen to enter feeding tube. Rate should be regulated to prevent sudden stomach distention, with possibility of vomiting and aspiration.
	Continue adding formula to syringe until desired volume has been absorbed. Then rinse tubing with 2–3 mL sterile water.	Rinsing tube ensures that infant receives all of formula. It is especially important to rinse tube if it is going to be left in place, because this decreases risk of clogging and bacterial growth in tube.
	Remove tube by loosening tape, folding tube over on itself, and quickly withdrawing it in one smooth motion. If tube is to be left in, position it so that infant is unable to remove it.	Folding tube over on itself minimizes potential for aspiration of fluid, which would otherwise flow from tubing as it passes epiglottis. A tube left in place should be replaced at least every 24 hours.
Maximize feeding pleasure of infant	Whenever possible, hold infant during gavage feeding. If it is too awkward to hold infant during feeding, be sure to take time for holding afterward.	Feeding time is important to infant's tactile sensory input.
	Offer a pacifier to infant during feeding.	Infants fed for long periods by gavage can lose their sucking reflex. Sucking during feeding comforts and relaxes infant, making formula flow more easily. One study showed that infants allowed to suck during feedings were able to switch to nipple feeding sooner and were discharged earlier than a control group who did not suck during tube feedings (Measel and Anderson, 1979).

An alternative method of feeding is transpyloric feeding. This feeding method should be done only in specially equipped and staffed high-risk nursuries since it can cause perforation of the stomach or intestines. Preterm infants who cannot tolerate any oral (enteral) feedings may be given nutrition by total parenteral nutrition (hyperalimentation).

Renal Physiology

The kidneys of the preterm infant are immature in comparison with those of the full-term infant. This situation poses clinical problems in the management of fluid and electrolyte balance. Specific characteristics of the preterm infant include the following:

1. The GFR is lower due to decreased renal blood flow. The more preterm the infant the less the GFR. Anuria and/or oliguria may be observed in the preterm infant after severe asphyxia with associated hypotension.

2. The kidneys of the preterm infant are limited in their ability to concentrate urine or to excrete excess amounts of fluid. This means that if excess fluid is administered, the infant is at risk for fluid retention and overhydration. If too little is administered, the infant will become dehydrated because of the inability to retain adequate fluid.

3. The kidneys of the preterm infant will begin excreting glucose (glycosuria) at a lower serum glucose level than occurs in the adult. Therefore, glycosuria with hyperglycemia is common (Oh, 1981).

4. The bicarbonate buffering capacity of the kidney is less, predisposing the infant to metabolic acidosis. Sodium bicarbonate is frequently required to treat metabolic acidosis.

5. The immaturity of the renal system affects the infant's ability to excrete drugs. Because excretion time is longer, many drugs are given at less frequent intervals in the preterm infant (that is, every 12 hours instead of every 8 hours). Urine output must be carefully monitored when the infant is receiving nephrotoxic drugs such as gentamicin, nafcillin, and others. In the event of poor urine output, drugs can become toxic in the infant much more quickly than in the adult.

Reactivity Periods and Behavioral States

Because of the immaturity of all systems in comparison to those of the full-term neonate, the preterm infant's periods of reactivity are delayed. The very ill infant may be hypotonic and unreactive for several days so these periods of reactivity may not be observed at all.

As the preterm newborn grows and the condition stabilizes, it becomes increasingly possible to identify behavioral states and traits unique to each infant. This is a very important part of nursing management of the high-risk infant. The nurse can help parents learn their infant's cues for interaction.

Preterm infants tend to be more disorganized in their sleep–wake cycles and are unable to attend as well to the human face and objects in the environment. Neurologically, their responses are weaker (sucking, muscle tone, states of arousal) than full-term infants' responses (Gorski et al., 1979).

Complications

The preterm neonate is at risk for many complications secondary to the immaturity of various body systems in addition to those already discussed. The most common of these complications are briefly described here and discussed in more detail later in the chapter:

1. *Apnea.* Cessation of breathing for more than 20–30 seconds. It is thought to be primarily a result of neuronal immaturity, a factor that contributes to the tendency for irregular breathing patterns in preterm infants. When cyanosis and bradycardia (heart rate less than 100 beats/min) are also present, these periods are called apneic episodes or spells (Avery, 1981).

2. *Patent ductus arteriosus.* Failure of ductus arteriosus to close due to decreased pulmonary arteriole musculature and hypoxemia.

3. *RDS.* For further discussion of RDS due to inadequate surfactant production, see p. 519.

4. *Intraventricular hemorrhage.* Up to 35 weeks' gestation the preterm's brain ventricles are lined by the germinal matrix, which is highly susceptible to hypoxic events. The germinal matrix is very vascular, and these blood vessels rupture in the presence of hypoxia.

5. *Hypocalcemia.* The preterm infant lacks adequate amounts of calcium secondary to early birth and growth needs. See p. 535.

6. *Hypoglycemia.* The preterm infant's decreased brown fat and glycogen stores and increased metabolic needs predisposes this infant to hypoglycemia, p. 532.

7. *Necrotizing enterocolitis.* This condition occurs when blood flow to the gastrointestinal tract is decreased secondary to shock or prolonged hypoxia. See p. 544 for discussion of necrotizing enterocolitis.

8. *Anemia.* The preterm infant is at risk for anemia because of the rapid rate of growth required, shorter red blood cell life, excessive blood sampling, decreased iron stores, and deficiency of vitamin E.

9. *Hyperbilirubinemia.* Immature hepatic enzymatic function decreases conjugation of bilirubin, resulting in increased bilirubin levels (p. 536).

10. *Infection.* The preterm infant is more susceptible to infection than term infants. Most of the neonate's immunity is acquired in the last trimester. Therefore the preterm infant has decreased antibodies available for protection.

Long-Term Needs and Outcome

The care of the preterm infant and the family does not stop upon discharge from the nursery. Follow-up care is extremely important because many developmental problems are not noted until the infant is older and begins to demonstrate motor delays or sensory disability.

Within the first year of life, preterm infants face higher mortality than term infants. Causes of death include sudden infant death syndrome

(SIDS) (which occurs about five times more frequently in the preterm infant), respiratory infections, and neurologic defects. Morbidity is also much higher among preterm infants, with those weighing less than 1500 g at highest risk for long-term complications.

The most common long-term problems observed in preterm infants include the following:

Retrolental fibroplasia (RLF) In spite of new technology and the ability to monitor arterial oxygen closely, RLF and resulting loss of eyesight continue to occur in the preterm infant.

Bronchopulmonary dysplasia (BPD) Long-term lung disease is a result of damage to the alveolar epithelium secondary to positive pressure respirator therapy and high oxygen concentration. These infants have long-term dependence on oxygen therapy and an increased incidence of respiratory infection during their first few years of life.

Speech defects The most frequently observed speech defects involve delayed development of receptive and expressive ability that may persist into the school years.

Neurologic defects The most common neurologic defects include cerebral palsy, hydrocephalus, seizure disorders, lower IQ scores, and learning disabilities. However, the socioeconomic climate and family support systems are extremely important influences on the child's ultimate intellectual ability in the absence of major neurologic defects (Fitzhardinge, 1976).

When evaluating the infant's abilities and disabilities, it is important for parents to understand that developmental progress must be evaluated from the expected date of birth, not from the actual date of birth. In addition, the parents need the consistent support of health care professionals in the long-term management of their infant to promote the highest quality of life possible.

Sensorineural hearing loss Preterm infants are still at risk for hearing loss, especially those with severe asphyxia or recurrent apnea in the neonatal period. Hyperbilirubinemia and ototoxic drugs such as gentamicin and furosemide (Lasix) are also known to contribute to hearing loss in the neonate.

Posterm Infant

The **postterm infant** is any infant delivered after 42 weeks' gestation. In the past, the terms *postterm* and *postmature* were used interchangeably. Currently the term *postmature* is used only when the infant is delivered after 42 weeks of gestation and demonstrates characteristics of the postmaturity syndrome (Hendriksen, 1985).

Prolonged pregnancy occurs in approximately 3.5%–10% of all pregnancies (Hobart and Depp, 1982). The cause of postterm pregnancy is not completely understood, but several factors are known to be associated with it, including primiparity, high multiparity mothers (greater than four), and a history of prolonged pregnancies (Affonso and Harris, 1980). Many postterm pregnancies are thought to be due to inaccurate obstetrical dates.

Modern obstetrical practice is faced with the dilemma of differentiating the postterm infant from one suffering with postmaturity syndrome. Antenatal management must be directed at distinguishing the postmaturity infant (alert; dry, cracking parchmentlike skin; long, thin arms and legs [Figure 22-7]; and some meconium staining) from a larger, well-nourished, equally alert counterpart who has experienced an equally long gestation (Table 22-1).

Prolonged pregnancy itself is not responsible for the postmaturity syndrome infant. The characteristics of the postmature infant are pri-

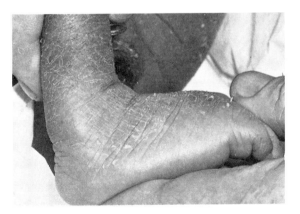

Figure 22-7
Postterm infant demonstrates deep cracking and peeling of skin. (From Dubowitz L, Dubowitz V: *Gestational Age of the Newborn.* Menlo Park, Calif.: Addison-Wesley, 1977.)

Table 22-1

Evaluation of Fetal Status in True Prolonged Pregnancy*

Clinical parameters	Positive	Guarded	Negative
Uterine size	Increasing	No increase	Decreasing
Amniotic fluid volume	Appropriate	Diminished	Oligohydramnios
Fetal activity	Unchanged	Diminished	Absent
Maternal weight	Increasing	Decreasing	
Estriol levels	Stable/increasing	Chronically low	Decrease $\geq$ 35%
Ultrasound (growth-adjusted sonographic age)	Maintenance of growth percentile	Decrease in growth percentile	Cessation of growth
Nonstress test	Reactive	Nonreactive: spontaneous variables	Spontaneous late deceleration
Oxytocin challenge test	Negative	Ambiguous: variable decelerations	Positive
Intrapartum monitoring	Baseline 100-140 beats/min, normal pattern, variability of 6-15 beats/min	Baseline > 150 beats/min, decreased variability, variable decelerations	Baseline > 150 beats/min, absent variability, repetitive late decelerations

*From Hobart JM, Depp R: Prolonged pregnancy. In *Gynecology and Obstetrics*. Vol. 3. Sciarra JJ (editor). Philadelphia: Harper & Row, 1982, p. 5.

marily due to advanced gestational age, placental insufficiency, and continued exposure to amniotic fluid (Clifford, 1957).

This postmature infant is at high risk for morbidity and has a mortality rate two to three times greater than term infants. The majority of deaths occur during labor, since by that time the fetus has used up necessary reserves. Because of decreased placental function, oxygenation and nutrition transport are impaired, leaving the fetus prone to hypoglycemia and asphyxia when the stresses of labor begin. Problems in surviving postmature infants are thus a result of inadequate placental function, decreased reserves, and the stress of labor. The most common disorders of the postmature infant are:

• Hypoglycemia, from nutritional deprivation and resultant depleted glycogen stores

• Meconium aspiration in response to hypoxia in utero

• Polycythemia due to increased production of RBCs in response to hypoxia

• Congenital anomalies of unknown cause

• Seizure activity because of hypoxic insult

• Cold stress because of loss or poor development of subcutaneous fat

Nursing interventions   Nursing interventions are primarily supportive measures. They include:

• Observation of cardiopulmonary status, since the stresses of labor are poorly tolerated and severe depression can ensue at birth

• Provision of warmth to balance poor response to cold stress and decreased liver glycogen and brown fat stores

• Frequent monitoring of blood glucose and initiation of early feeding (at 1 or 2 hours of age) or intravenous glucose per physician order

• Observation for the disorders identified earlier and appropriate management when possible.

Nursing attention also should be directed toward helping parents express feelings and fears regarding the infant's condition and long-term problems.

Large-for-Gestational-Age Infant

A **large-for-gestational-age (LGA)** neonate is one whose birth weight is at or above the ninetieth percentile on the intrauterine growth curve (at any week of gestation). The majority of infants categorized as LGA have been found to be so categorized because of miscalculation of dates due to postconceptual bleeding (Korones, 1981). The best-known condition leading to excessive fetal growth is maternal diabetes; however, only a minority of large infants are born to diabetic mothers. Certain factors or situations have also been found to correlate with the birth of LGA infants.

- Genetic predisposition is correlated to the prepregnancy weight and to weight gain during pregnancy. Large parents tend to have large infants.
- Multiparous women have three times the number of LGA infants as primigravidas.
- Male infants are traditionally larger than female infants.
- Infants with erythroblastosis fetalis, Beckwith-Wiedemann syndrome, or transposition of the great vessels are usually large.

The perinatal history, in conjunction with results of antenatal ultrasonic measurement of fetal skull and gestational age testing, is important in identifying an at-risk LGA newborn.

Characteristically the increase in the LGA infant's body size is proportional, although head circumference and body length are in the upper limits of intrauterine growth. The exception to this rule is the infant of the diabetic mother, whose body weight increases only in proportion to length.

Common disorders of the LGA infant include the following:

1. *Birth trauma because of CPD.* Because of their excessive size and biparietal diameter greater than 10 cm, there are more breech and shoulder dystocias, with resultant potential asphyxia, fractured clavicles, brachial palsy, facial paralysis, depressed skull fractures, and intracranial bleeding.

2. *Hypoglycemia.* This is most often seen with erythroblastosis fetalis, Beckwith-Wiedemann syndrome, and in IDMs. In these conditions the fetus is exposed to high levels of glucose, either because of breakdown of red blood cells in utero or increased circulating glucose from the mother, resulting in hyperplasia of the pancreatic islet cells and hyperinsulinemia.

3. *Polycythemia and hyperviscosity.* These conditions occur in the fetus when hemoglobin levels are elevated or when red blood cell mass increases (pathophysiologic mechanisms are not well known).

Essential components of the nursing assessment are monitoring vital signs and screening for hypoglycemia and polycythemia. For specific nursing interventions for common disorders of the LGA infant, see discussion of specific disorders in this chapter.

Small-for-Gestational-Age Infant

A **small-for-gestational-age (SGA)** infant is *any* infant who at birth is at or below the tenth percentile (intrauterine growth curve) on the Newborn Classification by Gestational Age and Birth Weight chart. An SGA infant may be preterm, term, or postterm. Other designations for a growth-retarded neonate include IUGR, small for dates (SFD), and dysmature.

Between 3%–7% of all pregnancies are complicated by IUGR. SGA infants have a five-fold increase in perinatal asphyxia and an eight-fold higher perinatal mortality than normal infants (Hobbins, 1982).

Etiology

IUGR may result from maternal, placental, or fetal causes or may result without apparent cause. Intrauterine growth steadily progresses in the normal pregnancy from approximately 28–38 weeks of gestation. After 38 weeks, growth is variable, depending on the growth potential of the fetus and placental functioning. The most commonly occurring causes of growth retardation are as follows:

Malnutrition   Maternal nutrition does not significantly influence the birth weight of the neonate unless starvation occurs during the last trimester of pregnancy. Before the third trimester, the nutritional supply to the fetus far exceeds its needs. Only in the third trimester is maternal nutrition a limiting factor in fetal growth.

Vascular complications   Complications associated with PIH (preeclampsia and eclampsia), chronic hypertensive vascular disease, and advanced diabetes mellitus cause diminished blood flow to the uterus.

Maternal disease   Maternal heart disease, alcoholism, narcotic addiction, sickle cell anemia, phenylketonuria, and asymptomatic pyelonephritis are associated with SGA.

Maternal factors   SGA is associated with such maternal factors as small stature, primiparity, grand multiparity, smoking, lack of prenatal care, age (very young or older), and low socioeconomic class—which usually results in poor health care, poor education, and poor living conditions.

Environmental factors   Such factors include high altitude, x-rays, and maternal use of drugs, such as antimetabolites, anticonvulsants, and trimethadione, which have teratogenic effects.

Placental factors   Placental conditions such as infarcted areas, abnormal cord insertions, placenta previa, or thrombosis may affect circulation to the fetus, which becomes more deficient with increasing gestational age.

Fetal factors   Congenital infections or malformations, multiple pregnancy (twins, triplets), sex (female neonate), chromosomal syndromes, and inborn errors of metabolism can predispose a fetus to IUGR.

Antenatal identification of fetuses suffering IUGR is the first step in the detection of common disorders of the SGA infant. (See Chapter 11 for antenatal diagnosis and management.) The perinatal history of maternal conditions and examination of the placenta and the newborn are important in determining this at-risk newborn.

Patterns of Intrauterine Growth Retardation

Growth occurs in two ways—increase in cell number and cell size. If insult occurs early during the critical period of organ development in the fetus, fewer new cells are formed, organs are small, and organ weight is subnormal. In contrast, growth failure that begins later in pregnancy does not affect the total number of cells but only their size. The organs are normal, but their size is diminished.

Two varying clinical pictures of SGA newborns have been described. They are characterized by either *symmetric* IUGR or *asymmetric* IUGR.

Symmetric IUGR is caused by long-term maternal conditions (such as chronic hypertension, severe malnutrition, chronic intrauterine infection, substance abuse, and anemia) or fetal genetic abnormalities (Bree and Mariona, 1980). Symmetric IUGR can be noted by ultrasound in the first half of the second trimester (Figure 22-8).

In symmetric IUGR there is chronic prolonged retardation of growth in size of organs, weight, length, and, in severe cases, head circumference. All body parts are in proportion but they are also below normal size for that gestational age. Therefore the head does not appear overly large or the length excessive in relation to the other body parts. These neonates are generally vigorous (Korones, 1981).

Asymmetric IUGR is caused by an acute compromise of uteroplacental blood flow. The growth retardation is usually not evident before the third trimester. Weight is decreased, yet length and head circumference remain appropriate for that gestational age. These neonates appear as follows:

- Head appears relatively large (although it approaches normal) because chest and abdominal size are decreased
- Loose dry skin
- Scarcity of subcutaneous fat, with emaciated appearance
- Long, thin in appearance
- Sunken abdomen

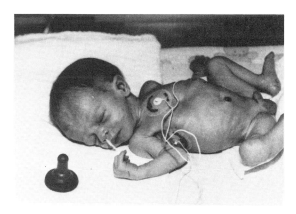

Figure 22-8 ▬▬▬▬▬▬

The infant with IUGR appears long, thin, and emaciated. The gestational age of the infant shown here is 41 weeks. He weighed approximately 1560 g at birth.

- Sparse scalp hair (may be more plentiful in postterm infants)
- Anterior fontanelle may be depressed
- May have vigorous cry and appear deceptively alert (this is attributed to chronic marginal hypoxia in utero)

Birth weight is reduced below the tenth percentile, whereas head size may be between the fifteenth and the nineteenth percentile.

Asymmetric SGA neonates are particularly at risk for perinatal asphyxia, pulmonary hemorrhage, hypocalcemia, and hypoglycemia in the neonatal period (Bree and Mariona, 1980).

Complications

The complications occurring most frequently in the SGA neonate are the following:

1. Perinatal asphyxia—because of chronic hypoxia in utero, which leaves little reserve to withstand the demands of labor and delivery and increases risk of intracranial bleeding and respiratory distress.

2. Aspiration syndromes—gasping secondary to in utero hypoxia can cause aspiration of amniotic fluid into the lower airways; or can lead to relaxation of the anal sphincter with passage of meconium. This results in meconium aspiration with first breaths after birth.

3. Heat loss—because of decreased ability to conserve heat resulting from diminished subcutaneous fat (used for survival in utero), depletion of brown fat in utero, and large surface area. The surface area is diminished somewhat because of the flexed position assumed by the SGA infant.

4. Hypoglycemia—caused by high metabolic rate (secondary to heat loss), poor liver glycogen stores and inhibited gluconeogenesis.

5. Hypocalcemia—secondary to birth asphyxia and preterm birth.

6. Polycythemia—thought to be a physiologic response to in utero chronic hypoxic stress.

Long-Term Outcome and Needs

Infants who have significant IUGR tend to have a poor prognosis, especially when born before 37 weeks' gestation. Factors contributing to poor outcome for these infants are as follows:

Congenital malformations　Usher (1970) found that congenital malformations occur 10 to 20 times more frequently in SGA infants than in AGA infants.

Continued poor growth　SGA infants will probably remain shorter and slimmer than other infants and children as they grow older.

Learning difficulties　Because SGA infants often have poor brain development and subsequent failure to catch up, minimal cerebral dysfunction is not uncommon. However, the environment of the SGA neonate can play a vital role in long-term outcome.

The long-term needs of the SGA neonate include scrupulous follow-up evaluation of patterns of growth and possible disabilities that may later interfere with learning or motor functioning. Long-term follow-up care is especially necessary for those infants with congenital malformations, congenital infections, and obvious sequelae from physiologic problems. In addition, the parents of the SGA neonate need support. As already pointed out, a positive atmosphere can enhance the neonate's growth potential and the child's ultimate outcome. (See Chapter 26 for further discussion of families facing childbearing crises.)

Infant of Diabetic Mother

An **infant of a diabetic mother (IDM)** is considered at risk and requires close observation the first few hours to the first few days of life. The typical IDM (type I, or White's classes B and C) is LGA (Figure 22-9). He or she is fat, macrosomic, and has a reddened complexion. The infant is not edematous since IDMs have decreased total body water, particularly in the extracellular spaces. Their excessive weight is due to visceral organomegaly, cardiomegaly, and increased body fat. The only organ not affected is the brain. IDMs are large in size but immature in physiologic functions, exhibiting many of the problems of the preterm infant. The cord and placenta are large. Mothers with severe diabetes or diabetes of long duration, associated with vascular complications, may give birth to infants who are SGA (type I or White's classes D–F).

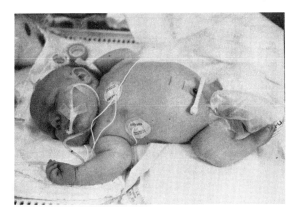

Figure 22-9
Macrosomic IDM. On x-ray film, this infant was noted to have caudal regression of the spine. (Courtesy Dr. Paul Winchester.)

The excessive fetal growth of the IDM is caused by high levels of maternal glucose, which readily crosses the placenta. The fetus responds to these high glucose levels with increased insulin production and hyperplasia of the pancreatic beta cells. Thus, insulin is an important regulator of fetal growth and metabolism.

After birth the most common problem of an IDM is hypoglycemia. Even though the high maternal glucose supply is lost, the fetus continues to produce high levels of insulin, which depletes the blood glucose within hours after birth. IDMs also have less ability to release glucagon and catecholamines. This normally stimulates glucagon breakdown and glucose release. The wide range in incidence of hypoglycemia is thought to be due to aspects of maternal care and success in controlling the diabetes, early versus late feedings of the infant, differences in maternal blood sugars at the time of delivery, length of labor, and the class of maternal diabetes.

In addition to hypoglycemia, other major problems may arise in the IDM during the first few hours and days of life. These include:

1. Hypocalcemia, with tremors the obvious clinical sign. This may be due to the IDM's increased incidence of prematurity and to the stresses of difficult pregnancy, labor, and delivery, which predispose any infant to hypocalcemia. Also, diabetic women tend to have higher calcium levels at term, causing possible secondary hypoparathyroidism in their infants.

2. Hyperbilirubinemia, which may be seen at 48–72 hours after birth, possibly due to slightly decreased extracellular fluid volume. This causes increased hematocrit level.

3. Birth trauma, as discussed in the section on LGA infants, p. 510.

4. Polycythemia, because of the decreased extracellular volume present in IDMs.

5. RDS, especially in newborns of classes A–C diabetic mothers. It is theorized that the high levels of fetal insulin interfere with the synthesis of the lecithin necessary for lung maturation. This does not appear to be a problem for infants born of class D–F diabetic mothers; instead the stresses of poor uterine blood supply may lead to increased production of steroids, resulting in acceleration of lung maturation.

6. Congenital birth defects, such as transposition of the great vessels, ventricular septal defect, and patent ductus arteriosus (common); neurologic defects; small left colon syndrome; and caudal regression syndrome (rare). Congenital malformations in LGA infants of diabetic mothers are more frequent because of the abnormal intrauterine environment due to diabetes and vascular complications and drugs taken by the mother during pregnancy (oral hypoglycemic agents).

Nursing management is based on early attention to the prenatal history and assessment of maternal diabetes throughout pregnancy to identify the infant at risk. An IDM should be treated as a preterm or high-risk infant, and close observation in an intensive care nursery should be instituted immediately after birth.

Drug- or Alcohol-Dependent Neonates

The newborn of an alcoholic or drug-dependent woman will also be alcohol- or drug-dependent. After birth, when an infant's connection with the maternal blood supply is severed, the neonate suffers withdrawal. In addition, the drugs ingested by the mother may be teratogenic, resulting in congenital anomalies.

Drug Dependency

Drug-dependent infants are predisposed to a number of problems. Since almost all narcotic drugs cross the placenta and enter the fetal circulation, the fetus can develop problems in utero and/or soon after birth.

The greatest risks to the fetus of the drug-dependent mother are:

- Intrauterine asphyxia—often a direct result of fetal withdrawal, secondary to maternal withdrawal. Fetal withdrawal is accompanied by hyperactivity with increased oxygen consumption, which, if not adequately compensated, can lead to fetal asphyxia. Moreover, narcotic-addicted women tend to have a higher incidence of PIH, abruptio placentae, and placenta previa, resulting in placental insufficiency and fetal asphyxia.

- Intrauterine infection—particularly sexually transmitted disease and hepatitis, is often connected with the pregnant addict's life-style. Such infections can involve the fetus.

- Alterations in birth weight—may depend on the type of drug the mother uses. Women using predominantly heroin have infants of lower birth weight who are SGA, whereas women maintained on methadone have higher-birth-weight infants, some of whom are LGA (Ostrea et al., 1978).

- Low Apgar scores—may be related to the intrauterine asphyxia or the medication the woman received during labor. The use of a narcotic antagonist (nalorphine or naloxone) to reverse respiratory depression is contraindicated, as it may precipitate acute withdrawal in the infant.

Problems of the neonate of a narcotic-addicted mother include:

- Respiratory distress—mainly aspiration pneumonia and transient tachypnea. Aspiration pneumonia is usually secondary to meconium aspiration and intrauterine asphyxia. The transient tachypnea may be secondary to the inhibitory effects of narcotics on the reflex clearing of fluid by the lungs.

- Jaundice—due to the higher incidence of prematurity in infants of drug-dependent mothers.

- Congenital malformations—slightly increased anomalies of the genitourinary and cardiovascular systems.

Clinical manifestations and nursing management Narcotic withdrawal symptoms usually occur within the first 72 hours after birth. In most cases, the withdrawal symptoms peak in the neonate about the third day and subside by the fifth to seventh day. Neonatal withdrawal can be classified in five groups.

1. Central nervous system signs
   a. Hyperactivity
   b. Hyperirritability (persistent high-pitched cry)
   c. Increased muscle tone
   d. Exaggerated reflexes
   e. Tremors
   f. Sneezing, hiccups, yawning
   g. Short, nonquiet sleep
   h. Fever
2. Respiratory signs
   a. Tachypnea
   b. Excessive secretions
3. Gastrointestinal signs
   a. Uncoordinated, vigorous suck
   b. Vomiting
   c. Drooling
   d. Sensitive gag reflex
   e. Hyperphagia
   f. Diarrhea
   g. Abdominal cramping
4. Vasomotor signs
   a. Stuffy nose
   b. Flushing
   c. Sweating
   d. Sudden, circumoral pallor
5. Cutaneous signs
   a. Excoriated buttocks
   b. Facial scratches
   c. Pressure point abrasions

Care of the newborn is based on reducing withdrawal symptoms and promoting adequate respiration, temperature, and nutrition. Specific nursery care measures include:

- Temperature regulation

- Careful monitoring of pulse and respirations every 15 minutes until stable; stimulation if apnea occurs.

- Small frequent feedings, especially in the presence of vomiting, regurgitation, and diarrhea

- Intravenous therapy as needed
- Medications as ordered, such as phenobarbital, paregoric, diazepam (Valium), or chlorpromazine hydrochloride (Thorazine); methadone should not be given because of possible neonatal addiction to it
- Proper positioning on side to avoid possible aspiration of vomitus or secretions
- Observation for problems of SGA or LGA infants
- Protection from injury
- Fostering positive mother–infant interaction to avoid potential negative feedback from infant because of abnormal sleep and nutrition patterns, inability to cuddle, and continuous crying.

At the time of discharge, the mother should be instructed to anticipate mild jitteriness and irritability in the infant, which may persist from 8–16 weeks, depending on the initial severity of the withdrawal.

Long-term outcomes   The incidence of SIDS is high (5.6%) among these infants. The occurrence of SIDS may be even higher in those infants who have had moderate-to-severe postnatal withdrawal (Ostrea et al., 1978).

For optimal fetal and neonatal outcome, the narcotic-addicted woman should receive complete prenatal care as soon as possible. In addition, she should be started on a methadone program with a reduction in dosage to 20 mg or less per day. The woman should not be withdrawn completely from narcotics while pregnant, since this induces fetal withdrawal with poor neonatal outcomes.

Alcohol Dependency

The **fetal alcohol syndrome** (FAS) described by Jones and colleagues (1973) refers to a series of malformations frequently found in infants born to women who have been chronic severe alcoholics. It has been estimated that the complete FAS syndrome occurs in 1 or 2 live births per 1000 with a partial expression frequency at about 3–5 live births per 1000 (Cohlan, 1980).

The characteristics of FAS infants include the following:

- Persistent postnatal growth deficiency for length, weight, and brain
- Facial abnormalities including short palpebral fissures, epicanthal folds, short upturned nose, maxillary hypoplasia, micrognathia, and thin upper lip.
- Cardiac defects such as primary septal defects
- Minor joint and limb abnormalities, including some restriction of movement and altered palmar crease patterns.

Controversy surrounds the exact cause of FAS. Although it is known that ethanol freely crosses the placenta to the fetus, it is still not known whether the alcohol alone or the breakdown products of alcohol cause the damage. Other factors in conjunction with alcohol may contribute to the teratogenic effects. The factors include drugs (diazepam), nicotine, and caffeine, in addition to poor diet and low socioeconomic status (Iosub et al., 1981).

The withdrawal symptoms of the alcohol-dependent neonate are similar to those exhibited by the mother: abdominal distention, tremors, agitation, arching of the back, sweating, and seizures. The infant often has a poor sucking reflex. Signs and symptoms often appear within 6–12 hours and at least within the first 24 hours (Ostrea et al., 1978). Seizures after the neonatal period are rare. Alcohol dependence in the infant is physiologic, not psychologic. Care of the alcohol-addicted newborn includes monitoring warmth, protection from injury during seizure, intravenous fluid therapy, reduction of environmental stimuli, and medication such as phenobarbital or diazepam to limit convulsions.

Long-term outcomes   The long-term prognosis for the FAS neonate is less than favorable. Most infants with FAS are growth-deficient at birth, and few infants have demonstrated catch-up growth. In fact, most FAS infants are evaluated for failure to thrive. Decreased adipose tissue is a constant feature of persons with FAS. Feeding problems are frequently present during infancy and preschool years.

CNS dysfunctions are the most common and serious problem associated with FAS. The brain is the organ that is most sensitive to damage from alcohol in the fetus. Most children exhibiting FAS are mildly to severely mentally retarded. The more abnormal the facial features, the lower the IQ scores. FAS children are often hyperactive and show a high incidence of speech and language abnormalities indicative of CNS disorders.

The most effective treatment of FAS is prevention, through early prenatal care for the pregnant woman with reduction in alcohol intake.

Asphyxia

Circulatory patterns that accompany asphyxia indicate an inability to make the transition to extrauterine circulation—in effect a return to fetal-like circulatory patterns. Failure of lung expansion and establishment of respiration rapidly produces hypoxia (decreased Pao_2), acidosis (decreased pH), and hypercarbia (increased Pco_2). These biochemical changes result in pulmonary vasoconstriction, with retention of high pulmonary vascular resistance, hypoperfusion of the lungs, and a large right-to-left shunt through the ductus arteriosus. The foramen ovale opens (as right atrial pressure exceeds left atrial pressure), and blood flows from right to left.

Biochemical changes that occur in asphyxia contribute to these circulatory changes. The most serious biochemical abnormality is a change from aerobic to anaerobic metabolism in the presence of hypoxia. This results in the accumulation of lactate and the development of metabolic acidosis. A concomitant respiratory acidosis may also occur due to a rapid increase in Pco_2 during asphyxia. In response to hypoxia and anaerobic metabolism, the amounts of free fatty acids and glycerol in the blood increase. Glycogen stores are also mobilized to provide a continuous glucose source for the brain. Rapid utilization of hepatic and cardiac stores of glycogen may occur during an asphyxial attack.

The neonate is supplied with the following protective mechanisms against hypoxial insults (Klaus and Fanaroff, 1979): a relatively immature brain and a resting metabolic rate less than that observed in the adult, an ability to mobilize substances within the body for anaerobic metabolism and use the energy more efficiently; and an intact circulatory system able to redistribute lactate and hydrogen ion in tissues still being perfused. Unfortunately, severe prolonged hypoxia will overcome these protective mechanisms, resulting in brain damage or death of the neonate.

Resuscitation

Knowledge of the perinatal history enables caregivers to anticipate the birth of a high-risk infant who will need resuscitative efforts. Need for resuscitation may be anticipated if the mother demonstrates the risk factors antepartally and intrapartally described in Tables 6-1 and 13-1. Neonatal risk factors for resuscitation are:

- Difficult delivery
- Fetal blood loss
- Apneic episode unresponsive to tactile stimulation
- Cardiac arrest
- Inadequate ventilation

Particular attention must be paid to at-risk pregnancies during the intrapartal period. Labor and delivery are asphyxiating processes and often the at-risk fetus has less tolerance to the stress of labor and delivery.

Nurse's Role

Identification of high-risk infants can be helped by communication between the prenatal office or clinic setting and the labor and delivery nurse. Upon arrival of the woman in the labor area, the nurse should have the antepartal record. Any contributory perinatal history factors and present fetal status are determined and recorded. As labor progresses, nursing assessments include ongoing monitoring of fetal heartbeat and its response to contractions, assisting with fetal scalp blood sampling, and observing for expulsion of meconium, thereby identifying fetal asphyxia and hypoxia. In addition, the nurse should alert the resuscitation team and the practitioner responsible for care of the neonate of any potential high-risk clients in the labor and delivery area.

Equipment and medications   After identification of possible high-risk situations, the next step in effective resuscitation is assembling the necessary equipment and ensuring proper functioning.

Systematic assembly and checking of equipment is essential for efficient resuscitation and for preventing "flail" efforts. Provision for pH and blood gas determination is desirable.

An adequate number of trained personnel must be in the delivery room for all deliveries. Resuscitation is at least a two-person effort. The nurse should call for assistance from trained personnel.

Necessary equipment includes the following:

- Radiant warmer to maintain a stable body temperature
- Open bed for easy access to newborn
- Newborn bag and mask
- Oxygen and flowmeter
- Laryngoscope
- Emergency cart and medications

Initial Resuscitative Management

The goals of resuscitation are to provide an adequate airway with expansion of the lungs, to decrease Pco_2 and increase the Po_2, to support adequate cardiac output, and to minimize oxygen consumption by reducing heat loss (Cloherty and Stark, 1981).

Appraisal of the infant's need for resuscitation begins at the time of birth. The time of the first gasp, first cry, and onset of sustained respirations should be noted in order of occurrence. The Apgar score (p. 311) is important in determining the severity of neonatal depression and the immediate course of necessary action (Table 22-2). During initial resuscitative management of the neonate, the infant should be kept in a head-down position prior to the first gasp to avoid aspirating oropharyngeal secretions, and must be suctioned immediately. After the first few breaths, the infant is kept in a flat position under a radiant heat source and dried quickly to maintain skin temperature at about 36.5C. Drying is also a good stimulation to breathing. Heat loss through evaporation is tremendous during the first few minutes of life. The temperature of a wet 1500 g baby in a 16C (62F) delivery room drops 1C every 3 minutes. Hypothermia increases oxygen consumption and in an asphyxiated infant increases the hypoxic insult and may lead to severe acidosis and development of respiratory distress.

Establish airway   A patent airway is established by clearing the nasal and oral passages of fluid that may obstruct the airway. Suctioning is always performed before resuscitation so that mucus, blood, meconium, or formula is not aspirated into the lungs.

Establish respirations   To establish the infant's breathing, the caregivers begin with the simplest form of resuscitative measures and, if unsuccessful, proceed to more complicated methods.

1. Simple stimulation is provided by rubbing the back.

2. If respirations have not been initiated or are inadequate (gasping or occasional respirations), the lungs must be inflated with positive pressure. The mask is positioned securely on the face (over nose and mouth; avoiding the eyes) with head in "sniffing" or neutral position (Figure 22-10). Hyperextension of the infant's neck will obstruct the trachea. An airtight seal is made between the infant's face and the mask (thus allowing the bag to inflate). The bag is squeezed rhythmically to inflate the lungs. Oxygen is then administered via the bag. In a crisis situation it is crucial that 100% O_2 be delivered with adequate pressure.

3. The rise and fall of the chest is observed for proper ventilation. The nurse should auscultate over both lungs for air entry and check

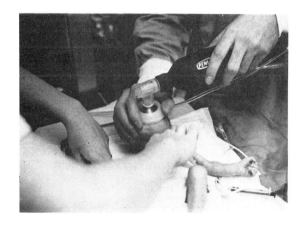

Figure 22-10 ▬▬▬▬▬▬

Resuscitation of infant with bag and mask. Note that the mask covers the nose and mouth, and the head is in a neutral position.

Table 22-2
Guidelines for Resuscitation of the Neonate

Apgar score	Heart rate	Appearance	Resuscitative measures
9 or 10	> 100	Regular respirations; flexed extremities; cries in response to flicking of soles of feet; may be dusky or show acrocyanosis	Place under radiant heat source and dry immediately; gently suction airway.
7 or 8	60-100	Limp, cyanotic, or dusky and dyspneic; respirations may be shallow, irregular, or gasping; heart rate is normal; fair response to flicking of sole	Dry and place under warmer; suction airway; give oxygen near face.
5 or 6	60-100	Same as for Apgar 7 or 8	Dry and place under warmer; clear airway and stimulate through drying process. If still not improved, place in "sniff" position, insert pharyngeal airway, and begin ventilation (100% O_2) with bag and mask, using pressure of 30 cm H_2O at rate of 30-50 per min. If difficulty persists, reevaluate maternal history of drug administration, especially if heart rate responds to ventilation but there is no spontaneous respiration. Give narcotic antagonist (Narcan) if indicated. Mildly depressed newborns will usually develop regular spontaneous respirations within 5 minutes. If tracheal aspiration reveals blood or meconium, directly visualize with laryngoscope and suction as needed before administering positive pressure.
3 or 4	< 60	Blue and limp, little or no respiratory effort. Jaw is slack during suctioning.	For Apgar 0-4: Dry under warmer; clear airway; consider immediate intubation. Hold O_2 near face during intubation. Ventilate after direct visualization with laryngoscope and appropriate suctioning. Check breath sounds. If heart rate remains low (0-40), immediately institute external cardiac massage. Correction of hypotension is usually via umbilical vein. Obtain blood gas values (pH, Pco_2, Po_2) and BP.
0 to 2	< 60	Same as for Apgar 3 or 4	

*Adapted from Korones, S. *High-Risk Newborn Infants: The Basis for Intensive Nursing Care.* 2nd ed. St. Louis: Mosby, 1981.

the heart rate. Manual resuscitation is coordinated with any voluntary efforts. The rate of ventilation should be between 30 and 50 per minute. Pressure should be less than 30 cm of H_2O. If ventilation is adequate, the chest moves with each inspiration, bilateral breath sounds are audible, and the lips and mucous membranes become pink. Distention of the stomach is controlled by inserting a nasogastric tube for decompression.

4. Intubation is rarely needed because most infants can be resuscitated by bag and mask.

Maintain circulation   Once breathing has been established, the heart rate should increase to over 100 beats/min. If the heart rate is less than 60 beats/min, external cardiac massage is begun. (Cardiac massage is started immediately if there is no detectable heartbeat.)

1. The infant is positioned *properly* on a firm surface.

2. The resuscitator uses two fingers or may stand at the foot of the infant and place both thumbs at the junction of the middle and lower third of the sternum, with the fingers wrapped around and supporting the back.

3. The sternum is depressed approximately two-thirds of the distance to the vertebral column (1.0–1.5 cm), at a rate of 80–100 beats/ min.

4. A 3:1 ratio of heartbeat to assisted ventilation is used.

Drug therapy   Drugs that should be available in the delivery room include those needed in the treatment of shock, cardiac arrest, and narcosis. Oxygen, because of its effective use in ventilation, is the drug most often used.

If by 5 minutes after delivery, the neonate has not responded to the resuscitation with spontaneous respirations and a heart rate above 100 beats/min, it may be necessary to correct the acidosis and provide the myocardium with glucose. Other medications that may be used during resuscitation are:

• Epinephrine or atropine to correct bradycardia

• 10% calcium gluconate to treat severe bradycardia, arrythmias, poor cardiac output, and hypocalcemia

• Dextrose to prevent or reverse hypoglycemia

• Naloxone hydrochloride to reverse narcotic depression

• Volume expanders (5% albumin, fresh frozen plasma, or blood) to correct shock

Respiratory Distress

One of the most severe conditions to which the neonate may fall victim is respiratory distress—an inappropriate respiratory adaptation to extrauterine life. Only with a clear understanding of this disease process and its implications can the nurse make appropriate observations concerning responses to therapy and development of complications.

Respiratory Distress Syndrome (Hyaline Membrane Disease)

Respiratory distress syndrome (RDS), also referred to as *hyaline membrane disease* (HMD), is a complex disease affecting primarily preterm infants. It accounts for 12,000 to 25,000 deaths per year in the United States alone. The factors causing the pathophysiologic changes of RDS have not been determined, but there are two main factors associated with the development of RDS:

1. *Prematurity*. All preterm infants and IDMs are at risk for RDS. The maternal and fetal factors resulting in preterm labor and delivery, complications of pregnancy, cesarean birth (indications for cesarean delivery rather than the type of delivery), and familial tendency are all associated with RDS.

2. *Asphyxia*. Asphyxia, with a corresponding decrease in pulmonary blood flow, may interfere with surfactant production.

Pathophysiology   Development of RDS indicates a failure to produce lecithin at a rate required to maintain alveolar stability. Upon expiration, this instability results in increasing atelectasis. The progressive atelectasis causes hypoxia, pulmonary vasoconstriction, and hypoperfusion and further inhibits surfactant production. These physiologic alterations result in:

1. Hypoxia causes vasoconstriction of the pulmonary vasculature, which increases pulmonary vascular resistance and further reduces pulmonary blood flow. Increased pulmonary vascular resistance may precipitate a return to fetal circulation as the ductus opens and blood flow is shunted away from the lungs (right-to-left shunt).

2. Hypoxia also causes impairment or absence of metabolic response to cold, reversion to anaerobic metabolism, and lactate accumulation (metabolic acidosis).

3. Pulmonary hypoperfusion and decreased alveolar ventilation result in hypercarbia (increased Pco_2) and respiratory acidosis.

4. Metabolic acidosis may also be the result of impaired delivery of oxygen at the cellular level.

The cycle of events of RDS leading to eventual respiratory failure is diagrammed in Figure 22-11.

Because of these pathophysiologic conditions, the neonate must expend increasing amounts of energy to reopen the collapsed

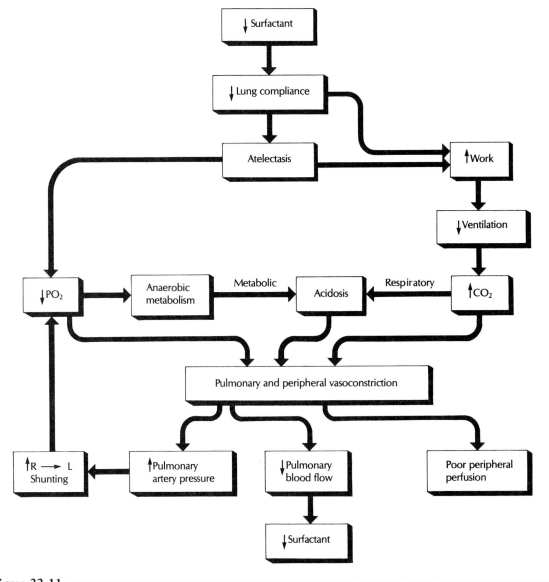

Figure 22-11

Cycle of events of RDS leading to eventual respiratory failure.

alveoli with every breath, so that each breath becomes as difficult as the first.

Clinical manifestations   The clinical manifestations are the result of the disease process and the newborn's efforts to compensate. Table 22-3 provides a review of clinical findings associated with respiratory distress.

The classic x-ray film of respiratory distress syndrome initially has a ground glass appearance (reticulogranular densities). Radiologic findings follow the pattern of disease process resolution and the timing of the reappearance of surfactant.

Table 22-3
Clinical Findings Associated with Respiratory Distress

Clinical picture	Significance
Skin	
Color	
Pallor or mottling	Represents poor peripheral circulation due to systemic hypotension and vasoconstriction and pooling of independent areas (usually in conjunction with severe hypoxia).
Cyanosis (bluish tint)	Depends on hemoglobin concentration, peripheral circulation, intensity and quality of viewing light, and acuity of observer's color vision; frankly visible in advanced hypoxia yet may be unobservable, because a large decrease in Pao$_2$ may be tolerated without signs of cyanosis.
Jaundice (yellow discoloration of skin and mucous membranes due to presence of unconjugated (indirect) bilirubin)	Metabolic aberrations (acidosis, hypercarbia, asphyxia) of respiratory distress predispose to dissociation of bilirubin from albumin-binding sites and deposition in the skin and central nervous system.
Edema (presents as slick, shiny skin)	Characteristic of preterm infant because of low total protein concentration with decrease in colloidal osmotic pressure and transudation of fluid; edema of hands and feet frequently seen within first 24 hours and resolved by fifth day in infant with severe RDS.
Respiratory system	
Tachypnea (normal respiratory rate 40-60/min; elevated respiratory rate 60+/min)	Increased respiratory rate is most frequent and easily detectable sign of respiratory distress after birth; a compensatory mechanism that attempts to increase respiratory dead space to maintain alveolar ventilation and gaseous exchange in the face of an increase in mechanical resistance. As a decompensatory mechanism it increases work load and energy output (by increasing respiratory rate), which causes increased metabolic demand for oxygen and thus increase in alveolar ventilation (of already over-stressed system). During shallow, rapid respirations, there is increase in dead space ventilation, thus decreasing alveolar ventilation.
Apnea (episode of nonbreathing of more than 25 sec in duration; periodic breathing, a common "normal" occurrence in preterm infants, is defined as apnea of 5-10 sec alternating with 10-15 sec periods of ventilation)	Poor prognostic sign; indicative of cardiorespiratory disease, central nervous system disease, and immaturity; physiologic alterations include decreased oxygen saturation, respiratory acidosis, and bradycardia.
Chest	Inspection of thoracic cage and measurement of anteroposterior diameter of chest may reveal decreased thoracic gas volume.
Labored respirations (Silverman-Andersen chart in Figure 22-12 indicates severity of retractions, grunting, and flaring, which are signs of labored respirations)	Indicative of marked increase in work of breathing.
Retractions (inward pulling of soft parts of chest cage—suprasternal, substernal, intercostal, subcostal—at inspiration)	Reflect significant increase in negative intrathoracic pressure necessary to inflate stiff, noncompliant lung; infants attempt to increase lung compliance by using accessory muscles;

Table 22-3
Clinical Findings Associated with Respiratory Distress (continued)

Clinical picture	Significance
	markedly decreases lung expansion; seesaw respirations are seen when chest flattens with inspiration and abdomen bulges; retractions increase work and O_2 need of breathing, so that assisted ventilation may be necessary due to exhaustion.
Flaring nares (inspiratory dilatation of nostrils)	Compensatory mechanism that attempts to lessen resistance of narrow nasal passage.
Expiratory grunt (Valsalva maneuver in which infant exhales against closed glottis, thus producing audible moan)	Produces increase in transpulmonary pressure, which decreases or prevents atelectasis, thus improving oxygenation and alveolar ventilation; intubation should not be attempted unless infant's condition is rapidly deteriorating, because it prevents this maneuver and allows aveoli to collapse.
Rhythmic movement of body with labored respirations (chin tug, head bobbing, retractions of anal area)	Result of utilization of abdominal and other respiratory accessory muscles during prolonged forced respirations.
Auscultation of chest reveals decreased air exchange with harsh breath sounds and fine inspiratory rales, posterior lung base	Decrease in breath sounds and distant quality may indicate air or fluid occupying chest.
Cardiovascular system Continuous systolic murmur may be audible	Patent ductus arteriosus is common occurrence with hypoxia, pulmonary vasoconstriction, right-to-left shunting, and congestive heart failure.
Heart rate usually within normal limits (fixed heart rate may occur with a rate of 110–120/min)	Fixed heart rate indicates decrease in vagal control.
Hypothermia	Inadequate functioning of metabolic processes that require oxygen to produce necessary body heat.
Muscle tone Flaccid, hypotonic, unresponsive to stimuli Hypertonia and/or seizure activity	May indicate deterioration in neonate's condition and possible CNS damage, due to hypoxia, acidemia, or hemorrhage.

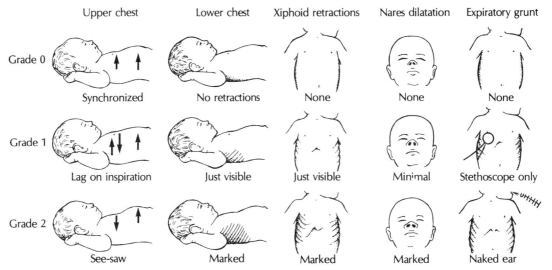

Figure 22-12

Evaluation of respiratory status using the Silverman-Andersen index. (From Ross Laboratories, Nursing Inservice Aid no. 2, Columbus, Ohio; and Silverman WA, Andersen DH: *Pediatrics* 1956; 17:1. Copyright © 1956 American Academy of Pediatrics.)

Interventions   The primary prenatal goal is the prevention of preterm delivery through aggressive treatment of premature labor and possible administration of glucocorticoids to enhance fetal lung development (see p. 355). Postnatally, supportive medical management consists of ventilatory therapy, transcutaneous oxygen monitoring (Cohen, 1984), correction of acid-base imbalance, environmental temperature regulation, adequate nutrition, and protection from infection. Ventilatory therapy is directed toward prevention of hypoventilation and hypoxia. Mild cases of RDS may require only increased humidified oxygen concentrations. Use of continuous positive airway pressure (CPAP) methods may be required in moderately afflicted infants. Severe cases of RDS require mechanical ventilatory assistance, with or without positive end-expiratory pressure (PEEP) (Figure 22-13).

The neonatal nurse bases the plan of care on the assessment of the clinical findings, implements therapeutic approaches to maintain physiologic homeostasis, and provides supportive care to the neonate with RDS (Nugent, 1983). (See the Nursing Care Plan—Respiratory Distress Syndrome.)

The nursing care of infants on ventilators or with umbilical artery catheters will not be discussed here. These infants have severe respiratory distress and are cared for in intensive care nurseries by nurses with special knowledge and training.

Transient Tachypnea of the Newborn (Type II Respiratory Distress Syndrome)

Some newborns, primarily AGA preterm, and near-term infants, develop progressive respiratory distress that resembles classic RDS. These infants have usually had some intrauterine or intrapartal asphyxia caused by maternal oversedation, cesarean delivery, maternal bleeding, prolapsed cord, breech delivery, or maternal diabetes. The resultant effect on the neonate is failure to clear the airway of lung fluid, mucus, and other debris or an excess of fluid in the lungs due to aspiration of amniotic or tracheal fluid.

Clinical manifestations—expiratory grunting, flaring of the nares, mild cyanosis, and tachypnea—occur during the first days of life. (The expiratory grunting is an attempt to eject as much of the trapped alveolar air as possible; in true RDS the grunt is an attempt to retain as much air as possible in an effort to maintain alveolar expansion.) Rales are absent but breath sounds are decreased. After 6 hours, symptoms progressively improve.

Text continued on p. 529.

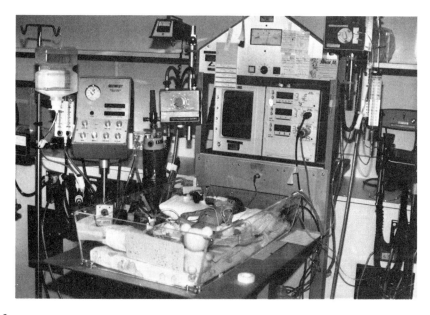

Figure 22-13
Infant on respirator.

NURSING CARE PLAN
Respiratory Distress Syndrome

PATIENT ASSESSMENT

History

Preterm delivery
Gestational history: recent episodes of fetal or intrapartal stress (that is, maternal hypotension, bleeding, maternal and resultant fetal oversedation), severe fetal lung circulation compromise
Neonatal history: birth asphyxia resulting in acute hypoxia, exposure to extremes of hypothermia
Familial tendency

Physical Examination

At birth or within 2 hours, rapid development initially of tachypnea (over 60 respirations/min), expiratory grunting (audible), or intercostal retractions
Followed by flaring of nares on inspiration, cyanosis and pallor, signs of increased air hunger (apneic spells, hypotonus), rhythmic movement of body and labored respirations, chin tug
Auscultation: initially breath sounds may be normal; then there is decreased air exchange with harsh breath sounds and, upon deep inspiration, rales; later there is a low-pitched systolic murmur indicative of patent ductus in infants
Increasing oxygen concentration requirements to maintain adequate Po_2 levels

Laboratory Evaluation

Arterial blood gases (indicating respiratory failure): PaO_2 less than 50 mm Hg while breathing 100% O_2 and PCO_2 above 70 mm Hg.
X-ray: diffuse reticulogranular density bilaterally, with air-filled tracheobronchial tube outlined by opaque lungs (air bronchogram); atelectasis/hypoexpansion is present; in severe cases, opacification of lung fields may be seen due to massive atelectasis, diffuse alveoli infiltrates, or pulmonary edema
Clinical course worsens first 24–48 hours after birth and persists for more than 24 hours

PLAN OF CARE

Nursing Priorities

1. Assure adequate oxygenation.
2. Provide for assisted ventilatory exchange.
3. Determine and correct acid-base imbalances.
4. Take supportive measures to maintain homeostasis—maintain neutral thermal environment, provide for adequate fluid, electrolyte and caloric requirements, prevent infection.
5. Provide for the emotional needs of the infant with respiratory distress without overstimulation and meet the needs of the family.
6. Observe possible complications of therapy and institute appropriate nursing interventions.

FAMILY EDUCATIONAL FOCUS

1. Discuss the significance of respiratory distress syndrome for the health of their newborn.
2. Explain treatment modalities and their rationale.
3. Explore possible long-term implications of RDS, such as need for prolonged hospitalizations even after acute episode, and possible complications of respiratory management, such as bronchopulmonary dysplasia and retrolental fibroplasia.
4. Refer parents to available resources and support groups.
5. Provide opportunities to discuss questions and individual concerns about their individual neonate.

Problem	Nursing interventions and actions	Rationale
Oxygen concentration	Maintain on respiratory and cardiac monitors—note rates every 30–60 min and when necessary. Check and calibrate all monitoring and measuring devices every 8 hr. Calibrate oxygen devices to 21% and 100% O_2 concentrations. Control and monitor oxygen concentrations at least every hour. Administer oxygen by: 1. Isolette (oxygen tubing is placed inside isolette). 2. Oxygen hood—a small transparent head hood that contains an inlet and carbon dioxide outlet (Figure 22-14).	Stable concentration of oxygen is necessary to maintain PaO_2 within normal limits (50–70 mm). Sudden increase or decrease in O_2 concentration may result in disproportionate increase or decrease in PaO_2 due to vasoconstriction in response to oxygen. Isolettes may reach 70% or more concentration but fluctuate when portholes are opened for caregiving Used when high concentration of oxygen (over 35%) is needed or when observations indicate that infant is unable to tolerate oxygen fluctuations. Provides a constant oxygen environment.

NURSING CARE PLAN (continued)
Respiratory Distress Syndrome

Problem	Nursing interventions and actions	Rationale
	Maintain infant in stable oxygen concentration by increasing or decreasing by 5%–10% increments and then obtain arterial blood gases.	
Fluctuation in oxygen environment	Response of infant to therapy is evaluated by arterial blood gases, transcutaneous oxygen monitoring and clinical assessment Observe for: 1. Pink color, cyanosis (central or acrocyanosis), duskiness, pallor 2. Respiratory effort (evaluation at rest), rate of respirations, patterns (apnea, periodic breathing), quality (easy, unlabored, abdominal, labored), auscultation (site of breath sounds—overall or part of lung fields—describe quality of breath sounds every 1–2 hr), accompanying sounds with respiratory effort (change from previous observations) 3. Activity—less active, flaccid, lethargic, unresponsive; increased activity, restless, irritable; inability to tolerate exertion, crying, sucking, or nursing care activity 4. Circulatory response (evaluate at rest), rate, regularity of rhythm of heart rate, periods of bradycardia, alterations of blood pressure Position infant with head slightly hyperextended. Observations of clinical condition are taken serially for comparison and for changes.	

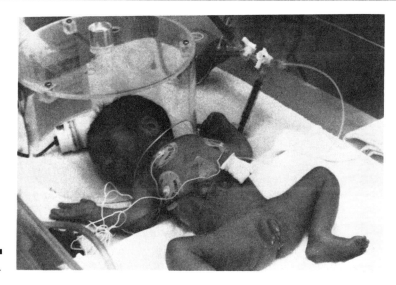

Figure 22-14 ■■■■
Infant in oxygen hood.

NURSING CARE PLAN (continued)
Respiratory Distress Syndrome

Problem	Nursing interventions and actions	Rationale
	Observations should be taken while infant is receiving oxygen and with any oxygen adjustment. Return O_2 concentration to previous levels if there is deterioration in neonate's condition or drop below desired tcm levels. Repeat arterial blood gases (keep PaO_2 50–70 mm Hg). Gases should be done within 15–20 min after any change in ambient O_2 concentration or after inspiratory or expiratory pressure changes. Record and report clinical observations and action taken.	Any deterioration of clinical condition with oxygen adjustments (usually a decrease in ambient oxygen concentration) indicates inability of neonate to compensate for hypoxia.
Humidification of inspired oxygen	Provide humidified oxygen.	Oxygen is dry gas and therefore irritating to airways. Evaporative water losses from skin and lungs are also decreased in high humidity (50%–65%).
	Pay careful attention to infection control by cleaning and replacing nebulizers/humidifiers at least every 24 hr; use sterile tubing and replace every 24 hr; use sterile distilled water.	The warm, moist environment found in Isolettes and with O_2 equipment promotes growth of microorganisms.
Warmed mist delivery	Provide heated mist (at the delivery site) 31–34C. Place a thermometer in the oxygen hood and monitor the temperature of the delivered oxygen. Oxygen hood and Isolette temperature should be maintained at the same temperature. Observe infant for temperature instability and signs of increased oxygen consumption (need for increased O_2 concentration) and metabolic acidosis.	Cold air/oxygen blown in face of newborn is source of cold stress and is stimulus for increased consumption of oxygen and increased metabolic rate.
Monitoring of arterial blood gas values	Maintain stable environment prior to collection of arterial blood gas sample: 1. Maintain constant O_2 concentration at least 15–20 min before sample. 2. Avoid any disturbances of infant 15 min before gases are drawn. Do not suction; if suction is absolutely necessary, delay blood sample. Maintain a warm temperature (pH should be measured at body temperature).	Accurate arterial blood determinations are essential in management of any infant receiving oxygen because presence or absence of cyanosis is unreliable. Values used to determine adequate oxygenation—normal PaO_2 50–70 mm Hg. Adequate ventilation—normal $PaCO_2$ 30–45 mm. Acid-base balance—normal pH 7.35–7.45. Crying or struggling may cause hyperventilation or breath holding and may increase shunting of blood.

NURSING CARE PLAN (continued)
Respiratory Distress Syndrome

Problem	Nursing interventions and actions	Rationale
	Provide arterial blood gas setup (a 3 mL syringe with heparinized solution and a heparinized tuberculin syringe) to obtain blood sample.	Use of temporal, radial, or brachial arteries takes skill and is time-consuming; total blood volume of infant is small; blood removed to clear umbilical catheter must be returned to prevent hypovolemia, anemia.
Inadequate ventilation	Initial observation of respiratory effort, ventilatory adequacy—observation of chest wall movement, skin, mucous membranes, color; estimation of degree and equality of air entry by auscultation, arterial blood gases, and pH determination. Assess need for assisted ventilatory measures. Criteria for assisted ventilation: 1. Apnea. 2. Hypoxia (Pao$_2$ 50 in 50%–60% oxygen). 3. Alert doctor if following criterion for assist is met: respiratory acidosis, pH 7.20.	Alveoli of normal infant remain stable during expiration due to presence of surfactant. Alveoli of infant with RDS lack surfactant and collapse with expiration. Grunting, a compensatory mechanism, increases transpulmonary pressure, overcomes high surface tension forces, and prevents atelectasis, and thus enables improved oxygenation and a rise in Pao$_2$. Application of CPAP or PEEP produces same stabilization force on alveoli as grunting does and produces same effect—improved oxygenation and rise in Pao$_2$.
Maintenance of homeostasis Thermoregulation	See p. 499	Increase in respiratory rate results in chemical thermogenesis (burning brown fat to maintain body temperature), which increases O$_2$ needs and insensible H$_2$O loss in already compromised infant.
Correction of acid-base imbalance Respiratory acidosis	Maintain adequate ventilation and excretion of returned CO$_2$ from the lungs by monitoring blood gases and regulating ventilatory assistance mechanisms per physician's orders.	Correction of acidosis is essential to maintain homeostasis. Acidosis is powerful pulmonary vasoconstrictor, decreases pulmonary blood flow, and may upset surfactant synthesis. Acidosis dissociates bilirubin from albumin binding sites and predisposes to kernicterus at low bilirubin levels. Acidosis is a central nervous system depressant that depresses respiratory center, which causes increase in CO$_2$ retention and hypoxia.
Metabolic acidosis	Treat with volume replacement and cautious administration of bicarbonate (see Drug Guide—Sodium Bicarbonate).	
Provision for adequate fluid, caloric, and electrolyte requirements	Maintain IV rate at prescribed level; record type and amount of fluid infused hourly. Use infusion pump. Observe vital signs for signs of too rapid infusion. Maintain normal urine output (1–3 mL/kg/hr). Maintain specific gravity of urine between 1.006 and 1.012. Take daily weights. Manage route of IV administration.	Fluids are provided to sick neonate by intravenous route and are calculated to replace sensible and insensible water losses as well as evaporative losses due to tachypnea. Overload of circulatory system by too much or too rapid administration of fluid causes pulmonary edema and cardiac embarrassment that may be fatal.

NURSING CARE PLAN (continued)
Respiratory Distress Syndrome

Problem	Nursing interventions and actions	Rationale
	Peripheral IV in scalp or extremity vein: Prepare equipment, insert IV in vein, and restrain infant.	Greater nutritional fluid is required because of energy needed to cope with stress. Stressed infants are predisposed to hypoglycemia because of increased metabolic demands as well as reduced glycogen stores and decreased ability to convert fat and protein to glucose.
	Vessel chosen is artery if it pulsates. Place peripheral IV in vein (which doesn't pulsate).	Very small arteries may not pulsate and arterial area will blanch if saline is infused.
	Maintain proper placement of IV. Advance as soon as possible from intravenous to oral feedings. Gavage or nipple feedings are used with IV as supplement (discontinued when oral intake is sufficient) (see Procedure 22-1). Provide adequate caloric intake: amount of intake, type of formula, route of administration, and need for supplementation of intake by other routes. Plan care for minimal energy and oxygen needs. Take daily weight measurement. Blood pH remains normal (no metabolic acidosis). Measure urine output and specific gravity.	Ability to aspirate blood and/or easily inject small amount of saline indicates patent IV. Infiltration is evaluated by area of edema and redness about site, inability to obtain blood on aspiration, or difficulty in injecting through IV line. Calories are essential to prevent catabolism of body proteins and metabolic acidosis due to starvation or inadequate caloric intake.
	Observe for hypocalcemia. Observe for hypoglycemia: Dextrostix below 45 mg. Observe for hyperglycemia. Dextrostix above 130 mg, urine screening: increased urine output (osmotic diuresis), sugar in urine with Dipstix and Clinitest. Treatment—glucose is highest priority (calcium is next). Usually 10% calcium gluconate is administered.	Hypocalcemia and hypoglycemia result from delayed or inadequate caloric intake and stress.
Prevention of infection	See section on sepsis nursing care, p. 546.	Decreased lung expansion predisposed to atelectasis and secondary superimposed infections.
Provision of stimulatory needs of infant .	Plan care to allow for rest periods to avoid exhausting infant.	
Support of family	Explain procedures to family. Facilitate parental participation in infant's care even if critically ill.	(See p. 633 for a discussion of parenting high-risk infants.)

NURSING CARE EVALUATION

Oxygen therapy is discontinued and no apnea, cyanosis, or other complications are evident.
Infant is afebrile and vital signs are stable.
Infant is gaining weight or stabilized at desired discharge weight and tolerating food and fluids.
Parent-infant bonding is appropriate.

Parents understand need for continued medical supervision.
Parents are aware of available parent groups for assistance after discharge.
Referral is completed to public health nurse and other community resources.

NURSING CARE PLAN (continued)
Respiratory Distress Syndrome

NURSING DIAGNOSES*	SUPPORTING DATA	NURSING ORDERS
Alterations in oral mucous membranes due to drying of mucous membranes secondary to intubation	Dry mucous membrane Accumulation of secretions on lips Dry, cracked lips Irritation of skin surrounding mouth	1. Gently wipe mouth and lips with moistened 4-by-4 gauze q shift. 2. Apply Vaseline or A and D ointment to lips. Note: Do *not* use oil-based lubricant if the infant is under phototherapy because it may result in burns to the area. 3. Devise and maintain a method of securing the infant's intubation tube so that: a. The tube is secure. b. The type of materials used takes the infant's skin condition into consideration.

*These are a few examples of nursing diagnoses that may be appropriate for an infant. It is not an inclusive list and must be individualized for each newborn.

Usually little or no difficulty is experienced at the onset of breathing. In room air, cyanosis may be noted and ambient O_2 concentrations as high as 70% may be required to correct the condition. Unlike infants with RDS, whose oxygen requirements increase in the first 48 hours, Type 2 infants are easily oxygenated during the first 8 hours and their oxygen requirements may decrease during this time.

Initial x-ray films may be identical to those showing HMD within the first 3 hours. The infants should be improving by 24–48 hours, except for modest O_2 dependence (less than 30%).

The duration of the clinical course of transient tachypnea is approximately 4 days (96 hours). Early acidosis, both respiratory and metabolic (as evidenced by a Pco_2 less than 50 mm), is easily corrected. Ventilatory assistance is rarely needed, and most of these infants survive. If progressive deterioration occurs to the extent that assisted ventilation is required, a diagnosis of superimposed sepsis should be considered and treatment measures initiated. For nursing actions, see the Nursing Care Plan on respiratory distress syndrome, p. 524.

Meconium Aspiration Syndrome

The presence of meconium in amniotic fluid often indicates asphyxial insult to the neonate. The physiologic response to asphyxia is increased intestinal peristalsis, relaxation of the anal sphincter, and passage of meconium into the amniotic fluid. Prolonged labor is also associated with meconium aspiration syndrome (MAS). MAS is a respiratory distress condition, primarily of term, SGA, and postterm infants. As the victims of intrauterine asphyxia, meconium-stained neonates or newborns who have aspirated meconium are often depressed at birth and require resuscitative efforts to establish adequate respiratory effort.

Management at delivery   The combined efforts of the obstetrician and pediatrician are needed to prevent MAS. The most effective form of preventive management is outlined here:

1. After the head of the neonate is delivered and the shoulders and chest are still in the birth canal, the nasopharynx and oropharynx are suctioned with a DeLee catheter. (The same procedure is followed with a cesarean delivery.)

2. Immediately after delivery of the neonate, the vocal cords should be visualized with a laryngoscope. If meconium is present, intubation and direct suctioning of the trachea through an endotracheal tube is performed.

Failure to suction the infant adequately when he or she is on the perineum or before the infant's respiratory or resuscitative efforts are begun pushes meconium into the airway and into the lungs. Stimulation of the neonate is avoided to minimize respiratory movements.

DRUG GUIDE
Sodium bicarbonate

OVERVIEW OF NEONATAL ACTION

Sodium bicarbonate is an alkalizing agent. It buffers hydrogen ions caused by accumulation of lactic acid from anaerobic metabolism occurring during hypoxemia. Sodium bicarbonate thereby raises the blood pH, reversing the metabolic acidosis. Sodium bicarbonate should *only* be used to correct severe metabolic acidosis in asphyxiated newborns once adequate ventilation has been established (Avery, 1981).

Note: Sodium bicarbonate dissociates in solution into sodium ion and carbonic acid, which can split into water and carbon dioxide. The carbon dioxide must be eliminated via the respiratory tract.

ROUTE, DOSAGE, FREQUENCY

For resuscitation and severe asphyxiation: intravenous push via umbilical vein catheter for quick infusion. Dosage is 2 mEq/K: 4 mL of 0.5 mEq/mL (4.2%) or 2 mL of 1 mEq/mL (8.4%). 8.4% solution diluted at least 1:1 with sterile water to decrease the osmolarity; infuse at rate no faster than 1 mEq/kg/min (Avery, 1981). Complete infusion should be given over a minimum of 10–15 minutes. Can repeat every 15 minutes if needed for total of 4 doses. For marked metabolic acidosis: a pH of less than 7.05 and a base deficit of 15 mEq/L should be corrected by 0.5 mEq/mL of sodium bicarbonate at a rate of 1 mEq/kg/min or slower.

NEONATAL CONTRAINDICATIONS

Inadequate respiratory ventilation that causes a rise in Pco_2 and decrease in pH

Presence of edema, metabolic or respiratory alkalosis, and hypocalcemia, anuria, or oliguria

NEONATAL SIDE EFFECTS

Hypernatremia, hyperosmolarity, fluid overload

Intracranial hemorrhage (rapid infusion of bicarbonate increases serum osmolarity, causing a shift of interstitial fluid into the blood and capillary rupture)

NURSING CONSIDERATIONS

Assess for any contraindications
Monitor intake and output rates

Assess adequacy of ventilation by monitoring respiratory status, rate, and depth; ventilate as necessary

Dilute bicarbonate prior to administration into umbilical vein catheter (for resuscitation) or peripheral IV to prevent sloughing of tissue

Evaluate effectiveness of drug by monitoring arterial blood gases for Pco_2, bicarbonate concentration, and pH determination
Incompatible with acidic solutions
Administration with calcium creates precipitates

DRUG GUIDE
Naloxone hydrochloride (Narcan)

OVERVIEW OF NEONATAL ACTION

Naloxone hydrochloride (Narcan) is used to reverse respiratory depression due to acute narcotic toxicity. It displaces morphinelike drugs from receptor sites on the neurons; therefore, the narcotics can no longer exert their depressive effects. Naloxone reverses narcotic-induced respiratory depression, analgesia, sedation, hypotension, and pupillary constriction (Berkowitz et al., 1981).

ROUTE, DOSAGE, FREQUENCY

Intravenous dose is 0.01 mg/kg, usually through umbilical vein, although naloxone can be given intramuscularly. Neonatal dose is supplied as 0.02 mg/mL solution (0.5 mL– 1 mL for preterms and 2 mL for full-terms). Reversal of drug depression occurs within 1–2 minutes and will last 1–2 hours. Dose may be repeated in 5 minutes. If no improvement after two or three doses, naloxone administration should be discontinued (Cloherty and Stark, 1981). If initial reversal occurs, repeat dose at 1–2 hour intervals as needed.

NEONATAL CONTRAINDICATIONS

Must be used with caution in infants of narcotic-addicted mothers as it may precipitate acute withdrawal syndrome. Respiratory depression resulting from nonmorphine drugs such as sedatives, hypnotics, anesthetics, or other nonnarcotic CNS depressants.

NEONATAL SIDE EFFECTS

Excessive doses may result in irritability and increased crying, and possibly prolongation of partial thromboplastin (PTT) (Benitz and Tatro, 1981).
Tachycardia

NURSING CONSIDERATIONS

Monitor respirations closely—rate and depth

Assess for return of respiratory depression when naloxone effects wear off and effects of longer-acting narcotic reappear

Have resuscitative equipment, O_2, and ventilatory equipment available

Monitor bleeding studies.

Because of incompatibilities, avoid alkaline solutions.

Further resuscitative efforts as indicated follow the same principles mentioned earlier in this chapter.

Clinical manifestations   Clinical manifestations of MAS include: (a) fetal hypoxia in utero a few days or a few minutes prior to delivery, and meconium staining of amniotic fluid. Signs of distress are also present at delivery, including pallor, cyanosis, apnea, slow heartbeat, and low Apgar scores (below 6) at 1 and 5 minutes. The literature indicates that passage of meconium in breech presentation *or* vertex presentation suggests fetal distress.

Presence of meconium in the lungs produces a ball-valve action (air is allowed in but not exhaled), so that alveoli overdistend; rupture with pneumomediastinum or pneumothorax commonly occurs. The meconium also initiates a chemical pneumonitis with oxygen and carbon dioxide trapping and hyperinflation. Secondary bacterial pneumonias are common. The chest x-ray film shows coarse, patchy infiltrates and hyperinflation. These infants have massive biochemical alterations, which include: (a) extreme metabolic acidosis resulting from the cardiopulmonary shunting and hypoperfusion; (b) extreme respiratory acidosis due to shunting and alveolar hypoventilation; and (c) extreme hypoxia, even in 100% O_2 concentrations and with ventilatory assistance. The extreme hypoxia is also caused by the cardiopulmonary shunting and resultant failure to oxygenate.

The infant may be depressed and have tachypnea at birth or show no respiratory distress for several hours. Symptoms of respiratory distress, when they appear, are usually severe. Infants have tachypnea, cyanosis, hyperexpanded chest, congestive heart failure (CHF), and irregular and gasping respirations (usually subsiding in 48 hours, although they may persist for 6–7 days).

Management in the nursery   Resuscitated neonates should be immediately transferred to the nursery for close observation and continuation of treatment. Treatment usually involves high ambient oxygenation, controlled ventilation, and antibiotic therapy. Treatment also includes chest physiotherapy (chest percussion, vibration, and postural drainage) to remove the debris. Mortality in term or postterm infants is very high because they are so difficult to oxygenate.

Nursing interventions after resuscitation should include temperature regulation at 37C, Dextrostix at 2 hours of age to check for hypoglycemia, observation of intravenous fluids, calculation of necessary fluids (which may be restricted in first 48–72 hours due to cerebral edema), and provision of caloric requirements.

Cold Stress

Cold stress is excessive heat loss resulting in compensatory mechanisms (increased respirations and nonshivering thermogenesis) to maintain core body temperature. Heat loss that results in cold stress occurs in the newborn through the mechanisms of evaporation, convection, conduction, and radiation. (See Chapter 19 for a detailed discussion on thermoregulation.) Heat loss at the time of delivery that leads to cold stress can play a significant role in the severity of RDS and the ultimate outcome of the infant.

The amount of heat loss to the environment by an infant depends to a large extent on the actions of the nurse or caretaker.

Both preterm and SGA infants are at risk for cold stress because they have decreased adipose tissue, brown fat stores, and glycogen available for metabolism.

As discussed in Chapter 19 the newborn infant's major source of heat production in nonshivering thermogenesis (NST) is brown fat metabolism. The ability of an infant to respond to cold stress by NST is impaired in the presence of hypoxemia, intracranial hemorrhage or any CNS abnormality, and hypoglycemia.

The metabolic consequences of cold stress can be devastating and potentially fatal to an infant. Oxygen requirements are raised, glucose use increases, and surfactant production decreases. The effects are graphically depicted in Figure 22-15.

Interventions   If cold stress occurs, the following nursing interventions are initiated:

1. The neonate is warmed slowly as rapid temperature elevation may cause apnea.

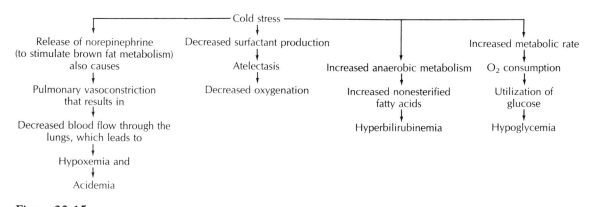

Figure 22-15
Cold stress schematic.

2. Skin temperature is observed every 15 minutes. Skin temperature assessments are used because initial response to cold stress is vasoconstriction resulting in a decrease in skin temperature.

3. The presence of hypoglycemia, which results from the metabolic effects of cold stress is assessed. Hypoglycemia is suggested by Dextrostix values below 45 mg/mL, tremors, irritability or lethargy, apnea, or seizure activity. See discussion of hypoglycemia.

4. The presence of anaerobic metabolism is assessed and interventions initiated for the resulting metabolic acidosis. Attempts to burn brown fat increase oxygen consumption, lactic acid levels, and metabolic acidosis.

Prolonged cold stress can deplete brown fat stores, interfere with normal temperature control, and result in infant death. Prevention is of the utmost importance and is achieved by careful temperature monitoring and maintenance of a neutral thermal environment.

Hypoglycemia

Hypoglycemia is the most common metabolic disorder occurring in LGA, SGA, and preterm AGA infants. The pathophysiology of hypoglycemia differs for each classification.

AGA preterm infants have not been in utero a sufficient time to store glycogen and fat. Therefore, they have very low glycogen and fat stores and a decreased ability to carry out gluconeogenesis (Fantazia, 1984). This situation is further aggravated by increased use of glucose by the tissues (especially the brain and heart) during stress and illness (chilling, asphyxia, sepsis, and RDS).

LGA infants, on the other hand, are often IGDMs or IDMs. These infants have increased stores of glycogen and fat. However, circulating insulin and insulin responsiveness are higher compared with other newborns. Because of the cessation of high in utero glucose loads at birth, the neonate experiences rapid and profound hypoglycemia.

SGA infants have used up their glycogen and fat stores because of intrauterine malnutrition. In addition, they have a weakened hepatic enzymatic response with which to carry out formation of glycogen from noncarbohydrate sources (gluconeogenesis).

Hypoglycemia in an infant is defined as a blood glucose below 30 mg/dL whole blood (below 35 mg in plasma or serum) in the first 3 days of life and below 40 mg/dL after the first 3 days. It may also be defined as a Dextrostix result below 45 mg/dL when corroborated with laboratory blood glucose value (Procedure 22-2).

No clinical symptoms or some or all of the following may occur:

- Lethargy, irritability
- Poor feeding
- Vomiting
- Pallor
- Apnea, irregular respirations, respiratory distress
- Hypotonia, possible loss of swallowing reflex
- Tremors, jerkiness, seizure activity
- High-pitched cry

PROCEDURE 22-2
Dextrostix

Objective	Nursing action	Rationale
Ensure quick, efficient completion of procedure	Gather the following equipment: 1. Lancet (do not use needles). 2. Alcohol swabs. 3. 2 × 2 sterile gauze squares. 4. Small Band-Aid. 5. Dextrostix and bottle.	All necessary equipment must be ready to ensure that blood sample is collected at time and in manner necessary. Do not use needles because of danger of nicking periosteum. Warm heel for 5–10 sec prior to heel stick with a warm wet towel to facilitate flow of blood.
	Select clear, previously unpunctured site. Cleanse site by rubbing vigorously with 70% isopropyl alcohol swab, followed by dry gauze square. Grasp lower leg and heel so as to impede venous return slightly.	Selection of previously unpunctured site minimizes risk of infection and excessive scar formation. Friction produces local heat, which aids vasodilatation. Impeding venous return facilitates extraction of blood sample from puncture site.
Minimize trauma at puncture site	Dry site completely before lancing.	Alcohol is irritating to injured tissue and may also produce hemolysis.
	With quick piercing motion, puncture lateral heel with blade, being careful not to puncture too deeply. Avoid the darkened areas in Figure 22-16. Toes are acceptable sites if necessary.	Lateral heel is site of choice because it precludes damaging posterior tibial nerve and artery, plantar artery, and important longitudinally oriented fat pad of the heel, which in later years could impede walking. This is especially important for infant undergoing multiple Dextrostix procedures. Optimal penetration is 4 mm.

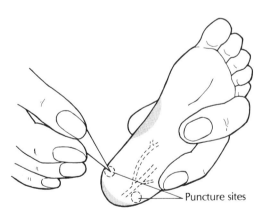

Figure 22-16
Dextrostix (heel prick).

Ensure accurate blood sampling	After puncture has been made, remove first drop of blood with sterile gauze square and proceed to collect subsequent drops of blood onto Dextrostix, ensuring that it is a stand-up drop of blood on Dextrostix (Figure 22-17).	First drop is usually discarded because it tends to be minutely diluted with tissue fluid from puncture.

Continued.

PROCEDURE 22-2 (continued)
Dextrostix

Objective	Nursing action	Rationale

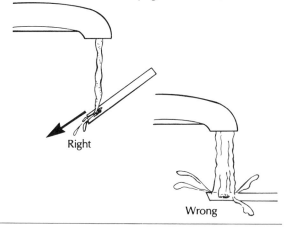

Figure 22-17
Dextrostix test strip.

	Wait one minute (apply Band-Aid while waiting), then rinse blood gently from stick under a steady stream of running water (Figure 22-18). Compare immediately against color chart on side of bottle.	For accurate results, directions must be followed closely, and reagent strips must be fresh. False low readings may be caused by:
		1. Timing.
	Record results on vital signs sheet or on back of graph. Report immediately any findings under 45 mg/dL or over 175 mg/dL.	2. Washing (chemical reaction can be washed off).
		3. Squeezing foot, causing tissue fluid dilution.
Prevent excessive bleeding	Apply folded gauze square to puncture site and secure firmly with bandage.	A pressure dressing should be applied to puncture site to stop bleeding.
	Check puncture site frequently for first hour after sample	Active infants sometimes kick or rub their dressings off and can bleed profusely from puncture site, especially if bandage becomes moist or is rubbed excessively against crib sheet.

Figure 22-18
Dextrostix test strip rinse.

Because the above clinical symptoms are also found in other complications of the newborn, such as sepsis, polycythemia, and hypocalcemia, identification of hypoglycemia is difficult.

Interventions Nursing interventions are based on knowledge of those at risk, observa-tion for symptoms, and screening for asymp-tomatic occurrence. Dextrostix, urine Dipstix (glucose), and urine volume (above 1–3 mL/kg/hr) are evaluated for osmotic diuresis and glycosuria.

Providing adequate caloric intake is impor-tant. Early formula feeding is a major preventative approach. If early feedings or intravenous glucose is started to meet the recommended fluid and caloric needs, the blood glucose is likely to remain above the hypoglycemic level.

When caring for a preterm AGA infant, blood glucose levels should be monitored using heel stick or laboratory determinations every 4–8 hours for the first day of life, and daily or as necessary thereafter. Intravenous infusions of a dextrose solution (5%–10%) begun immediately after birth should prevent hypoglycemia. However, in the very small AGA infant, infusions of 5%–10% dextrose solution may cause hyperglycemia to develop, requiring an alteration in the glucose concentration. Therefore, an intravenous glucose solution should be calculated based on body weight of the infant. Blood glucose determinations are performed to determine adequacy of the infusion treatment.

The LGA infant should be monitored hourly for the first several hours after birth as this is the time when dramatic falls in glucose are most likely. If immediate oral feedings containing glucose are not possible, intravenous dextrose should be administered until serum glucose levels have stabilized and the infant is able to take adequate amounts of formula or breast milk to maintain a normal blood sugar level. A rapid infusion of 25%–50% dextrose should not be used because it may lead to severe rebound hypoglycemia following an initial brief increase.

Hypoglycemia resulting from hyperinsulinemia may be helped by administration of long-acting epinephrine. Like glucagon, epinephrine promotes glycogen conversion to glucose; it is also an antiinsulin agent.

In the SGA infant, symptoms usually appear between 24 and 72 hours of age; occasionally they may begin as early as 3 hours of age. Infants who are below the tenth percentile on the intrauterine growth curve should have blood sugar assessments at least every 12 hours for 24 hours and every 8 hours until 4 days of age. Treatment is similar to that for preterm AGA infants.

In more severe cases of hypoglycemia, corticosteroids may be administered. It is thought that steroids enhance gluconeogenesis from noncarbohydrate protein sources (Avery, 1981).

The prognosis for untreated hypoglycemia is poor. It may result in permanent, nontreatable CNS damage or death.

Hypocalcemia

Calcium is transported across the placenta in increasing amounts during the third trimester of pregnancy. This predisposes the infant who is born preterm to have lower serum calcium levels in the neonatal period. This risk is increased in the presence of perinatal asphyxia, trauma, and hypotonia and with the use of bicarbonate in treating acidosis. IDMs and infants of mothers with hyperparathyroidism are also at higher risk for hypocalcemia. Hypocalcemia is a common occurrence in the intrapartally asphyxiated neonate in the first 2–3 days of life due to a delay in oral feedings, which results in less intestinal absorption of calcium. Hypocalcemia is also associated with the practice of administering low-calcium or calcium-free intravenous therapy management.

The symptoms of hypocalcemia are nonspecific and are seen in conjunction with other disorders. The signs and symptoms that may be observed are:

- Apnea
- Cyanotic episodes
- High-pitched cry
- Twitching, jitteriness
- Seizures (local or generalized)
- Abdominal distention
- Edema

Diagnosis and treatment Serum calcium levels should be monitored frequently in the at-risk neonate during the first few days of life. Normal serum calcium levels range from 8.0–10.5 mg/dL. Hypocalcemia refers to serum calcium levels less than 7 mg/dL.

Maintenance calcium (calcium chloride or calcium gluconate) will be given either parenterally or orally. High level of calcium chloride can cause gastric mucosal irritation and vomiting. Low-phosphorus milk may be used in the treatment of asymptomatic hypocalcemia.

Treatment for hypocalcemia is usually necessary for only 4 or 5 days unless other complications exist. Calcium levels should be monitored every 12–24 hours, tapering off gradually. By 1 week of age, normal calcium levels are maintained while receiving regular formula or breast milk without supplements.

Neonatal Jaundice _____

The most common abnormal physical finding in neonates is *jaundice* (icterus). Jaundice develops from deposit of the yellow pigment, *bilirubin*, in lipid tissues. Unconjugated bilirubin is a break-down product derived primarily from hemoglobin that is released from lysed red blood cells and heme pigments found in cell elements (nonerythrocyte bilirubin).

Fetal unconjugated bilirubin is normally cleared by the placenta in utero, so total bilirubin at birth is usually less that 3 mg/dL unless an abnormal hemolytic process has been present. Postnatally, the infant must conjugate bilirubin in the liver, producing a rise in serum bilirubin in the first few days of life. The bilirubin level at which an infant is harmed varies and depends on a number of factors; furthermore, many conditions can cause a more rapid rise in bilirubin and have the potential to produce permanent neurologic defects and even death.

Mechanism of Bilirubin Conjugation

Unconjugated bilirubin is normally transported in the plasma firmly bound to albumin, which makes it water soluble. Bilirubin not bound to albumin can cross the blood-brain barrier and damage the cells of the CNS and produce kernicterus.

Unconjugated albumin-bound bilirubin is taken up by the liver cells. The clearance and conjugation of bilirubin depends on the enzyme glucuronyl transferase system, which results in the attachment of unconjugated bilirubin to glucuronic acid (product of liver glycogen), producing conjugated bilirubin. It is excreted into the tiny bile ducts, then into the common duct and duodenum. It then progresses down the intestines, where bacteria transform it into urobilinogen, which is not reabsorbed and is excreted as a yellow-brown pigment in the stools.

When the amount of bilirubin in the vascular system overwhelms the clearing capabilities of the liver, jaundice develops. Conjugated bilirubin is cleared from the body after it is processed in the liver, excreted into the bile,

and eliminated with the feces. Unconjugated bilirubin is not in excretable form and is a potential toxin. Total serum bilirubin is the sum of conjugated and unconjugated bilirubin.

The rate and amount of conjugation depends on the rate of red blood cell destruction, on the maturity of the liver, and on albumin-binding sites. A normal, healthy, full-term infant's liver is usually sufficiently mature and is producing enough glucuronyl transferase so that total serum bilirubin levels do not reach pathologic levels (above 12 mg/dL blood). Elevation of bilirubin level may result from polycythemia (twin-to-twin transfusion, large placental transfer of blood), enclosed hemorrhage (cephalhematoma, bleeding into internal organs, ecchymoses), increased hemolysis (sepsis, hemolytic disease of the newborn), or an excessive dose of vitamin K.

Serum albumin-binding sites are usually sufficient to meet the usual demands. Certain conditions, such as fetal or neonatal asphyxia, hypothermia, and hypoglycemia, tend to decrease the sites available. Maternal use of sulfa drugs or salicylates interferes with conjugation or interferes with serum albumin-binding sites by competing with bilirubin for these binding sites.

The liver of the newborn infant, particularly that of the preterm infant, has relatively less glucuronyl transferase activity at birth and in the first few weeks of life than the adult. Some feel a substance in breast milk can inhibit bilirubin conjugation. A number of bacterial and viral infections (cytomegalic inclusion disease, toxoplasmosis, herpes, syphilis) can also affect the liver and produce jaundice.

Even after the bilirubin has been conjugated and bound, it can be converted back to unconjugated bilirubin by the enterohepatic process. This reconversion is prevalent in the newborn and particularly in preterm infants, who have very high β-glucuronidase activity levels, which deconjugate bilirubin; as well as delayed bacterial colonization of the gut.

Hyperbilirubinemia

Hyperbilirubinemia (increased serum bilirubin levels) of any origin must be considered pathologic if the following occur:

1. Serum bilirubin levels exceeding 6mg/dL within the first 24 hours or persisting beyond 7 days in the full-term infant and 10 days in the preterm infant

2. Serum bilirubin levels rising by more than 5 mg/dL a day or exceeding 12mg/dL in either full-term or preterm neonate

3. If conjugated (direct) bilirubin greater than 1.5–2.0 mg/dL

During pregnancy, women can be checked for conditions that may predispose to neonatal hyperbilirubinemia: hereditary spherocytosis, diabetes, intrauterine infections (TORCH) that stimulate production of maternal isoimmune antibodies, and drug ingestion (sulfas, salicylates, novobiocin, diazepam, oxytocin). The woman who is Rh-negative or who has blood type O should be asked about outcomes of any previous pregnancies and her history of blood transfusion. Prenatal amniocentesis with spectrophotographic examination may be indicated in some cases. Cord blood from neonates is evaluated for bilirubin level, which should not exceed 5 mg/dL. Neonates of these mothers are carefully assessed for appearance of jaundice and levels of serum bilirubin.

Some neonatal conditions predispose to hyperbilirubinemia: polycythemia (central hematocrit 65% or more), obstruction of GI tract, enclosed hemorrhage (cephalhematoma, large bruises), asphyxia neonatorum, hypothermia, acidemia, hypoglycemia. Hepatitis from intrauterine infections or metabolic liver disease elevates the level of conjugated bilirubin.

High serum bilirubin levels (hyperbilirubinemia), especially bilirubin in the unconjugated state, are dangerous to the neonate. The more premature the neonate the more susceptible to tissue damage. Since the cerebral cortex and thalamus are the last to be myelinated, the nuclei of these cells are more susceptible to being infiltrated by the unconjugated bilirubin, with subsequent brain damage.

The goal of the management of hyperbilirubinemia regardless of cause is to treat anemia if present, remove maternal antibodies and sensitized erythrocytes, increase serum albumin levels, and reduce the levels of serum bilirubin.

Methods include phototherapy, exchange transfusion, infusion of albumin, and drug therapy. (These treatment techniques are discussed on p. 539.)

Nursing Management

Primary nursing priorities are to identify factors that predispose to development of jaundice and to identify jaundice as soon as it is apparent. If jaundice appears, careful observation of the increase in depth of color and of the infant's behavior is mandatory. Should the infant require phototherapy (discussed on p. 541), the nurse provides the necessary care. The nurse assists with the exchange transfusion and observes the infant carefully after the procedure. The nurse working with the mother assists the parents in coping with the situation.

As the first step in identifying impending jaundice, the nurse reviews each neonate's prenatal and perinatal history for factors that predispose to hyperbilirubinemia. The neonate's blood type, Rh, and Coombs' test results (if done) are noted. The nurse assesses each neonate for gestational age and for cephalhematoma, and notes whether the infant is breast-fed or bottle-fed.

In the presence of one or more predisposing factors, laboratory determination should be made of serum bilirubin levels (direct, indirect, and total), serum albumin levels, and tests of bilirubin binding, if available. In addition, the nurse checks the neonate for jaundice about every 2 hours and records observations.

To check for jaundice, the nurse should blanch the skin over a bony prominence (forehead, sternum) by pressing firmly with the thumb. After pressure is released, if jaundice is present, the area appears yellow before normal color returns. The nurse should check oral mucosa and the posterior portion of the hard palate and conjunctival sacs for yellow pigmentation in darker-skinned neonates, because the underlying pigment of normal dark-skinned people can appear yellow. Assessment in daylight gives best results; pink walls and surroundings may mask yellowish tints; yellow colors make differentiation of jaundice difficult. The time of onset of jaundice is recorded and reported.

Kernicterus Unbound (unconjugated) bilirubin, although not soluble in body fluids, is capable of crossing cell membranes. **Kernicterus** (meaning "yellow nucleus") refers to the deposition of unconjugated bilirubin in the basal ganglia of the brain and to the symptoms of neurologic damage that follow untreated hyperbilirubinemia. Kernicterus (bilirubin encephalopathy) is most commonly found with blood-group incompatibility.

Kernicterus is associated with serum unconjugated bilirubin levels of over 20 mg/dL in normal term infants; safe levels for preterm infants or sick infants are lower and vary considerably. Sick preterm infants may develop kernicterus with unconjugated bilirubin levels as low as 10 mg/dL.

Determination of the (unbound) unconjugated portion of the total serum bilirubin is the most significant assessment of the potential for kernicterus. The neonate's behavior is assessed for neurologic signs of kernicterus, especially between days 3 and 10. Kernicterus never appears before 36 hours of age, even in severe cases of hemolytic disease. Clinical manifestations may range from diminished or absent Moro reflex, hypotonia, and lethargy to seizures, high pitched cry, and mental retardation.

Hemolytic Disease of the Newborn

Isoimmune hemolytic disease, also known as **erythroblastosis fetalis**, occurs after a maternal antibody that predisposes fetal and neonatal red blood cells to early destruction crosses the placenta. Jaundice, anemia, and compensatory erythropoiesis result and immature red blood cells—erythroblasts—are found in large numbers in the blood; hence the designation erythroblastosis fetalis.

Although there are more than 60 known red blood cell antigens, clinically significant hemolytic disease is associated with maternal–fetal incompatibility associated with the D factor in the Rh group and with the ABO blood types. The Rh incompatibility system is more complex.

Rh Incompatibility

Those whose red blood cells contain the Rh factor (antigen) are said to be positive; those who do not are negative. Isoimmunization occurs when an Rh-negative woman carries an Rh-positive (who has the Rh factor or antigen) fetus. When fetal Rh-positive antigens (an antigenic substance on the surface of the fetal red blood cell) leak in minute amounts into maternal circulation, maternal antibodies are produced, creating a sensitization reaction.

The leakage of fetal Rh antigens into the maternal circulation most commonly occurs at the time of delivery. Other obstetric factors known to increase the likelihood of maternal Rh sensitization are PIH, amniocentesis, version procedure, cesarean delivery, breech deliveries, abortion, abruptio placentae, and manual removal of the placenta (see Chapters 10 and 18). In subsequent pregnancies the maternal antibodies cross the placenta and cause immediate or delayed destruction (hemolysis) of the fetal red blood cells.

Hydrops fetalis, the most severe form of erythroblastosis fetalis, results when maternal antibodies attach to the Rh antigen of the fetal red blood cells, making them susceptible to destruction. The fetal system responds by increased erythropoiesis. Rapid and early destruction of erythrocytes results in a marked increase of immature red blood cells—erythroblasts—which do not have the functional capabilities of mature cells. If the anemia is severe, as seen in hydrops fetalis, cardiomegaly with severe cardiac decompensation and hepatosplenomegaly occur. Jaundice is not present until later because the bili pigments are being excreted through the placenta into the maternal circulation.

Severe anemia is also responsible for hemorrhage in lungs and other tissues. The hydropic hemolytic disease process also causes hyperplasia of the pancreatic islets, which predisposes the infant to neonatal hypoglycemia similar to that of IDMs. These infants also have increased bleeding tendencies due to associated thrombocytopenia and hypoxic damage to the capillaries. Hydrops is a frequent cause of intrauterine death among infants with Rh disease.

Laboratory data   If the hemolytic process is due to Rh sensitization, laboratory findings reveal the following:

- An Rh-positive neonate with a positive direct Coomb's test

- Increased erythropoiesis with many immature circulating red blood cells (nucleated blastocysts)
- Anemia, in most cases
- Elevated levels (5 mg/dL or more) of bilirubin in cord blood

Maternal data may include an elevated anti-Rh titer and spectrophotometric evidence of fetal hemolytic process. (See Chapter 10.)

ABO Incompatibility

ABO incompatibility, occurring in 20% of pregnancies, rarely results in hemolytic disease severe enough to be clinically diagnosed and treated. ABO incompatibility occurs when the woman carries a fetus with a blood type different from her own.

Anti-A and anti-B antibodies are naturally occurring; that is, women are naturally exposed to the A and B antigens through the foods they eat and through exposure to infection by gram negative bacteria. As a result, some women have high serum anti-A and anti-B titers before they become pregnant. Once the woman becomes pregnant, the maternal serum anti-A and anti-B antibodies cross the placenta and produce hemolysis of the fetal red blood cells. With ABO incompatibility the first infant is frequently involved. No relationship exists between the appearance of the disease and repeated sensitization from one pregnancy to the next.

The most common incompatibility occurs when the mother is type O (anti-A and anti-B antibodies) and the fetus is type A or B. A group B fetus of an A mother and a group A fetus of a B mother are only occasionally affected. Group O infants, because they have no antigenic sites on the red blood cells, are never affected regardless of the mother's blood type. The incompatibility occurs as a result of the maternal antibodies present in her serum and the interaction with the antigen sites on the fetal red blood cells.

Clinically, ABO incompatibility presents as jaundice and occasionally hepatosplenomegaly. Hydrops and stillbirth are rare.

Laboratory data   An increase in reticulocytes indicates the presence of a hemolytic process, but the resulting anemia is not significant during the neonatal period and is rare later on.

The direct Coombs' test may be negative or mildly positive, while the indirect Coombs' test may be strongly positive. Infants with a direct Coombs' positive test have increased incidence of jaundice with bilirubin levels in excess of 10 mg/dL. Increased numbers of spherocytes (spherical, plump, mature erythrocytes) are seen on a peripheral blood smear. Increased numbers of spherocytes are not seen on smears from Rh disease infants.

Neonatal Assessment

Hemolytic disease of the newborn is suspected if the placenta is enlarged (placental weight is usually only one-seventh of fetal weight), the neonate is edematous with pleural and pericardial effusion plus ascites, pallor or jaundice is noted during the first 24–36 hours, hemolytic anemia is diagnosed, or the spleen and liver are enlarged. Changes in the neonate's behavior or bleeding tendencies must be carefully assessed to determine the cause. Neonates who have received large doses of vitamin K or sulfonamides may have increased incidence of hyperbilirubinemia because these agents reduce the number of available bilirubin binding sites by competing for them.

Hyperbilirubinemia Treatment and Nursing Responsibilities

The management of the neonate is directed toward preventing anemia and hyperbilirubinemia (Figure 22-19). Exchange transfusion, phototherapy, and drug therapy are used. When determining the appropriate management of hyperbilirubinemia (exchange transfusion or phototherapy), three variables are considered: the serum bilirubin level; the neonate's birth weight; and the neonate's age in hours. If a neonate has hemolysis with an unconjugated bilirubin level of 14 mg/dL, weighs less than 2500 g (birth weight), and is 24 or less hours old, an exchange transfusion may be the best management. However, if that same neonate is over 24 hours of age, phototherapy is adequate to prevent the possible complication of kernicterus. It is generally accepted that if the neonate is preterm or at risk, phototherapy should be instituted when a bilirubin level is 10 mg/dL. Any neonate with a bilirubin level of 20 mg/dL or

Serum bilirubin mg/dL	Birth weight	<24 hrs.	24-48 hrs	49-72 hrs	> 72 hrs
<5	All				
5-9	All	Phototherapy if hemolysis			
10-14	<2500 g	Exchange if hemolysis	Phototherapy		
10-14	>2500 g	Exchange if hemolysis		Investigate bilirubin > 12 mg	
15-19	<2500 g	Exchange			Consider exchange
15-19	>2500 g	Exchange			Phototherapy
20 and +	All	Exchange			

☐ Observe   ▨ Investigate jaundice

Figure 22-19

Therapy for isoimmune hemolytic disease in the neonate. Phototherapy is used after any exchange transfusion. If the following conditions are present, treat the neonate as if in the next higher bilirubin category: perinatal asphyxia, respiratory distress, metabolic acidosis (pH 7.25 or below), hypothermia (temperature below 35C), low serum protein (5 g/dL or less), birth weight less than 1500 g, or signs of clinical or CNS deterioration. (From Avery GB: *Neonatology*, 2nd ed. Philadelphia: Lippincott, 1981, p. 511.)

above should have an exchange transfusion regardless of weight or age.

Exchange transfusion   Exchange transfusion is the withdrawal and replacement of the neonate's blood with donor blood. Early or immediate exchange transfusion is indicated in the presence of the following conditions:

- Anti-Rh titer of greater than 1:16 in the mother (see Chapter 10)
- Severe hemolytic disease in a previous newborn
- Clinical hemolytic disease of the newborn at birth or within the first 24 hours
- Positive direct Coomb's test
- Cord serum levels of conjugated (direct) bilirubin greater than 3.5 mg/dL in the first week
- Serum unconjugated bilirubin levels greater than 2.0 mg/dL in the first 48 hours
- Hemoglobin less than 12 g/dL or infants with hydrops at birth

Infants who are at greater risk for developing kernicterus receive an exchange transfusion at lower serum bilirubin levels.

Exchange transfusion is used to treat anemia with red blood cells that are not susceptible to maternal antibodies, remove sensitized red blood cells that would be lysed soon, remove serum bilirubin, and provide bilirubin-free albumin and increase the binding sites for bilirubin. In Rh incompatibility, fresh (under 2 days old) group O, Rh-negative whole blood, or packed red blood cells, is chosen. This type of blood contains no A or B antigens or Rh antigens; therefore the maternal antibodies still present in the neonate's blood will not cause hemolysis of the transfused blood. Packed cells are used if the infant is anemic. CPD (citrate-phosphate-dextrose) blood is preferred because it presents less of an acid load to the infant.

In case of ABO incompatibility, group O with Rh-specific cells and low titers of anti-A and anti-B donor blood is used, not the infant's blood type, since donor blood contains no antigens to further stimulate maternal antibodies.

Every 4–8 hours after the transfusion, bilirubin determinations are made. Repeat exchange may be necessary if the serum bilirubin level rises at a rate of 0.5–1.0 mg/dL/hr (Avery, 1981) or if the bilirubin level exceeds 20 mg/

dL. Daily hemoglobin estimates should be obtained until stable, and hemoglobin determinations every 2 weeks for 2 months are valuable.

Nursing interventions The nurse's responsibilities during an exchange transfusion are to:

• Assemble equipment (the necessary equipment varies with the hospital).

• Keep the neonate warm (under a radiant warmer) and NPO. Closely monitor vital signs during the procedure.

• Assist the physician during the procedure.

• Maintain a careful record of all events.

• Observe the neonate after the procedure for complications such as hypoglycemia and hypocalcemia from the transfusion.

• Observe for clinical signs of hyperbilirubinemia and neurologic damage.

Phototherapy Phototherapy may be used alone or in conjunction with exchange transfusion to reduce serum bilirubin levels. Exposure of the neonate to high-intensity light (a bank of fluorescent light bulbs or bulbs in the blue-light spectrum) decreases serum bili-

rubin levels in the skin. Unbound (unconjugated) bilirubin is thought to be photo-oxidized into nontoxic compounds that are excreted in the urine and feces (via bile). The newborn's entire skin area is exposed to the light. Phototherapy success is measured every 12 hours or with daily serum bilirubin levels. The lights must be turned off while drawing the serum bilirubin levels. Phototherapy plays an important role in preventing a rise in bilirubin levels but does not alter the underlying cause of jaundice, and hemolysis may continue and produce anemia (Blake, 1983).

Nursing interventions Because it is not known whether this light injures the delicate eye structures, particularly the retina, the nurse should apply eye patches over the neonate's closed eyes while the infant is receiving phototherapy (Figure 22-20). Phototherapy is discontinued, and the eye patches are removed at least once per shift to assess the eyes for the presence of conjunctivitis. Patches are also removed to allow eye contact during feeding (social stimulation) or when parents are visiting (parental attachment). Minimal covering is applied over the genitals and buttocks to expose maximum skin surface and to protect bedding.

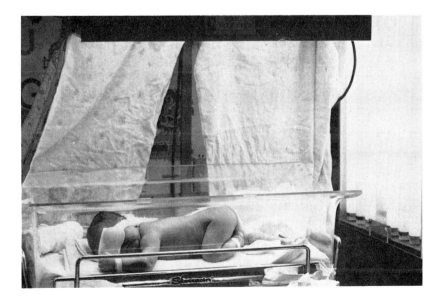

Figure 22-20 ▬▬▬▬▬▬▬

Infant receiving phototherapy. The phototherapy light is positioned over the Isolette. The infant is undressed to expose as much skin as possible. Bilateral eye patches are always used during phototherapy.

The neonate's temperature is monitored to prevent hyperthermia or hypothermia. The lights should be 18 inches above the neonate. The neonate will require additional fluids to compensate for the increased water loss through the skin and loose stools. Stools and urine are evaluated for green color and amount. Loose green stools are often seen with phototherapy, and skin care is essential.

Bronzing of the skin may occur, lasting about 3 weeks after therapy is discontinued, but with no long-term sequelae if the neonate has a healthy liver. "Tanning" or deeper pigmentation of Black infants has been reported during light exposure. As a side effect of phototherapy, some newborns develop a maculopapular rash.

In addition to assessing the neonate's skin color for jaundice and bronzing, the nurse examines the skin for developing pressure areas. The neonate should be repositioned at least every 2 hours to permit the light to reach all skin surfaces, to prevent pressure areas, and to vary the stimulation to the infant. The nurse keeps track of the number of hours each lamp is used so that lamps can be replaced before their effectiveness is lost.

Support of the Family

Many parents must face the mother's discharge while the neonate remains in the hospital for treatment of hyperbilirubinemia. The terms *jaundice*, *hyperbilirubinemia*, *exchange transfusion*, and *phototherapy* may sound frightening and threatening. Some parents may feel guilty that they have caused this situation to happen. The nurse must expect that the parents will need explanations repeated and clarified and that they may need help voicing their questions and fears. Early eye and tactile contact with the neonate is encouraged and planned so that the nurse can be present while the parents visit the neonate. Parents are kept informed of their infant's condition and are encouraged to return to the hospital or telephone at any time and to be involved in the care of their infant.

Neonatal Anemia

Neonatal anemia is often difficult to recognize by clinical evaluation alone. Normal hemoglobin in a full-term neonate is about 17 g/dL; infants with hemoglobin of less than 14 g/dL are usually considered anemic. The most common causes of neonatal anemia are blood loss, hemolysis, and impaired red blood cell production.

Blood loss (hypovolemia) occurs in utero from placental bleeding (placenta previa or abruptio placentae). Intrapartal blood loss may be twin-to-twin or the result of umbilical cord bleeding. Excessive hemolysis of red cells is usually a result of blood group incompatibilities but may be due to bacterial and nonbacterial infections. The most common cause of impaired red cell production is a deficiency in G-6-PD, which is genetically transmitted. Anemia and jaundice are the presenting signs.

A condition known as *physiologic anemia* exists as a result of the normal gradual drop in hemoglobin for the first 6–12 weeks of life. It is related to shorter neonatal red blood cell survival, reduced bone marrow activity, and the dilutional effect of expanded plasma on red blood cells.

Clinical manifestations and diagnosis Clinically, anemic infants are very pale in the absence of other symptoms of shock and usually are found to have abnormally low red blood cell counts. In acute blood loss, symptoms of shock may be present, such as pallor, low arterial blood pressure, and a decreasing hematocrit value. The initial laboratory workup should include hemoglobin and hematocrit measurements, reticulocyte count, examination of peripheral blood smear, bilirubin determinations, direct Coombs' test of infant's blood, and examination of maternal blood smear for fetal erythrocytes (Kleihauer–Betke test).

Management Hematologic problems can be anticipated based on the obstetric history and clinical manifestations. The age at which anemia is first noted is also of diagnostic value. Management depends on severity and whether blood loss is acute or chronic.

The infant should be placed on constant cardiac and respiratory monitoring. Mild or slow chronic anemia may be treated adequately with iron supplements alone or with iron-fortified formulas. Frequent determinations of hemoglobin, hematocrit, and bilirubin levels (in hemolytic disease) are essential. In severe cases of anemia, transfusions are the treatment of choice.

Nursing interventions   The nurse must be aware of and promptly report any symptoms and should assist in obtaining blood specimens and taking care of puncture sites. The amount of blood drawn for all laboratory tests is recorded so that total blood removed can be assessed and blood can be replaced by transfusion when necessary. Prophylactic measures carried out by the nurse include meticulous hand-washing and careful equipment cleaning to help prevent sepsis and subsequent hemolysis.

Polycythemia

Polycythemia is a condition in which blood volume and hematocrit values are increased. It is observed more commonly in SGA and full-term infants than in preterm neonates. An infant is considered polycythemic when the central venous hematocrit value is greater than 65%–70%, or the venous hemoglobin level is greater than 22 g/dL during the first week of life (Avery, 1981).

Several conditions predispose the neonate to polycythemia.

1. At the time of birth an excessive volume of placental blood may transfuse into the infant before the cord is cut, resulting in a blood volume increase.

2. During gestation an increased amount of blood may cross the placenta to the infant (maternofetal transfusion), resulting in increased blood volume after birth.

3. A twin-to-twin transfusion may occur, in which one twin receives less blood and becomes anemic, and the other twin receives an excess amount of blood resulting in polycythemia.

4. Increased red blood cell production may occur in utero in response to chronic fetal distress and may be seen in infants who are SGA or IDM.

Many infants are asymptomatic. If symptoms develop, they are related to the increased blood volume, hyperviscosity (thickness) of the blood, and decreased deformability of red blood cells, all of which result in poor perfusion of tissues. The most common symptoms observed include the following:

- Tachycardia and congestive heart failure due to the increased blood volume

- Respiratory distress with grunting, tachypnea, and cyanosis; increased oxygen need; or hemorrhage in respiratory system

- Hyperbilirubinemia due to increased numbers of red blood cell hemolysed

- Decrease in peripheral pulses, discoloration of extremities, alteration in activity or neurologic depression, renal vein thrombosis with decreased urine output, hematuria, or proteinuria due to thromboembolism

- Seizures due to decreased perfusion of the brain as a result of sluggish blood flow

The nurse should assess, record, and report symptoms and do initial screening of hematocrit on admission to the nursery.

Therapy   The goal of therapy is to reduce the central venous hematocrit to less than 60%. To achieve this, the symptomatic infant receives a partial exchange transfusion in which blood is removed from the infant and replaced milliliter for milliliter with fresh frozen plasma.

Hemorrhagic Disease

Several transient coagulation mechanism deficiencies normally occur in the first several days of a newborn's life. Foremost among these is a slight decrease in the levels of prothrombin, resulting in a prolonged clotting time during the initial week of life. For the liver to form prothrombin (factor II) and proconvertin (factor VII) for blood coagulation, vitamin K is required. Vitamin K, a fat-soluble vitamin, may be obtained from food, but it is usually synthesized by bacteria in the colon, and consequently, a dietary source is unnecessary.

Intestinal flora are practically nonexistent in newborns, so they are unable to synthesize vitamin K. Although cow's milk contains more vitamins than breast milk, neither is a rich source of K. Hemorrhagic disease of the newborn is more common in breast-fed babies, however. Bleeding due to vitamin K deficiency generally occurs on the second to third day of life, but it may occur earlier. Internal hemorrhage may occur. Bleeding from the nose, umbilical cord, circumcision site, gastrointestinal tract, and scalp, as well as generalized ecchymoses, may be seen.

This disorder may be completely prevented by the prophylactic use of an injection of vitamin K. A dose of 1 mg of AquaMEPHYTON is given as part of the immediate care of the newborn following delivery (see Drug Guide, p. 468). Larger doses are contraindicated because they may result in the development of hyperbilirubinemia.

Necrotizing Enterocolitis

With increased survival of severely ill infants, neonatologists are now facing a previously unknown disease, *necrotizing enterocolitis* (NEC). This disease occurs in the first weeks of life and may cause bowel perforation and ultimately death. The exact cause of NEC is not known, but some predisposing factors have been identified. The current concept is that the cause is multifocal involving mucosal damage, bacterial presence, and nutrient substrate available for proliferation of the organisms.

An ischemic attack to the intestine may be precipitated by conditions such as fetal distress, neonatal shock and asphyxia, low cardiac output syndrome, low Apgar score, RDS, umbilical arterial catheters, infusion of hyperosmolar solution, and prematurity.

Clinical Manifestations and Diagnosis
The neonatal nurse, providing constant bedside care, is often the first person to observe the subtle signs and symptoms of NEC. Onset usually occurs within the first 2–3 weeks of life, although NEC can be seen as early as the first day of life. Systemic symptoms are those associated with sepsis—temperature instability (often hypothermia), respiratory changes (apnea, labored respirations), cardiovascular collapse, and behavioral changes such as lethargy or irritability. Gastrointestinal symptoms include abdominal distention and tenderness,

feeding changes such as vomiting or increased gastric residual (bile-stained), poor feeding, abdominal wall cellulitis (development of an erythematous area on the abdominal wall), and blood (Hematest positive) and reducing substances in the stools.

Clinical findings are verified by radiographic findings. These include pneumatosis intestinalis (air in the bowel wall), paralytic ileus with stasis, bowel wall thickening and loops of unequal size with a bubbly appearance of the intestines, and pneumoperitoneum (free air in the portal vein). Serial radiographic evaluation is recommended every 4–6 hours to detect progression of the disease and determine complications indicating surgical intervention.

Interventions   Aggressive and early management may prevent the need for surgical intervention. Gastric decompression, fluid and electrolyte replacement, correction of acidosis, correction of temperature instability, and parenteral antibiotics are common treatments. Infusion of volume expanders such as fresh frozen plasma may be necessary to correct existing hypotension and to improve peripheral perfusion because large amounts of plasma protein are lost into the gut lumen and peritoneal cavity in the acute phase.

Intensive nursing management consists of supportive therapy and constant observation of the neonate's condition. The nurse must be prepared to stop oral feedings and to place a gastric tube for gastric decompression and drainage. Antibiotics may need to be instilled through the gastric tube. Parenteral fluids, calories via hyperalimentation, and antibiotics are started.

Arterial oxygenation must be maintained. Constant observation of vital signs, oxygen concentration, development of increasing abdominal girth, and worsening clinical condition is the responsibility of the nurse.

Recovery of the intestinal mucosa and return to proper small bowel functioning (in nutritional absorption) are delayed after enterocolitis (with or without surgical intervention). Meanwhile, parenteral hyperalimentation is used to maintain positive nitrogen balance and promote healing. After rest of the gastrointestinal tract, cautious feedings are begun, using elemental formulas to promote easy absorption.

Surgery is indicated for intestinal perforation with pneumoperitoneum, intestinal infarction without perforation, progressive abdominal ascites and/or bowel wall thickening, and clinical deterioration. Even small or subtle changes may indicate rapid progression and worsening of the disease and the need for immediate surgical intervention.

Surgical intervention consists of removal of those areas of bowel that are necrotic or perforated. The infant may return with a gastrostomy to decompress the intestinal tract and an ostomy for drainage. Meticulous nursing care is required for maintenance of skin integrity around the openings. Reestablishment of continuity of the intestines is done when the infant can tolerate oral feedings and when general health is improved.

Complications Complications or consequences of necrotizing enterocolitis include:

- Surgical removal of intestines leaving insufficient remaining small bowel to support life
- Stenosis of the intestinal tract that develops secondary to NEC or surgery
- Gastrointestinal dysfunction evidenced by recurring intolerance to oral feedings, with vomiting, abdominal distention, water loss diarrhea, and failure to gain weight
- Complications associated with prolonged hyperalimentation
- Prolonged hospitalization with separation from parents and possible lack of appropriate developmental stimuli

Infections

Sepsis Neonatorum

Neonates are particularly susceptible to infection, referred to as *sepsis neonatorum*, caused by organisms that do not cause significant disease in older children. Incidence of severe infection is 0.5 to 2 per 1000 live newborns.

Predisposing factors include prematurity because of immaturity of the immunologic system and increased number of invasive procedures such as intubation and umbilical catheterization. Even the full-term infant is susceptible because of an immature immunologic system. Another predisposing factor is intrapartal infections such as amnionitis.

At present in the neonatal period Gram-negative organisms (especially *Escherichia coli, Aerobacter, Proteus,* and *Klebsiella*) and the Gram-positive organism group B β-hemolytic streptococci are the most common causative agents. Pseudomonas is a common contaminant of equipment used for ventilatory support and oxygen therapy.

Clinical manifestations and diagnosis Sepsis neonatorum is characterized by positive blood cultures and generalized clinical manifestations of illness, which are subtle and nonspecific and may be caused by other problems. Early detection of sepsis is extremely important so that appropriate intervention is begun immediately.

Infants with a history of possible exposure to infection in utero (for example PROM more than 24 hours before delivery or questionable maternal history of infection) should have cultures (gastric aspirate and ear canal) taken as soon after birth as possible. The infant may deteriorate rapidly in the first 12–24 hours after birth if β-hemolytic streptococcal infection is present, with signs and symptoms mimicking RDS. On the other hand, the onset of sepsis may be more gradual with more subtle signs and symptoms. The most common symptoms observed include:

1. Subtle behavioral changes—the infant "isn't doing well" and is often lethargic or irritable (especially after first 24 hours) and hypotonic. Color changes may include pallor, duskiness, cyanosis, or a "shocky" appearance. Skin is cool and clammy.

2. Temperature instability, manifested by either hypothermia (recognized by a decrease in skin temperature) or hyperthermia (elevation of skin temperature) necessitating a corresponding increase or decrease in isolette temperature to maintain neutral thermal environment.

3. Poor feeding, evidenced by a decrease in total intake, abdominal distention, vomiting, poor sucking, lack of interest in feeding, and diarrhea.

4. Hyperbilirubinemia.

5. Onset of apnea.

Signs and symptoms may suggest CNS disease (jitteriness, tremors, seizure activity), respiratory system disease (tachypnea, labored respirations, apnea, cyanosis), hematologic disease (jaundice, petechial hemorrhages, hepatosplenomegaly), or gastrointestinal disease (diarrhea, vomiting, bile-stained aspirate, hepatomegaly). A differential diagnosis is necessary because of the similarity of symptoms to other more specific conditions.

Isolation of the causative agent is necessary to obtain the diagnosis of sepsis in a suspected case and to identify the drugs to which the pathogen is susceptible. The nurse must be prepared to assist in the aseptic collection of specimens for laboratory investigation (Siegel, 1985). Before antibiotic therapy is begun, cultures are obtained.

1. Two blood cultures are obtained from different peripheral sites.

2. Spinal fluid culture is done following a spinal tap.

3. Urine culture is best obtained from a specimen obtained by a suprapubic bladder aspiration.

4. Skin cultures are taken of any lesions or drainage from lesions or reddened areas.

5. Nasopharyngeal, rectal, ear canal, and gastric aspirate cultures may be obtained.

Other laboratory investigations include a complete blood count, chest x-ray examination, serology, and Gram stains of cerebrospinal fluid, urine, skin exudate, and umbilicus. White blood count with differential may indicate the presence or absence of sepsis. A level of 30,000 WBC may be normal in the first 24 hours of life, while a low WBC may be indicative of sepsis. A low neutrophil count and a high band count indicate that an infection is present. Stomach aspirate should be sent for culture and smear if a gonococcal infection or amnionitis are suspected. Serum IgM levels are elevated (normal level less than 20 mg/dL) in response to transplacental infections. Counterimmuno-electrophoresis tests for specific bacterial antigens, if available, are done. Evidence of congenital infections may be seen on skull x-ray films for cerebral calcifications (cytomegalovirus, toxoplasmosis), bone x-ray films (syphilis, cytomegalovirus), and serum-specific IgM levels (rubella). Cytomegalovirus infection is best diagnosed by urine culture.

Nursing management

Treatment Because neonatal infection causes high mortality, therapy is instituted before results of the septic workup are obtained. A combination of two broad spectrum antibiotics in large doses is given until culture with sensitivities is received.

After the pathogen and its sensitivities are determined, appropriate specific antibiotic therapy is begun. Combinations of penicillin or ampicillin and kanamycin have been used in the past, but new kanamycin-resistant enterobacteria and penicillin-resistant staphylococcus necessitate increasing use of gentamicin. Duration of therapy varies from 7–14 days. If cultures are negative and symptoms subside, antibiotics may be discontinued after 3 days.

In addition to antibiotic therapy, physiologic supportive care is essential in caring for a septic infant:

- Observe for resolution of symptoms or development of other symptoms of sepsis.

- Maintain neutral thermal environment with accurate regulation of humidity and oxygen administration.

- Provide respiratory support—administer oxygen and observe and monitor respiratory effort.

- Provide cardiovascular support—observe and monitor pulse and blood pressure; observe for hyperbilirubinemia, anemia, and hemorrhagic symptoms.

- Provide adequate calories intravenously if oral feedings are discontinued due to increased mucus, abdominal distention, vomiting, and aspiration.

- Provide fluids and electrolytes to maintain homeostasis.

- Detect and treat metabolic disturbances, a common occurrence.

- Observe for the development of hypoglycemia, hyperglycemia, acidosis, hyponatremia, and hypocalcemia.

Prevention   Protection of the newborn from infections starts prenatally and continues throughout pregnancy and delivery. Prenatal prevention should include maternal screening for venereal disease and monitoring of rubella titers in women who are negative. Intrapartally, sterile technique is essential, smears from genital lesions are taken, and placenta and amniotic fluid cultures are obtained if amnionitis is suspected. If genital herpes is present toward term, cesarean delivery may be indicated. Local eye treatment with silver nitrate or an antibiotic ophthalmic ointment is given to all newborns to prevent gonococcal damage.

In the nursery, environmental control and prevention of acquired infection is the responsibility of the neonatal nurse. Being the vanguard of infection control, the nurse must promote strict hand-washing technique for all who enter the nursery, including nursing colleagues; physicians; laboratory, x-ray, and inhalation technicians; and parents. Scrupulous care of equipment will prevent fomite contamination of infection-prone newborns. An infected neonate can be effectively isolated in an isolette and receive close observation. Visitation of the nursery area by unnecessary personnel should be discouraged. Restriction of visiting by parents has not been shown to have any effect on the rate of infection and may indeed be harmful for a newborn's psychologic development. With instruction and supervision from the nurse, both parents should be allowed to handle the baby and participate in the care, even inside the isolette.

Group B Streptococcus

Group B streptococcus (β-hemolytic streptococcus) has become a leading cause of septicemia in the newborn, and is a major cause of morbidity and mortality in the neonate. Pregnant women who carry group B streptococcus are asymptomatic but harbor the organism in the birth canal, resulting in exposure of the infant to the organism during the birth process.

Two clinical disease entities may result from group B streptococcus. One is an early onset form (first 24 hours) of acute septicemia. The other occurs later (several days to 3 months) as meningitis without respiratory distress. The early form carries a higher mortality risk (approximately 50%) than the later onset form (20%–40%) (Avery, 1981).

The *early onset* form of group B streptococcus usually occurs within the first 12–24 hours of life. The infant appears to be in severe respiratory distress (grunting and cyanosis), may become apneic, and may demonstrate symptoms of shock. The chest x-ray examination may show aspiration pneumonia or may appear similar to that seen in hyaline membrane disease. Early recognition of a group B streptococcal condition is essential to the infant's intact survival because the course is one of rapid deterioration. Cultures should be done immediately (blood, gastric aspirate, external ear canal, nasopharynx), and antibiotics should be started before results of the cultures are obtained. Antibiotic treatment usually involves aqueous penicillin or ampicillin. Some feel ampicillin combined with gentamicin is superior to ampicillin alone. It is the nurse's responsibility to be alert to all signs and symptoms suggesting sepsis, and to intervene as rapidly as possible when sepsis is suspected. There must be no delay in the administration of antibiotics, as this may determine the infant's ultimate survival.

Syphilis

Because congenital syphilis is difficult to detect at birth, all infants of syphilitic mothers should be screened to determine the necessity of treatment. Diagnostic serologic dilution tests are usually accurate between 3 and 6 months of age. Development and detection of the infant's own antibodies are essential for diagnosis.

The nursing management of these infants and their parents requires careful physical and psychologic care. Initially, nursing care includes use of isolation techniques. Drug treatment of choice is penicillin. After proper treatment for 48 hours, the infant should no longer be contagious, and general care may ensue. This would include basic assessment of axillary temperature every 3 to 4 hours; intake and output record; feedings; and infant's tolerances. Infants should be swaddled for comfort, and their hands should be covered to minimize trauma to their skin from scratching.

Support to the parents is crucial. They need to be informed of the infant's prognosis as treatment continues and to be involved in care as much as possible. They need to understand how the infection is transmitted. It is essential to avoid judging the parents, and to encourage positive parental involvement.

Gonorrhea

Gonorrhea may be contracted by the fetus during vaginal delivery and is usually manifested clinically as an eye infection, ophthalmia neonatorum. This is first diagnosed as a conjunctivitis that is indistinguishable from that caused by silver nitrate instillation. However, one clue is that chemical conjunctivitis disappears within 24 hours, whereas ophthalmia neonatorum becomes more readily apparent in the neonate on the third or fourth postnatal day. Other more severe clinical signs that develop are a purulent discharge and ulcerations of the cornea, which can be prevented if treatment is instituted promptly. In some cases, gonorrhea infection may be observed as temperature instability, poor feeding response, and/or hypotonia.

For neonates of all vaginal births, a 1% silver nitrate solution or antibiotic ophthalmic ointment is instilled in the conjunctiva of the infant's eyes to prevent infection. (See Drug Guide, p. 468.) Penicillin may also be administered topically and systemically in lieu of silver nitrate. If allergy to penicillin is suspected, erythromycin, tetracycline, or chloramphenicol may be substituted. If the infant's eyes are left untreated, partial or complete loss of vision may occur as a result of corneal ulceration.

Herpesvirus Type 2

A wide variety of clinical manifestations of herpesvirus hominis (HVH) type 2 are noted in the neonate. Signs and symptoms are present at birth or by 3–4 weeks of age. The disseminated form is seen as a bleeding tendency, hepatitis with jaundice, hepatosplenomegaly, and neurologic abnormalities. About one-third of affected infants exhibit vesicular skin lesions in small clusters all over the body. The more localized form includes convulsions (focal or generalized), abnormal muscle tone, opisthotonos, a bulging fontanelle, and lethargy or coma and

carries very high mortality rates. In the eyes, keratitis (cloudy corneas), conjunctivitis, and chorioretinitis are seen. Another form is asymptomatic at birth but infants can develop symptoms up to 12 days after birth. Frequently the skin lesions are the only diagnostic finding.

In the absence of skin lesions, diagnosis is difficult because the presenting clinical picture resembles septicemia (such as fever or subnormal temperature, respiratory congestion, dyspnea, cough, tachypnea, and tachycardia). It is therefore necessary to obtain cultures from the infant's lesions and throat and to identify the herpesvirus type 2 antibodies in the serum IgM assay. Positive cultures are observable within 24 to 48 hours.

Currently an antiviral drug acyclovir (Zovirax) is used for initial and recurrent mucosal and cutaneous herpes. Careful hand washing and adequate infection-control methods are essential. Isolation measures should be instituted for all infants born to mothers known to have had third-trimester infections.

Monilial Infection (Thrush)

Thrush (oral moniliasis) is caused by the fungus *Candida albicans*, contracted from a yeast-infected vagina during delivery. Clinically, it appears as white plaques distributed on the buccal mucosa, on the tongue, on the gums, inside the cheeks, and even on the lips. It can be distinguished from milk curds, which it resembles, by gently attempting to wipe away the patches with a cotton-tipped applicator. If the plaques are thrush, a raw bleeding area beneath them will be exposed. Involvement of the diaper area skin is seen as a bright red, well-demarcated eruption. On occasion, generalized moniliasis may be seen. Lesions are most frequently seen at about 5–7 days of age. However, infants receiving long-term antibiotic therapy are also susceptible to development of thrush, which may occur at any time in the hospitalization.

Care of the neonate infected with *Candida albicans* involves:

1. Maintaining cleanliness of hands, bedding, clothing, diapers, and feeding apparatus because *Candida albicans* is present in the oral secretions and in the stools. Breast-feeding mothers should be instructed on treating their nipples with topical nystatin; otherwise a cycle of reinfection as well as sore nipples with breakdown of nipple tissue will occur.

2. Administering drug therapy. Gentian violet (1%–2%) is swabbed on oral mucosa, usually an hour after feeding once or twice a day; or nystatin (Mycostatin) is instilled in the oral cavity with a medicine dropper. The mouth should be cleared of milk prior to instillation or swabbing of oral mucosa with the medication. Topical nystatin is used for skin involvement.

3. Discussing with the parents that gentian violet is a dye and will cause staining of the infant's mouth and possibly the infant's clothing if the saliva is gentian colored.

Infants with Congenital Heart Defects

The incidence of congenital heart defects is 7.5 per 1000 live births. They account for one third of deaths caused by congenital defects in the first year of life. Because accurate diagnosis and surgical treatment are now available, many such deaths can be prevented. Thus, it is crucial for the nurse to have comprehensive knowledge of congenital heart disease to detect deviations from normal and to initiate nursing interventions.

Overview of Congenital Heart Defects

Factors that might influence development of congenital heart malformation can be classified as environmental or genetic. Infections of the pregnant female, such as rubella, coxsackie B, and influenza, have been implicated. Thalidomide, steroids, alcohol, lithium, and some anticonvulsants have been shown to cause congenital malformations of the heart. Seasonal spraying of pesticides has also been linked to an increase in congenital heart defects.

Infants born with chromosomal abnormalities have a higher incidence of cardiovascular anomalies. Infants with Down syndrome and trisomy 13/15 and 16/18 frequently have heart lesions. Increased incidence and risk of recurrence of specific defects occur in families.

It is customary to divide congenital malformations of the heart into *acyanotic*—those that do not present with cyanosis—and *cyanotic*—those that do present with cyanosis. Normally, if an opening exists between the right and left sides of the heart, blood will flow from the area of greater pressure (left side) to the area of lesser pressure (right side). This process is referred to as left-to-right shunt and does not produce cyanosis because oxygenated blood is being pumped out to the systemic circulation. If pressure in the right side of the heart, due to obstruction of normal flow, exceeds that in the left side, unoxygenated blood will flow from the right side to the left side of the heart and out into the system. A right-to-left shunt is produced and causes cyanosis. If the opening is large, there may be a bidirectional shunt with mixing of blood in both sides of the heart, which also produces cyanosis.

The most common cardiac defects seen in the first 6 days of life are left ventricular outflow obstructions (mitral stenosis, aortic stenosis or atresia), hypoplastic left heart, and coarctation of the aorta, patent ductus arteriosus (PDA), transposition of the great vessels, tetralogy of Fallot, and large ventricular septal defect or atrial septal defects (see Figure 22-21). PDA is the most common cardiac defect.

Clinical Signs and Symptoms in the Neonate

General signs and symptoms of heart defects are as follows:

1. Tachypnea—reflects increased pulmonary blood flow
2. Dyspnea—caused by increased pulmonary venous pressure and blood flow, can also cause chest retractions, wheezing
3. Color—ashen, gray, or cyanotic
4. Difficulty in feeding—requires many rest periods before finishing even 1 or 2 oz
5. Diaphoresis—beads of perspiration over the upper lip and forehead, may accompany feeding fatigue
6. Stridor or choking spells
7. Failure to gain weight

Cyanotic

Complete Transposition of Great Vessels

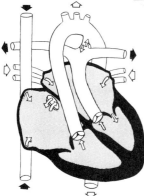

This anomaly is an embryologic defect caused by a straight division of the bulbar trunk without normal spiraling. As a result, the aorta originates from the right ventricle, and the pulmonary artery from the left ventricle. An abnormal communication between the two circulations must be present to sustain life.

Patent Ductus Arteriosus

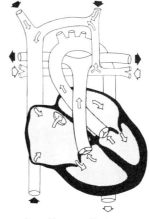

The patent ductus arteriosus is a vascular connection that, during fetal life, short circuits the pulmonary vascular bed and directs blood from the pulmonary artery to the aorta. Functional closure of the ductus normally occurs soon after birth. If the ductus remains patent after birth, the direction of blood flow in the ductus is reversed by the higher pressure in the aorta.

Coarctation of the Aorta

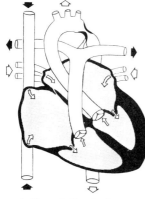

Coarctation of the aorta is characterized by a narrowed aortic lumen. It exists as a preductal or postductal obstruction, depending on the position of the obstruction in relation to the ductus arteriosus. Coarctations exist with great variation in anatomical features. The lesion produces an obstruction to the flow of blood through the aorta causing an increased left ventricular pressure and work load.

Anomalous Venous Return

Oxygenated blood returning from the lungs is carried abnormally to the right heart by one or more pulmonary veins emptying directly, or indirectly through venous channels, into the right atrium. Partial anomalous return of the pulmonary veins to the right atrium functions the same as an atrial septal defect. In complete anomalous return of the pulmonary veins, an interatrial communication is necessary for survival.

Tetralogy of Fallot - *Cyanotic*

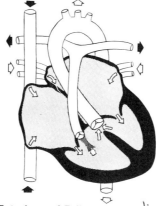

Tetralogy of Fallot is characterized by the combination of four defects: 1) pulmonary stenosis 2) ventricular septal defect 3) overriding aorta 4) hypertrophy of right ventricle. It is the most common defect causing cyanosis in patients surviving beyond two years of age. The severity of symptoms depends on the degree of pulmonary stenosis, the size of the ventricular septal defect, and the degree to which the aorta overrides the septal defect.

Ventricular Septal Defects

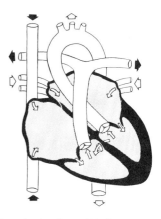

A ventricular septal defect is an abnormal opening between the right and left ventricle. Ventricular septal defects vary in size and may occur in either the membranous or muscular portion of the ventricular septum. Due to higher pressure in the left ventricle, a shunting of blood from the left to right ventricle occurs during systole. If pulmonary vascular resistance produces pulmonary hypertension, the shunt of blood is then reversed from the right to the left ventricle, with cyanosis resulting.

Atrial Septal Defects

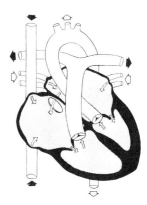

An atrial septal defect is an abnormal opening between the right and left atria. Basically, three types of abnormalities result from incorrect development of the atrial septum. An incompetent foramen ovale is the most common defect. The high ostium secundum defect results from abnormal development of the septum secundum. Improper development of the septum primum produces a basal opening known as an ostium primum defect, frequently involving the atrio-ventricular valves. In general, left to right shunting of blood occurs in all atrial septal defects.

Figure 22-21

Congenital heart abnormalities. (From Congenital heart abnormalities. Clinical Education Aid no. 7. Ross Laboratories, Columbus, Ohio.)

8. Heart murmur—may not be heard in left-to-right shunting defects since the pulmonary pressure in the newborn is greater than pressure in the left side of the heart in the early newborn period

9. Hepatomegaly—in right-sided heart failure caused by venous congestion in the liver

10. Tachycardia—pulse over 160, may be as high as 200

11. Cardiac enlargement—may be present

Nursing Assessment and Intervention

The primary goal of the neonatal nurse is early identification of cardiac defects and initiation of referral to the physician. The three most common manifestations of cardiac defect are cyanosis, detectable heart murmur, and congestive heart failure signs (tachycardia, tachypnea, diaphoresis, hepatomegaly, and cardiomegaly).

Care of infants with congestive heart failure has four major goals:

1. To reduce the energy requirements of the body

2. To increase cardiac efficiency

3. To increase oxygenation of the blood

4. To reduce retention of fluids in the tissues

Rest, with the use of a sedative may be required. Morphine sulfate, a dose of 0.05 mg/kg of body weight, can be used if the infant is markedly irritable (Graham and Bender, 1980). Morphine is thought to decrease peripheral and pulmo-nary vascular resistance, which results in decreased tachypnea. Infants in congestive heart failure are more comfortable in a semi-Fowler's position.

When the infant has dyspnea or cyanosis, oxygen must be given by an oxygen hood, tent, mask, cannula, or oxygen prongs. Mist is often ordered given with oxygen to infants, making the use of an oxygen hood or tent necessary. Oxygen administration should always be accompanied by humidity, and the air should be warmed to decrease the drying effects of cold, dry oxygen. Vital signs are carefully monitored for evidence of tachycardia, tachypnea, expiratory grunting, and retractions.

After the infant is stabilized and gaining weight, decisions can be made about ongoing care and surgical intervention. The family needs careful explanations and ongoing emotional support (see Chapter 26).

Other Congenital Anomalies

The birth of a baby with a congenital defect places both infant and family at risk. Many congenital anomalies can be life-threatening if not corrected within hours after birth; others are very visible and cause the families emotional distress. Some of the more common congenital disorders are listed in Table 22-4. Included in the discussion is the identification of the anomaly and its early management and nursing care in the neonatal period.

Table 22-4
Congenital Anomalies: Identification and Care in Newborn Period

Congenital anomaly	Clinical findings	Nursing interventions during neonatal period
Cleft lip	Unilateral or bilateral visible defect May involve external nares, nasal cartilage, nasal septum, and alveolar process Flattening or depression of midfacial contour (Figure 22-22)	Feed with special nipple. Burp frequently (increases the tendency to swallow air and reflex vomiting). Clean cleft with sterile water (prevents crusting on cleft prior to repair). Provide role model in interacting with infant (parents internalize other's responses to their newborn).

Continued.

Table 22-4 (continued)
Congenital Anomalies: Identification and Care in Newborn Period

Congenital anomaly	Clinical findings	Nursing interventions during neonatal period
Cleft palate	Fissure connecting oral and nasal cavity May involve uvula and soft palate May extend forward to nostril involving hard palate and maxillary alveolar ridge Difficulty in sucking Expulsion of formula through nose (Figure 22-23)	Place prone or in side-lying position to facilitate drainage. Suction nasopharyngeal cavity (prevent aspiration or airway obstruction). Feed with special nipple that fills cleft and allows sucking. Also decreases chance of aspiration through nasal cavity. During neonatal period, feed in upright position with head and chest tilted slightly backward (aids swallowing and discourages aspiration).
Tracheoesophageal fistula (type III)	History of maternal hydramnios Excessive mucous secretions Constant drooling Abdominal distention beginning soon after birth Periodic choking and cyanotic episodes Immediate regurgitation of feeding Clinical symptoms of aspiration pneumonia (tachypnea, retractions, rhonchi, decreased breath sounds, cyanotic spells) Failure to pass nasogastric tube (Figure 22-24)	Withhold feeding until esophageal patency is determined. Place on low intermittent suction to control saliva and mucus (prevent aspiration pneumonia). Place in warmed, humidified Isolette (liquefies secretions facilitating removal). Elevate head of bed 20° (prevent reflux of gastric juices). Keep quiet (crying causes air to pass through fistula to distend intestines causing respiratory embarrassment).
Diaphragmatic hernia	Difficulty initiating respirations Gasping respirations with nasal flaring and chest retraction Asymmetrical chest expansion Breath sounds absent usually on left side Heart sounds displaced to right Spasmodic attacks of cyanosis and difficulty in feeding Bowel sounds may be heard in thoracic cavity (Figure 22-25)	Immediately administer oxygen. Initiate gastric decompression. Place in high semi-Fowler's position (use gravity to keep abdominal organ's pressure off diaphragm). Turn to affected side to allow unaffected lung expansion. Carry out interventions to alleviate respiratory and metabolic acidosis.
Omphalocele	Herniation of abdominal contents into base of umbilical cord May have an enclosed transparent sac covering	Cover sac with moistened sterile gauze and place plastic wrap over dressing (prevent rupture of sac and infection). Initiate gastric decompression by insertion of nasogastric tube attached to low suction (prevent distention of lower bowel).
Myelomeningocele	Saclike cyst containing meninges, spinal cord, and nerve roots in thoracic and/or lumbar area (Figure 22-26) Myelomeningocele directly connects to subarachnoid space so hydrocephalus is often an associated defect No response or varying response to sensation below level of sac May have constant dribbling of urine. Incontinence or retention of stool Anal opening may be flaccid	Position on abdomen or on side and restrain (prevents pressure and trauma to sac). Meticulous cleaning of buttocks and genitals after each voiding and defecation (prevents contamination of sac and decreases possibility of infection). May put protective covering over sac (prevent rupture and drying). Observe sac for oozing of fluid or pus.

Table 22-4 (continued)
Congenital Anomalies: Identification and Care in Newborn Period

Congenital anomaly	Clinical findings	Nursing interventions during neonatal period
		Obtain occipital-frontal circumference baseline measurements, then measure head circumference once a day (detect hydrocephalus). Check fontanelle for bulging. Credé bladder as ordered (prevent urinary stasis).
Imperforate anus, congenital dislocated hip, and clubfoot	See discussion in Chapter 20	Early identification of defect and initiation of appropriate referral are key nursing interventions.

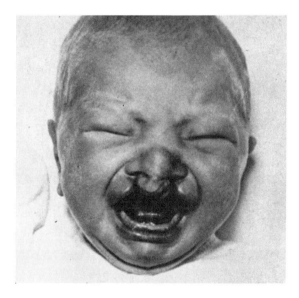

Figure 22-22
Bilateral cleft lip.

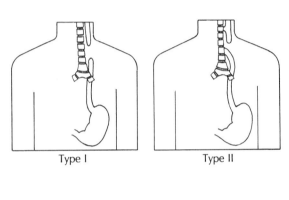

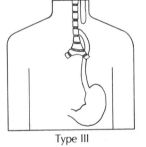

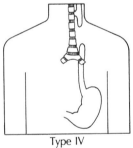

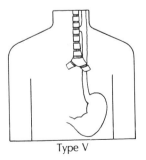

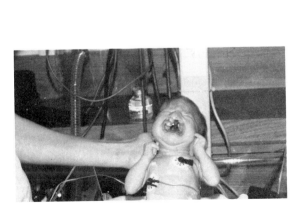

Figure 22-23
Cleft abnormality involving both hard and soft palate and unilateral cleft lip.

Figure 22-24
Five most frequently seen types of congenital tracheoesophageal fistula and esophageal atresia.

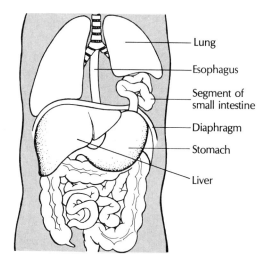

Figure 22-25
Diaphragmatic hernia. Note compression of the lung by the intestine on the affected side.

Lung

Esophagus

Segment of small intestine

Diaphragm

Stomach

Liver

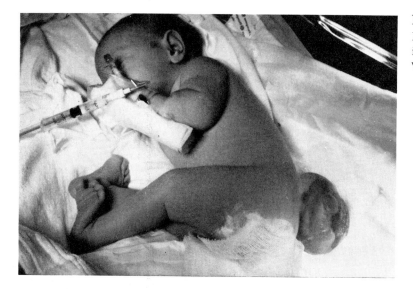

Figure 22-26
Infant with lumbar myelomeningocele. (Courtesy Dr. Paul Winchester.)

Summary

The high-risk neonate or neonate with a complication must be managed within narrow physiologic parameters. These parameters (respiratory and thermal regulation) will maintain physiologic homeostasis and prevent introduction of additional stress to the already stressed infant. Maintenance of this physiologic environment must begin immediately because lost ground is difficult or impossible to recover.

The nursing care of the neonate with special problems involves the understanding of normal physiology, the pathophysiology of the disease process, clinical manifestations, and supportive and corrective therapies. Only with this theoretical background can the nurse make appropriate observations concerning responses to therapy and development of further complications. Neonates communicate needs only by their behavior. The neonatal nurse, through objective observations and evaluations, must interpret this behavior into meaningful information about the neonate's condition.

References

Affonso DD, Harris TR: Postterm pregnancy: Implications for mother and infant, challenge for the nurse. *J Obstet Gynecol Neonatal Nurs* 1980; 9:139.

Avery GB (editor): *Neonatology*. Philadelphia: Lippincott, 1981.

Benitz WE, Tatio DS: *The Pediatric Drug Handbook*. Chicago: Year Book Medical Publishers, 1981.

Berkowitz RL et al: *Handbook for Prescribing Medications During Pregnancy*. Boston: Little, Brown, 1981.

Blake S: The bright side of phototherapy. *MCN* January/February 1983; 8:23.

Bree RL, Mariona FG: The role of ultrasound in the evaluation of normal and abnormal fetal growth. In: *Seminars in Ultrasound*. Raymond HW, Zwiebel WJ (editors). New York: Grune & Stratton, 1980.

Clifford S: Postmaturity. *Adv Pediatr* 1957; 9:13.

Cloherty JP, Stark AR (editors): *Manual of Neonatal Care*. Boston: Little, Brown, 1981.

Cohen MA: Transcutaneous oxygen monitoring for sick neonates. *MCN* September/October 1984; 9:324.

Cohlan SO: Drugs and pregnancy. In: *Progress in Clinical and Biological Research*. Young BK (editor). New York: Alan R. Less, Inc., 1980.

Fantazia D: Neonatal hypoglycemia. *JOGN* September/November 1984; 13(5):297.

Fitzhardinge PM: Follow-up studies on the low birth weight infant. *Clin Perinatol* 1976; 3:503.

Gorski PA et al: Stages of behavioral organization in the high-risk neonate: Theoretical and clinical considerations. *Semin Perinatol* 1979; 3:61.

Graham TP, Bender HW: Preoperative diagnosis and management of infants with critical congenital heart disease. *Ann Thorac Surg* 1980; 29(3):272.

Hendricksen A: Prolonged pregnancy—A review of the literature. *Journal of Nurse-Midwifery*, January/February 1985; 30(1):33.

Hobart JM, Depp R: Prolonged pregnancy. In: *Gynecology and Obstetrics*, Vol. 3. Sciarri JJ (editor). Philadelphia: Harper & Row, 1982.

Hobbins JC: Fetoscopy. In: *Protocols for High Risk Pregnancies*. Queenan JT, Hobbins JC (editors). Oradell, N. J.: Medical Economics Co., Inc., 1982.

Iosub S et al: Fetal alcohol syndrome revisited. *Pediatrics* October 1981; 68(4):475.

Jones KL et al: Pattern of malformation in offspring of chronic alcoholic mothers. *Lancet* June 1973; 1:1267.

Klaus MH, Fanaroff AA: *Care of the High-Risk Neonate*. Philadelphia: Saunders, 1979.

Korones SB: *High-risk Newborn Infants: The Basis for Intensive Care Nursing*, 3rd ed. St. Louis: Mosby, 1981.

McCormick A: Special considerations in the nursing care of the very low birth weight infant. *J Obstet Gynecol Neonatal Nurs* November/December 1984; 13(6):357.

Measel CP, Anderson GC: Non-nutritive sucking during tube feedings: Effect on clinical course in premature infants. *J Obstet Gynecol Neonatal Nurs* 1979; 8:265.

Noerr B: Nursing care to maintain neonatal thermoregulation. *Critical Care Nurse* March/April 1984; 4(2):103.

Nugent J: Acute respiratory care of the newborn. *J Obstet Gynecol Neonatal Nurs* (supplement) May/June 1983; 12:315.

Oh W: Renal functions and clinical disorders in the neonate. *Clin Perinatol* 1981; 4:321.

Ostrea EM et al: *The Care of the Drug Dependent Woman and Her Infant*. Michigan Department of Public Health, 1978.

Siegel JD: Neonatal sepsis. *Seminars in Perinatology* January 1985; 9(1):20.

Usher RH: Clinical and therapeutic aspects of fetal malnutrition. *Pediatr Clin North Am* February 1970; 17(1):169.

Additional Readings

Aylward GP: The developmental course of behavioral states in preterm infants: A descriptive study. *Child Dev* 1981; 52:564.

Bahr JE: Herpesvirus: Hominis type 2 in women and newborns. *MCN* January/February 1978; 3:16.

Baker CJ: Group B streptococcal infections in neonates. *Pediatrics in Review* 1979; 1:5.

Baumgart S et al: Fluid, electrolyte, and glucose maintenance in the very low birth weight infant. *Clin Pediatr* 1982; 21:199.

Brodish MS: Perinatal Assessment. *J Obstet Gynecol Neonatal Nurs* 1981; 10:42.

Canadian Pediatric Society. Nutrition Committee: Feeding the low-birthweight infant. *CMA Journal* 1981; 124:1301.

Collinge JM et al: Demand vs scheduled feedings for premature infants. *J Obstet Gynecol Neonatal Nurs* November/December 1982; 11:362.

Elsas TL: Family mental health care in the neonatal intensive care unit. *J Obstet Gynecol Neonatal Nurs* May/June 1981; 10(3):204.

Filston HC: *Surgical Problems in Children: Recognition and Referral.* St. Louis: Mosby, 1982.

Hansen FH: Nursing care in the neonatal intensive care unit. *J Obstet Gynecol Neonatal Nurs* January/February 1982; 11:17.

Mason TN: A hand ventilation technique for neonates. *MCN* November/December 1982; 7:366.

Noga KM: High-risk infants. The need for nursing follow-up. *J Obstet Gynecol Neonatal Nurs* 1982; 11:112.

Nugent J: Intra-arterial blood pressure monitoring in neonates. *J Obstet Gynecol Neonatal Nurs* September/October 1982; 11:281.

Ogata ES: Infant of the diabetic mother. In: *Gynecology and Obstetrics.* Vol. 3, Sciarri JJ (editor). Philadelphia: Harper & Row, 1982.

Smith KM: Congenital heart disease. Recognizing cardiac failure in neonates. *MCN* March/April 1979; 4(2):98.

Stephens CJ: The fetal alcohol syndrome: Cause for concern. *MCN* 1981; 6:4.

Trotter CW et al: Perinatal factors and the developmental outcome of preterm infants. *J Obstet Gynecol Neonatal Nurs* 1982; 11:83.

Whittemore R et al: Results of pregnancy in women with congenital heart defects. *Pediatr Res* 1980; 14:4.

Ziegler EE, Bega RL, Fomon SJ: Nutritional requirements of the premature infant. In: *Symposium on Pediatric Nutrition.* Suskind RM (editor). New York: Raven Press, 1983.

Romance fails us, and so do friendships, but the relationship of parent and child, less noisy than all others, remains indelible and indestructible, the strongest relationship on earth.

THEODOR REIK

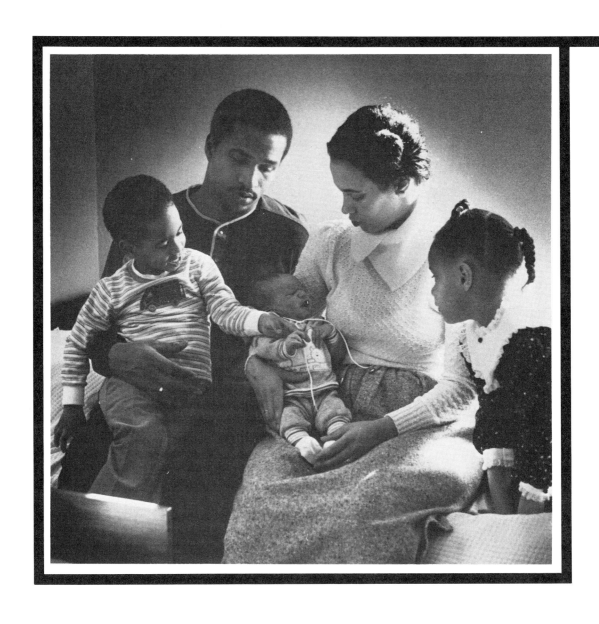

V

The Puerperium

23

Postpartal Adaptation and Nursing Assessment

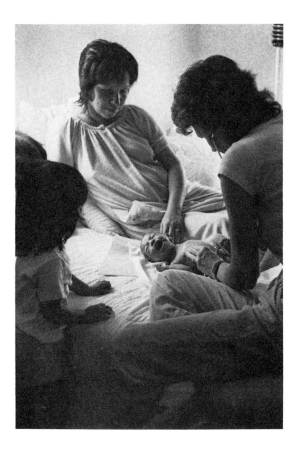

Chapter Contents

Objectives

- Describe the basic physiologic changes that occur in the postpartal period as a woman's body returns to its prepregnant state.

- Discuss the psychologic adjustments that normally occur during the postpartal period.

- Explore the factors that influence the development of attachment.

- Describe a normal postpartal assessment.

Key Terms

afterpains	lochia alba
diastasis recti	lochia rubra
abdominis	lochia serosa
en face	puerperium
engrossment	taking-hold phase
involution	taking-in phase
lochia	

The **puerperium**, or postpartal period, is the period during which the woman adjusts, physically and psychologically, to the process of childbirth. It begins immediately after delivery and continues for approximately 6 weeks or until the body has returned to a near prepregnant state. The puerperium is often referred to as the "fourth trimester." Although the time span is less than three months, this title demonstrates the idea of continuity.

This chapter describes the physiologic and psychologic changes that occur postpartally and the basic aspects of a thorough postpartal assessment.

Puerperal Physical and Psychologic Adaptations

Comprehensive nursing assessment is based on a sound understanding of the normal anatomic and physiologic processes of the puerperium. These processes involve the reproductive organs and other major body systems.

Reproductive organs

Involution of the uterus   Immediately following the delivery of the placenta, the uterus contracts to the size of a large grapefruit. The fundus is situated in the midline midway between the symphysis pubis and the umbilicus (Figure 23-1). The walls of the contracted uterus are in close proximity and the uterine blood

vessels are firmly compressed by the myometrium. Within 12 hours after delivery the fundus of the uterus rises to the level of the umbilicus or one finger breadth (1 cm) above it. A uterus that is higher than one finger breadth, or is deviated from the midline and is boggy, has probably been displaced by a distended bladder. Because the uterine ligaments are still stretched, the uterus can easily be moved by the bladder.

After delivery the uterus remains at the umbilicus level for about a day and then on each succeeding day descends into the pelvis approximately one finger breadth. If the mother is breast-feeding, the release of oxytocin from the posterior pituitary in response to suckling hastens this process. Within 2 weeks the uterus is again a pelvic organ and cannot be palpated abdominally. Barring complications, the uterus approaches its prepregnant size and location by 5–6 weeks.

The uterus gradually decreases in size as the cells grow smaller and the hyperplasia of pregnancy reverses. Protein material in the uterine wall is broken down and absorbed. The process is basically one of cell size reduction rather than a radical decrease in cell number.

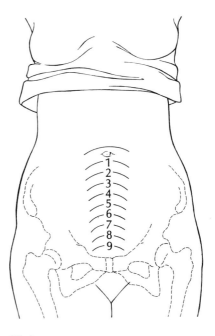

Figure 23-1

Involution of the uterus. The height of the fundus decreases about one fingerbreadth (approximately 1 cm) each day.

The term **involution** is used to describe this rapid reduction in size and the return of the uterus to a normal condition similar to its pre-pregnant state.

Following separation of the placenta, the decidua of the uterus is irregular, jagged, and varied in thickness. The spongy layer of the decidua is cast off as lochia while the inner layer forms the basis for the development of new endometrium. Except at the placental site, this process takes about 3 weeks. Bleeding from the larger uterine vessels of the placental site is controlled by compression of the retracted uterine muscle fibers. The clotted blood is gradually absorbed by the body. Some of these vessels are eventually obliterated and replaced by new vessels with smaller lumens.

Rather than forming a fibrous scar in the decidua, the placental site heals by a process of exfoliation. In this process, the site is undermined by the growth of the endometrial tissue both from the margins of the site and from the fundi of the endometrial glands left in the basal layer of the site. The infarcted superficial tissue then becomes necrotic and is sloughed off.

Exfoliation is a very important aspect of involution. If healing of the placental site left a fibrous scar, the area available for future implantation would be limited, as would the number of possible pregnancies.

Factors that retard uterine involution include prolonged labor, anesthesia or excessive analgesia, difficult delivery, grandmultiparity, a full bladder, and incomplete expulsion of the products of conception. Factors that enhance involution include an uncomplicated labor and delivery, complete expulsion of the products of conception, breast-feeding and early ambulation.

Lochia   The uterus rids itself of the debris remaining after delivery through a discharge called **lochia**, which is classified according to its appearance and contents. **Lochia rubra** is dark red in color. It occurs for the first 2–3 days and contains epithelial cells, erythrocytes, leukocytes, shreds of decidua, and occasionally fetal meconium, lanugo, and vernix caseosa. Lochia should not contain large clots; if it does the cause should be investigated without delay. **Lochia serosa** follows from about the third until the tenth day. It is a pinkish color and is composed of serous exudate (hence the name), shreds of degenerating decidua, erythocytes, leukocytes, cervical mucus, and numerous microorganisms. Gradually the red blood cell component decreases, and a creamy or yellowish discharge persists for an additional week or two. This final discharge is termed **lochia alba**, and is composed primarily of leukocytes, decidual cells, epithelial cells, fat, cervical mucus, cholesterol crystals, and bacteria. When the lochia stops, the cervix is considered closed, and chances of infection ascending from the vagina to the uterus decrease.

Like menstrual discharge, lochia has a musty, stale odor that is not offensive. Foul-smelling lochia suggest infection and should be assessed promptly.

The total volume of lochia is 240–270 mL and the daily volume gradually declines. Discharge is heavier in the morning due to pooling in the vagina and uterus. The amount of lochia may also be increased by exertion or breast-feeding.

Evaluation of lochia is necessary not only to determine the presence of hemorrhage but also to assess uterine involution. The type, amount, and consistency of lochia determine the stage of healing of the placental site, and a progressive change from bright red at delivery to dark red to pink to white/clear discharge should be observed. Persistent discharge of lochia rubra or a return to lochia rubra indicates subinvolution or late postpartal hemorrhage (see Chapter 25).

Cervical changes   Following delivery the cervix is flabby and formless and may appear bruised. The external os is markedly irregular and closes slowly. It admits two fingers for a few days following delivery, but by the end of the first week it will admit only a fingertip.

The shape of the external os is permanently changed by the first childbearing. The characteristic dimplelike os of the nullipara changes to the lateral slit (fish-mouth) os of the multipara. After significant cervical laceration or several lacerations, the cervix may appear lopsided.

Vaginal changes   Following delivery the vagina appears edematous and may be bruised. Small superficial lacerations may be evident and the rugae have been obliterated. The apparent bruising is due to pelvic congestion and will quickly disappear. The hymen, torn and jagged, heals irregularly leaving small tags called the *carunculae myrtiformes*.

The size of the vagina decreases and rugae return within 3 weeks. Tone and contractility of the vaginal orifice may be improved by perineal tightening exercises (Kegel's). The labia majora and labia minora are flabbier in the woman who has born a child than in the nullipara.

Perineal changes   During the early postpartal period the soft tissue in and around the perineum may appear edematous with some bruising. If an episiotomy is present, the edges should be drawn together. Occasionally ecchymosis occurs, and this may delay healing.

Recurrence of Ovulation and Menstruation

Approximately 40% of nonnursing mothers resume menstruation in 6 weeks, while 90% resume within 24 weeks after delivery. Of these, approximately 50% ovulate during the first cycle. At 12 weeks after delivery about 45% of the lactating primiparas are menstruating. Among nursing mothers 80% have one or more anovulatory cycles before the first ovulatory one (Danforth, 1982).

Abdomen

Following delivery the stretched abdominal wall appears loose and flabby, but it will respond to exercise within 2–3 months. In the grandmultipara, in the woman in whom overdistention of the abdomen has occurred, or in the woman with poor muscle tone before pregnancy, the abdomen may fail to regain good tone and remain flabby. **Diastasis recti abdominis**, a separation of the abdominal muscle, may occur with pregnancy, especially in women with poor abdominal muscle tone. If diastasis occurs, part of the abdominal wall has no muscular support but is formed only by skin, subcutaneous fat, fascia, and peritoneum. If rectus muscle tone is not regained, support may be inadequate during future pregnancies. This may result in a pendulous abdomen and increased maternal backache. Fortunately, diastasis responds well to exercise. (See p. 580 for a discussion of postpartal exercises.)

Striae (stretch marks), which are caused by stretching and rupture of the elastic fibers of the skin, are red to purple at delivery. These gradually fade and after a time appear as silver or white streaks.

Lactation

During pregnancy, breast development in preparation for lactation results from the influence of both estrogen and progesterone. After delivery, the interplay of maternal hormones leads to the establishment of milk production. This process is described in detail in the section on breast-feeding, p. 583.

Gastrointestinal System

Hunger following delivery is common, and the mother may enjoy a light meal. She may also be quite thirsty and will drink large amounts of fluid. This helps replace fluids lost in labor, in the urine, and through perspiration.

The bowels tend to be sluggish following delivery due to decreased abdominal muscle tone. Women who have had an episiotomy may tend to delay elimination for fear of increasing their pain or in the belief that their stitches will be torn if they bear down. In refusing or delaying the bowel movement, the woman may cause increased constipation and more pain when elimination finally occurs.

Urinary Tract

The postpartal woman has an increased bladder capacity, swelling and bruising of the tissue around the urethra, decreased sensitivity to fluid pressure, and a decreased sensation of bladder filling. Consequently, she is at risk for overdistention, incomplete emptying, and a buildup of residual urine. Women who have had an anesthetic block have inhibited neural functioning of the bladder and are more susceptible to bladder infections.

Puerperal diuresis causes rapid filling of the bladder. Thus adequate bladder elimination is an immediate concern. If stasis exists, chances increase that a urinary tract infection will develop. A full bladder may also increase the tendency toward uterine relaxation by displacing the uterus and interfering with contractility, which may lead to hemorrhage.

In the absence of infection, the dilated ureters and renal pelves will return to prepregnant size by the end of the sixth week.

Vital Signs

A temperature of 38C (100.4F) may occur after delivery as a result of the exertion and dehydration of labor. After the first 24 hours, the woman should be afebrile. Any temperature of 38C (100.4F) or greater would suggest infection.

Blood pressure readings should remain stable after delivery. A decrease may indicate physiologic readjustment to decreased intrapelvic pressure, or it may be related to uterine hemorrhage. Blood pressure elevations, especially when accompanied by headache, suggest PIH, and the woman should be evaluated further.

Puerperal bradycardia with rates of 50–70 beats/min commonly occurs during the first 6–10 days of the postpartal period. It may be related to decreased cardiac effort, the decreased blood volume following placental separation, contraction of the uterus, and increased stroke volume. Tachycardia occurs less frequently and is related to increased blood loss or difficult, prolonged labor and delivery.

Blood Values

The blood values should return to the prepregnant state by the end of the postpartal period. Pregnancy-associated activation of coagulation factors may continue for variable amounts of time. This condition, in conjunction with trauma, immobility, or sepsis, predisposes the woman to development of thromboembolism.

Leukocytosis often occurs, with white blood counts of 15,000–20,000. Hemoglobin and hematocrit values should approximate or exceed prelabor values within 2–6 weeks as normal concentrations are reached. As extracellular fluid is excreted, hemoconcentration occurs with a related rise in hematocrit.

Weight Loss

An initial weight loss of 10–12 lb occurs as a result of the delivery of infant, placenta, and amniotic fluid. Puerperal diuresis accounts for the loss of an additional 5 lb during the early puerperium. By the sixth to eighth week after delivery, the woman has returned to approximately her prepregnant weight if she has gained the average 25–30 pounds.

Postpartal Chill

Frequently the mother experiences a shaking chill immediately after delivery, which is related to a nervous response or to vasomotor changes. If not followed by fever, this chill is not of clinical concern, but it is uncomfortable for the woman. Many hospitals cover the woman with warmed bath blankets to alleviate the chill. The mother may also find a warm beverage helpful. Later in the puerperium, chill and fever indicate infection and require further evaluation.

Postpartal Diaphoresis

The elimination of excess fluid and waste products via the skin during the puerperium produces greatly increased perspiration. Diaphoretic episodes frequently occur at night, and the woman may awaken drenched with perspiration. This perspiration is not significant clinically, but the mother should be protected from chilling.

Afterpains

Afterpains more commonly occur in multiparas than primiparas and are caused by intermittent uterine contractions. Although the uterus of the primipara usually remains consistently contracted, the lost tone of the multiparous uterus results in alternate contraction and relaxation. This phenomenon also occurs if the uterus has been markedly distended, as with multiple pregnancies or hydramnios, or if clots or placental fragments were retained. These afterpains may cause the mother severe discomfort for 2–3 days following delivery. The administration of oxytocic agents stimulates uterine contraction and increases the discomfort of the afterpains. Because oxytocin is released when the infant suckles, breast-feeding also increases the severity of the afterpains. The nursing mother may find it helpful to take a mild analgesic approximately one hour before feeding her infant. An analgesic is also helpful at bedtime if the afterpains interfere with the mother's rest.

Psychologic Adaptations

Reva Rubin (1961) has identified two stages of emotional adjustment that occur in the postpartal period as the woman reverses the inward focus that characterized labor and slowly resumes her normal role and functions. During this period the woman also accepts the new responsibilities resulting from the birth of her child. The **taking-in phase** lasts for 2–3 days following delivery and is characterized by maternal passivity and dependence. The mother is hesitant about making decisions and somewhat preoccupied with her own needs. Food and sleep are major concerns for her.

The **taking-hold phase** begins on the second or third day after delivery as the mother resumes control of her life. She may be concerned about control of her bodily functions such as elimination. If she is breast-feeding she may worry about the quality of her milk and her ability to nurse her baby. She requires assurance that she is doing well as a mother. If her baby spits up following a feeding she may see this occurrence as a personal failure. She may also feel demoralized by the fact that nurses handle her baby proficiently while she still feels unsure and tentative.

A study by Martell and Mitchell (1984) suggests that today's new mothers tend to be less dependent and better able to assume self-care responsibilities early in the postpartum period. They suggest that nurses should examine Rubin's concepts carefully and more skeptically in light of current trends in maternity care. It will be interesting to see what further study brings to this subject.

The "postpartum blues" consist of a transient period of depression that often occurs during the first few days of the puerperium. It may be manifested by tearfulness, anorexia, difficulty in sleeping, and a feeling of letdown. This depression frequently occurs while the woman is still hospitalized, but it may occur at home, too. Psychologic adjustments and hormonal factors are thought to be the main cause, although fatigue, discomfort, and overstimulation may play a part.

Cultural Influences

Many cultures emphasize certain postpartal routines or rituals for mother and baby. Frequently, these are designed to restore harmony or the hot–cold balance of the body. For many Mexican Americans, Black Americans, and Orientals, cold is avoided after delivery. This prohibition includes cold air, wind, and all water (even if heated). Dietary changes also reflect the need to avoid cold foods and restore the balance between hot and cold (Horn, 1981).

The nurse caring for a mother during the postpartal period carefully assesses the family's beliefs and practices and adapts to them whenever possible. Family members can be encouraged to bring preferred food and drink, and client care can be modified somewhat to accommodate traditional beliefs.

The extended family frequently plays an essential role during the puerperium. The grandmother is often the primary helper to the mother and her newborn. She brings wisdom and experience, allowing the new mother time to rest, as well as giving her ready access to someone who can help with problems and concerns as they arise. It is imperative to include members who have authority in the family. Visiting rules may be waived to allow family members or authority figures access to the mother and newborn. These practices show respect, and the nurse may gain an ally in the care of the mother and baby, especially if the mother follows the advice of her cultural mentor. Nurses can work for a blending of old and new behaviors to meet the goals of all concerned.

Development of Attachment _____

A mother's first interaction with her infant is influenced by many factors, including participation in her family of origin, her relationships, the stability of her home environment, the communication patterns she developed, and the degree of nurturing she received as a child. These factors have shaped the self she has become. Certain characteristics of that self are also important:

- Level of trust. What level of trust has this mother developed in response to her life experiences? What is her philosophy of childrearing? Will she be able to treat her infant as a unique individual with changing needs that should be gratified as much as possible?

- Level of self-esteem. How much does she value herself as a woman and as a mother? Does she feel generally able to cope with the adjustments of life?

- Capacity for enjoying oneself. Is the mother able to find pleasure in everyday activities and human relationships?

- Interest in and adequacy of knowledge about childbearing and childrearing. What beliefs about the course of pregnancy, the capacities of newborns, and the nature of her emotions may influence her behavior at first contact with her infant and later?

- Her prevailing mood or usual feeling tone. Is the woman predominantly content, angry, depressed, or anxious? Is she sensitive to her own feelings and those of others? Will she be able to accept her own needs and to obtain support in meeting them?

- Reactions to the present pregnancy. Was the pregnancy planned? Did it go smoothly? Were there ongoing life events that enhanced her pregnancy or depleted her reserves of energy?

By the time of delivery each mother has developed an emotional orientation of some kind to the fetus based on these factors, as well as a physical awareness of the fetus within her and her fantasy images and perceptions. However, a large part of her postpartal adjustment relates to the new arrival in the family, who until the moment of birth is essentially an unknown factor in the equation.

Introductory Attachment

A fairly regular pattern of maternal behaviors is exhibited at first contact with a normal newborn (Klaus et al., 1970). In a progression of touching activities, the mother proceeds from fingertip exploration of the newborn's extremities toward palmar contact with larger body areas and finally to enfolding the infant with the whole hand and arms. The time taken to accomplish these steps varies from minutes to days, depending, it appears, on the timing of the first contact, the clothing barriers present, and the physical condition of the baby. Maternal excitement and elation tend to increase during the time of the initial meeting. The mother also increases the proportion of time spent in the

en face position (Figure 23-2). She arranges herself or the newborn so that she has direct face-to-face and eye-to-eye contact. There is an intense interest in having the infant's eyes open. When the eyes are open, the mother characteristically greets the newborn and talks in high-pitched tones to him or her.

In most instances the mother relies heavily on her senses of sight, touch, and hearing in getting to know what her baby is really like. She tends also to respond verbally to any sounds emitted by the newborn, such as cries, coughs, sneezes, and grunts. The sense of smell may also be involved, although this possibility has not yet been adequately studied.

In addition to acting on and interacting with the newborn, the mother is undergoing her own emotional reactions to the whole happening and, more specifically, to the baby as she perceives him or her. The frequency of the "I can't

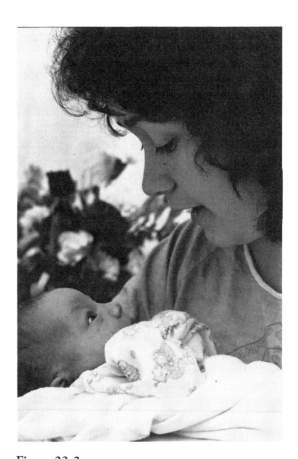

Figure 23-2
En face position.

believe" reaction leads to the speculation that human gains as well as losses may initially be met with a degree of shock, disbelief, and denial. A feeling of emotional distance from the newborn is quite common: "I felt he was a stranger." On the other hand, feelings of connectedness between the newborn and the rest of the family can be expressed in positive or negative terms: "She's got your cute nose, Daddy" or "Oh, God, no! He looks just like the first one, and he was an impossible baby." A mother's facial expressions or the frequency and content of her questions may demonstrate concerns about the infant's general condition or normality, especially if her pregnancy was complicated or if a previously delivered baby was not normal.

What are the characteristic behaviors of a newborn? Unless care is taken to effect a gentle birth, a number of harsh stimuli assault the senses of the newly born neonate. The newborn is probably suctioned, held with head down somewhat, exposed to bright lights and cool air, and in some way cleaned. The infant usually responds by crying. In fact, newborns are typically stimulated to cry to reassure the caretakers that they are well and normal. When newborns no longer need to concentrate most of their energy in physical and physiologic response to the immediate crisis of birth, they are able to lie quietly with eyes open, looking about, moving limbs occasionally, making sucking motions, possibly attempting to get hand to mouth. Placed in appropriate proximity to the mother, the neonate appears to focus briefly on her face and to attend to her voice repeatedly in the first moments. When their mother is talking and neonates are listening, they are likely to move parts of their body—arms, legs, fingers, eyelids—in an exact synchrony with their mother's minute voice changes (Condon and Sander, 1974). This synchrony between rhythms of speech and body movements of an infant can clearly be seen only with stop-frame analysis of films, but the mother probably has, at some level, an awareness of its occurrence.

During the first few days following her infant's birth, the new mother applies herself to the task of getting to know her baby. This is termed the *acquaintance phase*. If the infant gives clear behavioral cues about needs, the infant's responses to mothering will be predictable, which will make the mother feel effective and competent. Other behaviors that make an infant more attractive to caretakers are smiling, grasping a finger, nursing eagerly, cuddling, and being easy to console.

During this time the newborn is also becoming acquainted. Within a few days after birth, infants show signs of recognizing recurrent situations and responding to changes in routine. To the extent that the world is their mother, it can be said that they are actively acquainting themselves with her.

During the *phase of mutual regulation* mother and infant seek to deal with the issue of the degree of control to be exerted by each partner in their relationship. In this phase of adjustment, a balance is sought between the needs of the mother and the needs of the infant. The most important consideration is that each should obtain a good measure of enjoyment from the interaction. During the mutual adjustment phase negative maternal feelings are likely to surface or intensify. Because "everyone knows that mothers love their babies," these negative feelings often go unexpressed and are allowed to build up. If they are expressed, the response of friends, relatives, or health care personnel is often to deny the feelings to the mother: "You don't mean that." Some negative feelings are normal in the first few days following delivery, and the nurse should be supportive when the mother vocalizes these feelings.

When mutual regulation arrives at the point where both mother and infant primarily enjoy each other's company, reciprocity has been achieved. *Reciprocity* is an interactional cycle that occurs simultaneously between mother and infant (Brazelton et al., 1974). It involves mutual cuing behaviors, expectancy, rhythmicity, and synchrony. The development of reciprocity between a mother and her infant is evidence of the bond of attachment that has formed between them. It enables the mother to let go of the infant she knew as a fetus during pregnancy. A new relationship now develops with an individual who has a unique character and who evokes a response entirely different from the fantasy response of pregnancy. When reciprocity is synchronous, the interaction between mother and infant is mutually gratifying and is sought and initiated by both partners. They find pleasure and delight in each other's company and grow in mutual love.

Father–Infant Interactions

Traditionally, the primary role of the expectant father has been one of support for the pregnant woman. Commitment to family-centered maternity care, however, fostered interest in understanding the feelings and experiences of the new father. Evidence suggests that the father has a strong attraction to his newborn and that the feelings he experiences are similar to the mother's feelings of attachment (Figure 23-3). The characteristic sense of absorption, preoccupation, and interest in the infant demonstrated by fathers during early contact with their infants has been termed **engrossment** (Greenberg and Morris, 1974).

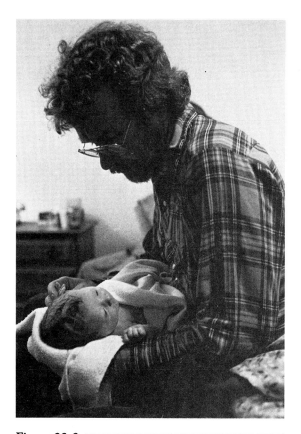

Figure 23-3 ▬▬▬▬▬▬▬
The bond between father and infant develops.

Siblings and Others

Recent work with infants has shown that they are capable of maintaining a number of strong attachments without loss of quality. These attachments may include siblings, grandparents, aunts, and uncles. The social setting and personality of the individual seem to be significant factors in the development of multiple attachments. The advent of open visiting hours and rooming-in permits siblings and grandparents to participate in the attachment process.

Postpartal Nursing Assessment ▬▬▬▬▬▬▬

Comprehensive care is based on a thorough assessment that identifies individual needs or potential problems. (See the accompanying Postpartal Physical Assessment Guide.)

Risk Factors

The emphasis on ongoing assessment and client education during the puerperium is designed to meet the needs of the childbearing family and to detect and treat possible complications. Table 23-1 identifies factors that may place the new mother at risk during the postpartal period. The nurse uses this knowledge during the assessment and is particularly alert for possible complications that may occur in an individual because of identified risk factors.

Physical Assessment

Several principles should be remembered in preparing for and completing the assessment of the postpartal woman.

- Select the time that will provide the most accurate data. Palpating the fundus when the woman has a full bladder, for example, may give false information about the progress of involution.

- An explanation of the purpose of regular assessment should be given to the woman.

- The woman should be relaxed, and the procedures should be done as gently as possible to avoid unnecessary discomfort.

- The data obtained should be recorded and reported as clearly as possible.

POSTPARTAL PHYSICAL ASSESSMENT GUIDE

Assess/normal findings	Alterations and possible causes*	Nursing responses to data†
VITAL SIGNS		
Blood pressure: Should remain consistent with baseline BP during pregnancy	High BP (PIH, essential hypertension, renal disease, anxiety) Drop in BP (may be normal; uterine hemorrhage)	Evaluate history of preexisting disorders and check for other signs of PIH Assess for other signs of hemorrhage
Pulse: 50–90 beats/min May be bradycardia of 50–70 beats/min	Tachycardia (difficult labor and delivery, hemorrhage)	Evaluate for other signs of hemorrhage
Respirations: 16–24/min	Marked tachypnea (respiratory disease)	Assess for other signs of respiratory disease
Temperature: 36.2–38C(98–100.4F)	After first 24 hr, temperature of 38C (100.4F) or above suggests infection	Assess for other signs of infection; notify physician
BREASTS		
General appearance: Smooth, even pigmentation, changes of pregnancy still apparent; one may appear larger	Reddened area (mastitis)	Assess further for signs of infection
Palpation: Depending on postpartal day—may be soft, filling, full or engorged	Palpable mass (caked breast, mastitis) Engorgement (venous stasis) Tenderness, heat, edema (engorgement, caked breast, mastitis)	Assess for other signs of infection: if blocked duct consider heat, massage, position change for breast-feeding See interventions for engorgement on pp. 584 and 589 Assess for further signs Report mastitis to physician
Nipples: Supple, pigmented, intact; become erect when stimulated	Fissures, cracks, soreness (problems with breast-feeding), not erectile with stimulation (inverted nipples)	Reassess technique; recommend appropriate interventions See p. 588 for appropriate interventions for nursing mothers
ABDOMEN		
Musculature: Abdomen may be soft, have a "doughy" texture; rectus muscle intact	Separation in musculature (diastasis rectus)	Evaluate size of diastasis; teach appropriate exercises for decreasing the separation
Fundus: Firm, midline; following appropriate schedule of involution	Boggy (full bladder, uterine bleeding)	Massage until firm; assess bladder and have woman void; attempt to express clots when firm If bogginess remains or recurs, report to physician
May be tender when palpated	Constant tenderness (infection)	Assess for evidence of endometritis
LOCHIA		
Scant to moderate amount, earthy odor; no clots	Large amount, clots (hemorrhage) Foul-smelling lochia (infection)	Assess for firmness, express additional clots; begin peri-pad count Assess for other signs of infection; report to physician
Normal progression: First 1–3 days—rubra Days 3–10—serosa (Alba seldom seen in hospital)	Failure to progress normally or return to rubra from serosa (subinvolution)	Report to physician
PERINEUM		
Slight edema and bruising in intact perineum	Marked fullness, bruising, pain (vulvar hematoma)	Assess size; apply ice glove; report to physician

*Possible causes of alterations are placed in parentheses.
†This column provides guidelines for further assessment and initial nursing actions.

POSTPARTAL PHYSICAL ASSESSMENT GUIDE (continued)

Assess/normal findings	Alterations and possible causes*	Nursing responses to data†
Episiotomy: No redness, edema, ecchymosis, discharge, edges well-approximated	Redness, edema, ecchymosis, discharge, or gaping stitches (infection)	Encourage sitz baths, review perineal care, appropriate wiping techniques
Hemorrhoids: None present; if present, should be small and nontender	Full, tender, inflamed hemorrhoids	Encourage sitz baths, side-lying position; tucks pads, anesthetic ointments, manual replacement of hemorrhoids; stool softeners, increased fluid intake
CVA TENDERNESS		
None	Present (kidney infection)	Assess for other symptoms of UTI; obtain clean catch urine; report to physician
LOWER EXTREMITIES		
No pain with palpation; negative Homan's sign	Positive findings (thrombophlebitis)	Report to physician
ELIMINATION		
Urinary output: Voiding in sufficient quantities at least every 4–6 hr; bladder not palpable	Inability to void (urinary retention) Symptoms of urgency, frequency, dysuria (UTI)	Employ nursing interventions to promote voiding; if not successful obtain order for catheterization Report symptoms of UTI to physician
Bowel elimination: Should have normal bowel movement by second or third day after delivery	Inability to pass feces (constipation due to fear of pain from episiotomy, hemorrhoids, perineal trauma)	Encourage fluids, ambulation, roughage in diet; sitz baths to promote healing of perineum; obtain order for stool softener

*Possible causes of alterations are placed in parentheses.
†This column provides guidelines for further assessment and initial nursing actions.

While the nurse is performing the physical assessment, she should also be teaching the woman. When the nurse is assessing breast milk production, the letdown reflex and breast self-examination can be discussed. Mothers are very receptive to instruction on postpartal abdominal tightening exercises when the nurse assesses the woman's fundal height and diastasis. The assessment also provides an excellent time to teach her about the body's physical and anatomic changes postpartally as well as danger signs to report. (See Essential Facts to Remember for information on common postpartal concerns.)

Breasts   Beginning with the breasts, the nurse should first assess the fit and support provided by the bra. A properly fitting bra provides support to the breasts and helps maintain breast shape by limiting stretching of supporting ligaments and connective tissue. If the mother is breast-feeding, the straps of the bra should be cloth, not elastic, and easily adjustable. The back should be wide and have at least three rows of hooks to adjust for fit. Traditional nursing bras have a fixed inner cup and a separate half cup that can be unhooked for breast-feeding while continuing to support the breast. Purchasing a bra one size too large during pregnancy will usually result in a good fit because the breasts increase in size with milk production.

The bra is then removed so the breasts can be examined. The nurse notes the size and shape of the breasts and any abnormalities, reddened areas or engorgement. The breasts are also lightly palpated for heat, engorgement, tenderness, or caking. The nipples are assessed for fissures, cracks, soreness, or inversion.

The nonnursing mother is assessed for evidence of breast discomfort, and relief measures are taken if necessary. (See discussion of lactation suppression in the nonnursing mother on p. 583.)

Table 23-1
Postpartal High-Risk Factors

Factors	Maternal implications
PIH (Preeclampsia-eclampsia)	↑ Blood pressure
	↑ CNS irritability
	↑ Need for bedrest → ↑ risk thrombophlebitis
Diabetes	Need for insulin regulation
	Episodes of hypoglycemia or hyperglycemia
	↓ Healing
Cardiac disease	↑ Maternal exhaustion
Cesarean birth	↑ Healing needs
	↑ Pain from incision
	↑ Risk infection
	↑ Length of hospitalization
Overdistention of uterus (multiple gestation, hydramnios)	↑ Risk hemorrhage
	↑ Risk anemia
	↑ Stretching of abdominal muscles
	↑ Incidence and severity of afterpains
Abruptio placentae or placenta previa	Hemorrhage → anemia
	↓ Uterine contractility after delivery → ↑ infection risk
Precipitous labor (<3 hours)	↑ Risk lacerations to birth canal → hemorrhage
Prolonged labor	Exhaustion
	↑ Risk hemorrhage
	Nutritional and fluid depletion
	↑ Bladder atony and/or trauma
Difficult delivery	Exhaustion
	↑ Risk perineal lacerations
	↑ Risk hematomas
	↑ Risk hemorrhage → anemia
Extended period of time in stirrups at delivery	↑ Risk thrombophlebitis
Retained placenta	↑ Risk hemorrhage
	↑ Risk infection

 ESSENTIAL FACTS TO REMEMBER

Common Postpartal Concerns

Several postpartal occurrences cause special concern for mothers. The nurse will frequently be asked about the following events.

Source of concern	Explanation
Gush of blood that sometimes occurs when she first arises	Due to pooling of blood in vagina. Gravity causes it to flow out when she stands.
Night sweats	Normal physiologic occurrence that results as body attempts to eliminate excess fluids that were present during pregnancy. May be aggravated by plastic mattress pad.
Afterpains	More common in multiparas. Due to contraction and relaxation of uterus. Increased by oxytocins, breast-feeding. Relieved with mild analgesics and time.
"Large stomach" after delivery and failure to lose all weight	Products of conception account for only a portion of the weight gained during pregnancy. The remainder takes approximately 6 weeks to lose. Abdomen also appears large due to ↓ tone. Postpartal exercises will help.

Abdomen and fundus   Before examination of the abdomen, the woman should void. This practice assures that a full bladder is not causing any uterine atony; if atony is present, other causes must be investigated.

The nurse determines the relationship of the fundus to the umbilicus and also assesses the firmness of the fundus. The nurse notes whether the fundus is in the midline or displaced to either side of the abdomen. The most common cause of displacement is a full bladder. Thus this finding requires further assessment. The results of the assessment should then be recorded. (See Procedure 23-1.)

Following the uterine assessment and prior to assessing the lochia, the nurse examines for diastasis recti. The separation in the rectus muscle is evaluated according to its length and width. The separation is palpated first just below the umbilicus, and the width is ascertained. Then the separation is palpated for length toward the symphysis pubis and toward the xiphoid process. If palpation is difficult due to abdominal relaxation, the woman is asked to lift her head unassisted by the nurse. This action contracts the rectus muscles and more clearly defines their edges.

Methods of charting these results vary from institution to institution. Some prefer recording the diastasis measured from the umbilicus down and then from the umbilicus up:

Diastasis: U ↓ 4 cm by 1 cm

U ↑ 2 cm by 1 cm

Others prefer recording the entire length:

Diastasis: 6 cm by 1 cm

Either method is acceptable.

In the woman who has had a cesarean birth, the abdominal incision should be inspected for any signs of infection, including drainage, foul odor, or redness.

Lochia   The next aspect to be evaluated is the lochia, which is assessed for character, amount, odor, and the presence of clots. During the first 1–3 days the lochia should be rubra. A few small clots are normal and occur as a result of blood pooling in the vagina. However, the passage of numerous or large clots is abnormal, and the cause should be investigated immediately. After 2–3 days, the lochia becomes serosa.

Lochia should never exceed a moderate amount, such as four to eight peri-pads daily, with an average of six. However, because this is influenced by an individual woman's pad-changing practices, she should be questioned about the length of time the current pad has been in use, whether the amount is normal, and whether any clots were passed prior to this examination, such as during voiding. If heavy bleeding is reported but not seen, the woman is asked to put on a clean perineal pad and is then reassessed in one hour. Clots and heavy bleeding may be caused by uterine atony or retained placental fragments and require further assessment. Because of the evacuation of the uterine cavity during cesarean delivery, women with such surgery have less lochia after the first 24 hours than mothers who deliver vaginally.

The odor of the lochia is nonoffensive and never foul. If foul odor is present, so is an infection.

The amount of lochia is charted first, followed by character. For example:

• Lochia: moderate amount rubra

• Lochia: small rubra/serosa

Perineum   The perineum is inspected with the woman lying in a Sims' position. The buttock is lifted to expose the perineum and anus. If an episiotomy was done or a laceration required suturing, the wound is assessed. The state of healing is evaluated by observing for redness, edema, ecchymosis, discharge, and approximation—the REEDA scale (Davidson, 1974). (See Table 25-1.)

After 24 hours some edema may still be present, but the skin edges should be "glued" together (well approximated) so that gentle pressure does not separate them. Gentle palpation should elicit minimal tenderness and there should be no hardened areas suggesting infection. Ecchymosis interferes with normal healing, as does infection.

Foul odors associated with drainage indicate infection. Further observation of the incision for separation should also be made.

The nurse next assesses the state of any hemorrhoids present around the anus for size, number, and pain or tenderness.

PROCEDURE 23-1
Assessing the Fundus

Objective	Nursing action	Rationale
Prepare woman	Explain procedure; have the woman void; position woman flat in bed with head comfortably positioned on a pillow; if the procedure is uncomfortable, woman may flex legs.	Having the woman void assures that a full bladder is not causing any uterine atony. Having woman flat prevents falsely high assessment of fundal height. Flexing the legs relaxes the abdominal muscles. The uterus may be tender if frequent massage has been necessary.
Determine uterine firmness	Gently place one hand on the lower segment of the uterus; using the side of the other hand, palpate the abdomen until the top of the fundus is located. Determine whether the fundus is firm. If it is not firm, massage until firm.	Provides support for uterus. Provides a larger surface for palpation and is less uncomfortable for the woman. A firm fundus indicates that the muscles are contracted and bleeding will not occur.
Determine the height of the fundus	Measure the height of the fundus in fingerbreadths. If the fundal height is more than one fingerbreadth in either direction, use additional fingers. (See Figure 23-4.)	Fundal height gives information about the progress of involution.
Ascertain position	Determine whether fundus is deviated from the midline.	Fundus may be deviated when bladder is full.
Record findings	Fundal height is recorded in fingerbreadths; example: 2 FB ↓ U; 1 FB ↑ U. If massage had been necessary it could be recorded as: Uterus: boggy → firm c̄ light massage	Allows for consistency of reporting among caregivers.

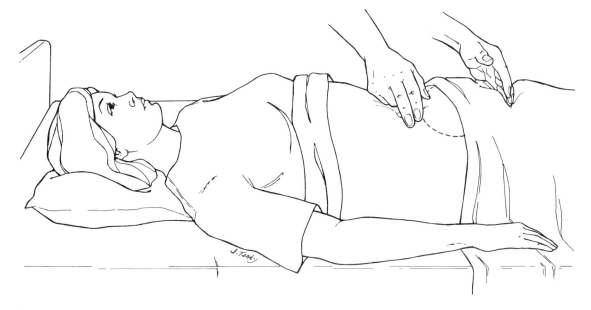

Figure 23-4
Measurement of descent of fundus. The fundus is located two fingerbreadths below the umbilicus.

Lower extremities   If thrombophlebitis occurs, the most likely site will be in the woman's legs. To assess for this, her legs should be stretched out straight and should be relaxed. The foot is then grasped and sharply dorsiflexed. No discomfort or pain should be present. If pain is elicited, the nurse–midwife or physician is notified that the woman has a positive Homan's sign (Figure 23-5). The pain is caused by inflammation of the vessel. The legs are also evaluated for edema. This may be done by comparing both legs, since usually only one leg is involved. Any areas of redness, tenderness, and increased skin temperature should also be noted.

Early ambulation is an important aspect in the prevention of thrombophlebitis. Most women are able to be up shortly after delivery. The cesarean birth client requires passive range of motion exercises until she is ambulating more freely.

Vital signs assessment   Alterations in vital signs may indicate complications, so they are assessed at regular intervals. The blood pressure should remain stable, while the pulse often shows a characteristic slowness that is no cause for alarm. Pulse rates return to prepregnant norms very quickly unless complications arise.

Temperature elevations (less than 38C (100.4F)) due to normal processes should last for only a few days and should not be associated with other clinical signs of infection. Any elevation should be evaluated in light of other signs and symptoms. The woman's history should also be carefully reviewed to identify other factors, such as PROM or prolonged labor, which might increase the incidence of infection in the genital tract.

Nutritional status   Determination of postpartal nutritional status is based primarily on information provided by the mother and on direct assessment. During pregnancy the recommended daily dietary allowances call for increases in calories, proteins, and most vitamins and minerals. After delivery, the nonnursing mother's dietary requirements return to prepregnancy levels (Food and Nutrition Board, 1980).

Visiting the mothers during mealtime provides an opportunity for unobtrusive nutritional assessment and counseling. The nonnursing mother should be advised about the need to reduce her caloric intake by about 300 cal and to return to prepregnancy levels for other nutrients. The nursing mother, on the other hand, should increase her caloric intake by

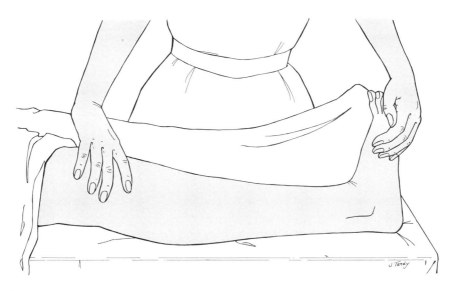

Figure 23-5

Homan's sign. While holding the woman's knee flat, the nurse dorsiflexes the woman's foot. Pain in the woman's foot or leg is indicative of a positive Homan's sign.

about 200 cal over the pregnancy requirements. Basic discussion will prove helpful, followed by referral as needed. In all cases, literature on nutrition should be provided so that the woman will have a source of information following discharge.

The dietitian should be informed of any mother whose cultural or religious beliefs require specific foods. Appropriate meals can then be prepared for her. Many women, especially those who gained excessively, are interested in losing weight after delivery. The dietitian can design weight-reduction diets to meet nutritional needs and food preferences. The nurse may also refer women with unusual eating habits or numerous questions about good nutrition to the dietitian.

New mothers are also advised that it is common practice to prescribe iron supplements for 4–6 weeks after delivery. The hematocrit is then checked at the postpartal visit to detect any anemia.

Elimination   During the hours after delivery the nurse carefully monitors a new mother's bladder status. A boggy uterus, a displaced uterus, or a palpable bladder are signs of bladder distention and require nursing intervention.

The postpartal woman should be encouraged to void every 4–6 hours. The bladder should be assessed for distention until the woman demonstrates complete emptying of the bladder with each voiding. The nurse may employ techniques to facilitate voiding, such as helping the woman out of bed to void or pouring warm water on the perineum. Catheterization is required when the bladder is distended and the woman cannot void or if no voiding has occurred in 8 hours. The cesarean birth mother may have an indwelling catheter inserted prophylactically. The same considerations should be made in evaluating bladder emptying once the catheter is removed.

During the physical assessment the nurse elicits information from the woman regarding the adequacy of her fluid intake, whether she feels she is emptying her bladder completely when she voids, and any signs of urinary tract infection she may be experiencing.

In the same way the nurse obtains information about the new mother's intestinal elimination and any concerns she may have about it. Many mothers fear that the first bowel movement will be painful and possibly even damaging if an episiotomy has been done. Stool softeners may be ordered to increase bulk and moisture in the fecal material and to allow more comfortable and complete evacuation. Constipation is avoided to prevent pressure on sutures that may increase discomfort. Encouraging ambulation, forcing fluids, and providing fresh fruits and roughage in the diet enhance bowel elimination and assist the woman in reestablishing her normal bowel pattern.

Rest and sleep status   As part of the postpartal assessment, the nurse evaluates the amount of rest a new mother is getting. If the woman reports difficulty sleeping at night, cause should be determined. If it is simply the strange hospital environment, a warm drink, backrub, or mild sedative may prove helpful. Appropriate nursing measures are indicated if the woman is bothered by normal postpartal discomforts such as afterpains, diaphoresis, or episiotomy or hemorrhoidal pain.

A daily rest period should be encouraged and hospital activities should be scheduled to allow time for napping.

Psychologic Assessment

Adequate assessment of the mother's psychologic adjustment is an integral part of postpartal evaluation. This assessment focuses on the mother's general attitude, feelings of competence, available support systems, and caregiving skills. It also evaluates her fatigue level, sense of satisfaction, and ability to accomplish her developmental tasks.

Fatigue is often a highly significant factor in a new mother's apparent disinterest in her newborn. Frequently the woman is so tired from a long labor and delivery that everything seems to be an effort. To avoid inadvertently classifying a very tired mother as one with a potential attachment problem, the nurse should do the psychologic assessment on more than one occasion. After a nap the new mother is often far more receptive to her infant and her surroundings.

Some new mothers have little or no experience with infants and may feel totally overwhelmed. They may show these feelings by asking questions and reading all available material or by becoming passive and quiet because they simply cannot deal with their feelings of inadequacy. Unless a nurse questions the woman about her plans and previous experience in a supportive, nonjudgmental way, one might conclude that the woman was disinterested, withdrawn, or depressed. Problem clues might include excessive continued fatigue, marked depression, excessive preoccupation with physical status and/or discomfort, evidence of low self-esteem, lack of support systems, marital problems, inability to care for or nurture the newborn, and current family crises (such as illness, unemployment, and so on). These characteristics frequently indicate a potential for maladaptive parenting, which may lead to child abuse or neglect (physical, emotional, intellectual) and cannot be ignored. Referrals to public health nurses or other available community resources may provide greatly needed assistance and alleviate potentially dangerous situations.

Assessment of Early Attachment

If attachment is accepted as a desired outcome of nursing care, a nurse in any of the various postpartal settings can periodically observe and note progress toward attachment. The following questions can be addressed in the course of nurse–client interaction:

1. Is the mother attracted to her newborn? To what extent does she seek face-to-face contact and eye contact? Has she progressed from fingertip touch, to palmar contact, to enfolding the infant close to her own body? Is attraction increasing or decreasing? If the mother does not exhibit increasing attraction, why not? Do the reasons lie primarily within her, in the baby, or in the environment?

2. Is the mother inclined to nurture her infant? Is she progressing in her interactions with her infant? Has she selected a rooming-in arrangement if it is available?

3. Does the mother act consistently? If not, is the source of unpredictability within her or her infant?

4. Is her mothering intelligently carried out? Does she seek information and evaluate it objectively? Does she develop solutions based on adequate knowledge of valid data? Does she evaluate the effectiveness of her maternal care and make appropriate adjustments?

5. Is she sensitive to the newborn's needs as they arise? How quickly does she interpret her infant's behavior and react to cues? Does she seem happy and satisfied with the infant's responses to her efforts? Is she pleased with feeding behaviors? How much of this ability and willingness to respond is related to the baby's nature and how much to her own?

6. Does she seem pleased with her baby's appearance and sex? Is she experiencing pleasure in interaction with her infant? What interferes with the enjoyment? Does she speak to the baby frequently and affectionately? Does she call him or her by name? Does she point out family traits or characteristics she sees in the newborn?

7. Are there any cultural factors that might modify the mother's response? For instance, is it customary for the grandmother to assume most of the child care responsibilities while the mother recovers from childbirth?

When these questions are addressed and the facts have been assembled by the nurse, the nurse's intuitive feelings and formal background of knowledge should combine to answer three more questions: Is there a problem in attachment? What is the problem? What is its source? Each nurse can then devise a creative approach to the problem as it presents itself in the context of a unique developing mother–infant relationship.

Summary

The postpartal period is a time of readjustment. A thorough knowledge of the physiologic and psychologic changes that occur during this time is essential if the nurse is to make accurate assessments and plan high-quality care. In addition, the nurse must be knowledgeable about each woman's history and the course of her pregnancy, labor, and delivery and the current status of the newborn. In this way the nurse will have the information necessary to individualize nursing care for each postpartal woman.

References

Brazelton TB et al: The origins of reciprocity: The early mother infant interaction. In: *The Effect of the Infant on Its Caregiver,* Lewis M, Rosenblum LA (editors). New York: Wiley, 1974.

Condon WS, Sander LW: Synchrony demonstrated between movements of the neonate and adult speech. *Child Dev* 1974; 45:456.

Danforth DN: *Obstetrics and Gynecology,* 4th ed. Philadelphia: Harper & Row, 1982.

Davidson N: REEDA: Evaluating postpartum healing. *J Nurse-Midwifery* 1974; 9(2):6.

Food and Nutrition Board, National Academy of Sciences—National Research Council: *Recommended Dietary Allowances,* 9th ed., Washington DC, 1980.

Greenberg M, Morris N: Engrossment: The newborn's impact upon the father. *Am J Orthopsychiatry* 1974; 44:520.

Horn BM: Cultural concepts and postpartal care. *Nurs Health Care* 1981; 2:516.

Klaus MH et al: Human maternal behavior at first contact with her young. *Pediatrics* 1970; 46:187.

Loebl S, Spratto G: *The Nurse's Drug Handbook,* 3rd ed. New York: John Wiley, 1983.

Martell LK, Mitchell SK: Rubin's puerperal change reconsidered. *J Obstet Gynecol Neonatal Nurs* May/June 1984; 13(3):145.

Rubin R: Puerperal change. *Nurs Outlook* 1961; 9:753.

Additional Readings

Dean PG, Morgan P, Towle JM: Making baby's acquaintance: A unique attachment strategy. *MCN* January/February 1982; 7:37.

Grace JT: Does a mother's knowledge of fetal gender affect attachment? *MCN* January/February 1984; 9:42.

Hangsleben KL: Transition to fatherhood: An exploratory study. *J Obstet Gynecol Neonatal Nurs* July/August 1983; 12(4):265.

Ketter DE, Shelton BJ: In-hospital exercises for the postpartal woman. *MCN* March/April 1983; 8:120.

Mitchell K, Mills NM: Is the sensitive period in parent-infant bonding overrated? *Pediatr Nurs* March/April 1983; 9:91.

Roberts F: Infant behavior and the transition to parenthood. *Nurs Res* July/August 1983; 32:213.

Sheehan F. Assessing postpartum adjustment: A pilot study. *J Obstet Gynecol Neonatal Nurs* January/February 1981; 10:19.

Wadd L: Vietnamese postpartum practices: Implications for nursing in the hospital setting. *J Obstet Gynecol Neonatal Nurs* July/August 1983; 12(4):252.

24

The Postpartal Family: Needs and Care

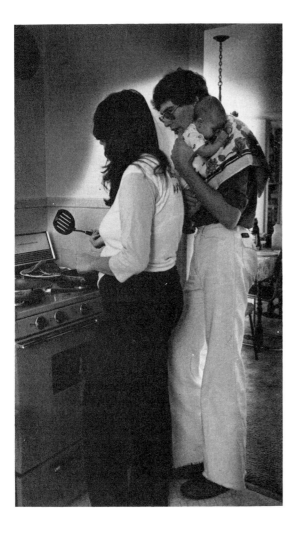

Objectives

• Discuss nursing management of the postpartal family.

• Delineate nursing responsibilities for client education about various newborn feeding methods.

• Describe contraceptive choices available to the postpartal family.

• Discuss the concept of the fourth trimester as it relates to the provision of nursing care for the postpartal family.

Key Terms

cervical cap

colostrum

condom

contraceptive sponge

diaphragm

fertility awareness
  methods

intrauterine devices

letdown reflex

oral contraceptives

oxytocin

prolactin

spermicides

tubal ligation

vasectomy

The information gained during the post-partal assessment enables the nurse to identify potential and existing problems of the postpartal woman and her family. Using this information the nurse is then able to plan more effective nursing care to assist the childbearing family.

Postpartal Nursing Care

The postpartal nursing plan of care is based on the following goals:

- Promotion of comfort and relief of pain
- Promotion of rest and graded activity
- Promotion of maternal psychologic well-being
- Promotion of successful infant feeding
- Promotion of effective parent education
- Promotion of family wellness
- Promotion of parent–infant attachment

Promotion of Comfort and Relief of Pain

Pain may be present to varying degrees in the postpartal woman. Potential sources of pain include an edematous perineum; an episiotomy, laceration, or extension; hematoma; or engorged hemorrhoids.

Women may be taught to tighten their buttocks before sitting to avoid direct trauma to the perineum. Lateral positions may also be more comfortable. Ice packs may be applied to the perineum during the first few hours following delivery. They help decrease edema and also relieve pain.

Perineal care after each elimination cleans the perineum and helps promote comfort. Many agencies provide "peri-bottles," which the woman can use to squirt warm water over the perineum following elimination. The woman should use toilet tissue in a blotting motion and should clean from front to back to prevent contamination of the vulva from the anal area. In addition, to prevent contamination, the perineal pad should be applied from front to back and should be changed after each elimination.

Sitz baths are especially useful with the severely traumatized perineum. Moist heat increases the circulation to decrease edema and promote healing. It also cleans the perineum and is soothing. Sitz baths are usually done at 105F for 20 minutes two to four times a day.

Dry heat in the form of a heat lamp is sometimes used. The perineum should be cleaned first to prevent drying of secretions on the perineum. Heat lamps are generally used for 20 minutes two or three times a day.

Topical anesthetics such as Dermoplast Aerosol Spray or Nupercainal Ointment may be used to relieve perineal discomfort. The woman is advised to apply the anesthetic following a sitz bath or perineal care. Because of the danger of tissue burns she must be cautioned not to apply anesthetic before using a heat lamp.

Afterpains are common postpartally, especially in multiparous and breast-feeding women. For greatest relief, analgesics are administered before the pain is too intense. For breast-feeding mothers, a mild analgesic administered an hour before feeding will promote comfort and enhance maternal–infant interaction.

Some mothers experience hemorrhoidal pain after delivery. Relief measures include the use of sitz baths, anesthetic ointments, rectal suppositories, or witch hazel pads applied directly to the anal area. The woman may be taught to digitally replace external hemorrhoids in her rectum. She may also find it helpful to maintain a side-lying position when possible and to avoid prolonged sitting. The mother is encouraged to maintain an adequate fluid intake, and stool softeners are administered to ensure greater comfort with bowel movements. The hemorrhoids usually disappear a few weeks after delivery if the woman did not have them prior to this pregnancy.

Discomfort may also be caused by immobility. The woman who has been in stirrups for any length of time may experience muscular aches from such extreme positioning. It is not unusual for women to experience joint pains and muscular pain in both arms and legs, depending on the effort they exerted during the second stage of labor.

Breast engorgement may be a source of pain for the postpartal woman. Specific nursing interventions for the bottle-feeding mother are discussed on p. 583. Nursing interventions for the breast-feeding mother with engorgement are discussed on p. 589.

Adequate personal hygiene also helps promote comfort. Because of postpartal diaphoresis a daily shower is refreshing and should be encouraged. The diaphoresis also leads to increased thirst. Thus the woman should have a filled pitcher of cold water on hand and should be offered milk and juice frequently.

Early ambulation is encouraged to help reduce the incidence of complications such as constipation and thrombophlebitis. It also helps promote a feeling of general well-being.

The nurse assists the woman the first few times she gets up during the postpartal period. Fatigue, effects of medications, loss of blood, and possibly even lack of food intake may result in feelings of dizziness or faintness when the woman stands up. Because this may be a problem during the woman's first shower, the nurse should remain in the room, check the woman frequently, and have a chair close by in case she becomes faint. During this first shower the nurse instructs the woman in the use of the emergency call button in the bathroom; if she becomes faint during a future shower, she can call for assistance.

Promotion of Rest and Graded Activity

Following delivery a woman may feel exhausted and in need of rest. In other cases she may be euphoric and full of psychic energy immediately after delivery, ready to relive the experience of birth repeatedly. The nurse can provide a period for airing of feelings and then encourage a period of rest.

Physical fatigue often affects other adjustments and functions of the new mother. For example, fatigue can reduce milk flow, thereby increasing problems with establishing breast-feeding. Energy is also needed to make the psychologic adjustments to a new infant and to assume new roles. Adjustments are most smoothly accomplished when adequate rest is obtained. Nurses can encourage rest by organizing their activities to avoid frequent interruptions for the woman. Rest times should be provided before encounters with the newborn if rooming-in is not used.

Postpartal exercises The woman should be encouraged to begin simple exercises while in the hospital and continue them at home. She is advised that increased lochia or pain means she should reevaluate her activity and make necessary alterations. Most agencies provide a booklet describing suggested postpartal activities. (Exercise routines vary for women undergoing cesarean birth or tubal ligation following delivery.) See Figure 24-1 for a description of some commonly used exercises.

Figure 24-1 ▬▬▬▬▬

Postpartal exercises. Begin with five repetitions two or three times daily and gradually increase to ten repetitions. First day: **A**, Abdominal breathing. Lying supine, inhale deeply, using the abdominal muscles. The abdomen should expand. Then exhale slowly through pursed lips, tightening the abdominal muscles. **B**, Pelvic rocking. Lying supine with arms at sides, knees bent and feet flat, tighten abdomen and buttocks and attempt to flatten back on floor. Hold for a count of ten, then arch the back, causing the pelvis to "rock." On second day add: **C**, Chin to chest. Lying supine with no pillow, legs straight, raise head and attempt to touch chin to chest. Slowly lower head. **D**, Arm raises. Lying supine, arms extended at 90° angle from body, raise arms so they are perpendicular and hands touch. Lower slowly. On fourth day add: **E**, Knee rolls. Lying supine with knees bent, feet flat, arms extended to the side, roll knees slowly to one side, keeping shoulders flat. Return to original position and roll to opposite side. **F**, Buttocks lift. Lying supine, arms at sides, knees bent, feet flat, slowly raise the buttocks and arch the back. Return slowly to starting position. On sixth day add: **G**, Abdominal tighteners. Lying supine, knees bent, feet flat, slowly raise head toward knees. Arms should extend along either side of legs. Return slowly to original position. **H**, Knee to abdomen. Lying supine, arms at sides, bend one knee and thigh until foot touches buttocks. Straighten leg and lower it slowly. Repeat with other leg. After 2–3 weeks, more strenuous exercises such as sit-ups and side leg raises may be added as tolerated. Kegel exercises, begun antepartally, should be done many times daily during postpartum to restore vaginal and perineal tone.

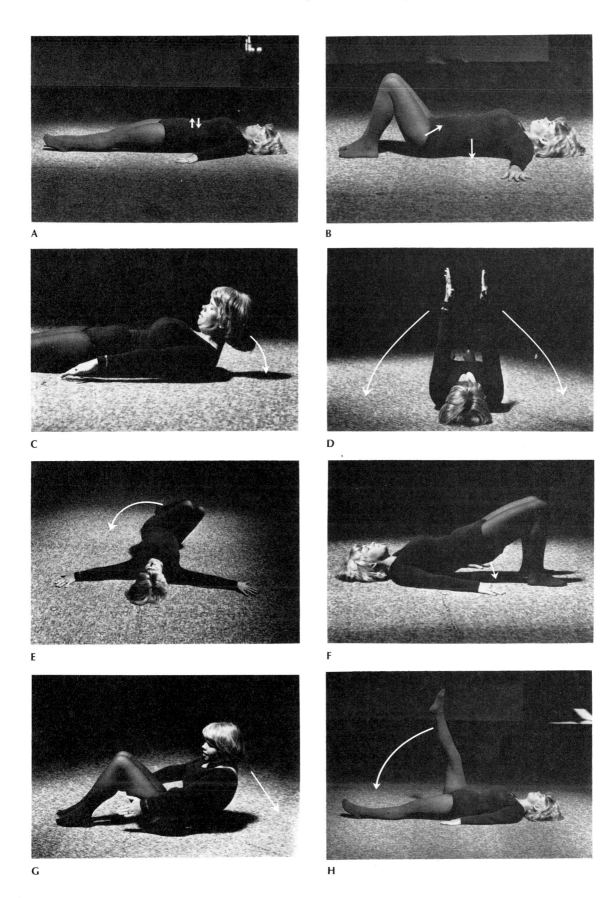

A

B

C

D

E

F

G

H

Resumption of activities   Ambulation and activity may gradually increase after discharge. The new mother should avoid heavy lifting, excessive stair climbing, and strenuous activity. One or two daily naps are essential and are most easily achieved if the mother sleeps when her baby does.

By the second week at home, light housekeeping may be resumed. Although it is customary to delay returning to work for 6 weeks, most women are physically able to resume practically all activities by 4–5 weeks. Delaying returning to work until after the final postpartal examination will minimize the possibility of problems.

Promotion of Maternal Psychologic Well-Being

The birth of a child, with the changes in role and the increased responsibilities it produces, is a time of emotional stress for the new mother. During the early puerperium she is emotionally labile, and mood swings and tearfulness are common.

Initially the mother may repeatedly discuss her experiences in labor and delivery. This allows the mother to integrate her experiences. If she feels that she did not cope well with labor, she may have feelings of inadequacy and may benefit from reassurance that she did well.

During this time the new mother must also adjust to the loss of her fantasized child and accept the child she has borne. This may be more difficult if the child is not of the desired sex or if he or she has birth defects.

During the taking-in period the mother is focused on bodily concerns and may not be fully ready to learn about personal and infant care. However, because early discharge is common, classes and information should be offered and printed handouts provided for reference as questions arise at home.

During the taking-hold phase the mother becomes concerned about her ability to be a successful parent. During this time the mother requires reassurance that she is effective. She also tends to be more receptive to teaching and demonstration designed to assist her in mothering successfully.

The depression and weepiness that characterizes the "postpartum blues" are often a surprise for the new mother. She requires reassurance that these feelings are normal, an explanation about why they occur, and a supportive environment that permits her to cry without feeling guilty.

Promotion of Successful Infant Feeding

Whether the mother has chosen to breast-feed or bottle-feed, the nurse can help the mother have a successful experience while in the hospital and during the early days at home. This is important because the mother's success or nonsuccess may influence her feelings about herself as an adequate mother. There are advantages and disadvantages to both breast-feeding and bottle-feeding and the nurse's primary role is to help the family achieve a positive result with the method they have chosen.

Before feeding, the mother should be made as comfortable as possible. Preparations may include voiding, washing her hands, and assuming a comfortable position.

The cesarean delivery mother needs support so that the infant does not rest on her abdomen for long periods. Thus she may prefer to breast-feed or bottle-feed her infant while lying on her side with a pillow behind her back and one between her legs. The infant may be propped on a pillow or supported by her arm. If she prefers to feed sitting up, a pillow may be placed on her lap for the infant. This avoids direct pressure on her incision. It may also be helpful to place a rolled pillow under the arm supporting the infant's head.

Depending on the newborn's level of hunger, the parents may use the time before feeding to get acquainted with their infant. The nurse should be available during part of the time to answer questions and reinforce effective parenting skills.

For a sleepy baby, a period of playful activity before feeding may increase alertness. Gently rubbing the feet and hands, or loosening coverings to expose the infant to room air may also help wake the infant so that he or she is ready for the feeding and will suck actively.

Cultural considerations in infant feeding   Breast-feeding has been the traditional feeding method for most cultures. However, bottle-feeding has become extremely popular, much to the dismay of older members of some cultures. Navajo elders, for instance, believe that breast-feeding ensures respect and obedience because the child remains close to the mother, while the bottle-fed infant will be more disobedient (Clark, 1981).

Western practices encourage the new mother to breast-feed as soon as possible, but in many cultures (for example, Mexican American, Navajo, Filipino, and Vietnamese) colostrum is not offered to the newborn. Breast-feeding begins only after the milk flow is established. Interestingly, a group of Vietnamese mothers who delayed breast-feeding until the third day after delivery had no difficulty breast-feeding (Ward, Pridmore, and Cox, 1981).

In many Oriental cultures the newborn is given boiled water until the mother's milk flows. The newborn is fed on demand and cries are responded to immediately. If the crying continues, evil spirits may be blamed and a priest's blessing may be necessary. In the Black American culture there is much emphasis on feeding. Solid foods are introduced early and may even be added to the infant's formula. For the traditional Mexican American, a fat baby is considered a healthy baby and infants are fed on demand. "Spoiling" is encouraged and a colicky baby may be given mint or olive oil for relief.

Lactation   The female breast is divided into 15 to 24 lobes separated from one another by fat and connective tissue. These lobes are subdivided into lobules, composed of small units called *alveoli* where milk is synthesized. The lobules have a system of lactiferous ductiles that join larger ducts and eventually open onto the nipple surface. During pregnancy, the increased levels of estrogen stimulate breast development in preparation for lactation.

Following delivery the levels of estrogen and progesterone drop rapidly, and the anterior pituitary begins to secrete **prolactin**. This hormone promotes milk production by stimulating the alveolar cells of the breast. **Oxytocin**, secreted by the posterior pituitary when the infant sucks on the mother's nipple, triggers the **letdown reflex** and a flow of milk results.

The letdown reflex can be stimulated by the newborn's sucking, presence, or cry, or even by maternal thoughts about her baby. Conversely, the mother's lack of self-confidence, fear of,

embarrassment about, or pain connected with breast-feeding may prevent the milk from being ejected into the duct system. Milk production is decreased with repeated inhibition of the letdown reflex. Failure to empty the breasts frequently and completely also decreases production. As milk accumulates and is not withdrawn, the buildup of pressure in the alveoli suppresses secretion.

Once lactation is well established, prolactin production decreases. Oxytocin and sucking continue to be the stimulators of milk production.

Colostrum, a creamy, yellowish fluid is the first milk produced by the breast. Thicker than later milk, it contains more protein, fat-soluble vitamins, and minerals. It also contains a high level of immunoglobulins, which may be a source of immunity for the infant. Colostrum usually lasts for 2–4 days, and then milk production begins. Mature milk has a high percentage of water and is similar in appearance to skim milk.

Suppression of lactation in the nonnursing mother   Lactation may be suppressed through drug therapy and mechanical inhibition. The drugs used are hormones that inhibit the secretion of prolactin. However, because many of these drugs, such as chlorotrianisene (TACE), are estrogen-based medications and are associated with an increased incidence of thromboembolic disease, most practitioners prescribe them much less frequently than formerly. A newer, nonhormonal lactation suppressant, bromocriptine mesylate (Parlodel) is now available. See the accompanying Drug Guide, p. 584.

The recognition of complications associated with drug therapy has led to renewed popularity for mechanical methods of lactation suppression. This is accomplished by applying a snug breast binder for 2–3 days postdelivery. The judicious use of analgesics and ice packs will alleviate some of the discomfort associated with tender full breasts. The mother is advised to avoid any stimulation of her breasts by her baby, herself, breast pumps, or her sexual partner until the sensation of fullness has passed, as this will increase milk production and delay the suppression process. Heat is avoided for the same reason, and the mother is encouraged to let shower water flow over her back rather than

DRUG GUIDE
Bromocriptine (Parlodel)

OVERVIEW OF OBSTETRIC ACTION

Bromocriptine is a dopamine agonist that acts to suppress lactation by stimulating the production of prolactin-inhibiting factor at the hypothalamic level. This results in decreased secretion of prolactin by the pituitary gland. The drug may also directly inhibit the pituitary by preventing the release of prolactin from the hormone-producing cells (Foster, 1982). When administered postpartally it helps suppress milk production and decrease breast leakage and pain. It may also be used for suppression after lactation has already begun.

ROUTE, DOSAGE, AND FREQUENCY

The usual dose is 2.5 mg orally two times per day. The total daily dose generally does not exceed 7.5 mg. The medication usually is taken for 2–3 weeks.

MATERNAL CONTRAINDICATIONS

Maternal hypotension, desire to breast-feed, pregnancy.

MATERNAL SIDE EFFECTS

Hypotension is the primary side effect. To prevent problems associated with hypotension, administration should be delayed until the new mother's vital signs are stable. Other side effects include nausea, headache, dizziness, and occasionally faintness and vomiting.

NURSING CONSIDERATIONS

Administration should be delayed until maternal blood pressure is stable. Blood pressure should be carefully monitored if bromocriptine is administered concurrently with any antihypertensives. Taking bromocriptine with meals may help decrease the possibility of nausea. Early resumption of ovulation has occurred in women taking bromocriptine; the woman should be informed of this and receive information about contraceptives (Foster, 1982).

her breasts. A well-fitting bra is worn continuously until lactation is suppressed. The bra provides support and eases the discomfort that may occur with tension on the breast tissue because of the fullness. In some agencies a supportive bra is recommended in lieu of breast binding, except in cases of marked engorgement and discomfort. The suppression process usually takes approximately 48–72 hours, but some milk may be produced up to a month after delivery (Benson, 1980).

Bottle-feeding The mother who has chosen to bottle-feed her infant is encouraged to assume a comfortable position with adequate arm support so she can easily hold her infant. Most women cradle their infants in the crook of the arm close to the body, which provides the intimacy and cuddling so essential to an infant.

The following important principles should be included in the teaching provided:

1. Bottles should always be held, not propped. Positional otitis media may develop when the infant is fed horizontally, because milk and nasal mucus may block the eustachian tube. Holding the infant provides a rest for the feeder, social and close physical contact for the baby, and an opportunity for parent–child interaction and bonding (Figure 24-2).

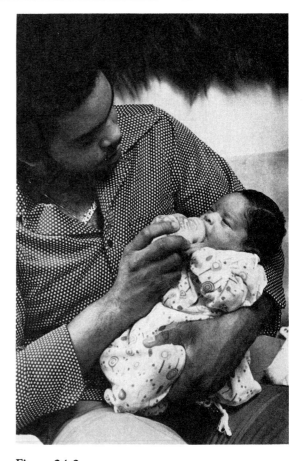

Figure 24-2
An infant is supported comfortably during bottle-feeding.

2. The nipple should have a hole big enough to allow milk to flow in drops when the bottle is inverted. Too large an opening may cause overfeeding or regurgitation because of too-fast feeding.

3. The nipple should be pointed directly into the mouth, and should be on top of the tongue. The nipple should be full of liquid at all times to avoid ingestion of extra air, which decreases the amount of feeding and increases discomfort.

4. The infant should be burped at intervals, preferably at the middle and end of the feeding. The infant who swallows a great deal of air while sucking may need more frequent burping. In addition, if the infant has cried before being fed, air may have been swallowed, and the infant should be burped before beginning to feed or after taking just enough to calm down.

5. Newborns frequently regurgitate small amounts of feedings and the mother may require reassurance that this is normal. Initially it may be due to excessive mucus and gastric irritation from foreign substances in the stomach from birth. Later, regurgitation may result when the infant feeds too rapidly and swallows air. It may also occur when the infant is overfed and the cardiac sphincter allows the excess to be regurgitated. Because this is a common occurrence, experienced mothers and nurses generally keep a "burp cloth" available. Although regurgitation is normal, vomiting or a forceful expulsion of fluid is not. When it occurs, further evaluation is indicated, especially if other symptoms are present.

6. A fat baby is not necessarily a healthy one. Parents should be encouraged to avoid overfeeding or feeding infants every time they cry. Infants should be encouraged but not forced to feed and should be allowed to set their own pace once feedings are established. Overfeeding results in infant obesity. During early feedings, however, the infant may need simple tactile stimulation—such as gently rubbing feet and hands, adjusting clothing, and loosening coverings—to maintain adequate sucking for a sufficient time to complete a full feeding.

Formula preparation and sterilization techniques usually concern parents. Cleanliness is essential, but sterilization is only necessary if the water source is questionable. (Procedure 24-1 describes methods of sterilization.) In most cases the bottles can be washed well, by hand or in a dishwasher. Nipples tend to become soft when washed in a dishwasher and should be done by hand. Powdered formulas, which are less expensive than liquid types, may be mixed with tap water. Usually one day's supply of formula is prepared at a time. Ready-to-use disposable bottles of formula are very convenient, but are also quite expensive.

Breast-feeding   Breast-feeding has many advantages for both the mother and her infant. Because suckling stimulates the release of oxytocin, uterine involution occurs more rapidly. Breast-feeding may also contribute to increased psychologic closeness between mother and infant. Breast-feeding is convenient and economical because there is no need to purchase and prepare formula on a routine basis; and breast-feeding may offer some antibody protection to the infant. Disadvantages and contraindications are primarily related to the mother and may include maternal illness, aversion to breast-feeding, and/or need to resume a full-time work schedule.

Beginning to breast-feed   The objectives of breast-feeding are (a) to provide adequate nutrition, (b) to establish an adequate milk supply, and (c) to prevent trauma to the nipples. All instructions are aimed toward these goals.

The newborn who is breast-feeding should be put to breast as soon as possible, depending on the situation of birth. Colostrum has sufficient nutrients to satisfy the infant until milk is established in 2–4 days. Establishment of lactation depends on the strength of the infant's suck and the frequency of nursing.

Positioning of the baby at the breast is a critical factor. The entire body of the infant should be turned toward the mother's breast, with the mouth adjacent to the nipple. The nipple should be directed straight into the mouth, and as much of the areola as possible should be included so that, as the baby sucks, the jaws compress the ducts that are directly beneath the areola (Figure 24-3). To do this the mother places her index finger above the nipple and her middle finger below. She then compresses the areolar area and guides the nipple into the

PROCEDURE 24-1
Methods of Bottle Sterilization

Terminal sterilization	Aseptic method of sterilization
Advantages:	**Advantages:**
1. Safest, most efficient method	1. May be modified for use with disposable bottles
2. More easily learned	**Disadvantages:**
Disadvantages:	1. Difficult to learn, contamination more likely
1. Prolonged cooling period (1–2 hr)	**Procedure:**
2. Not suitable for disposable bottles	1. Same as steps 1 and 2 of terminal method
Procedure:	2. Place all equipment needed (bottles, nipples, caps, can opener, tongs, measuring pitcher, and spoon) in a large kettle or sterilizer; cover with water and boil for 5 min
1. Assemble equipment and wash hands	3. In another pan boil the amount of water necessary to make the formula (boil for 5 min)
2. Thoroughly wash bottles, caps, and nipples in warm soapy water; squeeze some water through the nipple holes to rid them of accumulated milk; rinse well	4. Drain the water from the sterilizer pan and let the equipment cool for a few minutes
3. Wash the lid of the formula can (if using a liquid) and prepare formula according to directions	5. Remove the measuring pitcher, being certain to touch only the handle
4. Fill the bottles with the desired amount of formula and loosely apply the nipples and caps; one or two bottles of water may be prepared at the same time	6. Using the sterilized can opener, open a can of formula after first washing the lid with soapy water and rinsing well; pour the formula into the prepared measuring pitcher and add the correct amount of boiled water, mix with the prepared spoon
5. Place the prepared bottles in a large kettle or bottle sterilizer and add the appropriate amount of water (as specified on the sterilizer or 2–3 in. if a kettle is used)	7. Using tongs, remove the bottles from the sterilizer and fill them with the desired amount of formula; (one or two bottles of water may also be prepared by boiling enough additional water)
6. Cover the sterilizer, bring the water to a gentle boil and then boil for 25 min.	8. Using the tongs set the nipples on the bottles, then touching only the edges, apply the caps
7. Remove from heat but let the bottles remain in the sterilizer with the lid on until the sides of the pan are cool to the touch	9. Refrigerate until needed
8. Remove the bottles, tighten the lids, and refrigerate until needed	**To modify for disposable bottles:**
	Complete all steps as directed except *do not boil the bottles* with the other equipment and allow the water to cool for 15–20 min before preparing the formula (the plastic bag may melt if the formula is too hot)

infant's mouth. Through the rooting reflex, the infant can locate the nipple.

If the mother does not have a prominent or everted nipple, she may try rolling the nipple between her thumb and forefinger or stretching the nipple by pressing in and outward around the nipple prior to the feeding. Nurses should avoid the temptation to substitute a regular nipple shield to correct nipple positions. The shield tends to confuse the baby. The artificial nipples on the shields are softer and easier to feed from, and the baby may refuse the human nipple when it is reoffered. This problem, termed *nipple confusion*, may also be avoided if routine sterile water or dextrose and water feedings are not given to breast-feeding infants.

Breasts should be alternated at each feeding, beginning with 5 minutes on each side and progressing to 7–10 minutes by the third or fourth day and ultimately to 10 minutes on each side. Once feedings are established, length of nursing time on the second breast may be extended to meet the infant's oral needs, because the sucking reflex will not be as strong once the infant is partially satisfied with nourishment from the first breast. While nursing, the mother should press the breast away from the infant's nares to prevent obstruction of the nasal passageway.

The mother should be instructed in techniques for breaking suction prior to removing the infant from the breast. Inserting a finger into

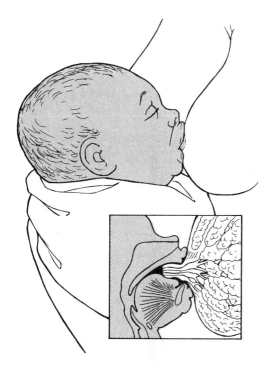

Figure 24-3 ▬▬▬▬▬▬▬▬▬▬

To nurse effectively, it is important that the infant's mouth covers the majority of the areola to compress the ducts below. (Reprinted with permission of Ross Laboratories, Columbus, Ohio.)

the infant's mouth beside the nipple will break the suction, and the nipple can be removed without trauma. The baby is burped between feedings on each breast and at the end of the feeding.

Initially more milk is produced than is required by the infant. Later the amount of milk will be produced to meet nutritional need, manifested through sucking. Milk may tend to leak until demand meets supply. The mother should expect and deal with this by using breast pads in her bra to absorb the secretions. She should be cautioned to remove wet pads frequently to avoid infection or irritation to the nipples.

The use of supplementary feedings for the breast-feeding infant may weaken or confuse the sucking reflex and interfere with successful outcome. Adequacy of intake may be easily determined. If the infant appears to gain weight and has six or more wet diapers a day, he or she is receiving adequate amounts of milk. Activity levels and intervals between feedings may also indicate how satisfied the infant is. Parents should know that, because breast milk is more easily digested than formulas, the breast-fed infant becomes hungry sooner. Thus the frequency of breast-feedings may be greater, particularly after discharge, when fatigue or excitement may decrease milk supply temporarily. Increasing the frequency of feedings alleviates problems during these periods. The parents may also expect the infant to demand more frequent nursing during periods when growth spurts are expected, such as 10 days to 2 weeks, 5–6 weeks, and 3 months. There is a lag in nursing due to increased activity and interest in surroundings at 4–6 months, 7 months, and 9 months to a year (Slattery, 1977).

The mother may be taught to express her milk manually and freeze it for bottle-feeding if she will be absent for a scheduled feeding. Breast milk should be frozen in plastic bottles; if glass bottles are used the antibodies will adhere to the sides of the bottle and their benefits will be lost. If the mother must go several hours without feeding, manual expression will relieve maternal discomfort and maintain the milk supply, which decreases unless the breasts are emptied regularly.

Many medications, when administered to the mother, are secreted in the milk. These include salicylates, bromides, antibiotics, most alkaloids, some cathartics, alcohol, and the majority of addicting drugs (Pritchard, MacDonald, and Gant, 1985). The mother should receive information about this and should also be instructed to inform her physician that she is nursing, should she require medical treatment at a later time.

See Appendix E for a list of the effects of drugs and substances on the breast-feeding mother and her newborn.

Pamphlets and organized La Leche League activities are available to parents to assist with successful breast-feeding. The breast-feeding mother needs the support of all family members, her pediatrician, her obstetrician, and nursing personnel. It is often the attitudes reflected by these people that ultimately lead the mother to success or failure.

Potential problems in breast-feeding Many women stop nursing because the problems they encounter seem overwhelming. When the nurse provides anticipatory guidance about possible problems, the mother is usually able to cope more successfully.

Abnormal nipples Nipple inversion is generally diagnosed during the prenatal period. When a nipple is inverted, pressure on the areola with the examiner's thumb and forefinger causes the nipple to retract. When recognized prenatally, the woman can begin Hoffman's (1953) exercises to increase nipple protractility (Figure 24-4). She may also wear special breast shields to correct the problem. These shields, worn the last 3–4 months of pregnancy, exert gentle pulling pressure on the edge of the areola, gently forcing the nipple through the center of the shield.

Nipple soreness The mother should be told that some soreness is common initially especially at the start of feeding. This will generally clear in a few days as the nipple becomes toughened. Feedings should not be delayed or shortened as this will only cause engorgement and more soreness. In fact, it is often helpful to increase the frequency of feedings. When this is done the baby is less "ravenous," and the suck will not be as vigorous.

Nipple soreness is especially pronounced during the first few minutes of the feeding. If the mother is not expecting this, she may become discouraged and quickly stop. The letdown reflex may take 3 minutes to activate and it may not occur if the mother stops nursing too quickly. The problem is compounded if the infant does not empty the mammary ducts; the infant is unsatisfied, and the possibility of engorgement for the mother increases.

The area of greatest stress to the nipple is in line with the newborn's chin and nose. Thus nipple soreness may be decreased by encouraging the mother to rotate positions when feeding the infant (Figure 24-5).

Substances such as lanolin or Massé® cream may be applied to the nipple between feedings to help prevent drying and cracking. They should be applied to a clean nipple and washed off with warm water prior to the next feeding.

Exposing the nipples to the air for 15–30 minutes after each feeding also helps prevent problems. Because dryness is essential to prevent skin breakdown, breast pads should be changed frequently. (Breast pads with plastic liners interfere with air circulation; the plastic should be removed before they are used.)

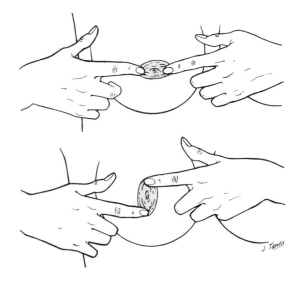

Figure 24-4 ▬▬▬
Hoffman's exercises are designed to increase nipple protractility. The woman is instructed to place her thumbs or index fingers opposite each other near the edge of the areola. She then presses into the breast and stretches outward to break any adhesions. This is done both horizontally and vertically.

Older remedies are receiving renewed acceptance. For instance, tea bags may be moistened in warm water and applied to the nipples. The tannic acid seems to help toughen the nipples and the warmth is soothing and promotes healing.

Cracked nipples Nipple soreness is frequently coupled with cracked nipples. If the baby is positioned correctly for feedings and cracks still exist, interventions are necessary. All the interventions described for sore nipples may be used. In addition, it may be helpful if the mother begins feeding on the less sore breast. This triggers the letdown reflex in both breasts. The infant does more vigorous sucking on the less tender breast, which helps avoid further trauma to the cracked nipple. A breast shield may also help protect the affected nipple.

In some cases the nipple is so traumatized that it bleeds. If this occurs the woman may be advised to skip one or two feedings on the affected breast and manually express the milk. This avoids trauma to the nipple and also prevents engorgement. In addition to the procedures previously discussed, the woman may also

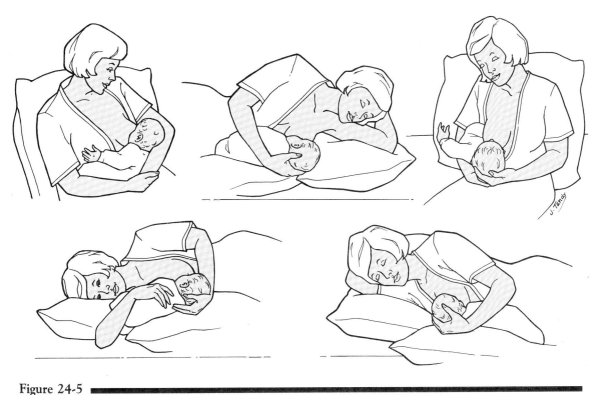

Figure 24-5
Examples of breastfeeding position changes to facilitate thorough breast emptying and prevent nipple soreness.

wish to expose her nipples to sunlight for brief periods once or twice daily.

Cracked nipples provide a route for infection and consequently the woman is more susceptible to mastitis. Thus, the need for careful handwashing before handling her breasts should be stressed.

Breast engorgement   About the time their milk initially comes in, many women complain of feelings of engorgement. Their breasts are hard, painful, and warm and appear taut and shiny. At first this fullness is caused by venous congestion due to the increased vascularity in the breasts. Later the problem may be compounded by the pressure of accumulating milk.

The mother should be encouraged to wear a well-fitting nursing bra 24 hours a day. Frequent nursing is also helpful in preventing or decreasing engorgement. Breast-feeding every 2–3 hours initially keeps the breasts emptied. It also increases the circulation in the breast and helps move the fluid that might lead to engorgement.

Because the breast is quite hard, nursing may be difficult for the infant and painful for the mother. Manual expression of milk or the use of a nontraumatic breast pump to initiate the flow may be helpful, as is the judicious use of analgesics. Warmth is often soothing, and the mother who has problems with engorgement may find a warm shower comforting. It is also useful in stimulating the letdown reflex. The mother may find it helpful to stand in the shower and manually express some milk before feeding. Warm, moist cloths may also be used for relief. The engorgement generally subsides within 12–24 hours.

Plugged ducts   Some mothers experience plugging of one or more ducts, especially in conjunction with or following engorgement. Manifested as an area of tenderness or "lumpiness" in an otherwise well woman, plugging may be relieved by the use of heat and massage. Frequent nursing will also help prevent the problem. In cases of repeatedly plugged ducts or caked breasts, the mother may need to limit her fat intake to polyunsaturated fats and to add lecithin to her diet (Lawrence, 1980).

Promotion of Effective Parent Education

Meeting the educational needs of the new mother and her family is one of the primary challenges facing the postpartum nurse. Each woman has educational needs that vary based on age, background, experience, and expectations. The steps of the nursing process provide a useful tool for identifying and meeting educational needs following delivery.

The nurse first assesses the learning needs of the new mother through observation and tactfully phrased questions. For example, "What plans have you made for handling things when you get home?" will elicit a response of several words and may provide the opportunity for some information sharing and guidance. Some agencies also use checklists of common concerns for new mothers. The woman can check those that are of interest to her.

Teaching should then be planned and implemented to provide learning experiences in a logical, nonthreatening way. Postpartal units use a variety of approaches, including handouts, formal classes, videotapes, and individual interaction. Regardless of the technique, timing is important. The new mother is more receptive to teaching during the taking-hold phase when she is ready to assume responsibility for her own care and that of her newborn. Unfortunately many women are discharged during the taking-in phase. Because of this many units provide printed material for new mothers to consult if questions arise at home.

Teaching should include information on role change and psychologic adjustments as well as skills. Anticipatory guidance can help prepare new parents for the many changes they experience with a new family member.

Information is also essential for women with specialized educational needs: the mother who has had a cesarean delivery, the parents of twins, the parents of an infant with congenital anomalies, and so on. Nurses who are attuned to these individual problems can begin providing guidance as soon as possible.

Evaluation may take several forms: return demonstrations, question and answer sessions, and even formal evaluation tools. Follow-up phone calls after discharge provides additional evaluative information and continues the helping process for the family.

Promotion of Family Wellness

The promotion of family wellness involves several areas of concern. These include a satisfactory maternity experience, the need for follow-up care for mother and infant, and birth control. The new or expanding family may also have needs for information about adjustment of siblings and resuming sexual relations.

Rooming-in   The emphasis on family-centered maternity care must be continued in the postpartal period. The practice of rooming-in provides increased opportunities for parent–child interaction.

In rooming-in the newborn shares the mother's unit, and they are cared for together. This enables the mother to have time to bond with her baby and learn to care for him or her in a supportive environment. Rooming-in is especially conducive to a self-demand feeding schedule for both breast-feeding and bottle-feeding babies. It also allows the father to participate in the care of his new child.

The rooming-in policy must be flexible enough to permit the mother to return the baby to the nursery if she finds it necessary because of fatigue or physical discomfort. Many agencies also return the infants to a central nursery at night so the mothers can get more rest.

Rooming-in provides an excellent opportunity for family bonds to grow. With rooming-in father, mother, infant, and often siblings can begin functioning as a family unit immediately.

Reactions of siblings   Sibling visitation helps meet the needs of both the siblings and their mother. A visit to the hospital reassures children that their mother is well and still loves them. It also provides an opportunity for the children to become familiar with the new baby. For the mother the pangs of separation are lessened as she interacts with her children and introduces them to the newest family member.

Although the parents have prepared their children for the presence of a new brother or sister, the actual arrival of the infant necessitates some adjustments. If small children are waiting at home, it is helpful if the father carries the baby inside. This practice keeps the mother's arms free to hug and touch her older children. Many mothers bring a doll home with them for an older child. The child cares for the doll alongside his or her mother or father, thereby identifying with the parent. This identification helps decrease anger and the need to regress for attention.

Parents may also provide supervised times when older children can hold the new baby and perhaps even help with a bottle-feeding. The older children feel a sense of accomplishment and learn tenderness and caring—qualities appropriate for both males and females. The nurse can help the parents come up with ways to show the other children that they, too, are valued and have their own places in the family.

Sexual relations   Previously couples were discouraged from engaging in sexual intercourse until 6 weeks postpartum. Currently the couple is advised to abstain from intercourse until the episiotomy is healed and the lochial flow has stopped (usually by the end of the third week). Because the vaginal vault is "dry" (hormone poor), some form of lubrication such as K-Y jelly may be necessary during intercourse. The female-superior or sidelying coital positions may be preferable because they allow the women to control the depth of penile penetration.

Breast-feeding couples should be forewarned that, during orgasm, milk may spurt from the nipples due to the release of oxytocin. Some couples find this pleasurable, others choose to have the woman wear a bra during sex. Nursing the baby prior to lovemaking may also decrease this.

Other factors may serve as deterrents to fully satisfactory sexual experience: the baby's crying may "spoil the mood"; the woman's changed body may be repulsive to some men and women; maternal sleep deprivation may interfere with a mutually satisfying experience; and the woman's physiologic response to sexual stimulation may be changed due to hormonal changes (this lasts about 3 months). With anticipatory guidance during the prenatal and postpartal periods, the couple can be forewarned of potential temporary problems. Anticipatory guidance is enhanced if the couple can discuss their feelings and reactions as they are experienced.

Family planning   Because many couples resume sexual activity before the postpartal examination, family-planning information should be made available before discharge. This enables a woman or a couple to select a method that is personally acceptable and physiologically appropriate.

The couple's decisions about contraception should be made voluntarily, with full knowledge of options, advantages, disadvantages, effectiveness, side effects, and long-range effects. Many outside factors influence a couple's choice, including cultural influences, religious beliefs, personality, cost, effectiveness, misinformation, practicability of method, and self-esteem. Different methods of contraception may be appropriate at different times in the couple's life.

Fertility awareness methods   **Fertility awareness methods**, formerly called natural family-planning, are based on an understanding of the changes that occur throughout a woman's ovulatory cycle. All these methods require periods of abstinence and recording of certain events throughout the cycle; hence cooperation of the partner is important. Advantages of the natural methods include an increased awareness of the body and avoidance of artificial substances.

The *basal body temperature method* to detect ovulation requires that the woman take her BBT every morning and record the readings on a temperature graph. Intercourse is avoided on the day of temperature rise and for the following 3 days. Not all temperature curves are interpretable, however, so many abstain from intercourse for an extended period of time, between days 12 and 18 in a cycle, to ensure safety.

The *calendar rhythm method* requires the recording of each menstrual cycle for at least 6 months so that the shortest and longest cycles can be identified. The first day of menstruation is the first day of the cycle. The fertile phase is calculated from the 18th day before the end of the shortest recorded cycle through the 11th day from the end of the longest recorded cycle (Hatcher et al., 1984). For example, if a woman's cycle lasts from 24–28 days, the fertile phase would be calculated as day 6 through 17. Once this information is obtained, the woman can identify the fertile and infertile phases of her cycle. For effective use of the method, she must abstain from intercourse during the fertile phase.

Rhythm is a variation of the calendar rhythm method. It is based on identification of the "unsafe period" of a menstrual cycle, which is a period of time immediately before and after ovulation. Theoretically, conception may occur on only 3 days in each cycle, but women who have irregular cycles find it difficult to pinpoint the time of ovulation.

The *ovulation method*, sometimes called the *Billings method*, involves the assessment of cervical mucus changes that occur during the menstrual cycle. The amount and character of cervical mucus change as a result of the influence of estrogen and progesterone. At the time of ovulation the mucus (type E) is clearer, more stretchable (spinnbarkeit), and is more permeable to sperm. It also shows a characteristic fern pattern when placed on a glass slide and allowed to dry.

During the luteal phase the cervical mucus is thick and sticky and forms a network that traps sperm, making their passage more difficult—type G mucus.

To use the ovulation method, the woman abstains from intercourse for the first menstrual cycle. Cervical mucus is assessed daily for amount, ferning, and spinnbarkeit as the woman becomes familiar with varying characteristics. After the pattern has been established the woman abstains from intercourse whenever the mucus is type E and for 4 days after ovulation.

The *symptothermal method* consists of various assessments that are made and recorded by the couple. This includes information regarding cycle days, coitus, cervical mucus changes, and secondary signs such as increased libido, abdominal bloating, mittelschmerz, and basal body temperature. Through the various assessments, the couple learns to recognize signs that

indicate ovulation. This combined approach tends to improve the effectiveness of fertility awareness birth control approaches.

Situational contraceptives also fall under the heading of natural family planning. These methods involve no prior preparation of the couple but involve motivation to abstain from intercourse or to interrupt the sexual act prior to the ejaculation of the sperm into the vagina. *Coitus interruptus*, or withdrawal, is the oldest method of contraception but has limited effectiveness as a pregnancy preventive.

Mechanical contraceptives Mechanical contraceptive methods act either as barriers preventing the transport of sperm to the ovum or by preventing implantation of the ovum/zygote. **Condoms** offer a viable means of contraception when used consistently and properly (Figure 24-6). Acceptance has been increasing as a growing number of men are assuming responsibility for regulation of fertility. The condom is applied to the erect penis, rolled from the tip to the end of the shaft, before vulvar or vaginal contact. A small space must be left at the end of the condom to allow for collection of the ejaculate so that the condom will not break at the time of ejaculation. Vaginal jelly should be used if the condom or vagina are dry to prevent irritation

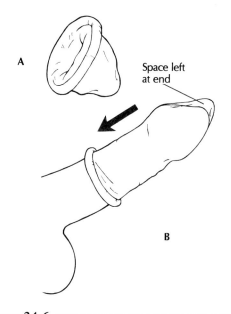

Figure 24-6

A, Condom. **B**, Condom applied to penis. Note space left at end to allow collection of ejaculate.

and possible condom breakage. Care must be taken in removing the condom after intercourse. For optimum effectiveness, the penis should be withdrawn from the vagina while still erect and the condom rim held to prevent spillage. If after ejaculation the penis becomes flaccid while still in the vagina, the male should hold onto the edge of the condom while withdrawing from the vagina to avoid spilling the semen and to prevent the condom from slipping off. The effectiveness of condoms is largely determined by their use. The condom is small, lightweight, disposable, and inexpensive; has no side effects; requires no medical examination or supervision; offers visual evidence of effectiveness; and protects against venereal diseases. Breakage, displacement, possible perineal or vaginal irritation, and dulled sensation are possible disadvantages.

The **diaphragm** (Figure 24-7) offers a good level of protection from conception, especially when used with spermicidal creams or jellies. The woman must be fitted with a diaphragm and instructions given by trained personnel. The diaphragm should be rechecked for correct size after each childbirth and if a client has a weight gain or loss of 15–20 pounds or more.

The diaphragm must be inserted prior to intercourse, with approximately 1 teaspoonful (or 1½ inches from the tube) of spermicidal jelly placed around its rim and in the cup. This serves as a chemical barrier to supplement the mechanical barrier of the diaphragm itself. The diaphragm is inserted through the vagina and covers the cervix. The last step in insertion is to push the edge of the diaphragm under the symphysis pubis, which may result in a "popping" sensation. When fitted properly and correctly in place, the diaphragm should not cause discomfort to the woman or her partner. Correct placement of the diaphragm can be checked by touching the cervix with a fingertip through the cup. The cervix feels like a small rounded structure and has a consistency similar to that of the tip of the nose. The center of the diaphragm should be over the cervix. Women who have chronic urinary tract infections or those who object to manipulation of the genitals for insertion, determination of correct placement, and removal may find this method offensive. If more than 4 hours elapse between insertion of the diaphragm and intercourse, additional spermi-

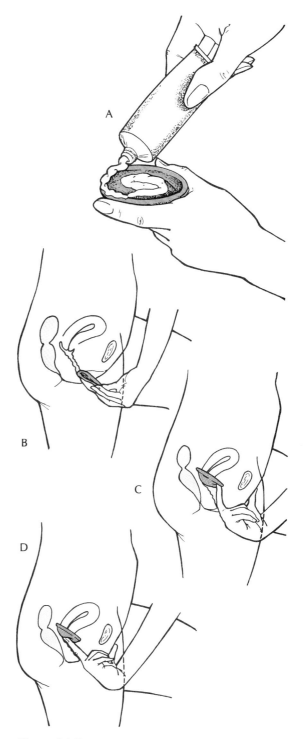

Figure 24-7

A, Diaphragm and jelly. Jelly is applied to the rim and center of the diaphragm. **B**, Insertion of the diaphragm. **C**, Rim of diaphragm is pushed under the symphysis pubis. **D**, Checking placement of diaphragm. Cervix should be felt through the diaphragm.

cidal cream should be used. It is necessary to leave the diaphragm in for 6 hours after coitus. Some couples feel that the use of a diaphragm interferes with the spontaneity of intercourse. It can be suggested that the partner insert the diaphragm as part of the foreplay to overcome this idea. If intercourse is again desired within the next 6 hours, another type of contraception must be used or additional spermicidal jelly placed in the vagina with an applicator, taking care not to disturb the placement of the diaphragm. The diaphragm should be periodically held up to a light and inspected for tears or holes.

Diaphragms are an excellent contraceptive means for women who cannot or do not desire to use the pill (hormonal contraceptives), who wish to avoid exposure to the increased risk of pelvic inflammatory disease associated with intrauterine devices, or who wish to be sexually active for several years prior to starting their families (Hatcher et al, 1984).

The **cervical cap** is a cup-shaped "diaphragm" placed over the cervix that stays in place by suction. The degree of suction depends on the tightness of the fit between the cap and the cervix. The fitting must be meticulous, with best results from custom-made cups. Since pregnancies have occurred without cup displacement, spermicidal jelly should be used in the cup. It can remain in place for one or more days. At present the FDA prohibits their use outside specific test sites, and the only manufacturer is in Great Britain (Tatum and Connell-Tatum, 1981).

Contraceptive sponges were approved by the FDA for use in 1983. The contraceptive sponge, available without prescription, is a small pillow-shaped polyurethane sponge with a concave cupped area on one side designed to fit over the cervix. The sponge currently available, Today® Vaginal Contraceptive Sponge, contains spermicide. Although the sponge is slightly less effective than the diaphragm, it is easier to use (Rosenfield, 1985). The sponge is moistened with water prior to use and inserted into the vagina so that the cupped area fits snugly over the cervical os. This decreases the chance of the sponge dislodging during intercourse.

Advantages of the sponge are: professional fitting not required as for the diaphragm; may be used for multiple coitus up to 48 hours unlike the single-use condom; one size fits all; and it is both barrier and spermicide. Problems associated with sponge use include difficulty removing the sponge, cost (approximately one dollar per sponge), and irritation or allergic reactions. Some women also report that vaginal dryness is sometimes a problem because the sponge absorbs vaginal secretions. Women with a history of toxic shock syndrome should not use vaginal sponges (Hatcher et al., 1984).

Intrauterine devices (IUDs) primarily work by producing a local sterile inflammatory reaction in the uterus. Consequently, even if fertilization occurs, implantation is inhibited.

Possible adverse reactions to the IUD include discomfort to the wearer, increased bleeding during menses, pelvic inflammatory disease, perforation of the uterus, intermenstrual bleeding, dysmenorrhea, expulsion of the device, and ectopic pregnancy. Advantages include convenience, no coital-related activity, and duration of effectiveness.

The IUD is inserted into the uterus with its string or tail protruding through the cervix into the vagina. Types currently in use include Lippes loop, copper 7, and copper T. The copper 7 and the T-shaped IUDs are smaller and have a lower incidence of pain after insertion, and therefore are used more frequently in nulliparous women (Figure 24-8).

The copper 7 continuously releases a small amount of copper and has to be replaced every 3 years. Plastic IUDs may also have to be replaced on a regular basis. When they have been in place more than a year, calcium salts may become deposited on the plastic. This forms a rough surface that irritates the endometrium and can cause ulceration and bleeding. If these symptoms occur, the IUD should be removed and replaced.

An IUD may be inserted at the 4–6 week postpartum check or during a menstrual period. After insertion, the woman should be instructed to check for the presence of the string once a week for the first month and then after each menses. She is told that she may have some cramping and/or bleeding intermittently for 2–6 weeks and her first few menses may occur in an irregular fashion. Follow-up examination is suggested 4–8 weeks after insertion.

Oral contraceptives   The use of hormones, specifically the combination of estrogen and

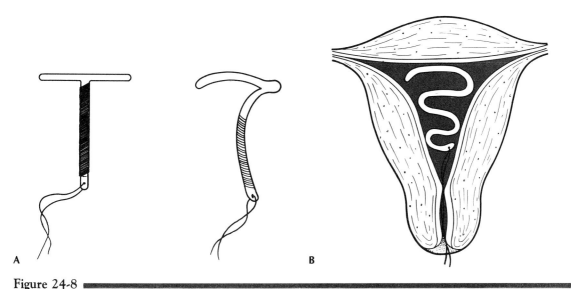

Figure 24-8

A, Types of intrauterine devices. *Left*, copper T; *right*, copper 7. **B**, Lippes loop in place within uterus.

progesterone, is a very successful birth control method. **Oral contraceptives** work by inhibiting the release of an ovum and by maintaining type G mucus, which is hostile to sperm. Numerous oral contraceptives are available. The "pill" is taken daily for 21 days beginning on the Sunday after the first day of the menstrual cycle. Seven days after completing her last pill, the woman restarts the pill. Thus the woman always begins the pill on the same day. Some companies offer a 28-day pack with seven "blank" pills so that the woman never stops taking a pill. The pill should be taken at approximately the same time each day—usually upon arising or before retiring in the evening.

Although highly effective, oral contraceptives may produce side effects ranging from break-through bleeding to thrombus formation. The majority of the side effects are related to the dosage. The use of dosages 50 mcg or lower has reduced many of the side effects, but the threat of potential risk deters some women from using oral contraceptives.

Contraindications of the use of oral contraceptives include pregnancy, previous history of thrombophlebitis or thromboembolic disease, acute or chronic liver disease of cholestatic type with abnormal function, presence of estrogen-dependent carcinomas, undiagnosed uterine bleeding, heavy smoking, hypertension, diabetes, PIH, age over 40, lack of regular menstrual cycles for at least 1–2 years in adolescents, and

hyperlipoproteinemia. In addition, women with the following conditions who use oral contraceptives should be examined every 3 months: migraine headaches, epilepsy, depression, oligomenorrhea, and amenorrhea. Women who choose this method of contraception should be fully advised of potential side effects. See Table 24-1 for side effects of oral contraceptives.

Following delivery a nonnursing mother may begin taking oral contraceptives 3–4 weeks postpartum. This reduces the risk of thromboembolism associated with estrogen use in the early postpartal period. Mothers who have received bromocriptine to suppress lactation should start by the 14th day because ovulation may occur earlier for them.

Because estrogen suppresses lactation and will cross into the breast milk, mothers are advised not to take oral contraceptives until weaning their child.

Spermicides   A variety of creams, jellies, foams, and suppositories, inserted into the vagina prior to intercourse, destroy sperm or neutralize vaginal secretions and thereby immobilize sperm. **Spermicides** that effervesce in a moist environment offer more rapid protection and coitus may take place immediately after they are inserted. Suppositories may require up to 30 minutes to dissolve and will *not* offer protection until they do so. The woman should be instructed to insert these spermicide preparations high in the vagina and maintain a supine

Table 24-1
Side Effects of Oral Contraceptives*

ESTROGEN COMPONENT

Nausea, bloating
Edema and cyclic weight gain
Irritability, nervousness
Venous or capillary engorgement (spider nevi)
Breast tenderness or engorgement
Chloasma
Altered clotting factors—thrombophlebitis
Altered carbohydrate metabolism
Hypertension
Excessive menstrual flow
Headache
Leukorrhea, cervical erosion, or polyposis
Altered convulsive threshold
Altered lipid metabolism

PROGESTIN COMPONENT

Oligomenorrhea
Amenorrhea
Acne
Hirsutism
Breast regression
Anabolic weight gain
Increased appetite
Fatigue
Depression and altered libido
Moniliasis
Loss of hair

*Modified from Nelson JH: Selecting the optimum oral contraceptive. *J Reprod Med* 11:135, 1973.) Reproduced with permission from Kreutner AKK: Contraception, in AKK Kreutner and DR Hollingsworth (eds): *Adolescent Obstetrics and Gynecology*. Copyright ©1978 by Year Book Medical Publishers, Inc. Chicago, IL.

position. Spermicides are minimally effective when used alone, but in conjunction with a diaphragm or condom, their effectiveness increases. They provide a high degree of protection from exposure to several sexually transmitted diseases, especially gonorrhea (Tatum and Connell-Tatum, 1981).

Operative sterilization   Before sterilization is performed on either partner, a thorough explanation of the procedure should be given to both. Each should understand that sterilization is not a decision to be taken lightly or entered into when psychologic stresses, such as separation or divorce, exist. Even though both male and female procedures are theoretically reversible, the permanency of the procedure should be stressed and understood.

Male sterilization is achieved through a relatively minor procedure called a **vasectomy**. This involves severing of the vas deferens in both sides of the scrotum. Side effects of vasectomy include hematoma, sperm granulomas, and spontaneous reanastomosis.

Female sterilization is most frequently accomplished by **tubal ligation**. The tubes are located through a small subumbilical incision or by minilaparotomy techniques and are crushed, ligated, or plugged (in the newer, reversible procedures).

The postpartal period is an ideal time to perform a tubal ligation because the tubes are somewhat enlarged and easily located. Usually the woman remains in the hospital one extra day. Most hospitals require that the consent for tubal ligation be completed prior to admission for delivery to avoid hasty, later-regreted, decisions.

Complications of female sterilization procedures include coagulation burns on the bowel, bowel perforation, infection, hemorrhage, and adverse anesthesia effects. Reversal of a tubal ligation depends on many factors, including the portion of the tube excised, the presence or absence of the fimbriae, and the length of the tube remaining. With microsurgical techniques, a pregnancy rate of approximately 70% is possible (Silber and Cohen, 1980).

Promotion of Parent–Infant Attachment

Nursing interventions to enhance the quality of parent–infant attachment should be designed to promote feelings of well-being, comfort, and satisfaction. Following are some suggestions for ways of achieving this:

1. Determine the childbearing and child-rearing goals of the infant's mother and father and adapt them wherever possible in planning nursing care for the family. This includes giving the parents choices about their labor and delivery experience and their initial time with their new infant.

2. Postpone eye prophylaxis to facilitate eye contact between parents and their newborn.

3. Provide time in the first hour after delivery for the new family to become acquainted with as much privacy as possible.

4. Arrange the health care setting so that the individual nurse–client relationship can be developed and maintained. A primary nurse can develop rapport and assess the mother's strengths and needs.

5. Encourage the parents to involve the siblings in integrating the infant into the family by bringing them to the hospital for sibling visits.

6. Use anticipatory guidance from conception through the postpartal period to prepare the parents for expected problems of adjustment.

7. Include parents in any nursing intervention, planning, and evaluation. Give choices whenever possible.

8. Initiate and support measures to alleviate fatigue in the parents.

9. Help parents to identify, understand, and accept both positive and negative feelings related to the overall parenting experience.

10. Support and assist parents in determining the personality and unique needs of their infant. Whenever possible rooming-in should be available. This practice gives the mother a chance to learn her infant's normal patterns and develop confidence in caring for him or her. It also allows the father more uninterrupted time with his infant in the first days of life. If mother and baby are doing well and if help is available for the mother at home, early discharge permits the family to begin establishing their life together.

——————— CASE STUDY ———————

Elena Rodriguez was an 18-year-old, Spanish-speaking only, primipara who had recently moved to the United States from Mexico with her husband, Raoul, age 20. Raoul spoke English fairly well and acted as interpreter for Elena. Elena's sister, Theresa, and her husband, Joseph Gallegos, a native of Arizona, were sponsors for the couple. Joseph had a small, but successful construction company, and Raoul worked there as a carpenter. Theresa and Raoul attended the delivery of Ramon Joseph Rodriguez and both provided great support for Elena.

County Hospital, where Elena delivered, was a large urban teaching hospital. The city had a sizable Spanish-speaking population, and many of the staff spoke the language.

Alice Warren, a nursing student who spoke Spanish fluently, was assigned to care for Elena on the morning following Elena's delivery. Alice soon noted that, although Elena was polite and answered Alice's questions, she seemed upset and distracted. Finally Elena blurted out that the preceding evening she had been examined by several male doctors on rounds. When Elena had walked in the halls earlier she noticed that many doctors were on the floor. Elena had been extremely embarrassed to be examined by so many men and was afraid that it would happen again. Alice realized that Elena was modest and had indeed been very embarrassed. She quickly discussed the situation with her instructor and team leader. The three decided that Alice should discuss the situation with the chief resident, Tim Erikson. Tim was sensitive to Elena's need and agreed with Alice's suggestion that one physician, preferably a woman, be assigned to Elena. Tim had second-year resident Sandy Ryan take the case and skipped Elena on rounds.

Elena was quite relieved, and, as she relaxed, became very responsive to teaching. Alice helped her with breast-feeding and showed her how to diaper Ramon.

When Theresa arrived she sought out Alice's instructor and told the instructor how much she appreciated all Alice had done to provide good care for Elena. She told the instructor that Elena and her family would be living with the Gallegos until they were able to afford a place of their own. Theresa had arranged to take a few days off from work to be home with Elena, so things were well-organized at home.

The following morning Alice reviewed the items on the postpartum teaching list a final time and also gave Elena some postpartum literature printed in Spanish. She then had Elena do a return demonstration of basic aspects of infant care such as bathing. Alice and Elena spent time discussing potential problems such as fatigue. Alice also tactfully included information about sexual issues.

When Raoul arrived to get Elena, he told Alice that Elena had been very afraid of having her baby in a "foreign" hospital. However, the experience had been wonderful, and she felt confident of her ability to care for her son.

Postpartal Nursing Care after Cesarean Birth _____

After a cesarean birth the new mother has postpartal needs similar to those of her counterparts who delivered vaginally. Because she has undergone major abdominal surgery, the woman's nursing care needs are also similar to those of other surgical patients.

The chances of pulmonary infection are increased due to immobility after the use of narcotics and sedatives, and because of the altered immune response in postoperative patients. For this reason, the woman is encouraged to cough and deep breathe every 2–4 hours while awake for the first few days following cesarean delivery.

Leg exercises are also encouraged every two hours until the woman is ambulating. They increase circulation and help prevent thrombophlebitis and also aid intestinal mobility by tightening abdominal muscles.

Monitoring and management of the woman's pain experience is carried out during the postpartum period. Sources of pain include incisional pain, gas pain, referred shoulder pain, periodic uterine contractions (afterbirth pains), and pain from voiding, defecation, or constipation.

Nursing interventions are oriented toward preventing or alleviating pain or helping the woman cope with pain. The nurse should undertake the following measures:

- Administer analgesics as needed, especially during the first 24–72 hours. Their use will relieve the woman's pain and enable her to be more mobile and active.
- Offer comfort through proper positioning, backrubs, oral care, and the reduction of noxious stimuli such as noise and unpleasant odors.
- Encourage the presence of significant others, including the newborn. This practice provides distraction from the painful sensations and helps reduce the woman's fear and anxiety.
- Encourage the use of breathing, relaxation, and distraction (for example, stimulation of cutaneous tissue) techniques taught in childbirth preparation class.

Abdominal distention may produce marked discomfort for the woman during the first postpartal days. Measures to prevent or minimize gas pains include leg exercises, abdominal tightening, ambulation, avoiding carbonated or very hot or cold beverages, avoiding the use of straws, and providing a high-protein, liquid diet for the first 24–48 hours. Medical intervention for gas pain includes the use of suppositories and enemas and encouraging the woman to lie on her left side. Lying on the left side allows the gas to rise from the descending colon to the sigmoid colon so that it can be expelled more readily.

The nurse can minimize discomfort and promote satisfaction as the mother assumes the activities of her new role. Instruction and assistance in assuming comfortable positions when holding and/or breast-feeding the infant will do much to increase her sense of competence and comfort.

Signs of depression, anger, or withdrawal may indicate a grief response to the loss of the fantasized birth experience. Fathers as well as mothers may experience feelings of "missing out," guilt, or even jealousy toward another couple who had a vaginal birth. The cesarean birth couple needs the opportunity to tell their story repeatedly to work through these feelings. The nurse can provide factual information about their situation and support the couple's effective coping behaviors.

By the second or third day the cesarean birth mother moves into the taking-hold phase and is usually receptive to learning how to care for herself and her infant. Special emphasis should be given to home management. She should be encouraged to let others assume responsibility for housekeeping and cooking. Fatigue not only prolongs recovery but, interferes with breast-feeding and mother–infant interaction.

The cesarean birth mother usually does extremely well postoperatively. Most women are ambulating by the day after the surgery. Usually by the third postpartal day the incision can be covered with plastic wrap so the woman can shower, which seems to provide a mental as well as physical lift. Most are discharged by the fifth or sixth postoperative day, although some go home as early as the fourth day after delivery.

Parent-Infant Interaction after Cesarean Birth

Many factors associated with cesarean birth may hinder successful and frequent maternal-infant interaction. These include the physical condition of the mother and newborn and maternal reactions to stress, anesthesia, and medications. The mother and her infant may be separated after birth because of hospital routines, prematurity, or neonatal complications. A healthy infant born by uncomplicated cesarean delivery is no more fragile than a vaginally delivered newborn. However, some agencies automatically place cesarean-delivered infants in the high-risk nursery for a time, thereby causing anxiety for the parents and interfering with parent-infant interaction.

The presence of the father or significant other during the birth process positively influences the woman's perception of the birth event (Marut and Mercer, 1979). Not only does his or her presence reduce the woman's fears, but it enhances her sense of control. It also enables the couple to share feelings and respond to one another with touch and eye contact. Later, they have the opportunity to relive the experience and fill in any gaps or missing pieces. This is especially valuable if the mother has had general anesthesia. The father or significant other can take pictures, hold the infant, and foster the discovery process by directing the mother's attention to the details of the infant.

The perception of and reactions to a cesarean birth experience depend on how the woman defines that experience. Her reality is what she perceives it to be. If the woman's attitude is more positive than negative, successful resolution of subsequent stressful events is more likely. Because the definition of events is transitory in nature, the possibility of change and growth is present. Often the mothering role is perceived as an extension of the childbearing role. Inability to fulfill expected childbearing behavior (vaginal birth) may lead to parental feelings of role failure and frustration. The nurse can help families alter their negative definitions of cesarean birth, and bolster and encourage positive perceptions. (See the list of resource groups at the end of this chapter.)

The Postpartal Adolescent

The adolescent mother has special postpartal needs, depending on her level of maturity, support systems, and cultural background. The nurse needs to assess maternal–infant interaction, roles of support people, plans for discharge, knowledge of childrearing, and plans for follow-up care. It is imperative to have a community health service be in touch with the woman shortly after discharge.

Contraception counseling is an important part of teaching. The incidence of repeat pregnancies during adolescence is high. The younger the adolescent, the more likely she is to become pregnant again.

The nurse has many opportunities for teaching the adolescent about her newborn in the postpartal unit. Because the nurse is a role model, the manner in which she handles the newborn greatly influences the young mother. The father should be included in as much of the teaching as possible.

A newborn examination done at the bedside gives the adolescent information about her baby's health and shows her proper methods of handling an infant. Because adolescent mothers tend to focus their interaction in the physical domain, they need to learn the importance of verbal, visual, and auditory stimulation as well. The nurse can also use this time to give information about infant behavior. Parents who have some idea of what to expect from their infant will be less frustrated with the newborn's behavior.

The adolescent mother appreciates positive feedback about her fine newborn and her developing maternal responses. This praise and encouragement will increase her confidence and self-esteem.

Group classes for adolescent mothers should include infant care skills, information about growth and development, infant feeding, well-baby care, and danger signals in the ill newborn.

Ideally, teenage mothers should visit adolescent clinics where mother and newborn are assessed for several years after birth. In this way, the woman's enrollment in classes on parenting, need for vocational guidance, and school attendance can be followed closely. School systems offering classes for young mothers are an excellent way of helping adolescents finish school and learn how to parent at the same time.

Discharge Information _____

Ideally, preparation for discharge begins from the moment a woman enters the hospital to deliver her baby. Nursing efforts should be directed toward assessing the couple's knowledge, expectations, and beliefs and then providing anticipatory guidance and teaching accordingly. Since teaching is one of the primary responsibilities of the postpartum nurse, many agencies have elaborate teaching programs and classes. Before the actual discharge, however, the nurse should spend time with the couple to determine if they have any last-minute questions. In general, discharge teaching should include at least the following information:

1. The woman should contact her caregiver if she develops any of the signs of possible complications. (See Essential Facts to Remember—Signs of Postpartal Complications.)

 ESSENTIAL FACTS TO REMEMBER

Signs of Postpartal Complications

After discharge, a woman should contact her physician if any of the following develop:

- Sudden persistent or spiking fever
- Change in the character of the lochia—foul smell, return to bright red bleeding, excessive amount
- Evidence of mastitis, such as breast tenderness, reddened areas, malaise
- Evidence of thrombophlebitis, such as calf pain, tenderness, redness
- Evidence of urinary tract infection, such as urgency, frequency, burning on urination
- Continued severe or incapacitating postpartal depression

2. The woman should review the literature she has received that explains recommended postpartum exercises, the need for adequate rest, the need to avoid overexertion initially, and the recommendation to abstain from sexual intercourse until lochia has ceased. The woman may take either a tub bath or shower and may continue sitz baths at home if she desires.

3. The woman should be given the phone number of the postpartum unit and encouraged to call if she has any questions, no matter how simple.

4. The woman should receive information on local agencies and/or support groups, such as La Leche League and Mothers of Twins, that might be of particular assistance to her.

5. Both breast-feeding and bottle-feeding mothers should receive information geared to their specific nutritional needs. They should also be told to continue their vitamin and iron supplements until their postpartal examination.

6. The woman should have a scheduled appointment for her postpartal examination and for her infant's first well-baby examination before they are discharged.

7. The mother should clearly understand the correct procedure for obtaining copies of her infant's birth certificate.

8. The new parents should be able to provide basic care for their infants and should know when to anticipate that the cord will fall off; when the infant can have a tub bath; when the infant will need his or her first immunizations; and so on. They should also be comfortable feeding and handling the baby, and should be aware of basic safety considerations including the need for using a car seat whenever the infant is in a car.

9. The parents should also be aware of signs and symptoms in the infant that indicate possible problems and who they should contact about them (see p. 486 for a discussion of this).

The nurse can also use this final period to reassure the couple of their ability to be successful parents. She can stress the infant's need to feel loved and secure. She can also urge parents to talk to each other and work together to solve any problems that may arise.

The Fourth Trimester _____

The first several postpartal weeks have been termed *the fourth trimester* to stress the idea of continuity as the family adjusts to having a new member and as the woman's body returns to an essentially prepregnant state. During this period the woman must accomplish certain physical and developmental tasks (Gruis, 1977):

- Restoring physical condition

- Developing competence in caring for and meeting the needs of her infant

- Establishing a relationship with her new child

- Adapting to altered life-styles and family structure resulting from the addition of a new member.

The new mother may have an inadequate or incorrect understanding of what to expect during the early postpartal weeks. She may be concerned with restoring her figure and surprised because of continuing physical discomfort from sore breasts, episiotomy, or hemorrhoids. Fatigue is perhaps her greatest yet most underestimated problem during the early weeks. This may be aggravated if she has no extended family support or if there are other young children at home.

Developing skill and confidence in caring for an infant may be especially anxiety provoking for a new mother. As she struggles to establish a mutually acceptable pattern with her baby, small unanticipated concerns may seem monumental. The woman may begin to feel inadequate and, if she lacks support systems, isolated.

Nursing Management

Nurses have been in the forefront of health providers in attempting to improve the care currently existing during the postpartal period. Many obstetricians and nurse practitioners now routinely see all postpartal women 1–2 weeks after delivery in addition to the routine 6-week checkup. This extra visit provides an opportunity for physical assessment as well as assessment of the mother's psychologic and informational needs.

Follow-up Care

Follow-up care for the postpartal woman may be accomplished by home visits, follow-up phone calls, or postpartal classes. A home visit 2–3 days after discharge permits accurate assessment and teaching. It is especially useful for women who took advantage of early discharge policies and left the hospital after 24 hours or less.

The follow-up telephone call is usually initiated by a nurse from the postpartal unit of the agency where the mother delivered. It is made during the first week after discharge and is designed to provide assessment and care if necessary, to reinforce knowledge and provide additional teaching, and to make referrals if indicated (Donaldson, 1977).

Postpartal classes are becoming more common as caregivers recognize the continuing needs of the childbearing family. A series of structured classes may focus on topics such as parenting, postpartal exercise, or nutrition, or there may be loosely structured group sessions that address concerns of mothers as they arise. Such classes offer chances for the new mother to socialize, share her concerns, and receive encouragement. Because babysitting arrangements may be difficult or expensive, it is desirable to provide child care for newborns and siblings, or in some instances, infants may remain with mothers in the class.

Two- and Six-Week Examinations

The routine physical assessment, which can be made rapidly, focuses on the woman's general appearance, breasts, reproductive tract, bladder and bowel elimination, and any specific problems or complaints. (See the accompanying Postpartal Physical Assessment Guide.) In addition, conversation is used to determine nutrition patterns, fatigue level, family adjustment, and psychologic status of the mother (see the Psychologic Assessment Guide on p 604). Any problems with child care are explored, and referral to a pediatric nurse practitioner or pediatrician is made if needed. Available community resources, including Public Health

Text continued on p. 605.

POSTPARTAL PHYSICAL ASSESSMENT GUIDE: 2 WEEKS AND 6 WEEKS AFTER DELIVERY

Assess/normal findings	Alterations and possible causes*	Nursing responses to data†
VITAL SIGNS		
Blood pressure: Return to normal prepregnant level	Elevated blood pressure (anxiety, essential hypertension, renal disease)	Review history, evaluate normal baseline; refer to physician if necessary.
Pulse: 60–90 beats/min (or prepregnant normal rate)	Increased pulse rate (excitement, anxiety, cardiac disorders)	Count pulse for full minute, note irregularities; marked tachycardia or beat irregularities require additional assessment and possible physician referral.
Respirations: 16–24/min	Marked tachypnea or abnormal patterns (respiratory disorders)	Evaluate for respiratory disease; refer to physician if necessary.
Temperature: 36.2C–37.6C (98F–99.6F)	Increased temperature (infection)	Assess for signs and symptoms of infection or disease state.
WEIGHT		
2 weeks: probable weight loss of 14–20+ lb	Little or no weight loss (fluid retention, subinvolution, poor dietary habits)	Evaluate dietary habits and nutritional state; review blood pressure to evaluate fluid retention or blood losses.
6 weeks: returning to normal prepregnant weight	Retained weight (poor dietary habits)	Determine amount of daily exercise. Refer to dietitian if necessary for dietary counseling.
	Extreme weight loss (excessive dieting)	Discuss appropriate diets; refer to dietitian if necessary.
BREASTS		
Nonnursing:		
2 weeks: may have mild tenderness; small amount of milk may be expressed; breasts returning to prepregnant size 6 weeks: soft, with no tenderness; return to prepregnant size	Some engorgement (incomplete suppression of lactation) Redness; marked tenderness (mastitis) Palpable mass (tumor)	Engorgement usually seen only when no medication has been given to suppress lactation; advise client to wear a supportive well-fitted bra, avoid hot showers, etc. (see p. 583); evaluate for signs and symptoms of mastitis (rare in nonnursing mothers).
Nursing:		
Full, with prominent nipples; lactation established	Cracked, fissured nipples (feeding problems) Redness, marked tenderness, or even abcess formation (mastitis) Palpable mass (full milk duct, tumor)	Counsel about nipple care (see p. 588). Evaluate client condition, evidence of fever; refer to physician for initiation of antibiotic therapy, if indicated. Opinion varies as to value of breast examination for nursing mothers; some feel a nursing mother should examine her breasts monthly, after feeding, when breasts are empty; if palpable mass is felt, refer to physician for further evaluation. For breast inflammation instruct the mother to: 1. Keep breast empty by frequent feeding 2. Rest when possible 3. Take aspirin for pain

*Possible causes of alterations are placed in parentheses.
†This column provides guidelines for further assessment and initial nursing interventions.

POSTPARTAL PHYSICAL ASSESSMENT GUIDE: 2 WEEKS AND 6 WEEKS AFTER DELIVERY (continued)

Assess/normal findings	Alterations and possible causes*	Nursing responses to data†
		4. Force fluids If symptoms persist for more than 24 hours, instruct her to call her physician.
ABDOMINAL MUSCULATURE 2 weeks: improved firmness, although "bread dough" consistency is not unusual, especially in multipara	Marked diastasis recti (relaxation of muscles)	Evaluate exercise level; provide information on appropriate exercise program.
Striae pink and obvious Cesarean incision healing	Drainage, redness, tenderness, pain, edema (infection)	Evaluate for infection; refer to physician if necessary.
6 weeks: muscle tone continues to improve; striae may be beginning to fade, may not achieve a silvery appearance for several more weeks; linea nigra fading		
ELIMINATION PATTERN Urinary tract: Return to prepregnant urinary elimination routine	Urinary incontinence, especially when lifting, coughing, laughing, and so on (urethral trauma, cystocele)	Assess for cystocele; instruct in appropriate muscle tightening exercises; refer to physician.
	Pain or burning when voiding, urgency and/or frequency, pus or WBC in urine, pathogenic organisms in culture (urinary tract infection)	Evaluate for urinary tract infection; obtain clean catch urine; refer to physician for treatment if indicated.
Routine urinalysis within normal limits (proteinurea disappeared)	Sugar or ketone in urine—may be some lactose present in urine of breast-feeding mothers (diabetes)	Evaluate diet; assess for signs and symptoms of diabetes; refer to physician.
Bowel habits: 2 weeks: may still be some discomfort with defecation, especially if client had severe hemorrhoids or 3° extension	Severe constipation or pain when defecating (trauma or hemorrhoids)	Discuss dietary patterns; encourage fluid, adequate roughage. Continue use of stool softener if necessary to prevent pain associated with straining; continue sitz baths, periods of rest for severe hemorrhoids; assess healing of episiotomy and/or lacerations; severe constipation may require administration of laxatives, stool softeners, and an enema.
6 weeks: return to normal prepregnancy bowel elimination	Marked constipation	See above.
	Fecal incontinence or constipation (rectocele)	Assess for evidence of rectocele; instruct in muscle tightening exercises; refer to physician.
REPRODUCTIVE TRACT Lochia: 2 weeks: lochia alba, scant amounts, fleshy odor	Foul odor, excessive in amounts (infection) Return to lochia rubra or persistence of lochia rubra or serosa	Assess for evidence of infection and/or subinvolution; culture lochia; refer to physician.

*Possible causes of alterations are placed in parentheses.
†This column provides guidelines for further assessment and initial nursing interventions.

POSTPARTAL PHYSICAL ASSESSMENT GUIDE: 2 WEEKS AND 6 WEEKS AFTER DELIVERY (continued)

Assess/normal findings	Alterations and possible causes*	Nursing responses to data†
6 weeks: no lochia, or return to normal menstruation pattern	See above	See above.
Pelvic examination:		
2 weeks: uterus no longer palpable abdominally; external os closed; uterine muscles still somewhat lax and uterus may be displaced; introitus of vagina still lacking tone—gapes when intraabdominal pressure is increased by coughing or straining	External cervical os open, uterus not decreasing appropriately (subinvolution, infection) Evidence of redness, tenderness, poor tissue approximation in episiotomy and/or laceration (wound infection)	Assess for evidence of subinvolution and/or infection; refer to physician if indicated.
Episiotomy and/or lacerations healing; no signs of infection		
6 weeks: almost returned to prepregnant size with almost completely restored muscle tone	Continued flow of lochia, some opening of cervical os, failure to decrease appropriately in size (subinvolution)	Assess for evidence of subinvolution and/or infection; refer to physician for further evaluation and for dilatation and curettage if necessary.
Cervix completely closed with only transverse slit apparent		
Good return of muscle tone to pelvic floor	Marked relaxation of pelvic floor muscles (uterine prolapse)	Assess for evidence of uterine prolapse; discuss appropriate perineal exercises; refer to physician if indicated.
Papanicolaou test: Negative	Test results show atypical cells	Refer to physician for further evaluation and treatment.
HEMOGLOBIN AND HEMATOCRIT LEVELS		
6 weeks: Hgb 12 g/dL Hct 37% ± 5%	Hgb < 12 g/dL Hct 32% (anemia)	Assess nutritional status, begin (or continue) supplemental iron; for marked anemia (Hgb 9 g/dL) additional assessment and/or physician referral may be necessary.

*Possible causes of alterations are placed in parentheses.
†This column provides guidelines for further assessment and initial nursing interventions.

POSTPARTAL PSYCHOLOGIC ASSESSMENT GUIDE

Assess/normal findings	Alterations and possible causes*	Nursing response to data†
ATTACHMENT		
Bonding process demonstrated by soothing, cuddling, and talking to infant; appropriate feeding techniques; eye-to-eye contact; calling infant by name.	Failure to bond demonstrated by lack of behaviors associated with bonding process, calling infant by nickname that promotes ridicule, inadequate infant weight gain, infant is dirty, hygienic measures are not being maintained, severe diaper rash, failure to obtain adequate supplies to provide infant care (malattachment).	Provide counseling; refer to public health nurse for continued home visits.

*Possible causes of alterations are placed in parentheses.
†This column provides guidelines for further assessment and initial nursing interventions.

POSTPARTAL PSYCHOLOGIC ASSESSMENT GUIDE (continued)

Assess/normal findings	Alterations and possible causes*	Nursing response to data†
ADJUSTMENT TO PARENTAL ROLE		
Parents are coping with new roles in terms of division of labor, financial status, communication, readjustment of sexual relations, and adjusting to new daily tasks.	Inability to adjust to new roles (immaturity, inadequate education and preparation, ineffective communication patterns, inadequate support, current family crisis)	Provide counseling; refer to parent groups.
EDUCATION		
Mother understands self-care measures.	Inadequate knowledge of self-care (inadequate education)	Provide education and counseling.
Parents are knowledgeable regarding infant care.	Inadequate knowledge of infant care (inadequate education)	
Siblings are adjusting to new baby.	Excessive sibling rivalry	
Parents have chosen a method of contraception.	Birth control method not chosen	

*Possible causes of alterations are placed in parentheses.
†This column provides guidelines for further assessment and initial nursing interventions.

Department follow-up visits, are mentioned when appropriate. If not already discussed, teaching about family planning is appropriate at this time, and information regarding birth control methods is provided.

In ideal situations a family approach involving the father, infant, and possibly other siblings would permit a total evaluation and provide an opportunity for all family members to ask questions and express concerns. In addition, disturbed family patterns might be more readily diagnosed and therapy instituted to prevent future problems of neglect or abuse.

Summary

During the puerperium the new mother is adjusting physically and psychologically to the birth of her child. In addition the entire family is adjusting to a reordered and restructured family unit. These changes may be stressful for the new family.

Through an understanding of expected changes and assessment of numerous physical and psychologic factors, the nurse can intervene appropriately and help the new family take on the parenting role. In these times of increased mobility and lack of family members in close proximity, the new family looks to the nurse as a resource person who can assist them in learning their new tasks.

Resource Groups

Cesarean Association for Research, Education, Support and Satisfaction in Birthing (CARESS) (Burbank, CA 91510).
Cesarean Birth Council (San Jose, CA 95101).
Cesarean/Support, Education and Concern (C/Sec., Inc.) (Dedham, MA 02026).
La Leche League (9616 Minneapolis Avenue, Franklin, IL 60131).
Parent Education Resource Center (Box 94, Metropolitan State College, 1006 11th Street, Denver, CO 80204).

References

Benson RC: *Handbook of Obstetrics and Gynecology*. Los Altos, Calif.: Lange Medical Publications, 1980.
Clark AL: *Culture and Childrearing*. Philadelphia: Davis, 1981.
Donaldson NE: Follow-up at home. *Am J Nurs* 1977; 77(7):1176.
Foster S. Bromocriptine: Suppressing lactation. *MCN* March/April 1982; 7:99.
Gruis M: Beyond maternity: Postpartum concerns of mothers. *MCN* May/June 1977; 2(3):182.
Hatcher RA et al: *Contraceptive Technology 1984–1985*, 12th ed. New York: Irvington Publishers, 1984.
Hoffman JB: A suggested treatment for inverted nipples. *Am J Obstet Gynecol* 1953; 66:346.
Lawrence RA: *Breastfeeding: A Guide for the Medical Profession*. St. Louis: Mosby, 1980.

Marut J, Mercer R: Comparison of primiparas' perceptions of vaginal and cesarean births. *Nurs Res* May 1979; 28:260.

Pritchard JA, MacDonald PC, Gant NF: *Williams Obstetrics*, 17th ed. New York: Appleton-Century-Crofts, 1985.

Rosenfield AG: Contraception: Where are we in 1985? *Contemp Ob/Gyn* February 1985; 25(2):79.

Silber SJ, Cohen R: Microsurgical reversal of female sterilization: Role of tubal length. *Fertil Steril* 1980; 33(6):598.

Slattery, JS: Nutrition for the normal healthy infant. *MCN* March/April 1977; 12(2):105.

Tatum HJ, Connell-Tatum EB: Barrier contraception. *Fertil Steril* July 1981; 36(1):1.

Ward BG, Pridmore BR, Cox LW: Vietnamese refugees in Adelaide: An obstetric analysis. *Med J Aust* 1981; 1:72.

Additional Readings ───────

Bartosch JC: Oral contraceptives: Selection and management. *The Nurse Pract* May 1983; 8:56.

Brooten DA et al: A comparison of four treatments to prevent and control breast pain and engorgement in nonnursing mothers. *Nurs Res* July/August 1983; 32:225.

Darney PD: What's new in contraception. *Contemp Ob/Gyn* June 1984; 23:117.

Dickerson J: Oral contraceptives: Another look. *Am J Nurs* October 1983; 83(10):1392.

Ketter DE, Shelton BJ: In-hospital exercises for the postpartal woman. *MCN* March/April 1983; 8:120.

Leonard LG: Breastfeeding twins: Maternal-infant nutrition. *J Obstet Gynecol Neonatal Nurs* May/June 1982; 11:148.

MacDonald J: The working mother and her breastfeeding infant. *The Canad Nurse* March 1983; 79:21.

Oakley A: Does maternal work harm children? *Contemp Ob/Gyn* April 1984; 23:122.

Renaud MT: Effects of discontinuing cover gowns on a postpartal ward upon cord colonization of the newborn. *J Obstet Gynecol Neonatal Nurs* November/December 1983; 12:399.

Riordan J, Riordan M: Drugs in breast milk. *Am J Nurs* March 1984; 84:328.

Schlegel AM: Observation on breastfeeding technique: Facts and fallacies. *MCN* May/June 1983; 8:204.

25

Complications of the Puerperium

Chapter Contents

Postpartal Hemorrhage and Hematoma
Postpartal Hemorrhage
Hematomas

Puerperal Infections
Causative Factors
Pathophysiology
Interventions and Nursing Care
Discharge Planning

Thromboembolic Disease
Superficial Leg Vein Disease
Deep Leg Vein Disease
Pulmonary Embolism

Postpartal Cystitis and Pyelonephritis
Overdistention
Cystitis
Pyelonephritis
Interventions and Nursing Care

Disorders of the Breast
Mastitis
Breast Abscess

Puerperal Psychiatric Disorders

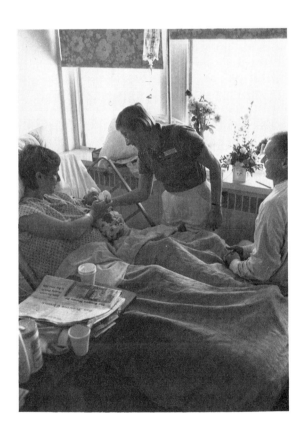

Objectives

• List the causes of and nursing interventions for hemorrhage during the postpartal period.

• Discuss the causative factors, pathophysiology, and nursing interventions for puerperal infections.

• Discuss causative factors, pathophysiology, and nursing interventions for thromboembolic disease of the puerperium.

- Describe puerperal cystitis and pyelonephritis and the implications for maternal nursing care.

- Differentiate disorders of the breast and complications of lactation.

- Identify the possible precipitating factors associated with puerperal psychiatric disorders.

Key Terms

endometritis	puerperal morbidity
mastitis	salpingitis
oophoritis	subinvolution
pelvic cellulitis	

The puerperium is usually viewed as a smooth, uneventful transition time, and often it is. However, the nurse must be aware of problems that may develop postpartally and their implications for the childbearing family. This chapter deals with complications that may occur during the puerperium and appropriate nursing interventions and care.

Postpartal Hemorrhage and Hematomas

Postpartal Hemorrhage

Postpartal hemorrhage has been divided into early and late postpartal hemorrhage. Early postpartal hemorrhage (or immediate postpartal hemorrhage) occurs when blood loss is greater than 500 mL in the first 24 hours after delivery. Late postpartal hemorrhage (delayed postpartal hemorrhage) occurs after the first 24 hours.

Early hemorrhage   The main causes of early postpartal hemorrhage are uterine atony, lacerations of the vagina and cervix, and retained placental fragments. Certain factors predispose to hemorrhage:

- Overdistention of the uterus due to hydramnios, a large infant, or multiple gestation
- Grandmultiparity
- Use of anesthetic agents (especially halothane) to relax the uterus

- Trauma due to obstetric procedures such as intrauterine manipulation or forceps rotation
- An abnormal labor pattern, either hypotonic or hypertonic
- Use of oxytocin to induce or augment labor
- Maternal malnutrition, anemia, PIH, or history of hemorrhage

In most cases the clinician can predict which woman is at risk for hemorrhage. The key to successful management is prevention. (See Essential Facts to Remember—Signs of Postpartal Hemorrhage.)

Prevention begins with adequate nutrition, good prenatal care, and early diagnosis and management of any complications that may arise. Traumatic procedures should be avoided, and delivery should take place in a facility that has blood immediately available.

During delivery excessive kneading of an already contracted fundus should be avoided because it may cause incomplete placental separation and increased blood loss. After delivery the uterus and birth canal should be carefully inspected for any retained placental fragments or lacerations, and the placenta should be examined for intactness. (For further discussion of appropriate care see the Nursing Care Plan on hemorrhage on p. 368.)

Periodic assessment for evidence of bleeding is a major nursing responsibility on the postpartal unit. After the fourth stage of labor most hemorrhage is caused by retained cotyledons, retained fetal membranes, or subnormal or abnormal involution of the placental site.

 ESSENTIAL FACTS TO REMEMBER

Signs of Postpartal Hemorrhage

The nurse must suspect postpartal hemorrhage or hematoma formation if a woman complains of any of the following:

- Excessive or bright red bleeding
- A boggy fundus that does not respond to massage
- Abnormal clots
- Any unusual pelvic discomfort or backache
- High temperature

Careful observation and documentation of vaginal bleeding (by counting or weighing peripads) is important. A boggy uterus that does not stay contracted without constant massage is atonic, whereas a uterus that does not involute appropriately is investigated for possible retained placental tissue and infection. The most common intervention is a continuous infusion of fluids and oxytocin. If the woman is normotensive, methylergonovine maleate or ergonovine maleate may be used. If this treatment is not effective or if a placental fragment is retained for several days, curettage is usually indicated, together with the administration of antibiotics to prevent puerperal infection.

Late hemorrhage Occasionally, late postpartal hemorrhage occurs around the fifth to the fifteenth day after delivery when the woman is home and recovering. Bleeding most often is caused by retained placental fragments or abnormal involution of the placental site. This type of hemorrhage is usually treated with the administration of oxytocics, curettage if necessary, and prophylactic antibiotics.

Subinvolution **Subinvolution** of the uterus occurs when the uterus fails to follow the normal pattern of involution and remains enlarged. Retained placental fragments or infection are the most frequent causes. With subinvolution the fundus is higher in the abdomen than expected. In addition, lochia often fails to progress from rubra to serosa to alba. Lochia may remain rubra or return to rubra after several days postpartum. Leukorrhea and backache may occur if infection is the cause.

Subinvolution is most commonly diagnosed during the routine postpartal examination at 4–6 weeks. The woman may relate a history of irregular or excessive bleeding, or describe the symptoms listed previously. Diagnosis is made when an enlarged, softer-than-normal uterus is palpated with bimanual examination. Treatment involves oral administration of methylergonovine maleate (Methergine) or ergonovine maleate (Ergotrate) 0.2 mg every 3–4 hours for 24–48 hours (see Drug Guide below). When metritis is present, antibiotics are also administered. If this treatment is not effective or if the cause is believed to be retained placental frag-

DRUG GUIDE
Methylergonovine Maleate (Methergine)

OVERVIEW OF OBSTETRIC ACTION

Methylergonovine maleate is an ergot alkaloid that stimulates smooth muscle. Because the smooth muscle of the uterus is especially sensitive to this drug, it is used postpartally to stimulate the uterus to contract. This contraction clamps off uterine blood vessels and prevents hemorrhage. In addition, the drug has a vasoconstrictive effect on all blood vessels, especially on the larger arteries. This may result in hypertension, particularly in a woman whose blood pressure is already elevated.

ROUTE, DOSAGE, AND FREQUENCY

Methergine has a rapid onset of action and may be given intramuscularly, orally, or intravenously.

Usual IM dose: 0.2 mg following delivery of the placenta. The dose may be repeated every 2–4 hours if necessary.

Usual oral dose: 0.2 mg every 4 hours (six doses).

Usual IV dose: Because the adverse effects of Methergine are far more severe with IV administration, this route is seldom used. If Methergine is given intravenously, the rate should *not* exceed 0.2 mg/min and the client's blood pressure should be monitored continuously.

MATERNAL CONTRAINDICATIONS

Pregnancy, induction of labor, hepatic or renal disease, threatened spontaneous abortion, uterine sepsis, cardiac disease, hypertension, and obliterative vascular disease contraindicate this drug's use (Loebl and Spratto, 1983).

MATERNAL SIDE EFFECTS

Hypertension (particularly when administered IV), nausea, vomiting, headache, bradycardia, dizziness, tinnitus, abdominal cramps, palpitations, dyspnea, chest pain, and allergic reactions may be noted.

EFFECTS ON FETUS/NEONATE

Because Methergine has a long duration of action and can thus produce tetanic contractions it should never be used during pregnancy as it may result in fetal trauma or death.

NURSING CONSIDERATIONS

1. Monitor fundal height and consistency and the amount and character of the lochia.
2. Assess the blood pressure before administration.
3. Observe for adverse effects or symptoms of ergot toxicity.

ments, curettage is indicated (Pritchard, Mac-Donald, and Gant, 1985).

Hematomas

Hematomas are usually the result of injury to a blood vessel without noticeable trauma to the superficial tissue. Hematomas occur following spontaneous as well as forceps deliveries.

The most frequently observed hematomas are of the vagina and vulva. The soft tissue in the area offers no resistance, and hematomas containing 250–500 mL of blood develop rapidly. The woman complains of severe vulvar pain (pain that seems out of proportion or excessive), usually from her "stitches," or of severe rectal pressure. On examination, the large hematoma appears as a unilateral, tense, fluctuant bulging mass at the introitus or encompassing the labia majora. With smaller hematomas the nurse may note unilateral bluish or reddish discoloration of the skin of the perineum. The area feels firm and is painful to the touch. The nurse should estimate the size of the hematoma so that increasing size will be quickly noted.

Hematomas can develop in the upper portion of the vagina. In this case, besides pain the woman may have difficulty voiding because of pressure on the urethra or meatus. Diagnosis is confirmed through careful vaginal examination.

Hematomas may also occur upward into the broad ligament, which may be more difficult to diagnose. The woman may complain of severe lateral uterine pain, flank pain, or abdominal distention. Occasionally the hematoma can be discovered with high rectal examination or with abdominal palpation. If the bleeding continues, signs of anemia may be noted.

Small vulvar hematomas may be treated with the application of ice packs and continued observation. Large hematomas generally require surgical intervention to evacuate the clot and to achieve hemostasis. General anesthesia is usually required. If the hematoma is not accessible vaginally, a laparotomy must be performed.

Continuous assessment of the vaginal bleeding is required after surgery to treat vaginal hematomas. If the hematoma was of the vulva or perineum, the nurse should check for recurrence.

Puerperal Infections

Puerperal infection is an infection of the reproductive tract associated with childbirth. Because infection accounts for a large percentage of postpartal morbidity, it is useful to remember the definition of **puerperal morbidity** published by the Joint Committee on Maternal Welfare:

> Temperature of 100.4F (38.0C) or higher, the temperature to occur on any two of the first ten postpartum days, exclusive of the first 24 hours, and to be taken by mouth by a standard technique at least four times a day.

Recent research (Filker and Monif, 1979) suggests that a temperature greater than 38.3C (101F) in the first 24 hours is also "highly indicative of ensuing infection."

Causative Factors

The vagina and cervix of pregnant women generally contain pathogenic bacteria sufficient to cause infection. Generally, other factors must be present, however, for infection to occur. PROM allows organisms to ascend into the uterus and is a major factor in the development of infection postpartally. In addition, the placental site, episiotomy, lacerations, abrasions, and any operative incisions are all potential portals for bacterial entrance and growth. Hematomas are easily infected and enhance the possibility of sepsis. Tissue that has been compromised through trauma is less able to marshal the necessary forces to combat infection. Other factors predisposing the woman to infection include frequent vaginal examinations, lapses in aseptic technique, anemia, intrauterine manipulation, hemorrhage, cesarean delivery, retained placental fragments, and faulty perineal care.

Approximately 70% of puerperal infections are caused by anaerobic bacteria. The most common anaerobes involved include bacteriodes (all species), peptococcus, and *Clostridium perfringens*.

Aerobic bacteria are also responsible for postpartal infection. *Escherichia coli* may be introduced as a result of contamination of the vulva or reproductive tract from feces during labor and delivery. Group A beta hemolytic streptococci may be transmitted from the skin or nasopharynx of the woman herself, or more probably from an external source such as personnel or equipment. Other aerobic bacteria implicated in puerperal infections include *Klebsiella*, *Proteus mirabilis*, *Pseudomonas*, *Staphylococcus aureus*, and *Neisseria gonorrhoeae* (Eschenbach and Wager, 1980).

Pathophysiology

Localized infections   A less severe complication of the puerperium is a localized infection of the episiotomy or of lacerations to the perineum, vagina, or vulva. Wound infection of the abdominal incision site following cesarean delivery is also not infrequent. The skin edges become reddened, edematous, firm, and tender. The skin edges then separate, and purulent material, sometimes mixed with sanguineous liquid, drains from the wound (Table 25-1). The woman may complain of localized pain and dysuria and may have a low-grade fever (less than 38.3C or 101F). If the wound abscesses or is unable to drain, high temperature and chills may result.

Prevention is, of course, the first clinical goal, and is accomplished by aseptic technique, client teaching about correct perineal care, and the use of sitz baths or heat lamps to facilitate healing (see Nursing Care Plan for further discussion). The woman's perineum should be inspected at least twice each day for early signs of developing infection. When a localized infection develops, it is treated with antibiotic creams, sitz baths, and analgesics as necessary for pain relief. If an abscess has developed or a stitch site is infected, the suture is removed and the area allowed to drain.

Endometritis   After delivery of the placenta, the placental site provides an excellent culture medium for bacterial growth. The remaining portion of the decidua is also susceptible to pathogenic bacteria because of its thinness and hypervascularity. The cervix may also become a bacterial breeding ground because of the multiple small lacerations that occur with normal labor and delivery.

In mild cases the woman will generally have discharge that is scant (or profuse), bloody, and foul smelling. In more severe cases, the symptoms may include uterine tenderness and jagged, irregular temperature elevation, usually between 38.3C (101F) and 40C (104F). Tachycardia, chill, and evidence of subinvolution may be noted. Although foul-smelling lochia is cited as a classic sign of **endometritis**, with infection caused by beta hemolytic streptococcus the lochia may be scant and odorless (Pritchard, MacDonald, and Gant, 1985).

Table 25-1
REEDA Scale Used to Evaluate Healing*

Points	Redness	Edema	Ecchymosis	Discharge	Approximation
0	None	None	None	None	Closed
1	Within 0.25 cm of incision bilaterally	Perineal, less than 1 cm from incision	Within 0.25 cm bilaterally or 0.5 cm unilaterally	Serum	Skin separation 3 mm or less
2	Within 0.5 cm of incision bilaterally	Perineal and/or vulvar, between 1 to 2 cm from incision	Between 0.25 to 1 cm bilaterally or between 0.5 to 2 cm unilaterally	Serosanguineous	Skin and subcutaneous fat separation
3	Beyond 0.5 cm of incision bilaterally	Perineal and/or vulvar, greater than 2 cm from incision	Greater than 1 cm bilaterally or 2 cm unilaterally	Bloody purulent	Skin, subcutaneous fat, and fascial layer separation
Score:	_____	_____	_____	_____	_____
					Total _____

*From Davidson N: REEDA: Evaluating postpartum healing. *J Nurs-Midwifery* 19:2, Summer 1974. Reprint permission granted by the American College of Nurse Midwives ©.

Text continued on p. 615.

NURSING CARE PLAN
Puerperal Infection

CLIENT ASSESSMENT

History

1. Predisposing health factors include:
   a. Malnutrition
   b. Anemia
   c. Debilitated condition

2. Predisposing factors associated with labor and delivery include:
   a. Prolonged labor
   b. Hemorrhage
   c. Premature and/or prolonged rupture
   d. Soft tissue trauma
   e. Invasive techniques
   f. Operative procedures

Physical Examination

1. Localized episiotomy infections may present the following signs and symptoms:
   a. Complaints of unusual degree of discomfort
   b. Reddened edematous lesion
   c. Purulent drainage
   d. Failure of skin edges to approximate
   e. Fever (generally below 38.3C or 101F)
   f. Dysuria

2. Endometritis
   a. Mild case may be asymptomatic or characterized only by low-grade fever, anorexia, and malaise
   b. More severe cases may demonstrate:
      (1) Fever of 101–103F+
      (2) Anorexia, extreme lethargy
      (3) Chills
      (4) Rapid pulse
      (5) Lower abdominal pain or uterine tenderness
      (6) Lochia—appearance varies depending on causative organism: may appear normal, be profuse, bloody, and foul smelling, may be scant and serosanguineous to brownish and foul smelling
      (7) Severe afterpains

3. Pelvic cellulitis (parametritis)
   a. Signs and symptoms of severe infection (see previous discussion of endometritis)
   b. Severe abdominal pain, usually lateral to the uterus on one or both sides and apparent with both abdominal palpation and pelvic examination

4. Puerperal peritonitis
   a. Symptoms just described plus severe abdominal pain
   b. Abdominal rigidity, guarding, rebound tenderness
   c. Possible vomiting and diarrhea
   d. Tachycardia, shallow respirations, anxiety
   e. Marked bowel distention if paralytic ileus develops

Laboratory Evaluation

1. Elevated white blood count (WBC), although it may be within normal puerperal limits (5000–15,000/mm^3) initially

2. Culture of intrauterine material to reveal causative organism

3. Urine culture to rule out an asymptomatic urinary tract infection (should be normal)

PLAN OF CARE

Nursing Priorities

1. Promote healing of perineum, uterus, and pelvic area without exposure to infectious agents.

2. Assess signs and symptoms of impending infections with prompt interventions.

3. Implement an appropriate client education program based on the specific needs of the woman and her partner.

Client/Family Educational Focus

1. Provide the woman and her partner with information about the signs and symptoms, course of the condition, treatment methods, self-care measures to ensure cleanliness and promote tissue healing, and home care routines for postpartal infections.

2. Provide opportunities for the couple to ask questions, express concerns and make plans for home and infant management depending on the seriousness of the infection and the amount of assistance available at home.

NURSING CARE PLAN (continued)
Puerperal Infection

Problem	Nursing interventions and actions	Rationale
Wound infection	Promote normal wound healing by using: 1. Sitz baths 2–4 times daily for 10–15 min 2. Peri-light 2–3 times daily for 10–15 min 3. Peri-care following elimination 4. Frequent changing of peri-pads 5. Early ambulation 6. Diet high in protein and vitamin C 7. Fluid intake to 2000 mL/day Evaluate degree of healing by applying REEDA scale (Table 25-1). Observe, record, and report signs and symptoms of wound infection, including: 1. Redness 2. Edema 3. Excessive pain 4. Inadequate approximation of wound edges 5. Purulent drainage 6. Fever, anorexia, malaise Obtain culture from wound site and administer antibiotics, per physician order. Increase wound drainage by: 1. Assisting physician in opening wound for drainage, when indicated 2. Anticipating packing of a cavity greater than 2–3 cm with iodoform gauze Assess pain level and administer analgesics per physician orders if pain is not relieved through nursing measures. Prevent spread of infection through: 1. Careful hand-washing techniques by staff, patient, and visitors 2. Special disposal of infected materials such as disposable bed chux, peri-pads, and contaminated linen Promote and maintain mother-infant interaction by: 1. Encouraging mother to continue feeding her infant 2. Reassuring mother that infant is not likely to become infected by her localized infection	Warm water is cleansing, promotes healing through increased vascular flow to affected area, and is soothing to woman. Peri-care promotes removal of urine and fecal contaminants from perineum. Changing pads frequently decreases the media for bacterial growth. These nutrients are essential for satisfactory wound healing. REEDA scale provides consistent, objective tool for evaluation of wound healing. Wound infection produces characteristic signs and symptoms. Antibiotic therapy based on knowledge of causative organism is treatment of choice for localized infection. Abscesses may develop when infected material accumulates in closed body cavity Iodoform packing maintains patency of opening so drainage can continue. Success at feeding infant generally enhances the woman's outlook, encourages mother-infant interaction, and prevents woman from dwelling on herself to exclusion of infant. Breast-feeding is not affected by localized infection and should be encouraged. Some institutions still insist on separation of the mother and infant if an infection is present; the mother must be instructed in pumping her breasts (if breast-feeding) and will need support during this separation.
Metritis/endometritis	Care of the patient is essentially the same as for wound infections, including antibiotics, analgesics, and careful cleansing techniques.	

NURSING CARE PLAN (continued)
Puerperal Infection

Problem	Nursing interventions and actions	Rationale
	Newborn: Assess breast-feeding infant's mouth for signs of thrush, which is a common side effect of antibiotics ingested by infant in mother's milk. Treatment should be initiated but breast-feeding need not be stopped.	Thrush, a monilial infection caused by *Candida albicans*, often occurs when normal oral flora are destroyed by antibiotic therapy.
Pelvic cellulitis	Observe, record, and report signs and symptoms of severe infection, including: 1. Fever spiking to 38.9C–40C (102F–104F) 2. Elevated white blood count 3. Chills 4. Extreme lethargy 5. Lower abdominal pain, especially lateral to uterus 6. Nausea and vomiting	Infection produces characteristic signs and symptoms.
	Administer IV fluids and antibiotics as ordered.	IV fluids maintain proper hydration of woman.
	Assist physician in pelvic examination for detection of abscess; be prepared for surgical incision and drainage if necessary; in cases where all management fails, removal of infected uterus, tubes, and ovaries may be necessary. Promote patient comfort through: 1. Adequate periods of rest 2. Emotional support 3. Judicious use of antibiotics 4. Maintenance of cleanliness and warmth 5. Maintenance of semi-Fowler's position	Position promotes comfort and helps prevent spread of infection.
Peritonitis	Observe, record, and report signs and symptoms of severe infection, such as nausea, vomiting, and abdominal rigidity.	Paralytic ileus is frequently associated with peritonitis.
	Maintain continuous nasogastric suction per physician order.	Continuous nasogastric suction is used to decompress bowel when paralytic ileus complicates clinical course.
	Administer IV fluids and antibiotics as ordered. Monitor intake and output, urine specific gravity, vital signs, and level of hydration. Provide narcotic analgesics for alleviation of severe pain, per physician order.	Vigorous fluid and electrolyte therapy is necessary not only because of vomiting and diarrhea, but also because both fluid and electrolytes become sequestered in lumen and wall of bowel.
	Transfer patient to intensive care or provide critical care services by skilled registered nurse.	Patient with peritonitis is in critical condition, and quality of nursing care this patient receives will weigh the balance between recovery and demise.
	Provide emotional support, including: 1. Anticipate maternal depression. 2. Provide opportunities for mother to see, touch, and hold infant when possible, taking proper precautions to protect infant.	Critically ill patient may become very depressed not only from disease process but also because her anticipated postpartal course is now denied to her, and she may interpret this as a failure of her ability to mother her infant.

NURSING CARE PLAN (continued)
Puerperal Infection

Problem	Nursing interventions and actions	Rationale
	3. Assist breast-feeding mothers to pump breasts in order to maintain milk production.	
	4. Encourage partner/family/support persons to become involved with patient's care and with infant.	
	5. Take pictures of the infant for the mother's bedside.	

NURSING CARE EVALUATION

Purulent drainage, odor, edema, elevated temperature, and wounds are controlled or relieved.	Woman understands condition, treatment regimen, prevention of spread of infection, infant care, and necessity of continued medical supervision.
Wound is healing.	
Woman is ambulating.	

NURSING DIAGNOSIS*	SUPPORTING DATA	NURSING ORDERS
Potential for injury related to spread of infection	Increased temperature Chills Vaginal discharge Malaise	Decrease potential for spread of infection: 1. Use aseptic technique. 2. Instruct patient in safe hand-washing. 3. Isolate contaminated materials.
Knowledge deficit related to the condition and its treatment	Expressed concerns or questions about specific aspects of care Inadequate hygiene practices	Increase patient knowledge base: 1. Assess knowledge base. 2. Provide teaching for identified informational needs.

*These are examples of nursing diagnoses that may be appropriate for a person with this condition. It is not an inclusive list and must be individualized for each woman.

Salpingitis and oophoritis Occasionally, bacteria may spread into the lumen of the fallopian tubes, producing infection in the tubes (**salpingitis**) and ovaries (**oophoritis**). Most often caused by a gonorrheal infection, such infection generally becomes apparent between the ninth and fifteenth postpartal day. Symptoms include bilateral (or unilateral) lower abdominal pain, high temperature, and tachycardia. If tubal closure results, sterility may ensue (Vorherr, 1982). Treatment is basically the same as that described in the next section on parametritis.

Pelvic cellulitis (Parametritis) and Peritonitis) Pelvic cellulitis (parametritis) refers to infection involving the connective tissue of the broad ligament and, in more severe forms, the connective tissue of all the pelvic structures. It is generally spread by way of the lymphatics in the uterine wall, but may also

occur if pathogenic organisms invade a cervical laceration that extends upward into the connective tissue of the broad ligament. This laceration then serves as a direct pathway that allows the pathogens already in the cervix to spread into the pelvis. *Peritonitis* refers to infection involving the peritoneum.

Pelvic abscess may form and most commonly is found in the uterine ligaments, Douglas' cul-de-sac, and subdiaphragmatic space.

A woman suffering from parametritis may demonstrate a variety of symptoms, including marked high temperature (38.9–40C or 102–104F), chills, malaise, lethargy, abdominal pain, subinvolution of the uterus, tachycardia, and local and referred rebound tenderness. If peritonitis develops, the woman will be acutely ill with severe pain, marked anxiety, high fever, rapid, shallow respirations, pronounced tachycardia, excessive thirst, abdominal distention, nausea, and vomiting.

Interventions and Nursing Care

Assessment of an infection that is no longer simply a localized infection requires careful assessment of presenting signs and symptoms. During the first 24–48 hours symptoms may be minimal: often a temperature no higher than 38.3C–38.9C (101F–102F) may occur, while a white blood count remains in the normal range. As the infection progresses, the patient has a sustained temperature elevation and may manifest other symptoms such as pain, tenderness, malaise, anorexia, and urinary complaints. Diagnosis of the infection site and causative pathogen is accomplished by a complete physical examination, blood work, cultures (particularly of lochia), and urinalysis.

Antibiotic therapy usually is implemented based on the culture and sensitivity results. A broad-spectrum antibiotic effective against the most commonly occurring causative organisms is used in the interim. The antibiotics are administered intravenously.

The development of an abscess is frequently heralded by the presence of a palpable mass and may be confirmed with ultrasound. An abscess usually requires incision and drainage to avoid rupture into the peritoneal cavity and development of possibly fatal peritonitis.

The Nursing Care Plan on puerperal infection presents the nursing management for infections. General and specific aspects of nursing care are identified for the major patient problems.

Discharge Planning

The woman with a severe puerperal infection may need assistance when she is discharged from the hospital. The community health/visiting nurse service can be contacted as soon as puerperal infection is diagnosed so that the nurse can meet with the mother for a family and home assessment and development of a home care plan.

The mother should be instructed regarding activity, rest, medications, diet, and signs and symptoms of complications, and she should be scheduled for a return medical examination.

Thromboembolic Disease _____

Thromboembolic disease occurs in approximately 1% of spontaneously delivered women and in 2%–10% of women undergoing cesarean birth (Vorherr, 1982). Although the disease may also occur antepartally, it is generally considered a postpartal complication. *Venous thrombosis* refers to thrombus formation in a superficial or deep vein with the accompanying risk that a portion of the clot might break off and result in pulmonary embolism. When the thrombus is formed in response to inflammation in the vein wall, it is termed *thrombophlebitis*. In this type of thrombosis the clot tends to be more firmly attached and therefore is less likely to result in embolism. In *noninflammatory venous thrombosis* (also called phlebothrombosis) the clot tends to be more loosely attached, and the risk of embolism is greater. The main factors responsible for this type of thrombosis are venous stasis, vascular anoxia, and endothelial damage (Vorherr, 1982).

The following factors contribute directly to the development of thromboembolic disease postpartally:

- Increased amounts of certain blood-clotting factors
- Postpartal thrombocytosis (increased quantity of circulating platelets and their increased adhesiveness)
- Release of thromboplastin substances from tissue of the decidua, placenta, and fetal membranes
- Increased amounts of fibrin inhibitors

Superficial Leg Vein Disease

Superficial thrombophlebitis is far more common postpartally than during pregnancy. Often the clot involves the saphenous veins. This disorder is more common in women with preexisting varices, although it is not limited to these women. Symptoms usually become apparent about the third or fourth postpartal day: tenderness in a portion of the vein, some local heat and redness, absent or low-grade fever, and occasionally, slight elevation of the pulse.

Treatment involves application of local heat, elevation of the affected limb, bed rest, analgesics, and the use of elastic support hose. Anticoagulants are usually not necessary unless complications develop. Pulmonary embolism is extremely rare. Occasionally the involved veins have incompetent valves, and as a result, the problem may spread to the deeper leg veins, such as the femoral vein.

Deep Leg Vein Disease

Deep venous thrombosis is more frequently seen in women with a history of thrombosis. Certain obstetric complications such as hydramnios, PIH, and operative delivery are associated with an increased incidence.

Clinical manifestations may include edema of the ankle and leg, and an initial low-grade fever, often followed by high temperature and chills. Depending on the vein involved, the woman may complain of pain in the popliteal and lateral tibial areas (popliteal vein), entire lower leg and foot (anterior and posterior tibial veins), inguinal tenderness (femoral vein), or pain in the lower abdomen (iliofemoral vein). The Homan's sign (Figure 23-5) may or may not be positive, but pain often results from calf pressure. Because of arterial spasm, sometimes the limb is pale and cool to the touch—the so-called milk leg or *phlegmasia alba dolens*—and peripheral pulses may be decreased.

Because cases are seldom clearcut, diagnosis involves a variety of approaches, such as client history and physical examination, occlusive cuff impedence phlebography (IPG), Doppler ultrasonography, and contrast venography. In questionable cases, contrast venography provides the most accurate diagnosis of deep venous thrombosis. Unfortunately, venography is not practical for multiple examinations or prospective screening and may, in itself, induce phlebitis.

Treatment involves the administration of intravenous heparin, using an infusion pump to permit continuous, accurate infusion of medication. Bed rest is required, and analgesics are given as necessary to relieve discomfort. If fever is present, deep thrombophlebitis is suspected and the woman is also given antibiotic therapy. The nurse monitors the woman closely for signs of pulmonary embolism, the most severe complication of deep venous thrombosis. Nurses must observe for any signs of bleeding while the woman is receiving the heparin. In most cases thrombectomy is not necessary.

Once the symptoms have subsided (usually in a few days), the woman may begin ambulation while wearing elastic support stockings. She is instructed to avoid prolonged standing or sitting, and to avoid crossing her legs. The knee gatch on the bed should never be used. Women who have deep venous thrombosis often are given warfarin therapy and need careful instruction about its use, side effects, implications for breast-feeding, and possible interactions with other medications.

Pulmonary Embolism

A sudden onset of dyspnea accompanied by sweating, pallor, cyanosis, confusion, systemic hypotension, and increased jugular pressure may indicate the possibility of a pulmonary embolism. Chest pain that mimics heart attack, coupled with the woman's verbalized fear of imminent death and complaint of pressure in the bowel and rectum, should alert the nurse to the extensive size of the embolus. Smaller emboli may present with only transient syncope, tightness of the chest, or unexplained fever.

Even x-ray films and ECG changes and laboratory data are not always reliable diagnostic methods. If a case of pulmonary embolism is suspected, prompt treatment should begin even in the absence of collaborative data. If the embolism is small and heparin therapy is begun quickly, the chance of survival is excellent. However, when a large thrombus occludes a major pulmonary vessel, death may occur before therapy can even begin.

Therapy involves the administration of a variety of intravenous medications, such as meperidine hydrochloride to relieve the pain, lidocaine for the correction of any arrhythmias, and drugs such as papaverine hydrochloride and aminophylline to reduce spasms of the bronchi and coronary and pulmonary vessels (Vorherr, 1982). Oxygen is administered and heparin infusion is begun. In severe cases an embolectomy may be necessary, although fibrinolytic therapy with medications (such as streptokinase) that lyse clots may be tried first.

For nursing management of thrombophlebitis and pulmonary embolism, see the accompanying Nursing Care Plan.

Text continued on p. 621.

NURSING CARE PLAN
Thrombophlebitis and Pulmonary Embolism

CLIENT ASSESSMENT

History

1. Predisposing factors include:
   a. Increased maternal age
   b. Obesity
   c. Increased parity
   d. Prolonged labor with associated pressure of the fetal head on the pelvic veins
   e. PIH
   f. Heart disease
   g. Hypercoagulability of the early puerperium
   h. Anemia
   i. Immobility
   j. Hemorrhage
   k. Previous history of venous thrombosis

2. Initiating factors may include:
   a. Trauma to deep leg veins due to faulty positioning for delivery
   b. Operative delivery, including cesarean
   c. Abortion
   d. Postpartal pelvic cellulitis

Physical Examination

1. Superficial thrombophlebitis
   a. Tenderness along the involved vein
   b. Areas of palpable thrombosis
   c. Warmth and redness in the involved area

2. Deep vein thrombosis
   a. Positive Homan's sign (pain occurs when foot is dorsiflexed while leg is extended)
   b. Tenderness and pain in affected area
   c. Fever (initially low, followed by high fever and chills)
   d. Edema in affected extremity
   e. Pallor and coolness in affected limb
   f. Diminished peripheral pulses

3. Pulmonary embolism
   a. Sudden onset of dyspnea, sweating, pallor, cyanosis, confusion, chest pain, and verbalized anxiety and feelings of impending doom
   b. Possible systemic hypotension and increased jugular pressure
   c. Gallop heart rhythm

Laboratory Evaluation

1. Thrombophlebitis
   a. Doppler ultrasonography demonstrates increased circumference of affected extremity
   b. Occlusive cuff IPG
   c. Venography confirms diagnosis

2. Pulmonary embolism
   a. Electrocardiogram may reveal indications of right-sided heart strain
   b. Lung scan or pulmonary angiography may reveal evidence of pulmonary embolism but may not be definitive
   c. SGOT and LDH may be elevated

PLAN OF CARE

Nursing Priorities

1. Prevent circulatory stasis through correct positioning in delivery stirrups, early ambulation, leg exercise, applications of support stockings, and avoiding crossing legs.

2. Maintain maternal–infant interactions.

3. Perform daily assessments to recognize the development of vascular complications and implement appropriate nursing care if they develop.

4. Promote mental health through woman's expressions of fears, acceptance of change in body image, and alternatives to infant care when activities are restricted.

Client/Family Educational Focus

1. Provide information about the cause of the condition, the treatment regimen, medications, infant care, necessity of continued medical supervision, and means to avoid circulatory stasis.

2. Carefully review the implications, rationale, side effects, and possible problems that may develop with warfarin therapy following discharge.

3. Provide opportunities for the couple to ask questions and express concerns about the diagnosis and its implications.

Problem	Nursing interventions and actions	Rationale
Thrombophlebitis	Initiate and maintain actions to prevent development of thrombophlebitis, including: 1. Careful positioning of woman in stirrups for delivery 2. Early active ambulation 3. Use of support stockings following operative deliveries	Prolonged pressure, resulting in venous stasis and trauma to the vein wall, is contributing factor to development of thrombophlebitis. Movement and support encourage venous return and decrease tendency to venous stasis.

NURSING CARE PLAN (continued)
Thrombophlebitis and Pulmonary Embolism

Problem	Nursing interventions and actions	Rationale
	4. Instruction as to necessity for doing leg exercises regularly when confined to bed	
	5. Instruction not to elevate knee gatch in bed	
	Observe, record, and report signs and symptoms of thrombophlebitis.	
	Maintain bed rest and warm, moist soaks as ordered.	Bed rest is ordered to decrease possibility that portion of clot will dislodge and cause pulmonary embolism. Warmth promotes blood flow to affected area. Heparin does not dissolve clot but is administered to prevent further clotting. It is safe for breast-feeding mothers because heparin is not excreted in mother's milk.
	Administer analgesics for relief of pain per physician order.	
	Administer intravenous heparin as ordered, by continuous intravenous drip, heparin lock, or subcutaneously, including:	
	1. Monitor IV or heparin lock site for signs of infiltration.	
	2. Obtain Lee-White clotting times or partial thromboplastin time (PTT) per physician order and review prior to administering heparin.	
	3. Observe for signs of anticoagulant overdose with resultant bleeding, including: a. Hematuria b. Epistaxis c. Ecchymosis d. Bleeding gums	
	4. Provide protamine sulfate, per physician order, to combat bleeding problems related to heparin overdosage.	Protamine sulfate is heparin antagonist, given intravenously, which is almost immediately effective in counteracting bleeding complications caused by heparin overdose.
	5. Initiate progressive ambulation following the acute phase; provide properly fitting elastic stockings prior to ambulation.	Elastic stockings or "Teds" help prevent pooling of venous blood in lower extremities.
	6. Obtain prothrombin time (PT) and review prior to beginning warfarin. Repeat periodically per physician order.	PT is the test most commonly used to monitor the blood of clients receiving warfarin.
	7. Discuss the use of warfarin, its side-effects, implications for breast-feeding and possible interactions with other medications.	Such discussion helps woman understand medication and its implications.
Pulmonary embolism	Observe, record, and report signs and symptoms of pulmonary embolism, including: 1. Sudden onset of severe chest pain, often located substernally 2. Apprehension and sense of impending catastrophe 3. Cough (may be accompanied by hemoptysis) 4. Tachycardia 5. Fever	Signs and symptoms may occur suddenly and require immediate emergency treatment; prognosis is related to size and location of embolism.

NURSING CARE PLAN (continued)
Thrombophlebitis and Pulmonary Embolism

Problem	Nursing interventions and actions	Rationale

	6. Hypotension
	7. Diaphoresis, pallor, weakness
	8. Shortness of breath
	9. Neck vein engorgement
	10. Friction rub and evidence of atelectasis upon auscultation
	Initiate or support emergency treatment and additional treatment, including:
	1. Combat hypoxia:
	  a. Administer oxygen.
	  b. Assist physician with tracheal intubation if necessary.
	2. Monitor vital signs, ECG.
	3. Administer medications as ordered:
	  a. Sedative
	
	  b. Digitalis
	4. Prepare patient for embolectomy if ordered.
	5. Additional treatment involves anticoagulants, bed rest, and analgesics and is similar to treatment for thrombophlebitis.
		
		Sedation is used to control pain and anxiety.
		
		Digitalis is administered to improve myocardial function.

Prevention of maternal/ infant deprivation	Maintain mother–infant attachment when mother is on bed rest: 1. Provide frequent contacts for mother and infant; modified rooming-in possible if crib placed tangent to mother's bed or if Baby Bonding Crib is used. 2. Encourage continuation of breast-feeding or pump breasts for acutely ill patients. 3. Provide photos of infant if contact limited.	Evidence indicates that first few days of life may be crucial to development of maternal–infant bonds, and separation during this period should be avoided. Flow of milk is contingent on emptying of breast, either by placing infant to breast or pumping milk from breast; many institutions use milk pumped from mother's breasts for feeding infant.

NURSING CARE EVALUATION

Presenting signs and symptoms are relieved or controlled.

Patient is stabilized on anticoagulant medication.

No inflammatory process is evident.

Patient is ambulatory without pain.

Patient applies elastic stocking correctly.

Patient knows to avoid constrictive clothing; to avoid placing legs in dependent positions; purposes of medications, including dosage, untoward effects of anticoagulant medications, frequency, symptoms to report to physician; and necessity of continued medical supervision.

Maternal–infant bonding is established.

NURSING DIAGNOSIS*	SUPPORTING DATA	NURSING ORDERS
Potential alteration in tissue perfusion secondary to deep vein thrombosis	Reddened, edematous, painful area Cool extremity below inflamed area Edema of extremity Decreased peripheral pulses	Increase peripheral circulation 1. Elevate extremity. 2. Prevent pressure by instructing patient not to use knee gatch in bed. 3. Assess peripheral pulses.

NURSING CARE PLAN (continued)
Thrombophlebitis and Pulmonary Embolism

NURSING DIAGNOSIS*	SUPPORTING DATA	NURSING ORDERS
Potential fluid deficit related to bleeding from anticoagulant therapy	Lab data in excess of therapeutic range Bruising Bleeding gums GI bleeding	**Prevent Bleeding Episodes** 1. Protect from injury that might precipitate bruising. 2. Assess labortaory data. 3. Assist patient in using soft tooth brush.

*These are examples of nursing diagnoses that may be appropriate for a person with this condition. It is not an inclusive list and must be individualized for each woman.

Postpartal Cystitis and Pyelonephritis

The postpartal woman is at increased risk of developing urinary tract problems due to the normal postpartal diuresis, increased bladder capacity, decreased bladder sensitivity from stretching and/or trauma, and possible inhibited neural control of the bladder following the use of general anesthesia.

Emptying the bladder is vital. Women who are not sufficiently recovered from the effects of anesthesia cannot void spontaneously, and catheterization is necessary.

Retention of residual urine, bacteria introduced at the time of catheterization, and a bladder traumatized by delivery combine to provide an excellent environment for the development of cystitis.

Overdistention

The overdistended bladder appears as a large mass, reaching sometimes to the umbilicus and displacing the uterine fundus upward. There is increased vaginal bleeding, a boggy fundus, and the woman may complain of cramping as the uterus attempts to contract.

Diligent monitoring of the bladder during the recovery period and preventive health measures greatly reduce the chances for overdistention of the bladder. Encouraging the mother to void spontaneously and assisting her to use the toilet, if possible, or the bedpan, if she has received conductive anesthesia, prevent the largest percentage of overdistention.

If discovered in the recovery room, overdistention is often managed by draining the bladder with a straight catheter as a one-time measure. If the overdistention recurs or is diagnosed later in the postpartal period, an indwelling catheter is generally ordered for 24 hours.

Cystitis

E. coli causes 73%–90% of the cases of postpartal cystitis and pyelonephritis (Vorherr, 1982). In most cases the infection ascends the urinary tract from the urethra to the bladder and then to the kidneys because vesiculoureteral reflux forces contaminated urine into the renal pelvis.

Symptoms of cystitis (bladder inflammation) often appear 2–3 days after delivery. The initial symptoms may include frequency, urgency, dysuria, and nocturia. Hematuria and suprapubic pain may also be present. The temperature may be slightly elevated but often there are no systemic symptoms.

When cystitis is suspected in the puerperium, a clean-catch midstream urine sample is obtained for microscopic examination, culture, and sensitivity tests. Taking a catheterized specimen is avoided when possible because of the increased risk of infection. When the bacterial concentration is greater than 100,000 microorganisms per milliliter of fresh urine, infection is generally present; counts between 10,000 and 100,000 are suggestive, particularly if clinical symptoms are noted.

Pyelonephritis

When a urinary tract infection progresses to pyelonephritis, systemic symptoms usually occur, and the woman becomes acutely ill. Symptoms include chills, high fever, flank pain (unilateral or bilateral), nausea, and vomiting, in addition to all the signs of lower urinary tract infection. Costovertebral pain (CVA tenderness) also may be elicited. If untreated, the renal cortex may be damaged and kidney function may be impaired.

Interventions and Nursing Care

Prevention is important in dealing with urinary tract infection. Regular, complete bladder emptying, instruction on proper wiping techniques to avoid fecal contamination of the meatus, good perineal care, and frequent changing of perineal pads all decrease chances of infection.

When cystitis is suspected, treatment is delayed until the culture and sensitivity reports are available. The appropriate antibiotic medication is then begun. In the case of pyelonephritis, bed rest, forced fluids, and broad-spectrum antibiotics are prescribed even before the culture results are available. If nausea and vomiting are severe, fluids are administered intravenously. Antispasmodics and analgesics are also given to relieve discomfort. The woman usually continues to take antibiotics for 2–4 weeks after clinical and bacteriologic response. A routine clean-catch urine culture should be obtained 2 weeks after completion of therapy and then periodically for the next 2 years.

Continuation of breast-feeding during therapy is acceptable and is only limited by the degree of the mother's malaise and clinical discomfort. For the breast-feeding mother the antibiotic chosen should be selected carefully to avoid problems for the infant via the milk. The mother is encouraged to be as actively involved with her new baby as possible to promote the maternal–infant bond and help distract the woman from her problems.

Disorders of the Breast

Mastitis

Mastitis refers to an inflammation of the breast generally caused by *Staphylococcus aureus* and primarily seen in breast-feeding mothers. Because symptoms seldom occur before the second to fourth week postpartally,

nurses often are not fully aware of how uncomfortable and acutely ill the woman may be.

The infection usually begins when bacteria invade the breast tissue. Often the tissue has been traumatized in some way (fissured or cracked nipples, overdistention, manipulation, or milk stasis) and is especially susceptible to pathogenic invasion. The most common sources of the bacteria are the infant's nose and throat, although other sources include the hands of the mother or hospital personnel or the woman's circulating blood.

Once the infection develops, the woman may have a high temperature, chills, tachycardia, and headache. The breasts may be very tender, have a reddened and warm area, feel firm to the touch, or show areas of lumpiness (Figure 25-1). Diagnosis is usually based on the symptoms, physical examination, and a culture and sensitivity test of the breast milk.

Prevention is far simpler than therapy. Meticulous hand-washing by all personnel is the primary measure in preventing epidemic nursery infections and subsequent maternal mastitis. Prompt attention to mothers who have blocked milk ducts eliminates the stagnant milk as a growth medium for bacteria. Frequent breast-feeding of the infant usually prevents mastitis.

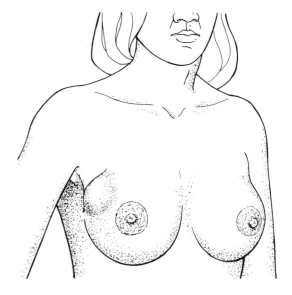

Figure 25-1

Mastitis. Erythema and swelling are present in the upper outer quadrant of the breast. Axillary lymph nodes are enlarged and tender.

If the mother finds that one area of her breast feels distended (caked), she can rotate the position of her infant for nursing, manually express milk remaining in the breast after nursing (or use a nontraumatic breast pump), or massage the caked area toward the nipple as the infant nurses.

Mastitis is treated by administration of appropriate antibiotics, use of analgesics to relieve discomfort, and local application of heat.

Opinion varies about whether breast-feeding should be discontinued in the presence of mastitis. Those advocating cessation of breast-feeding suggest that a vicious cycle of reinfection may develop as the infant ingests infected milk, becomes reinfected, and in turn, reinfects the mother. Those favoring continuation of breast-feeding raise several points in support of their beliefs.

1. If the milk contains bacteria, it also contains the antibiotic that the mother is taking.
2. If infants are the initial carriers of the infection, they should also be under treatment.
3. Sudden cessation of lactation will certainly cause caking and severe engorgement, which may be much more painful than continuing to breast-feed.
4. Breast-feeding stimulates circulation and moves bacteria-containing milk out of the breast, instead of leaving the affected milk to stagnate in the breast.

A third option, advocated by many agencies, involves the temporary cessation of breast-feeding from the involved breast during the acute phase. The milk from that breast can be manually expressed to avoid engorgement. Nursing can be resumed when the mother is afebrile and has received antibiotics for a time. To prevent recurrence the mother must continue taking the antibiotic for the full 10 days of therapy.

Breast Abscess

Occasionally the process of mastitis continues and a frank abscess develops. The mother's milk and any drainage from the nipple is then cultured and antibiotic therapy instituted. In addition, it is usually necessary to incise and drain the area and pack it with sterile gauze. The packing is gradually decreased to permit proper healing. Breast-feeding is usually suspended until the incision is healed. Then careful breast-feeding may resume, closely supervised by the experienced nurse.

Puerperal Psychiatric Disorders

Many different types of psychiatric problems may be encountered in the puerperium but only rarely is the disorder serious. Approximately 60% of women experience a transient depression during the first week, most commonly on the third postpartal day (Danforth, 1982). This transient depression is usually accompanied by tearfulness and is a self-limiting, brief episode.

The DSM-III (Diagnostic and Statistical Manual III) does not have a definitive heading for postpartum psychosis per se. In some instances the clinical picture will meet the criteria for Schizophreniform Disorder, Paranoid Disorder, Affective Disorder, or Organic Mental Disorder. If not, it is included under 298.20, Atypical Psychosis.

When psychiatric illness occurs after delivery, one or several of the following signs are usually present: depression, delusions, confusion, mania, delirium, hallucinations, anxiety, and sexual dysfunction (Hamilton, 1982). Occasionally, violent behavior forms part of the clinical picture; sometimes this violence is directed against the infant. Approximately 1 in 1000 term pregnancies is followed by psychiatric problems sufficiently severe to require hospitalization (Hamilton, 1982).

It is important to consider contributing factors to postpartal psychiatric disorders because one-fourth of women with a history of postpartal mental illness experience recurrence after a subsequent pregnancy. Contributing factors include the following (Barglow, 1982):

- A chronic history of inability to deal with crisis without decompensating
- A traumatic relationship with the woman's own mother, especially during childhood
- Self-defensive or conflicting motives for the pregnancy itself

- External variables, such as prolonged infertility prior to pregnancy, physical complications during the pregnancy or labor and delivery, and problems or abnormalities with the infant
- Concomitant life stresses, such as poverty, a recent family member's death, or home or job change

Prevention is the main goal. The clinician should be familiar with the woman and her partner, the woman's background, family, and personal history, social adjustment, level of maturity, and attitudes toward pregnancy and childrearing (Danforth, 1982). Frank and frequent discussion between the woman and her caregiver helps permit early intervention. In addition, active participation in the entire delivery process helps the woman achieve a sense of mastery.

Mild postpartal psychiatric disorders are usually treated on an outpatient basis, although medication or hospitalization is indicated in some cases. If the mother appears to have rejected her infant, it is never wise to compel her to care for him or her. This forces the woman to deal with feelings of guilt, shame, and hostility that may overwhelm her and endanger the infant.

It is important to identify problems before they become major obstacles to the woman's or her infant's emotional health. Psychiatric problems often are noted first by a nurse, obstetrician, or family member. If caregivers have any doubts about the woman's stability, a referral may be made to the public health service so that follow-up care is possible.

Summary

The normal puerperium is a dynamic period during which major physiologic changes must take place in order for the body to return to its nonpregnant state. When nurses are keenly aware of these normal physiologic changes, they can quickly assess whether deviations occur in the involutional process. These deviations place additional stress on the body, creating a risk situation for the mother that necessitates immediate intervention and evaluation.

References

Barglow P: Postpartum mental illness: Detection and treatment. In: *Gynecology and Obstetrics*. Vol. 2. Sciarra JJ (editor). Philadelphia: Harper & Row, 1982.

Danforth DN (editor): *Obstetrics and Gynecology*, 4th ed. Philadelphia: Harper & Row, 1982.

Eschenbach D, Wager G: Puerperal infections. *Clin Obstet Gynecol* 1980; 23(4):1003.

Filker R, Monif G: The significance of temperature during the first 24 hours postpartum. *Obstet Gynecol* March 1979; 53(3):358.

Hamilton JA: Puerperal psychoses. In: *Gynecology and Obstetrics*. Vol. 2. Sciarra JJ (editor). Philadelphia: Harper & Row, 1982.

Loebl S, Spratto G: *The Nurse's Drug Handbook*, 3rd ed. New York: Wiley, 1983.

Pritchard JA, MacDonald PC, Gant NF: *Williams Obstetrics*, 17th ed. New York: Appleton-Century-Crofts, 1985.

Vorherr H: Puerperium: Maternal involutional changes—management of puerperal problems and complications. In: *Gynecology and Obstetrics*. Vol. 2. Sciarra JJ (editor). Philadelphia: Harper & Row, 1982.

Additional Readings

Droegmueller W: Cold sitz baths for relief of postpartum perineal pain. *Clin Obstet Gynecol* 1980; 23(4):1039.

Faro S: Group B beta hemolytic streptococci and puerperal infections. *Am J Obstet Gynecol* 1981; 139(6):686.

Friedman C: Maternal infections: Problems and prevention. *Nurs Clin North Am* 1980; 15(4):817.

Ott WJ: Primary cesarean section: Factors related to postpartum infection. *Obstet Gynecol* 1981; 57(2):171.

Petrick J: Postpartum depression: Identification of high-risk mothers. *J Obstet Gynecol Neonatal Nurs* January/February 1984; 13:37.

Tentoni SC, High KA: Culturally induced postpartum depression. *J Obstet Gynecol Neonatal Nurs* July/August 1980; 9(4):246.

Vanden Bergh RL: Postpartum depression. *Clin Obstet Gynecol* 1980; 23(4):1105.

Wager GP, Martin DH, Koutsky L et al: Puerperal infectious morbidity: Relationship to route of delivery and to antepartum chlamydia trachomatis infection. *Am J Obstet Gynecol* 1980; 138:1028.

Watson P: Postpartum hemorrhage and shock. *Clin Obstet Gynecol* 1980; 23(4):985.

26

Families in Crisis and the Role of the Nurse

Chapter Contents

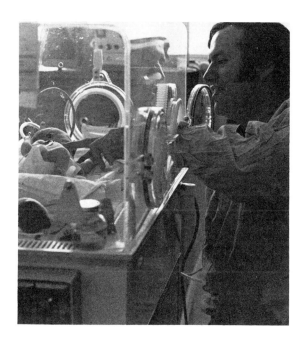

Objectives

- Compare the process of crisis intervention to the nursing process.

- Identify specific assessment strategies to predict which families will need additional support to avert or resolve a crisis.

- Describe the stages of the grieving process.

- Discuss the effects on the family of complications during pregnancy or birth.

- Discuss the nurse's role in assisting the family that loses an infant.

- Identify the needs of and nursing support for family members who must deal with the birth of a high-risk infant or infant with a defect.

- Discuss the role of the nurse in the resolution of the following postpartal crises: malattachment, relinquishment of the infant, adolescent parenting, child abuse, and single-parent families.

Key Terms

acute grief	grief work
chronic grief	loss
crisis	modeling
crisis intervention	reciprocal inhibition
grief	

Many experiences of a family are predictable, such as graduation from school, marriage, childbearing, and retirement. When a family cannot or does not prepare for these events, a **crisis** may result.

Unpredictable life events also occur within families, including unexpected death or a serious illness of a member, natural disasters resulting in personal or financial loss, stillbirth, or birth of an infant with congenital anomaly or a potentially fatal disease. Experiences like these can place so much stress on a family that normal coping mechanisms are not adequate and a crisis ensues.

The postpartal family must deal with several stress-producing events simultaneously. The stress of adjusting to the new family member, learning new roles and responsibilities, and adapting to rearranged daily schedules and lifestyle changes can bring about disruption within a family. When a diagnosis of high-risk pregnancy is made, a couple faces a unique set of problems. The uncertainty of the outcome leads them to view the pregnancy with anxiety and ambivalence rather than confidence. If other factors, such as economic problems, are present, the family may not be able to cope with the situation. These crises can prevent a family from properly performing the task of nurturing its members.

A crisis is potentially growth promoting or emotionally destructive for those involved. How a family meets a crisis depends on the personalities of those involved, the family structure, and previously existing problems. It is also determined by the family's experience with crises and patterns of problem solving.

The Role of the Maternity Nurse During Family Crises

Maternity nurses deal with families suffering from a variety of crises, ranging from birth of a child with a congenital anomaly to unwanted pregnancy and relinquishment of the child. The nurse who is familiar with the signs of crisis and methods of intervention can help identify and avert or resolve the crises of individuals and families. Nurses who are able to identify crisis situations can make referrals as well as explain a woman's situation to other members of the health care team. In addition to being a therapeutic agent, the nurse can serve as the primary coordinator of the intervention program for the family.

Identifying Families at Risk and Developing an Intervention Plan

Through the process of assessment, nurses and other health care professionals are responsible for identifying families at risk. Assessment should reveal crisis or precrisis states, and by further questioning, professionals can determine the family's ability to cope with the crisis. The information obtained from careful assessment becomes the basis for the plan of intervention. The answers to the following questions will help determine the effects of the crisis on the family:

- To what extent has the crisis disrupted the family's normal life pattern?

- Has the family's economic status been affected?

- Can family members handle the responsibilities involved in the activities of daily living—for example, eating or personal hygiene.

- Does the family or a family member seem to be on the brink of despair?

- Has the high level of tension distorted one or more individual's perception of reality?

- Is the family's usual support system present, absent, or exhausted?
- What are the resources of the nurse or agency in relation to the family's assessed needs?

Essential data are identified from the answers to these and related questions. This information is used to determine the goals of the intervention plan.

An effective intervention plan has the following features (Hoff, 1984):

- Focuses on the immediate concrete problem
- Considers the family's functional level and dependency needs
- Is appropriate to the family's culture and lifestyle
- Includes all family members and significant others
- Is practical, has a specified time frame, and is concrete
- Is dynamic and renegotiable
- Includes an arrangement for follow-up contact

Methods of Intervention

Depending on the family's ability to accept and adjust to the situation causing the crisis, the nurse may find one or more of the following intervention methods helpful.

Anticipatory guidance   Anticipatory guidance of both expectant families and families with newborns can help prevent crisis (Clausen, 1979; McCabe, 1979). Whether the pregnancy and infant are normal or high risk, anticipatory guidance can give families the knowledge they need to understand and cope with the situation. Clients will feel more in control if they know what to expect.

The nurse's role as health educator is good preparation for this intervention. Before birth, parents may need to discuss the emotional and physical changes that accompany pregnancy. They want to know what to expect during labor and delivery, and, if the pregnancy is high risk, how to prevent further complications and increase the infant's chances for survival and health. Postpartal families are more concerned with infant care. If the child is not healthy, they want information about special problems to expect and medical care that is required.

Modeling   **Modeling** is introducing the behaviors of others as examples by role playing or having the client talk with someone who has mastered a similar crisis. This is an especially effective strategy if the crisis concerns a mother feeling inadequate about her parenting skills. As the mother watches the nurse caring for the infant in a relaxed and comfortable manner, she is encouraged to incorporate these behaviors into her way of functioning.

Relaxation techniques   Relaxation techniques are especially valuable for parents who respond to stress with increased tension, feelings of helplessness, withdrawal from caretaking responsibilities, or abusive behaviors. Relaxation techniques are based on the principle of **reciprocal inhibition**, meaning that it is impossible to feel relaxed and tense at the same time. With guidance from the nurse, clients can learn to do relaxation exercises on their own.

The three primary components of relaxation techniques are breathing techniques, muscle relaxation, and imagery. A relaxation exercise may incorporate one or more of these components.

Crisis intervention   **Crisis intervention** is perhaps the most important skill that a nurse can use to help families at risk. Crisis intervention is a form of psychotherapy that focuses on the immediate crisis. It is not necessary to know the history or personalities of the people involved. The therapist's role is direct, active, and participating.

The techniques of crisis intervention are relatively simple and do not require extensive training. Since most crises last no longer than 4–6 weeks, usually one to four crisis intervention sessions are enough.

The primary goals of crisis intervention are to help the client deal with the crisis, regain his or her equilibrium, grow from the experience, and improve coping skills (Getz et al., 1974). The specific problem-solving steps involved in crisis intervention as outlined by Aguilera and Messick (1982) are similar to the steps of the nursing process: assessment, planning of therapeutic intervention, intervention, and evaluation.

The first objective in *assessment* is to define the situation clearly and identify the crisis-precipitating event. Assessment is then made of the client's perception of the event (whether realistic or distorted), the person's support system, and his or her coping skills.

When the assessment is complete, a *plan of intervention* is developed. This plan is based on how much the crisis has disrupted the individual's or family's life and the feelings of those involved. Tentative approaches are proposed to the individual and examined for their usefulness.

The type of *intervention* used by the maternity nurse depends on the nurse's knowledge base about crisis and on his or her flexibility, creativity, and interpersonal skills. The nurse should be aware of the limit of his or her skills and should refer the client to appropriate professionals when the limit is reached.

Therapeutic aspects of crisis counseling include:

- Empathetic listening
- Exploring a client's coping mechanisms
- Identifying and expanding the client's support system
- Encouraging release of tension through nondestructive means such as crying or physical activity

The nurse should be able to assess the potential for destructive behavior toward self or others. This information should be obtained in a gentle but direct way. Using words such as *suicide* will not suggest ideas that are not already being entertained by someone in crisis. If the nurse believes that the client is at risk for destructive behavior, the nurse must notify appropriate agencies who can help the client.

Intervention may include one or more of the following techniques:

- Interpretation and confrontation
- Encouraging the person to express and explore his or her feelings
- Reassurance and feedback about progress
- Self-disclosure by the counselor
- Assistance in problem solving

Group therapy may be an effective way to avert or resolve a client's crisis. The nurse working with maternity clients does not have to be a trained psychotherapist to use groups effectively. Groups are often an ideal format in which to provide anticipatory guidance about child care or allow parents to express their concerns. Parents who have a preterm infant or child with a congenital anomaly often find the support and shared information from a group of parents in the same situation absolutely invaluable.

No matter how well trained in crisis intervention techniques, a nurse cannot perceive the meaning of a crisis to an individual unless he or she has some understanding of that person's world. Awareness of sociocultural values and attitudes will make any intervention more effective.

Evaluation is an ongoing process throughout planning and intervention. Various approaches are tried and discarded or modified depending on their success. The adaptive coping mechanisms that the client has used successfully are reinforced.

Loss and Grief

Many crises affecting families postpartally involve loss and grief. **Loss** is a state of being deprived of, or being without, something one has had. The most serious loss is the loss of a loved one by death, but such a loss can also occur through divorce or separation. One can also lose an aspect of "self." Loss of health, body parts, pride, and independence are examples of loss of self.

Grief is an emotional state, a reaction to loss. Studies have shown that the grief reaction is similar whether the loss is of a loved one or a body part or function (Schoenberg et al., 1970).

Grief work is the inner process of working through or managing the bereavement (Schoenberg et al., 1974). There are five stages in the process:

1. *Disbelief*—In this stage, the person may say, "No, no ... it can't be."

2. *Questioning*—The person who suffers the loss looks for reasons for the death, asking "What happened?" and "How?"

3. *Anger*—The person may express anger at God, asking "Why did this happen?"

4. *Anger combined with desperation*—The person seems resigned, dismayed, and in despair.

5. *Resolution*—The person accepts the loss.

The duration of the grief process may last up to a year, but the **acute grief** should be over in 1 or 2 months. The best indicator of the resolution of acute grief is a gradual return to the preloss level of functioning.

People who do not successfully complete the grief work may have prolonged or distorted grief reactions. For example, delayed grief may occur if affected persons are maintaining the morale of others and therefore are repressing their own reactions.

Chronic grief is a response that represents a denial of the reality of the loss. There can be no resolution if there is no acceptance. One manifestation of chronic grief is retaining the lost loved one's belongings as they were during his or her lifetime.

Anticipatory grief reactions are seen when there is a threat of death or separation (Lindemann, 1944). Because the dynamics of anticipatory grief have much in common with those of acute grief, one might expect that working through anticipatory grief would diminish the acute grief when the loss finally does occur. This may be the case for some, but most people cannot work through the feelings of denial, and hope that the loss will not actually occur.

Those close to the dying person often have ambivalent feelings about the loved one that they find difficult to recognize or accept. The ambivalence may be interpreted as a death wish—which is too unacceptable to admit—and so these feelings are repressed.

Grief work can be helped or hindered by a person's emotional status and by the ability of family members or significant others to allow the expression of grief. The stable family, with healthy coping mechanisms and strong support, both within the family structure and from friends and other ties, can weather the crisis of loss. However, the high-risk family that does not have either the internal strength or support from extended family and friends may need help and support from other sources, including the health care team.

The maternity nurse may be involved with clients who are grieving for a loss. Parents grieve after the birth of an infant with a congenital anomaly and mourn the loss of the normal infant they dreamed would be theirs. Intense grief usually attends the death of a newborn. Even parents who had a strong preference for the sex of their unborn child may experience a brief period of sorrow after the birth of the "wrong sex" infant.

Occasionally a nurse may become frustrated with parents who mourn a minor anomaly or the gender of a child. The nurse may feel that the parents should be happy they have a healthy child. It is important to realize, however, that parents must mourn the idealized infant before they can begin to form a strong attachment with their actual infant. The nurse's acceptance and support promote attachment between the parents and child.

In the remainder of this chapter, selected high-risk perinatal situations are considered and methods of nursing management are described.

Complicated Childbirth

Complicated childbirth is a crisis situation that can test the coping mechanisms of every person involved. The family may respond to the crisis in relatively typical ways or in disturbed ways.

During the antepartal period, the family may have ambivalent feelings toward a complicated pregnancy. Fear and anxiety about the health and welfare of both fetus and mother may be exhibited as hostile behaviors and guilt feelings. The expectant mother may feel that she is inadequate as a woman and a childbearer. The father may blame himself for impregnating his partner. The family may accuse the health care team of poor management.

During labor and delivery, unexpected problems can ensue. Even if complications had been diagnosed before labor began, the health care team may need to take unexpected or extraordinary measures to ensure the well-being of mother and child. The tension of the staff and atmosphere of emergency may increase the fear and anxiety already felt by the expectant parents. The couple may feel powerless, and their responses can range from emotional paralysis to hostility toward the health care team.

Nursing management   When a labor is complicated, the woman must have consistent support. The partner should be encouraged to remain, and the nurse can provide emotional support as well as observe the woman by being present. Thoughtful comfort measures such as ice chips, clean chux, and judicious use of analgesics also demonstrate a caring attitude (Kowalski and

Osborn, 1977). If emergency and/or operative measures are necessary, the nurse should explain to the couple and other support persons why these measures are necessary and what they are.

Loss of Newborn

The loss of a newborn evokes intense mourning reactions whether the baby lives an hour or several days, or is stillborn; whether the baby is a nonviable 500 g fetus or a full-term 4000 g infant; whether the baby is planned or not. Both parents show the same grief reactions (Klaus and Fanaroff, 1979), although the father may have more difficulty expressing his grief. He may be suppressing his own feelings and delaying his grief work while supporting and comforting the mother.

The couple dealing with the loss of a newborn will feel anger, guilt, pain, and sadness. However, because they have had little or no time to know the child as a person, the soothing part of the mourning process—"identification" built on memories, shared experiences, and living together—is absent (Furman, 1978).

The following case study of Mary, a woman who lost her newborn and then later had two healthy children, relates some of the feelings associated with the loss of an infant.

CASE STUDY

One day I was working, feeling happy and healthy, and the next day I found myself in the hospital, having given birth to our baby almost 3 months early. There were no warning signs. On all my prenatal visits the doctor assured me "everything was fine." I started bleeding in the morning and when it didn't stop, the doctor advised that I be admitted to the hospital. I was terrified because I knew if I went into labor now, the baby might not live. As I lay there on the bed, with blood infusing in one arm and an intravenous line in the other, thoughts were racing through my head. Primarily I thought about whether the baby was going to live or die through all this. Certain things in my environment seemed to fade into oblivion and other things became very intense. One of the nurses caring for me had a terrible cold, and I kept thinking "I wish she would leave the room" because I was sure that

on top of everything else I would catch that cold. I was feeling very vulnerable.

The bleeding continued, and contractions started. After it became obvious that the baby would be born, my concerns changed. I began to worry about whether the baby would be all right if it lived. I thought that if the baby was going to be retarded or deformed, I wanted it to die instead. I remember feeling very guilty about these thoughts, especially after Beth did not live. I wondered if we could afford long hospitalizations and care if it would be needed. During the entire time, my husband was supportive and comforting, although seemingly overwhelmed by everything.

When I was taken into the delivery room, it was as if I were progressing through a normal delivery. After Beth was born, they let me look at her and touch her very briefly before rushing her off for special care. I remember saying "She's so beautiful." That moment was the highlight of the entire experience for me. I recapture the sight frequently. The next day the doctor told me that the baby's weight was a positive factor (slightly over 3 lb), but that her lungs were not well developed. It was too early for him to talk about her prognosis. When I asked if I could go in to see her, he said he preferred that I did not. How I wish I would have had the assertiveness to take the matter into my own hands and insist, but I had no self-direction and seemed to be waiting for others to tell me what to do next. This feeling was in sharp contrast to my normal way of functioning.

In the morning the woman who takes the baby pictures came in to get permission from mothers to photograph babies. I was very excited about the prospect, but when she learned the baby wasn't in the regular nursery, she said it probably wouldn't be possible to photograph her. I was so disappointed. The mother in the bed next to me was receiving her baby for feedings, and I felt so alone and so empty during those times. We named our baby and started hoping and believing that she was going to be all right. The ambivalence was overwhelming—wanting to hold and love her, but knowing that if we became too attached, the hurt would be greater if we lost her.

I felt very angry that everyone else seemed to be having healthy babies. I was an intelligent, competent woman. Why was I so inadequate at this? When friends and relatives called I tried to tell them what a beautiful baby we had but that she was born early. My husband visited her, and I pried every bit of information out of him that I could about her progress.

Later that day, the doctor came in and told me that Beth had died. My husband came and we cried and cried. Other than having him there, nothing seemed to comfort. One of the staff came in and asked what we wanted to do with her body. That came as a shock. Somehow I never thought of having to make a decision like that. We decided to bury her near my grandparents. It was critically important to me that she had been baptized, and the nurses assured me that she had been baptized shortly after delivery.

My husband took me home from the hospital empty-armed. My feelings were very confusing. I felt guilty—thinking that perhaps if I had stopped working earlier or had called the doctor earlier things would have been different. I was angry. I was sad. I wondered if we would ever have other children. A neighbor had hand-crocheted some beautiful white baby clothes before I went to the hospital, and she told me to keep them—that was very meaningful and I got them out and looked at them many times. When I got back to work, people who knew I was pregnant but hadn't heard the outcome asked about the baby. I had to tell them.

Nursing management The death of an infant evokes powerful reactions in both parents and health care professionals. Sadness, shock, and anger may be felt by parents and staff alike. However, it is imperative that nurses learn to deal with their feelings so that they can be supportive of the family.

When a diagnosis of intrauterine death is made before or during labor, shock and disbelief plus the physical discomfort of labor produce overwhelming stresses. Denial is maintained by most women up to the moment of delivery, often combined with anger, bargaining, and depression (Kübler-Ross, 1969). Allowing the woman to express her feelings helps her to work through her acute grief in a healthy manner when the death is confirmed at delivery.

The laboring woman should not be left alone. For emotional support and continuity of care, one caregiver should attend the woman throughout the labor and delivery and into the immediate postpartal period. (See the Nursing Care Plan on Stillbirth.)

Infant death may occur after the discharge of the mother from the hospital or after both mother and infant have been at home for some time and the attachment process with the family has been progressing. Parents may be expecting the death, as in the case of terminal illness or fatal congenital defect. In other cases, the death may be unexpected, as in SIDS. In either situation, the loss is an overwhelming experience for the family. Nursing interventions can help the family resolve feelings of grief, anger, confusion, guilt, and depression.

If the infant dies while hospitalized and the parents are not present at the time of death, they are usually notified by the physician. Privacy should be provided for them at the hospital. The parents may want to be alone or may prefer that the nurse stay with them for a while. The nurse should encourage them not to hold back their feelings—to cry if they feel like it. Unless they are told what reactions to expect, their feelings may worry them and interfere with their relationship.

When the death of a child is inevitable, open honest discussion about their dying child is important to parents. Occasionally parents of a dying child refuse to visit the nursery. However, most parents are interested in the newborn's progress, visit regularly, and telephone when they are unable to visit. It is important for parents to touch their infant and to take photographs even if the child is surrounded by technical equipment (Wooten, 1981). Parents frequently want to cradle the baby in their arms at the time of death.

Being certain that a dying infant is baptized is of great importance to some parents. All nurses who work in the delivery room or nursery should know how to perform a baptism in the event that the hospital chaplain is not available. If spiritual support is requested by parents, the nurse should be prepared to contact appropriate clergy.

Research indicates that most mothers want to see and touch their dead babies (Seitz and Warrick, 1974; Kowalski and Osborn, 1977). Allowing mothers to see and touch their dead infants seems to aid grief work because acceptance and resolution follow more smoothly. If parents wish to see the child and are denied their wish, they may imagine something far worse than the reality.

NURSING CARE PLAN
Stillbirth

CLIENT ASSESSMENT

History

1. Prenatal history
   a. Uneventful? High risk?
   b. Fetal death before labor? During labor? Totally unexpected?
2. Family history
   a. Interactions, communications—are they mutually supportive? Blaming?
   b. Grief response—are normal reactions manifested?

PLAN OF CARE

Nursing Priorities

1. Facilitate the normal grief process.

Client/Family Educational Focus

1. Explain the grief process and its psychologic impact.
2. Provide names of local support groups the couple might find helpful when they are ready.
3. Provide close family and friends with information about ways in which they can help the grieving couple cope with their loss.

Problem	Nursing interventions and actions	Rationale
Communications between couple	Encourage them to express feelings, to cry. Provide support.	Disturbance in communication can delay resolution of grief and cause possible long-range disturbances within family.
Father's needs	Include father in intervention.	Both parents have same grief responses; each needs support of the other.
Acceptance of reality of the situation	Listen; correct any misconceptions, answer questions. Make it possible for couple to see infant; explain the reasons for the infant's death, if known; prepare them fully for the experience.	Misconceptions reinforce guilt feelings and lower self-esteem. Acceptance is facilitated and resolution will follow more smoothly.

NURSING CARE EVALUATION

There is evidence that normal grief work is in process.

Disbelief phase has been worked through, followed by questioning and anger; feelings have been expressed freely, and acceptance has begun.

Because crisis lasts 4–6 weeks, resolution will not be evident in the hospital; further support may be needed to help parents cope because acute grief can be recurrent; referral can be made to community mental health agency, to appropriate parent groups, or to visiting community health nurse.

A month or 6 weeks after the stillbirth, parents are regaining their equilibrium to precrisis level; their coping skills have been strengthened, and family relationships are even closer than before.

Without resolution, guilt feelings and lack of communication between parents may lead not only to abnormal grief reactions (delayed or chronic grief) but also to disorganization of family unit.

Parents find the experience less stressful if they are prepared by hearing a description of the infant's appearance and explanations of what happened when there is evidence of trauma. All normal and positive aspects of the infant may be pointed out. Mothers who have seen their dead babies (even those who are macerated or deformed) have stated that the reality was not so bad as what they had imagined.

If parents do not wish to see their infant, the nurse should support their decision. For the mother unable to face the task, some benefit may be derived from answering her questions about the delivery and the infant.

A major goal of the nurse is to aid and encourage communication between parents who have lost a newborn. The nurse also should watch for feelings of shame and guilt in the mother. Women often blame themselves for the infant's death. Because these feelings are destructive to the woman's self-esteem and can delay her grief work, the nurse must clarify these misperceptions.

NURSING CARE PLAN (continued)
Stillbirth

NURSING DIAGNOSIS*	SUPPORTING DATA	NURSING ORDERS
Grieving related to actual loss	Crying Inability to cry Anger Denial Withdrawal Resolution	Provide support during grieving process: 1. Arrange time to be with mother and father and listen to them. 2. Respond to their concerns and questions in an honest caring manner. 3. Provide an opportunity for them to see the baby. 4. Provide privacy when desired, but do not isolate them from support. 5. Help them obtain answers to their questions. 6. Provide names of resources as needed and desired. 7. Maintain open environment so support persons can come and go as needed.

*This is an example of a nursing diagnosis that might be appropriate for a couple experiencing this loss. It is not necessarily inclusive and must be individualized for each person experiencing this crisis.

The nurse must be as positive as possible but should avoid such meaningless phrases as "Don't worry" or "Everything will be fine." It is especially important to avoid comments on future pregnancies, such as, "You are young; you can have other babies." Such remarks negate the present baby; effective crisis intervention focuses on the immediate problem.

Siblings of a dying or dead infant need special consideration from the family and nurse. During bereavement, parents may become so consumed by their own reactions that they seem detached from the other children. The children perceive this withdrawal as abandonment. Loneliness engulfs the siblings just when their needs for love and reassurance are very strong. Children—especially young children who use magical thinking—may respond to the death of a brother or sister with guilt feelings (Williams, Rivara, and Rothenberg, 1981). They feel responsible for the death and need reassurance that they are not to blame. Young children may also view the cause of death as communicable and may develop symptoms similar to those of the deceased child. An in-depth knowledge of child development helps the nurse plan appropriate interventions with siblings.

If the family needs assistance with funeral arrangements, body or organ donation, autopsy requests, or legal problems, the nurse can refer the parents to the appropriate departments or agencies. The nurse should also refer parents to community agencies or support groups if continuing assistance is needed. Parent support groups are especially helpful for parents who have lost an infant to SIDS.

Health professionals must clarify their own feelings about death before they can work effectively with others. Nurses may be shocked at their own feelings of anger and despair, but it is important that they not suppress these feelings. Nurses who suppress or deny their reactions tend to remove themselves from the situation, increase their physical and psychologic distance from clients, and thus reduce their effectiveness. Each nurse must assess personal reactions: How am I expressing my anger? Am I venting my anger on my peers or my family? Am I being nonjudgmental, helpful, and approachable with my client?

Structured peer groups may help resolve the professional's conflicts about death. Support groups may be especially helpful for nurses in intensive care nurseries where death may be more frequent.

Birth of a High-Risk Infant or Infant with a Congenital Anomaly

The birth of a preterm or ill infant or an infant with a congenital anomaly is a serious crisis situation for a family. Acute grief reactions follow the loss of the perfect baby they have fantasized.

In the case of a preterm birth, the mother is denied the last few weeks of pregnancy that seem to prepare her psychologically for the stress of birth and the attachment process. Attachment at this time is fragile, and interruption of the process by separation can affect the future mother-child relationship.

Feelings of guilt and failure also plague the mother regarding the onset of premature labor or delivery. She asks herself, "Why did labor start? What did I do (or not do)?" She may have guilt fantasies ("Was it because I had sexual intercourse with my husband recently?") and wonders if she is being punished for something she did in the past.

Table 26-1 illustrates the maternal emotional and situational differences between term and preterm births. The factors listed are commonly found in mothers but are by no means universal. These factors may be influenced by the woman's experiences, personality, and educational background and the support she received.

The birth of an infant with a congenital anomaly creates a devastating crisis. Not only is the expected normal child lost, but also the par-ents feel a severe loss of self-esteem and self-confidence. Guilt and ambivalent feelings are overwhelming. As in the birth of a preterm infant, the woman in particular may entertain ideas of personal guilt: "What did I do (or not do) to cause this?" "Am I being punished for something?" Parents of an infant with severe birth defects or disabilities are often faced with difficult and painful decisions about treatment of their child. The benefits of the treatment besides merely sustaining life and the quality of their child's life during and as a result of that treatment must be considered.

Olshansky (1962) calls the grief reaction of parents of children with congenital anomalies or mental retardation *chronic sorrow*. The parents begin this process with the birth of the child, and the grieving or sorrow continues throughout the life span. As long as the child lives, there can be no resolution of grief. As time elapses, however, the unresolved grief becomes less intense.

Adjustment   The birth of a preterm or ill infant or infant with a congenital anomaly requires major adjustments by parents. They must grieve the loss of their idealized child. Simultaneously

Table 26-1
Comparison of Maternal Emotional and Situational Factors in Term and Preterm Births*

Factors	Term birth	Preterm birth
Emotional factors at time of birth	More likely to be regarded as rewarding experience	May be regarded as less than rewarding experience; frustration and a sense of missing something
	More likely to have good self-image regarding body functioning	May have poor self-image regarding imperfectly functioning body
	Pleasurable experience	Anxiety-producing experience
	Confident in ability to give birth with good outcome	Not confident in ability to give birth with good outcome
	Little fear of danger to infant	Great fear of danger to infant
	Great sense of achievement; pride in success	Little sense of achievement; no pride in failure; guilt
	Emotionally prepared for outcome as planned and expected	Shocked; emotionally unprepared for outcome, which is different from plans and expectations
	Previous pregnancy and birth experience likely to have been considered favorable	Previous pregnancy and birth experience probably considered unfavorable if previous reproductive failure occurred
	Happiness and joy	Unhappiness and grief
	Meets expectations	Disappointment; does not meet expectations

*Copyright © 1980, Lauri Lowen, Chairman of Parents of Prematures, Seattle, Washington.

Table 26-1
Comparison of Maternal Emotional and Situational Factors in Term and Preterm Births
(continued)

Factors	Term birth	Preterm birth
Situational factors at time of birth	Able to choose option of active role in birth	Possibly forced to play passive role by circumstances
	More in control of situation; more opportunity for voluntary decisions	Less in control of situation; decisions often made for her
	More opportunity to be independent	Dependent
	Nonemergency atmosphere	Emergency and crisis atmosphere
Postpartal emotional factors	Pleased at appearance of newborn	Shocked at appearance of newborn
	Identifies with other mothers in her chosen role	Does not identify with other mothers; did not choose this strange role; does not know exactly what her role is
	Loss of fantasized child; replaced by different but probaby equally acceptable child	Loss of fantasized child; replaced by less acceptable sick or imperfect child
	Usually under less than severe stress	Under severe stress
	Happy with successful completion of pregnancy	Regrets unsuccessful completion of pregnancy; feels ``empty''
	Less anxious about newborn's health than mother of preterm infant	Very anxious about infant's health
	Sees newborn as better than average; feels proud	Sees infant as better than average preterm baby but not as good as average term baby; may feel envious
	Confident in ability to care for child	Not confident in ability to care for child
	Naturally inclined and eager to increase attachment to child	Naturally inclined to increase attachment to child, but may be hindered by question of infant's survival
	Attachment process free of many obstacles	Attachment process more difficult, with more obstacles
	Realistic expectations	May have unrealistic expectations; less able to anticipate outcome
	Infant seems to be parents' possession	Newborn seems to be hospital's possession
Postpartal situational factors	Infant is responsive to mother	Newborn is less responsive to mother
	Major caregiver; role as major caregiver begins early; caregiving requires moderate energy and effort	Not major caregiver; role as major caregiver begins late; caregiving requires more energy and effort
	Recognition by others of identity as mother	Less recognition by others of identity as mother
	Gives pregnancy up in exchange for possessing infant	Gives pregnancy up but cannot possess newborn
	Many opportunities for contact with infant	Fewer opportunities for contact with infant
	Information about parents' situation readily available	Information about parents' situation not readily available
	Family unit can be together	Family unit may be divided due to hospitalization of infant

they must adopt the less-than-perfect child as the new love object. Parental responses to an infant at high-risk or with a congenital anomaly may be viewed as a staged process (Klaus and Kennell, 1982):

1. *Shock* at the reality of the birth of a child with congenital anomalies

2. *Denial* of the reality of the situation, characterized by a refusal to believe the child is less than perfect or at risk

3. *Depression* about the situation possibly accompanied by anger

4. *Acceptance* characterized by a decrease in emotional reactions of the parents

5. *Reorganization* of the family to deal with the child's problems

The family can adjust to the situation in adaptive or maladaptive ways. Maladaptive responses include overwhelming guilt or denial. Persistent denial can make it almost impossible to care for the infant. The mother who feels extremely guilty may spend all her time with the affected child, ignoring her other children. Marriages or relationships often break down under the tremendous strain of the situation.

Attachment   As discussed in Chapter 24, the period immediately after birth is extremely important for the attachment process. The development of maternal bonding and effective mothering is highly influenced by the mother's ability to see and touch her baby immediately after delivery. Research suggests that interference with this acquaintance process (for example, separation because of the need for resuscitation) may disturb the developing relationship between a mother and her newborn.

Klaus and Kennell (1982) have demonstrated a significant difference in the amount of eye contact and touching behaviors of mothers of normal newborns and mothers of preterm infants. Whereas mothers of normal newborns progress within minutes to palm contact of the infant's trunk, the mother of a preterm infant is slower to progress from fingertip to palm contact and from the extremities to the trunk. The progression to palm contact with the infant's trunk may take several visits to the nursery.

Although the reactions and steps of attachment are altered by the birth of an infant at high-risk or with a congenital anomaly, a healthy parent–child relationship can occur. Kaplan and Mason (1974) have identified four psychologic tasks that must be completed for successful resolution of the crisis:

1. Anticipatory grief as psychologic preparation for possible loss of the child, while still hoping for its survival

2. Acknowledgment of maternal failure to produce a term infant, expressed as anticipatory grief and depression until the chances of survival seem secure

3. Resumption of the process of relating to the infant, which has been interrupted by the threat of nonsurvival

4. Understanding the special needs and growth patterns of the infant

The best indicator for healthy or unhealthy outcomes in the parent-child relationship is the frequency of parental visits to the child in the nursery (Caplan et al., 1965). These visits indicate acceptance of the child's condition, as well as concern and caring.

Developmental consequences   The infant who is born prematurely, is ill, or has a congenital malformation or disability is at risk for emotional, intellectual, and physical development problems. The risk is directly proportional to the seriousness of the problem and the length of treatment. For example, resolution of meconium plug syndrome during the expected hospital stay, allowing the infant to be discharged with the mother, is not expected to alter the child's developmental course. However, the physical appearance, immediate and repeated surgeries, and complex rehabilitation problems of exstrophy of the bladder or myelomeningocele preclude a normal development course for the child.

Mothers of gravely ill newborns are often unable to risk an emotional investment in their child. Even after a woman is told that her child will survive, she may be unable to develop maternal feelings. She may reject the infant or overcompensate because of underlying guilt feelings. The child may then be further handicapped by inability to relate well to others and by seeing the world as unsatisfying and painful.

Parents must have a clear picture of the reality of the child's disability and the types of developmental hurdles ahead (West, 1984). Unexpected behaviors and responses caused by the defect or disorder can be upsetting and frightening. For example, parents find it difficult to cope with an infant's lack of motor or social responsiveness and tend to interpret the lack as a form of rejection. The parents may in turn respond with rejection, and an unfortunate cycle is begun.

The demands of care of the child strain family relationships. One or more family members may make a scapegoat of the child. Another may become the youngster's champion to the exclusion of others. Parents or siblings may feel that their own needs (emotional, material, freedom of movement) are being set aside while all resources and energy go to support the child's needs.

The parents and child must confront daily a society that values normality. If the parents cannot develop a positive attitude toward the child, the child may also have a negative self-image, perhaps even feel responsible for the predicament.

Nursing management As soon as possible after birth, the nurse must ensure that the mother is reunited with her infant so that:

1. She knows that her baby is alive.

2. She knows what the infant's real problems are. Fantasies of the infant's problems may be more devastating than the reality.

3. She can begin the grief work over the loss of the idealized child and the process of attachment with the real child.

4. She can share the experience of the infant's problems with the father.

If the newborn must be moved to a regional center, the nurse should ensure that the mother sees the infant before transport. When the infant reaches the referral center, a staff member should call the parents with information about the infant's condition during transport, safe arrival at the center, and present condition.

Occasionally the mother may be unable to see the infant before transport, for example, if she is still under general anesthesia or is experiencing complications such as shock, hemorrhage, or seizures. In these cases, the infant should be photographed before being transferred. The photograph is given to the mother, along with an explanation of the infant's condition, problems, and a detailed description of the infant's characteristics. These measures will facilitate the attachment process until the mother can visit the child.

Before parents see their child, the nurse must prepare them to see their newborn. It is important that a realistic but positive attitude be presented to the parents. An overly negative, fatalistic attitude further alienates the parents from the infant and retards attachment behaviors. If the child has a congenital anomaly, the parents should be prepared to see both the defect and the normal aspects of their infant. All infants have strengths as well as deficiencies. For example, the nurse may say to parents of a preterm infant "Your baby is small, about the length of my two hands. She weighs 2 pounds, 3 ounces but is very active and cries when we disturb her. She is having some difficulty breathing but is breathing without assistance and is in only 35% oxygen."

The equipment being used for the high-risk neonate should be described and explained before the parents enter the intensive care unit. The primary physician and nurse caring for the newborn should be with the parents when they first visit the child. Upon entering the unit, parents may be overwhelmed by the sounds of monitors, alarms, and respirators. Provision of chairs and time to regain composure will assist the parents. Slow, complete, and simple explanations—first about the infant and then about the equipment—reduce fear and anxiety.

As parents attempt to deal with the initial stages of shock and grief, they may fail to grasp new information. Misconceptions about equipment, its placement on the infant, and its potential harm are common. The parents may need repeated explanations in order to accept the reality of the situation, procedures, equipment, and the infant's condition on subsequent visits.

Concern about the infant's physical appearance is common but may remain unvoiced. Such questions need to be anticipated and addressed by the nurse. Showing pictures, such as of an infant after cleft lip repair, may be reassuring to doubting parents. Knowledge of the development of a "normal" preterm infant will allow the nurse to reassure parents that their child is normal for his or her level of maturity.

The tone of the neonatal intensive care unit is set by the nursing staff. Development of a safe, trusting environment depends on viewing the parents as essential caregivers, not as visitors or nuisances in the unit. Pleasant, relaxed physical surroundings convey the sense of hospitality and encourage parents to "be at home here."

Parenting behavior toward an infant in intensive care occurs in stages, with touching being the first stage (Figure 26-1). Touching helps parents get to know their infant and thus establish a bond with the child. Parents visiting a small or sick infant may need several visits to become comfortable and confident in touching the infant. Barriers such as isolettes, incisions, monitor electrodes, and tubes may intimidate parents. By supporting, reassuring, and encouraging them, the nurse can help parents overcome their fears and increase their confidence about physical contact with the infant.

Caretaking may be delayed for the mother of a high-risk newborn. The variety of equipment needed for life support is hardly conducive to anxiety-free caretaking by the parents. However,

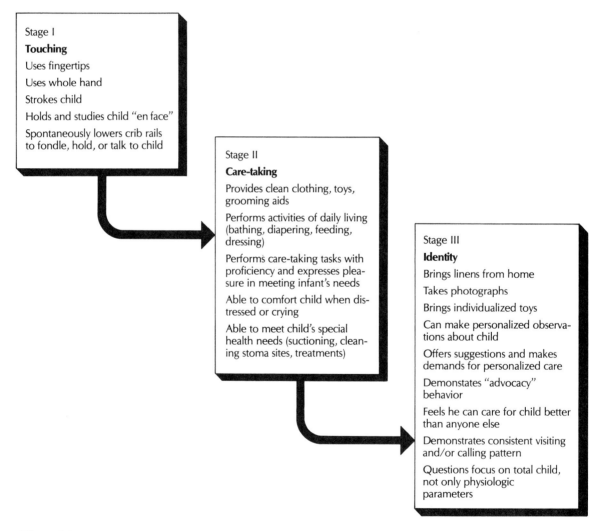

Figure 26-1

Stages of parenting behavior toward infant in intensive care. (Adapted from the work of Rubin, Schaeffer, Jay, and Schraeder by Schraeder BD: Attachment and parenting despite lengthy intensive care. *MCN* January/February 1980; 5:38. Reprinted with permission from the American Journal of Nursing Company, ©1980.)

the parents can contribute to the care of even the sickest infant. The nurse can ask the parents to change the infant's diaper, give skin or oral care, or help turn the infant. As parents become more comfortable and confident in caretaking, they receive satisfaction from the child's reactions and their ability to "do something." Being part of the team increases the parents' self-esteem, which has received recent blows of guilt and failure. The mother in particular feels less futile if she can do something useful and positive. If the child dies, detachment is easier because the parents know they did all they could for their child while he or she was alive.

A trusting relationship between parents and nursing staff is essential, and collaboration in the care of the neonate is critical. Powell (1981) suggests several positive strategies that increase the effectiveness of nursing interventions with parents:

- Problem solve with the family rather than giving advice.
- View the child as a total individual rather than emphasizing the problem.
- Observe the uniqueness of the child rather than stereotyping or labeling the child as slow, unmanageable, etc.
- Avoid labeling parents as inadequate, rejecting, or angry.
- Stress the child's similarities to other children.
- Stress strengths and competence of parents.
- Help parents realize that they are in charge of their children and themselves.
- Be aware of the needs of all members of the family, including siblings.

Often mothers of high-risk infants have ambivalent feelings toward the nurse. As the mother watches the nurse competently perform the caretaking tasks, she feels both grateful for the nurse's abilities and expertise and jealous of the nurse's ability to care for her infant. These feelings may be acted out in criticism of the care being received by the infant, manipulation of staff, or personal guilt. Instead of fostering (by silence) these inferiority feelings within mothers, nurses should recognize such feelings and intervene appropriately to enhance mother–infant bonding.

Nurses who are understanding and secure will be able to support the parents' egos instead of collecting rewards for themselves. To reinforce positive parenting behaviors, professionals must first believe in the importance of the parents. The nurse can hardly convince doubting parents of their importance to the infant unless the nurse really believes it. Both attitudes and words must say: "You are a good mother/father. You have an important contribution to make to the care of your infant." For example, a nurse can encourage a mother to supply breast milk to her high-risk infant. Positive remarks, such as "Breast milk is something that only you can give your baby," reinforce the mother's feelings that she is necessary to her child's well-being.

The nurse can also encourage parents to meet their newborn's need for stimulation. Stroking, rocking, cuddling, singing, and talking should be an integral part of the parents' caretaking responsibilities.

A primary role of the nurse is to identify high-risk parents. Visiting and caregiving patterns help indicate the level of or lack of parental attachment. A record of visits, caretaking procedures, displays of affection toward the newborn, and telephone calls is essential. Serial observations must be obtained.

Grant (1978) has developed a conceptual framework depicting adaptive and maladaptive responses to parenting of a preterm infant or one with congenital anomaly (Figure 26-2). If a pattern of distancing behaviors evolves, appropriate intervention should be instituted. Follow-up studies have found that a significant number of preterm or sick infants or those with congenital anomalies suffer from failure to thrive, battering, or other disorders of parenting. Early detection of these problems may prevent irreparable damage.

The parents should be encouraged to use their support system during the crisis. The nurse must search out relatives and friends with close relationships to the family and help them understand the situation so that they can provide support to the parents.

The nurse should encourage open communication among family members, particularly between spouses. Open communication is especially important when the mother is hospitalized apart from the infant. Because of her anxiety and

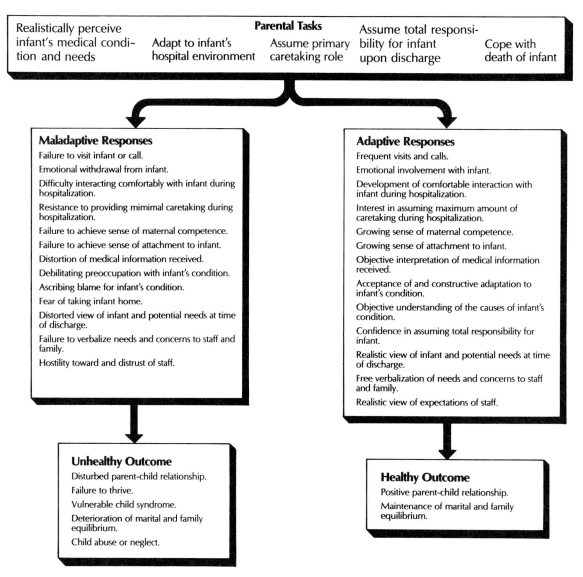

Parental Tasks

Realistically perceive infant's medical condition and needs | Adapt to infant's hospital environment | Assume primary caretaking role | Assume total responsibility for infant upon discharge | Cope with death of infant

Maladaptive Responses

Failure to visit infant or call.

Emotional withdrawal from infant.

Difficulty interacting comfortably with infant during hospitalization.

Resistance to providing mimimal caretaking during hospitalization.

Failure to achieve sense of maternal competence.

Failure to achieve sense of attachment to infant.

Distortion of medical information received.

Debilitating preoccupation with infant's condition.

Ascribing blame for infant's condition.

Fear of taking infant home.

Distorted view of infant and potential needs at time of discharge.

Failure to verbalize needs and concerns to staff and family.

Hostility toward and distrust of staff.

Adaptive Responses

Frequent visits and calls.

Emotional involvement with infant.

Development of comfortable interaction with infant during hospitalization.

Interest in assuming maximum amount of caretaking during hospitalization.

Growing sense of maternal competence.

Growing sense of attachment to infant.

Objective interpretation of medical information received.

Acceptance of and constructive adaptation to infant's condition.

Objective understanding of the causes of infant's condition.

Confidence in assuming total responsibility for infant.

Realistic view of infant and potential needs at time of discharge.

Free verbalization of needs and concerns to staff and family.

Realistic view of expectations of staff.

Unhealthy Outcome

Disturbed parent-child relationship.

Failure to thrive.

Vulnerable child syndrome.

Deterioration of marital and family equilibrium.

Child abuse or neglect.

Healthy Outcome

Positive parent-child relationship.

Maintenance of marital and family equilibrium.

Figure 26-2

Maladaptive and adaptive parental responses during crisis period showing unhealthy and healthy outcomes. (Reprinted from Grant P: Psychosocial needs of families of high risk infants. *Fam Comm Health* 1978; 11:93, by permission of Aspens Systems Corporation, © 1978.)

isolation, she may mistrust all those who provide information (the father, nurse, physician, or extended family) until she can see the infant for herself. This can put tremendous stress on the relationship between spouses. The parents (and family) should be given information together. This practice helps overcome misunderstandings and misinterpretations and promotes mutual "working through" of problems.

Families with children in the newborn inten-

sive care unit often become friends and support one another, and many units have established parent groups. Most groups make contact with families within a day or two of the infant's admission to the unit, either through telephone calls or visits to the hospital. This personalized method gives the grieving parents an opportunity to express personal feelings about the situation with others who have experienced the same feelings (Elsas, 1981).

The needs of siblings should not be overlooked. They have been looking forward to the new baby, and they too suffer a degree of loss. Young children may react with hostility and older ones with shame at the birth of an infant with an anomaly. Both reactions make them feel guilty. Parents, preoccupied with working through their own feelings, often cannot give the other children the attention and support they need. Sometimes another child becomes the focus of family tension. Anxiety thus directed can take the form of finding fault or of overconcern. It is a form of denial; the parents cannot face the real worry—the infant at risk. After assessing the situation, the observant nurse could see that another family member or friend steps in and gives the needed support to the siblings of the affected baby.

Predischarge planning begins once the infant's condition becomes stable and indications suggest the newborn will survive. Adequate predischarge teaching will help the parents to transform their feelings of inadequacy and competition with the nurse into feelings of self-assurance and attachment. From the beginning the parents should be taught about their infant's special needs and growth patterns. The nurse's responsibility is to provide instructions in an optimal environment for parental learning. Learning should take place over time, not in a bombardment of instructions on the day or hour before discharge (Figure 26-3).

Many intensive care units provide facilities for parents to room-in with their infants for a few days before discharge. This allows parents a degree of independence in the care of their infant with the security of nursing help nearby. This practice is particularly helpful for anxious parents, parents who have not had the opportunity to spend extended time with their infant, or parents who will be giving complex physical care at home, such as tracheostomy care.

The basic elements of predischarge care are as follows:

1. Teaching parents routine well-baby care, such as bathing, temperature taking, formula preparation, breast-feeding

2. Training parents to do special procedures as needed by the newborn, such as gavage or gastrostomy feedings, tracheostomy or enterostomy care, and medication administration

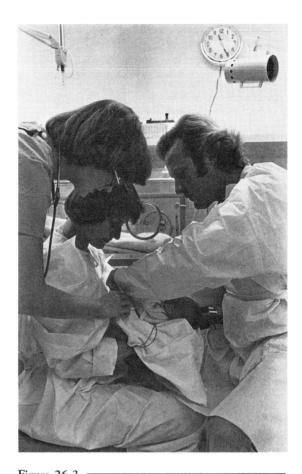

Figure 26-3
The parents of a preterm infant learning how to take care of their child.

3. Referrals to community health and support organizations

4. Teaching parents about growth and developmental needs of their infant

5. Arranging medical follow-up care

6. Placing necessary special equipment or supplies for infant care (such as a respirator, oxygen, and apnea monitor) in the home

Further evaluation after the infant has gone home is useful in determining whether the crisis has been resolved satisfactorily. The parents are usually given the intensive care nursery's telephone number to call for support and advice. It is suggested that the staff follow up each family with visits or telephone calls at intervals for several weeks to assess and evaluate the infant's (and parents') progress.

Attachment Problems _____

In the prenatal period, warning signs that may indicate lack of acceptance and a potential for malattachment include the following (Helfer and Kempe, 1976):

- Negative maternal self-perception
- Excessive mood swings or emotional withdrawal
- Failure to respond to quickening
- Excessive maternal preoccupation with appearance
- Numerous physical complaints
- Failure to prepare for the infant during the last trimester

At delivery, signs of maladaptive responses include:

- Lack of interest in seeing or holding the infant
- Withdrawal, sadness, or disappointment
- Negative comments ("She's so ugly.")
- Expressions of marked dissappointment when told of the infant's sex

The mother may also avoid asking questions about the infant or talking to the infant and may suddenly decide that she does not want to breast-feed (Johnson, 1979).

During the postpartal period, the following maternal behaviors are evidence of maternal maladaptive parenting:

- Limited handling of or smiling at the infant
- Lack of preparation or questions about the infant's needs and care
- Failure to snuggle the newborn to her neck and face
- Negative or hostile comments about the newborn

The father also may exhibit signs of malattachment to his infant. Examples of maladaptive paternal behaviors are inattentiveness and indifference toward the child; rough or inappropriate handling; and tense, rigid posture. He may also show no protective behavior toward the infant (Johnson, 1979).

A serious sign of malattachment may be exhibited by the infant in the form of nonorganic failure to thrive. Most authorities agree that nonorganic failure to thrive is caused by disturbed or lack of nurturing maternal behaviors (Yoos, 1984).

Nursing management   Promotion of healthy parent–infant attachment should begin during the prenatal period. The health history should include questions that provide caregivers with some initial understanding of the parents' attitudes, support systems, fears, and knowledge. As the pregnancy progresses, the nurse can elicit further information and begin teaching. During the third trimester, caregivers should look for evidence that the parents have started to prepare for the infant. After delivery, mother, father, and newborn must have time alone together whenever possible to begin getting acquainted.

When maladaptive behaviors are identified, various interventions can be used. A team approach involving all three nursing shifts is advised. Any positive behaviors are communicated so that each staff member can continue to offer support and encourage further development of such behaviors.

Parents need a supportive, understanding person they can interact with as they work through their feelings about the baby. Occasionally, in the presence of severe emotional disorders, a referral to a psychologist or psychiatrist may be necessary. Referral to community agencies such as the Public Health Department is advised so that follow-up can be established.

When infants require lengthy intensive care, special efforts by the nurse may facilitate attachment. It is important that the parents believe that the child belongs to them rather than to the health care team. The parents should be encouraged to participate in care and to give suggestions about that care. If there is a specific problem with the feeding schedule or technique, for example, the parents might be encouraged to work with the nurses to help establish the care plan.

Personal or telephone contact may be maintained after discharge so that the parents can continue to have contact with a supportive person with whom they are already acquainted. They should be encouraged to call the postpartal unit or newborn nursery if they have questions.

Unwanted Pregnancy and Relinquishment

Sometimes a pregnancy is unwanted. The expectant woman may be an adolescent, unmarried, or economically restricted. She may dislike children or the idea of being a mother. She may feel that she is not emotionally ready for the responsibilities of parenthood. Her partner may disapprove of the pregnancy. These and many other reasons may cause the woman to continue to reject the idea of her pregnancy. An emotional crisis arises as she attempts to resolve the problem. She may choose to have an abortion, to carry the fetus to term and keep the baby, or to have the baby and relinquish it for adoption.

Many mothers who choose to give their infants up for adoption are young and/or unmarried. More young women choose to keep the child than to give it up, however. Approximately two-thirds of children born out of wedlock are raised by their mothers alone.

The decision of a mother to relinquish her infant is an extremely difficult one. Harvey (1977) reports that there are social pressures against giving up one's child. Some women may want to prove to themselves that they can manage on their own by keeping their infants.

The mother who chooses to let her child be adopted usually experiences intense ambivalence. These feelings may heighten just before delivery and upon seeing her baby. After childbirth, the mother will need to complete a grieving process to work through her loss.

Nursing management The woman with an unwanted pregnancy must make the difficult decision: whether to have the child or have an abortion. If she decides to complete the pregnancy, she must decide whether to keep the baby. During this difficult time, the expectant woman may look to others, such as the nurse, for help in making these decisions. The woman should be given information rather than direct advice during this time, and be allowed to discuss her situation and problem solve.

The mother who decides to relinquish the child usually has made considerable adjustments in her life-style to give birth to this child. She may not have told friends and relatives about the pregnancy and so lacks an extended support system.

During the prenatal period, the nurse can help her by encouraging her to express her grief, loneliness, guilt, and other feelings.

When the relinquishing mother is admitted to the maternity unit, the staff should be informed about the mother's decision to relinquish the infant. Any special requests for delivery should be respected and the woman encouraged to express her emotions (Harvey, 1977). After the delivery the mother should be allowed access to the infant; she will decide whether she wants to see the newborn. Seeing the newborn often aids the grieving process. When the mother sees her baby, she may feel strong attachment and love. The nurse needs to assure the woman that these feelings do not mean that her decision to relinquish the child is a wrong one; relinquishment is often a painful act of love (Arms, 1984). Postpartal nursing management also includes arranging ongoing care for the relinquishing mother.

Initial denial of pregnancy by women usually moves into acceptance of the pregnant state. Occasionally, however, a nurse may encounter a woman who denies she is pregnant even as she is admitted to the maternity unit. It may seem impossible that a woman who is so obviously pregnant could maintain this delusion. Because of this denial, the woman has not sought prenatal care. Preparation for the birth experience may be incomplete, and the mother and infant may be at risk.

The nurse must establish a trusting relationship with this woman. While building rapport with the woman, the nurse should gently guide the mother-to-be to accept reality.

In the event that a woman decides to keep an unwanted child, the nurse should be aware of the potential for parenting problems. Families with unwanted children are more crisis prone than others, although in many cases, parents grow to love their child after attachment occurs. The nurse should be ready to initiate crisis strategies or make appropriate referrals as the need arises.

Child Abuse

Child abuse is the physical, emotional, or sexual harming of a child by parents, siblings, or other caretakers. Among the many serious effects of child abuse are physical handicaps, poor self-image, inability to love others, antisocial or violent behavior in later life, and death.

A small number of abusing parents have serious mental illnesses, but most abusing parents have less serious problems. The parents of an abused child rarely hate or bear the child ill will. Most often the abusing parents suffer from low self-esteem and guilt, and many have been victims of abuse as children.

It may be necessary to remove children temporarily from the parents' home during therapy, but the goal of treatment is to help parents and their children live together.

Nursing management The health professional is required by law to report cases of suspected child abuse. The law not only protects the nurse who in good faith reports a case of suspected child abuse that is mistaken, but also holds an individual liable if a case of abuse is known and not reported.

Nurses who work in prenatal and postnatal settings are in a unique situation to help prevent child abuse by identifying families who show the potential for emotional and physical abuse. Some of the signs that can alert the nurse to the possibility of child abuse are:

- Parents express distaste or rejection the first time they see the infant.
- Mother seems unduly concerned about the "correct" appearance of the baby.
- Parents are extremely unhappy with the sex of the baby.
- Mother has extremely unrealistic views of motherhood.
- Parents give the child a derisive or cruel name or fail to name the baby for an extended period of time.
- Parents make many comments about "not spoiling" the baby or "controlling bad behavior."
- Mother repeatedly refers to her infant as "bad," "impossible," or other disparaging terms.
- Parents were abused as children or abuse each other.
- Parents abuse alcohol or drugs.

Once they have identified a family at risk for child abuse, primary caregivers can develop an intensive interdisciplinary approach to prevention involving both public health nurses and social workers (Christensen et al., 1984). The nurse can begin intervention by encouraging the parents to express their feelings about the situation. The nurse must understand the parents' emotional needs to provide the proper intervention. It is particularly valuable to involve the parents in planning the medical care for the child so they feel that they are doing something positive and perhaps "making up" for the harm.

The nurse's attitudes are critically important in the development of a therapeutic nurse–client relationship. Empathy, warmth, and understanding are essential. The nurse who is repulsed by the parents' behavior and projects blame or rejection will increase the parents' guilt and further lower their self-esteem. The child may bear the brunt of the parents' frustration and self-hate.

The nurse should explain to the parents the function of the child welfare authorities, pointing out that they are there to help the parents. The nurse can also help by referring the parents for appropriate counseling or to self-help groups such as Parents Anonymous.

Adolescent Parent

As mentioned in Chapter 5, pregnancy and the birth of a child are normal developmental crises for a family. When the parents are very young or immature, the crisis situation may be compounded.

The adolescent mother may be faced with many factors that complicate her situation. She may have used pregnancy to escape from an intolerable situation at home. She may come from a family in which emotional or physical abuse or incest took place. Economic conditions and poverty may be a problem. Emotional support may be lacking. The adolescent may not have told her parents about the pregnancy for fear of rejection. She may feel shame and lack of self-esteem. There may be pressure for her to marry the father. Career and education plans may be threatened by the responsibility and expense of being a parent.

The adolescent may view the new baby as an object—a toy or plaything—by which she can increase her own self-esteem and solidify her role identity. When the infant does not fulfill these needs, frustration and abuse may result.

Nursing management   The nurse who plans to be involved with adolescent parents should develop a complete understanding of the developmental needs of both adolescents and infants. The teenager often lacks knowledge about normal infant growth and development as well as information about child care.

The nurse may use role modeling to demonstrate infant care to the mother, rather than merely telling her. Having the teenager repeat the procedure is important so that the nurse can give positive feedback about her skills and abilities. As the teenage mother's confidence in her ability to care for the infant increases, her self-esteem rises.

Whenever possible the father of the child should be involved both before and after the infant is born. The nurse may offer contraceptive counseling to the young couple. Referrals to community agencies may be appropriate, depending on the specific problems of the young parents. Supportive grandparents can also provide assistance. If possible, adolescent parents should be encouraged to finish high school.

Single-Parent Families

In the United States, about 20% of all children under 18 years of age live with one parent—about 90% with their mothers and the remainder with their fathers. Single-parent homes most commonly are a result of divorce, desertion, or death of a spouse. Single-parent families also occur when the child's parents are unmarried and the child lives with either the mother or father.

Some older unmarried women are choosing to have children without a partner. As these women near the end of their reproductive years, they decide that childbearing and childrearing are experiences they desire.

Single-parent homes may also occur as a result of adoption. This phenomenon, although still relatively rare, is increasing.

Hazards to successful childrearing do exist for single-parent families. As children pass through certain developmental stages, they must be provided with opportunities to relate to individuals of the same and opposite sex to learn sex roles. In a single-parent family, these opportunities may not be readily available, and substitute experiences must be provided. An additional drawback in a single-parent family is the lack of opportunities for the child to observe parental man–woman interactions. Furthermore, the parent in a single-parent situation is usually employed outside the home and must handle the demands of both job and family alone.

Nursing management   Nurses will be able to counsel the single parent more effectively if they understand the stresses and demands of parenting a child. A single parent is more likely to have minimal support.

The nurse can begin by assessing the parent's educational needs and providing information as needed. Interventions may include investigation of the availability of child care facilities and referral to single-parent support groups, such as Parents Without Partners.

Summary

The nurse is often the first one in contact with a family in a crisis brought on by health care problems. The premature birth of an infant, the birth of an infant with a congenital anomaly, and the death of an infant are types of crises that may be seen in maternity nursing. Other causes of family crises are unwanted pregnancy, child abuse, adolescent or single parenthood, and attachment problems.

Recognition of the dynamics of loss and grief is important for the nurse with clients who are experiencing these situations. An important part of nursing care is to assess the emotional turmoil of a client and plan intervention to help the client return to an adaptive level of functioning.

Successful coping on the part of the maternity client and her family can be promoted by nurses armed with a variety of skills, especially in crisis intervention. Even if nurses are unsure of their crisis intervention skills, they may be in the best position to make a referral for a family in crisis. Recognizing the stresses that contribute to a crisis and making a referral to a skilled crisis intervention counselor can be a positive nursing intervention for a grieving or otherwise troubled individual or family.

Resource Groups

Local chapters of Trisomy 13 Clubs, March of Dimes Birth Defects Foundation, Handicapped Children's Services, Teen Mother and Child Programs and parent support groups.

National Association for Mental Health (1800 North Kent Street, Arlington, Va. 22209).

National Committee for Prevention of Child Abuse (Box 2866, Chicago, Il. 60690).

National Organization of Mothers of Twins Clubs (5402 Amberwood Lane, Rockville, Md. 20853).

National Sudden Infant Death Syndrome Foundation (Dept. N83, 2 Metro Plaza, Suite 205, 8240 Professional Place, Landover, Md. 20785).

National Women's Health Network (2025 I Street NW, Suite 105, Washington, D.C. 20006).

Parents Anonymous (22330 Hawthorne Boulevard, Suite 208, Torrance, Ca. 90505).

Parents Without Partners, Inc. (80 Fifth Avenue, New York, N.Y. 10011).

Resolve Through Sharing (La Crosse Lutheran Hospital, 1910 South Ave., LaCrosse, Wi. 54601). An in-hospital bereavement counseling center offering training for staff caring for families experiencing perinatal loss.

SHARE (St. John's Hospital, 800 East Carpenter St., Springfield, Il. 62769). Interdisciplinary support group for families grieving a perinatal loss.

References

Aguilera DC, Messick JM: *Crisis Intervention: Theory and Methodology*, 4th ed. St. Louis: Mosby, 1982.

Arms S: *To Love and Let Go*. New York: Knopf, 1984.

Caplan G et al: Four studies of crisis in parents of prematures. *Community Mental Health J* 1965; 1:149.

Christensen ML, Schommer BL, Valasquez J: An interdisciplinary approach to preventing child abuse. *MCN* March/April 1984; 9:108.

Clausen JP: Anticipatory guidance of the expectant family. In: *Family Health Care*, Vol. 2, *Developmental and Situational Crises*, 2nd ed. Hymovich DP, Barnard MV (editors). New York: McGraw-Hill, 1979.

Elsas TL: Family mental health care in the neonatal intensive care unit. *J Obstet Gynecol Neonatal Nurs* May/June 1981; 10:204.

Furman E: The death of a newborn: Care of the parents. *Birth Fam J* Winter 1978; 5:214.

Getz W et al: *Fundamentals of Crisis Counseling*. Lexington, Mass.: D. C. Heath, 1974.

Grant P: Psychosocial needs of families of high-risk infants. *Fam Com Health* November 1978; 1(3):91.

Harvey R: Caring perceptively for the relinquishing mother. *MCN* January/February 1977; 2:24.

Helfer RE, Kempe CH: *Child Abuse and Neglect: The Family and the Community*. Cambridge, Mass.: Ballinger, 1976.

Hoff LA: *People in Crisis: Understanding and Helping*, 2nd ed. Menlo Park, Calif.: Addison-Wesley, 1984.

Johnson SH: *High-Risk Parenting: Nursing Assessment and Strategies for the Family at Risk*. Philadelphia: Lippincott, 1979.

Kaplan DM, Mason EA: Maternal reactions to premature birth viewed as an acute emotional disorder. In: *Crisis Interventions*, Parad HJ (editor). New York: Family Services Association of America, 1974.

Klaus MH, Fanaroff AA: *Care of the High-Risk Neonate*, 2nd ed. Philadelphia: Saunders, 1979.

Klaus MH, Kennell JH: *Parent-Infant Attachment*, 2nd ed. St. Louis: Mosby, 1982.

Kowalski K, Osborn MR: Helping mothers of stillborn infants to grieve. *MCN* January/February 1977; 2:29.

Kübler-Ross E: *On Death and Dying*. New York: Macmillan, 1969.

Lindemann E: Symptomatology and management of acute grief. *Am J Psychiatry* 1944; 101:141.

McCabe SN: Anticipatory guidance for families with infants. In *Family Health Care,* Vol. 2. *Developmental and Situational Crises*, 2nd ed. Hymovich DP, Barnard MV (editors). New York: McGraw-Hill, 1979.

Olshansky S: Chronic sorrow: A response to having a mentally defective child. *Soc Casework* 1962; 43:109.

Powell ML: *Assessment and Management of Developmental Changes and Problems in Children*, 2nd ed. St. Louis: Mosby, 1981.

Schoenberg B et al: *Loss and Grief: Psychological Management in Medical Practice*. New York: Columbia University Press, 1970.

Schoenberg B et al: *Anticipatory Grief*. New York: Columbia University Press, 1974.

Seitz PM, Warrick LH: Perinatal death: The grieving mother. *Am J Nurs* 1974; 74:2028.

West M: The mother, the developmentally disabled child, and the nurse. *Topics Clin Nurs* October 1984; 6:19.

Williams HA, Rivara FP, Rothenberg MB: The child is dying: Who helps the family? *MCN* July/August 1981; 6:121.

Wooten B: Death of an infant. *MCN* July/August 1981; 6:257.

Yoos L: Taking another look at failure to thrive. *MCN* January/February 1984; 9:32.

Additional Readings

Barnes B, Coplon J: *The Single-Parent Experience: A Time for Growth*. New York: Family Service Association of America, 1980.

Bascom L: Women who refuse to believe: Persistent denial of pregnancy. *MCN* May/June 1977; 2:174.

Boro S, Lasker J: *When Pregnancy Fails*. Boston: Beacon Press, 1981.

Gonda TA, Ruark JE: *Dying Dignified: The Health Professional's Guide to Care*. Menlo Park, Calif.: Addison-Wesley, 1984.

Harris DM, Karrow L, Phillips PJ: Adolescent parenthood. In: *Family Health Care*, Vol. 2. *Developmental and Situational Crisis*, 2nd ed. Hymovich DP, Barnard MU (editors). New York: McGraw-Hill, 1979.

Hawkins-Walsh E: Diminishing anxiety in parents of sick newborns. *MCN* January/February 1980; 5:30.

Hughes CP: The single father. *Topics in Clin Nurs* October 1984; 6:1.

Kennell JH: Birth of a malformed baby: Helping the family. *Birth Fam J* Winter 1978; 5:219.

Selye H: *Stress Without Distress*. Philadelphia: Lippincott, 1974.

Appendices

A
The Pregnant Patient's Bill of Rights*

The Pregnant Patient has the right to participate in decisions involving her well-being and that of her unborn child, unless there is a clearcut medical emergency that prevents her participation. In addition to the rights set forth in the American Hospital Association's "Patient's Bill of Rights," the Pregnant Patient, because she represents TWO patients rather than one, should be recognized as having the additional rights listed below.

1. *The Pregnant Patient has the right*, prior to the administration of any drug or procedure, to be informed by the health professional caring for her of any potential direct or indirect effects, risks or hazards to herself or her unborn or newborn infant which may result from the use of a drug or procedure prescribed for or administered to her during pregnancy, labor, birth or lactation.

2. *The Pregnant Patient has the right*, prior to the proposed therapy, to be informed, not only of the benefits, risks, and hazards of the proposed therapy but also of known alternative therapy, such as available childbirth education classes which could help to prepare the Pregnant Patient physically and mentally to cope with the discomfort or stress of pregnancy and the experience of childbirth, thereby reducing or eliminating her need for drugs and obstetric intervention. She should be offered such information early in her pregnancy in order that she may make a reasoned decision.

3. *The Pregnant Patient has the right*, prior to the administration of any drug, to be informed by the health professional who is prescribing or administering the drug to her that any drug which she receives during pregnancy, labor and birth, no matter how or when the drug is taken or administered, may adversely affect her unborn baby, directly or indirectly, and that there is no drug or chemical which has been proven safe for the unborn child.

4. *The Pregnant Patient has the right* if cesarean birth is anticipated, to be informed prior to the administration of any drug, and preferably prior to her hospitalization, that minimizing her and, in turn, her baby's intake of nonessential preoperative medicine will benefit her baby.

5. *The Pregnant Patient has the right*, prior to the administration of a drug or procedure, to be informed of the areas of uncertainty if there is NO properly controlled follow-up research which has established the safety of the drug or procedure with regard to its direct and/or indirect effects on the physiological, mental and neurological development of the child exposed, via the mother, to the drug or procedure during pregnancy, labor, birth, or lactation—(this would apply to virtually all drugs and the vast majority of obstetric procedures).

6. *The Pregnant Patient has the right*, prior to the administration of any drug, to be informed of the brand name and generic name of the drug in order that she may advise the health professional of any past adverse reaction to the drug.

*Prepared by Doris Haire, Chair, Committee on Health Law and Regulation, International Childbirth Education Association, Inc., Rochester, N.Y.

7. *The Pregnant Patient has the right* to determine for herself, without pressure from her attendant, whether she will accept the risks inherent in the proposed therapy or refuse a drug or procedure.

8. *The Pregnant Patient has the right* to know the name and qualifications of the individual administering a medication or procedure to her during labor or birth.

9. *The Pregnant Patient has the right* to be informed, prior to the administration of any procedure, whether that procedure is being administered to her for her or her baby's benefit (medically indicated) or as an elective procedure (for convenience, teaching purposes or research).

10. *The Pregnant Patient has the right* to be accompanied during the stress of labor and birth by someone she cares for, and to whom she looks for emotional comfort and encouragement.

11. *The Pregnant Patient has the right* after appropriate medical consultation to choose a position for labor and for birth which is least stressful to her baby and to herself.

12. *The Obstetric Patient has the right* to have her baby cared for at her bedside if her baby is normal, and to feed her baby according to her baby's needs rather than according to the hospital's regimen.

13. *The Obstetric Patient has the right* to be informed in writing of the name of the person who actually delivered her baby and the professional qualifications of that per-

son. This information should also be on the birth certificate.

14. *The Obstetric Patient has the right* to be informed if there is any known or indicated aspect of her or her baby's care or condition which may cause her or her baby later difficulty or problems.

15. *The Obstetric Patient has the right* to have her and her baby's hospital medical records complete, accurate and legible and to have their records, including Nurses' Notes, retained by the hospital until the child reaches at least the age of majority, or to have the records offered to her before they are destroyed.

16. *The Obstetric Patient*, both during and after her hospital stay, has the right to have access to her complete hospital medical records, including Nurses' Notes, and to receive a copy upon payment of a reasonable fee and without incurring the expense of retaining an attorney.

It is the obstetric patient and her baby, not the health professional, who must sustain any trauma or injury resulting from the use of a drug or obstetric procedure. The observation of the rights listed above will not only permit the obstetric patient to participate in the decisions involving her and her baby's health care, but will help to protect the health professional and the hospital against litigation arising from resentment or misunderstanding on the part of the mother.

B

Common Abbreviations in Maternity Nursing

ABC	Alternative birthing center *or* airway, breathing, circulation	cm	centimeter
Accel	Acceleration of fetal heart rate	CNM	Certified nurse-midwife
		CNS	Central nervous system
		CPAP	Continuous positive airway pressure
AC	Abdominal circumference	CPD	Cephalopelvic disproportion *or* Citrate-phosphate-dextrose
ACTH	Adrenocorticotrophic hormone		
AFP	α-fetoprotein	CPR	Cardiopulmonary resuscitation
AFV	Amniotic fluid volume		
AGA	Average for gestational age	C-R	Crown-to-rump length
AID or AIH	Artificial insemination donor (H designates mate is donor)	C/S	Cesarean section or C-section
		CST	Contraction stress test
ARBOW	Artificial rupture of bag of waters	CVA	Costovertebral angle
		CVP	Central venous pressure
AROM	Artificial rupture of membranes	D&C	Dilatation and curettage
		dec	deceleration of fetal heart rate
BAT	Brown adipose tissue (brown fat)		
		DIC	Disseminated intravascular coagulation
BBT	Basal body temperature		
BL	Baseline (fetal heart rate baseline)	dil	dilatation
		DM	Diabetes mellitus
BMR	Basal metabolic rate	DRG	Diagnostic related groups
BOW	Bag of waters	DTR	Deep tendon reflexes
BP	Blood pressure	EDC	Estimated date of confinement
BPD	Biparietal diameter *or* Bronchopulmonary dysplasia		
		EFM	Electronic fetal monitor
		ELF	Elective low forceps
BSST	Breast self-stimulation test	epis	Episiotomy
CC	Chest circumference *or* Cord compression	FAD	Fetal activity diary
		FAS	Fetal alcohol syndrome
cc	cubic centimeter	FBM	Fetal breathing movements
C-H	Crown-to-heel length	FBS	Fetal blood sample *or* fasting blood sugar test
CHF	Congestive heart failure		
CID	Cytomegalic inclusion disease	FFA	Free fatty acids
		FHR	Fetal heart rate
CMV	Cytomegalovirus	FHT	Fetal heart tones

FL	Femur length	LH	Luteinizing hormone
FM	Fetal movement	LHRH	Luteinizing hormone–releasing hormone
FMD	Fetal movement diary		
FPG	Fasting plasma glucose test	LMA	Left-mentum-anterior
FRC	Female reproductive cycle	LML	Left mediolateral episiotomy
FSH	Follicle-stimulating hormone		
		LMP	Last menstrual period *or* Left-mentum-posterior
FSHRH	Follicle-stimulating hormone–releasing hormone		
		LMT	Left-mentum-transverse
		LOA	Left-occiput-anterior
FSI	Foam stability index	LOF	Low outlet forceps
GDM	Gestational diabetes mellitus	LOP	Left-occiput-posterior
		LOT	Left-occiput-transverse
GFR	Glomerular filtration rate	L/S	Lecithin/sphingomyelin ratio
GI	Gastrointestinal		
GnRF	Gonadotrophin-releasing factor	LSA	Left-sacrum-anterior
		LSP	Left-sacrum-posterior
GnRH	Gonadotrophin-releasing hormone	LST	Left-sacrum-transverse
		MAS	Meconium aspiration syndrome
grav	gravida		
HAI	Hemagglutination-inhibition test	MCT	Medium chain triglycerides
		mec	Meconium
HC	Head compression	mec st	Meconium stain
hCG	Human chorionic gonadotrophin	M & I	Maternity and Infant Care Projects
hCS	Human chorionic somatomammotrophin (same as hPL)	ML	Midline (episiotomy)
		MLE	Midline echo
		MUGB	4-methylumbelliferyl quanidinobenzoate
HMD	Hyaline membrane disease		
hMG	Human menopausal gonadotrophin	multip	Multipara
		NANDA	North American Nursing Diagnosis Association
hPL	Human placental lactogen		
HVH	Herpes virus hominis	NEC	Necrotizing enterocolitis
IDDM	Insulin-dependent diabetes mellitus (Type I)	NGU	Nongonococcal urethritis
		NIDDM	Noninsulin-dependent diabetes mellitus (Type II)
IDM	Infant of a diabetic mother		
IGT	Impaired glucose tolerance	NP	Nurse practitioner
IGTT	Intravenous glucose tolerance test	NPO	Nothing by mouth
		NST	Nonstress test *or* nonshivering thermogenesis
IPG	Impedance phlebography		
IUD	Intrauterine device		
IUFD	Intrauterine fetal death	NSVD	Normal sterile vaginal delivery
IUGR	Intrauterine growth retardation		
		OA	Occiput anterior
JCAH	Joint Commission on the Accreditation of Hospitals	OCT	Oxytocin challenge test
		OF	Occipitofrontal (diameter)
LADA	Left-acromion-dorsal-anterior	OFC	Occipitofrontal circumference
LADP	Left-acromion-dorsal-posterior	OGTT	Oral glucose tolerance test
		OM	Occipitomental (diameter)
LBW	Low birth weight	OP	Occiput posterior
LGA	Large for gestational age	p	Para

PBI	Protein-bound iodine	SFD	Small for dates
PDA	Patent ductus arteriosus	SGA	Small for gestational age
PEEP	Positive end-expiratory pressure	SIDS	Sudden infant death syndrome
PG	Phosphatidyglycerol *or* Prostaglandin	SOAP	Subjective data, objective data, analysis, plan
PI	Phosphatidylinositol	SOB	suboccipitobregmatic diameter
PID	Pelvic inflammatory disease		
PIH	Pregnancy-induced hypertension	SMB	Submentobregmatic diameter
Pit	Pitocin	SRBOW	Spontaneous rupture of the bag of waters
PKU	Phenylketonuria		
PMI	Point of maximal impulse	SROM	Spontaneous rupture of the membranes
POR	Problem-oriented record		
Preemie	Premature infant	STD	Sexually transmitted disease
Primip	Primipara		
PROM	Premature rupture of membranes	STH	Somatotrophic hormone
		STS	Serologic test for syphilis
PTT	Partial thromboplastin test	SVE	Sterile vaginal exam
RADA	Right-acromion-dorsal-anterior	TC	Thoracic circumference
		TCM	Transcutaneous monitoring
RADP	Right-acromion-dorsal-posterior	TNZ	Thermal neutral zone
		TORCH	Toxoplasmosis, rubella, cytomegalovirus, herpesvirus hominis type 2
RBC	Red blood cell		
RDA	Recommended dietary allowance		
		TPAL	Term, preterm, abortion, living; a system of recording maternity history
RDS	Respiratory distress syndrome		
REM	Rapid eye movements	ū	Umbilicus
RIA	Radioimmune assay	u/a	Urinalysis
RLF	Retrolental fibroplasia	UC	Uterine contraction
ROA	Right-occiput-anterior	UPI	Uteroplacental insufficiency
ROP	Right-occiput-posterior	U/S	Ultrasound
ROM	Rupture of membranes	UTI	Urinary tract infection
ROT	Right-occiput-transverse	VBAC	Vaginal birth after cesarean
RMA	Right-mentum-anterior	VDRL	Venereal Disease Research Laboratories
RMP	Right-mentum-posterior		
RMT	Right-mentum-transverse	WBC	White blood cell
RRA	Radioreceptor assay	WIC	Supplemental food program for Women, Infants, and Children
RSA	Right-sacrum-anterior		
RSP	Right-sacrum-posterior		
RST	Right-sacrum-transverse		

C
Conversion of Pounds and Ounces to Grams

Conversion of Pounds and Ounces to Grams

POUNDS	OUNCES 0	1	2	3	4	5	6	7	8	9	10	11	12	13	14	OUNCES 15
0	–	28	57	85	113	142	170	198	227	255	283	312	340	369	397	425
1	454	482	510	539	567	595	624	652	680	709	737	765	794	822	850	879
2	907	936	964	992	1021	1049	1077	1106	1134	1162	1191	1219	1247	1276	1304	1332
3	1361	1389	1417	1446	1474	1503	1531	1559	1588	1616	1644	1673	1701	1729	1758	1786
4	1814	1843	1871	1899	1928	1956	1984	2013	2041	2070	2098	2126	2155	2183	2211	2240
5	2268	2296	2325	2353	2381	2410	2438	2466	2495	2523	2551	2580	2608	2637	2665	2693
6	2722	2750	2778	2807	2835	2863	2892	2920	2948	2977	3005	3033	3062	3090	3118	3147
7	3175	3203	3232	3260	3289	3317	3345	3374	3402	3430	3459	3487	3515	3544	3572	3600
8	3629	3657	3685	3714	3742	3770	3799	3827	3856	3884	3912	3941	3969	3997	4026	4054
9	4082	4111	4139	4167	4196	4224	4252	4281	4309	4337	4366	4394	4423	4451	4479	4508
10	4536	4564	4593	4621	4649	4678	4706	4734	4763	4791	4819	4848	4876	4904	4933	4961
11	4990	5018	5046	5075	5103	5131	5160	5188	5216	5245	5273	5301	5330	5358	5386	5415
12	5443	5471	5500	5528	5557	5585	5613	5642	5670	5698	5727	5755	5783	5812	5840	5868
13	5897	5925	5953	5982	6010	6038	6067	6095	6123	6152	6180	6209	6237	6265	6294	6322
14	6350	6379	6407	6435	6464	6492	6520	6549	6577	6605	6634	6662	6690	6719	6747	6776
15	6804	6832	6860	6889	6917	6945	6973	7002	7030	7059	7087	7115	7144	7172	7201	7228
16	7257	7286	7313	7342	7371	7399	7427	7456	7484	7512	7541	7569	7597	7626	7654	7682
17	7711	7739	7768	7796	7824	7853	7881	7909	7938	7966	7994	8023	8051	8079	8108	8136
18	8165	8192	8221	8249	8278	8306	8335	8363	8391	8420	8448	8476	8504	8533	8561	8590
19	8618	8646	8675	8703	8731	8760	8788	8816	8845	8873	8902	8930	8958	8987	9015	9043
20	9072	9100	9128	9157	9185	9213	9242	9270	9298	9327	9355	9383	9412	9440	9469	9497
21	9525	9554	9582	9610	9639	9667	9695	9724	9752	9780	9809	9837	9865	9894	9922	9950
22	9979	10007	10036	10064	10092	10120	10149	10177	10206	10234	10262	10291	10319	10347	10376	10404

D
Clinical Estimation
of Gestational Age

Brazie and Lubchenco's "Clinical Estimation of Gestational Age Chart" is one of the assessment tools available to nurses to evaluate a newborn's gestational age. The form used to guide the physical examination appears on p. 657. The neurologic examination form appears on p. 658. (This assessment tool is reproduced courtesy of Mead Johnson Laboratories, Evansville, Indiana.)

CLINICAL ESTIMATION OF GESTATIONAL AGE
An Approximation Based on Published Data*

► Examination First Hours

PHYSICAL FINDINGS		20	21	22	23	24	25	26	27	28	29	30	31	32	33	34	35	36	37	38	39	40	41	42	43	44	45	46	47	48
																	WEEKS GESTATION													
VERNIX					APPEARS		COVERS BODY, THICK LAYER											ON BACK, SCALP, IN CREASES		SCANT, IN CREASES		NO VERNIX							
BREAST TISSUE AND AREOLA			AREOLA & NIPPLE BARELY VISIBLE NO PALPABLE BREAST TISSUE				FLAT, SHAPELESS								AREOLA RAISED		1-2 MM NODULE	3-5 MM	5-6 MM	7-10 MM			?12 MM					
EAR	FORM															BEGINNING INCURVING SUPERIOR		INCURVING UPPER 2/3 PINNAE			WELL-DEFINED INCURVING TO LOBE							
	CARTILAGE				PINNA SOFT, STAYS FOLDED										CARTILAGE SCANT RETURNS SLOWLY FROM FOLDING		THIN CARTILAGE SPRINGS BACK FROM FOLDING					PINNA FIRM, REMAINS ERECT FROM HEAD							
SOLE CREASES					SMOOTH SOLES Š CREASES							1-2 ANTERIOR CREASES			2-3 AN- TER- IOR CREA- SES	CREASES ANTERIOR 2/3 SOLE		CREASES INVOLVING HEEL				DEEPER CREASES OVER ENTIRE SOLE						
SKIN	THICKNESS & APPEARANCE		THIN, TRANSLUCENT SKIN, PLETHORIC, VENULES OVER ABDOMEN EDEMA										SMOOTH THICKER NO EDEMA				PINK		FEW VESSELS	SOME DES- QUAMATION PALE PINK			THICK, PALE, DESQUAMATION OVER ENTIRE BODY				
	NAIL PLATES		AP- PEAR										NAILS TO FINGER TIPS										NAILS EXTEND WELL BEYOND FINGER TIPS					
HAIR			APPEARS ON HEAD		EYE BROWS & LASHES			FINE, WOOLLY, BUNCHES OUT FROM HEAD										SILKY, SINGLE STRANDS LAYS FLAT				?RECEDING HAIRLINE OR LOSS OF BABY HAIR SHORT, FINE UNDERNEATH					
LANUGO			AP- PEARS		COVERS ENTIRE BODY					VANISHES FROM FACE						PRESENT ON SHOULDERS			NO LANUGO							
GENITALIA	TESTES								TESTES PALPABLE IN INGUINAL CANAL						IN UPPER SCROTUM					IN LOWER SCROTUM							
	SCROTUM								FEW RUGAE						RUGAE, ANTERIOR PORTION				RUGAE COVER			PENDULOUS					
	LABIA & CLITORIS								PROMINENT CLITORIS LABIA MAJORA SMALL WIDELY SEPARATED					LABIA MAJORA LARGER NEARLY COVERED CLITORIS					LABIA MINORA & CLITORIS COVERED							
SKULL FIRMNESS					BONES ARE SOFT					SOFT TO 1" FROM ANTERIOR FONTANELLE					SPONGY AT EDGES OF FON- TANELLE CENTER FIRM			BONES HARD SUTURES EASILY DISPLACED			BONES HARD, CANNOT BE DISPLACED					
POSTURE	RESTING		HYPOTONIC LATERAL DECUBITUS			HYPOTONIC					BEGINNING FLEXION THIGH		STRONGER HIP FLEXION		FROG-LIKE		FLEXION ALL LIMBS			HYPERTONIC			VERY HYPERTONIC					
RECOIL - LEG				NO RECOIL											PARTIAL RECOIL					PROMPT RECOIL							
	ARM			NO RECOIL											BEGIN FLEXION NO RE- COIL		PROMPT RECOIL MAY BE INHIBITED				PROMPT RECOIL AFTER 30" INHIBITION							

Confirmatory Neurologic Examination to be Done After 24 Hours

Mead Johnson LABORATORIES

WEEKS GESTATION: 20 21 22 23 24 25 26 27 28 29 30 31 32 33 34 35 36 37 38 39 40 41 42 43 44 45 46 47 48

TONE

Physical Finding	Findings across weeks gestation
HEEL TO EAR	NO RESISTANCE (≈20–28) · SOME RESISTANCE (≈30) · IMPOSSIBLE (≈34)
SCARF SIGN	NO RESISTANCE (≈23–31) · ELBOW PASSES MIDLINE (≈32–34) · ELBOW AT MIDLINE (≈36–37) · ELBOW DOES NOT REACH MIDLINE (≈44–46)
NECK FLEXORS (HEAD LAG)	ABSENT (≈30–31) · HEAD IN PLANE OF BODY (≈38–39) · HOLDS HEAD (≈44–45)
NECK EXTENSORS	HEAD BEGINS TO RIGHT ITSELF FROM FLEXED POSITION (≈32–33) · GOOD RIGHTING CANNOT HOLD IT (≈36) · HOLDS HEAD FEW SECONDS (≈38–39) · KEEPS HEAD IN LINE c̄ TRUNK >40'' (≈41) · TURNS HEAD FROM SIDE TO SIDE (≈45)
BODY EXTENSORS	STRAIGHTENING OF LEGS (≈33) · STRAIGHTENING OF TRUNK (≈36) · STRAIGHTENING OF HEAD & TRUNK TOGETHER (≈42)
VERTICAL POSITIONS	WHEN HELD UNDER ARMS, BODY SLIPS THROUGH HANDS (≈29) · ARMS HOLD BABY LEGS EXTENDED (≈34–35) · LEGS FLEXED GOOD SUPPORT c̄ ARMS (≈38)
HORIZONTAL POSITIONS	HYPOTONIC ARMS & LEGS STRAIGHT (≈28–29) · ARMS AND LEGS FLEXED (≈36–37) · HEAD & BACK EVEN FLEXED EXTREMITIES (≈40) · HEAD ABOVE BACK (≈42)

FLEXION ANGLES

Physical Finding	Findings across weeks gestation
POPLITEAL	NO RESISTANCE (≈24) · 150° (≈28) · 110° (≈32) · 100° (≈34–35) · 90° (≈38) · 80° (≈40)
ANKLE	45° (≈32) · 20° (≈36) · 0° (≈40) · A PRE-TERM WHO HAS REACHED 40 WEEKS STILL HAS A 40° ANGLE (≈44)
WRIST (SQUARE WINDOW)	90° (≈29) · 60° (≈32) · 45° (≈36) · 30° (≈38) · 0° (≈40)

REFLEXES

Physical Finding	Findings across weeks gestation
SUCKING	WEAK NOT SYNCHRONIZED c̄ SWALLOWING (≈26) · STRONGER SYNCHRONIZED (≈33) · PERFECT (≈35–36) · PERFECT (≈45)
ROOTING	LONG LATENCY PERIOD SLOW, IMPERFECT (≈27–28) · HAND TO MOUTH (≈30) · BRISK, COMPLETE, DURABLE (≈34) · PERFECT HAND TO MOUTH (≈38) · COMPLETE (≈45)
GRASP	FINGER GRASP IS GOOD STRENGTH IS POOR (≈27–28) · STRONGER (≈34) · CAN LIFT BABY OFF BED INVOLVES ARMS (≈39) · HANDS OPEN (≈46)
MORO	BARELY APPARENT (≈25) · WEAK NOT ELICITED EVERY TIME (≈27–28) · STRONGER (≈33) · COMPLETE c̄ ARM EXTENSION OPEN FINGERS, CRY (≈34–35) · ARM ADDUCTION ADDED (≈39) · ?BEGINS TO LOSE MORO (≈46)
CROSSED EXTENSION	FLEXION & EXTENSION IN A RANDOM, PURPOSELESS PATTERN (≈27–28) · EXTENSION BUT NO ADDUCTION (≈32) · STILL INCOMPLETE (≈36) · COMPLETE (≈45)
AUTOMATIC WALK	MINIMAL (≈30) · BEGINS TIPTOEING GOOD SUPPORT ON SOLE (≈32–33) · FAST TIPTOEING (≈36) · HEEL-TOE PROGRESSION WHOLE SOLE OF FOOT (≈40) · A PRE-TERM WHO HAS REACHED 40 WEEKS WALKS ON TOES (≈43–45) · ?BEGINS TO LOSE AUTOMATIC WALK (≈46)
PUPILLARY REFLEX	ABSENT (≈24) · APPEARS (≈30) · PRESENT (≈42)
GLABELLAR TAP	ABSENT (≈25) · APPEARS (≈33) · PRESENT (≈40)
TONIC NECK REFLEX	ABSENT (≈25) · APPEARS (≈35) · PRESENT AFTER 37 WEEKS (≈42)
NECK-RIGHTING	ABSENT (≈27) · APPEARS (≈37)

*Brazie, J.V., and Lubchenco, L.O.: The Estimation of Gestational Age Chart, in Kempe, Silver and O'Brien: Current Pediatric Diagnosis and Treatment, ed. 3, Los Altos, California, Lange Medical Publications, 1974, chapter 3.

E
Actions and Effects of Selected Drugs During Breast-Feeding*

Drugs	Comments
Antibiotics	
Ampicillin	Very small amounts excreted in the milk
Penicillin	Infant may develop "allergic" sensitization and candidal diarrhea
Amoxicillin	
Tetracycline	Effects are dose-related; amount the infant receives from breast-feeding is too small to cause discoloration of the teeth
Chloramphenicol[†]	Neonate may be unable to conjugate the drug; potential infant bone marrow suppression leading to anemia, shock and death
Metronidazole	Concentrated in the milk; potential adverse neurologic or hematologic effects; nursing may be resumed 48 hours after last dose
Sulfonamides	May cause jaundice in the neonatal period May cause hemolytic anemia in infants with glucose-6-phosphate dehydrogenase (G6PD) deficiency
Anticoagulants	Contraindicated, except with heparin; may cause bleeding episodes in the infant
Anticholinergics	
Atropine	May interfere with milk production
Antihistamines	Not appreciably excreted in the milk, but large doses may affect the milk supply
Antineoplastics	Generally contraindicated; some agents excreted in measurable amounts in the milk
Cyclophosphamide[†]	
Antithyroids	
Thiouracil[†]	May cause goiter or agranulocytosis
Methimazole[†]	
Cardiac agents	
Quinidine[†]	Contraindicated; may cause arrhythmia in the infant
Diuretics	May interfere with milk production
Heavy metals	
Bismuth[†] (contained in some dermatologic preparations)	Contraindicated for nipple care; dangerous if ingested
Mercury[†]	Excreted in the milk and hazardous to infant

*Modified from Palma, P. A., and Adcock, III, E. W. July 1981. Human milk and breastfeeding. *American Family Physician.* 24:179; and Sahu, S. Dec. 1981. Drugs and the nursing mother. *American Family Physician* 24:138.
[†]Indicates drugs that are absolutely contraindicated.

Drugs	Comments
Hormones	
Diethylstilbestrol[†]	Contraindicated; inhibits milk secretion
Oral contraceptives	May cause reduction of milk supply
	Progestins can produce feminization of the male infant
	Avoid or use with close observation for side effects
Laxatives	
Cascara	Can cause diarrhea in the infant
Narcotics	Use with caution; can cause sedation in the infant
Radioactive materials for testing	
Gallium citrate (^{67}G)	Insignificant amount excreted in breast milk; no nursing for 2 weeks
Iodine[†]	Contraindicated; may affect infant's thyroid gland
^{125}I	Discontinue nursing for 48 hours
^{131}I	Nursing should be discontinued until excretion is no longer significant; after a test dose, nursing may be resumed after 24 to 36 hours; after a treatment dose, nursing may be resumed after 2 to 3 weeks
^{99}Technetium	Discontinue nursing for 48 hours (half-life = 6 hours)
Recreational drugs	
Cannabis	No data on effects in infant
	Impaired formation of DNA and RNA in animals
Cocaine	No data; more study needed
Polyhalogenated biphenyls[†] (e.g., PCB$_5$, PBB$_5$)	Contraindicated; may interfere with mother's caretaking abilities
p-Lysergic acid[†] (LSD)	
Sedatives and tranquilizers	
Lithium carbonate[†]	Contraindicated; definitely toxic
Barbiturates	May produce sedation
Phenothiazines	May produce sedation
Diazepam	May produce sedation

[†] Indicates drugs that are absolutely contraindicated.

Selected Drugs Used During the Maternity Cycle— Generic and Trade Names

Acyclovir (Zovirax)*
Aluminum hydroxide (Amphojel)
Ampicillin (Omnipen, Polycillin)
Atropine (Atropisol)
Betamethasone (Celestone Solupan)
Bromocriptine (Parlodel)
Bupivacaine (Marcaine)
Calcium carbonate (Caltrate, Tums)
Calcium gluconate (none)
Chloramphenicol (Chloromycetin)
Chloroprocaine (Nesacaine)
Chlorotrianisene (TACE)
Chlorpromazine hydrochloride (Thorazine)
Clomiphene citrate (Clomid)
Clotrimazole (Mycelex)
Danocrine (Danazol)
Dexamethasone (Decadron)
Diazepam (Vallium)
Epinephrine (Adrenalin chloride)
Ergonovine maleate (Ergotrate)
Erythromycin (Ilotycin, Erythrocin)
Furosemide (Lasix)
Gentamicin sulfate (Garamycin)
Glucagon (none)
Heparin (none)
Hydralazine hydrochloride (Apresoline)
Hydroxyzine hydrochloride (Vistaril)
Isoxsuprine hydrochloride (Vasodilan)
Kanamycin sulfate (Kantrex)
Magnesium hydroxide (Maalox)
Magnesium sulfate (none)
Meperidine hydrochloride (Demerol)

Mepivacaine hydrochloride (Carbocaine)
Methadone (Dolophine)
Methylergonovine maleate (Methergine)
Metronidazole (Flagyl)
Miconazole (Monistat)
Morphine sulfate (none)
Nafcillin (Unipen)
Nalorphine hydrochloride (Nalline)
Naloxone hydrochloride (Narcan)
Nitrofurantoin (Furadantin)
Novobiocin (Albamycin)
Nystatin (Mycostatin)
Oxytocin (Pitocin)
Paregoric; camphorated opium tincture (none)
Penicillin (Bicillin)
Phenobarbital (Luminal)
Procaine (Novocaine)
Promethazine (Phenergan)
Protamine sulfate (none)
Phytonadione (AquaMEPHYTON)
$Rh_o(D)$ immune globulin (RhoGAM)
Ritodrine (Yutopar)
Salicylates; acetylsalicylic acid (Aspirin)
Silver nitrate (none)
Sodium bicarbonate (none)
Sulfisoxazole (Gantrisin)
Terbutaline sulfate (Brethine)
Tetracaine (Pontocaine)
Tetracycline hydrochloride (Achromycin)

*Trade name is in parentheses.

Glossary

abdominal effluerage   light abdominal stroking, which relieves mild to moderate pain during uterine contractions.

abortion   loss of pregnancy before the fetus is viable outside the uterus; miscarriage.

abruptio placentae   premature separation, partially or totally, of a normally implanted placenta.

acceleration   periodic increase in the baseline fetal heart rate.

acrocyanosis   cyanosis of the extremities.

active acquired immunity   formation of antibodies by the pregnant woman in response to illness or immunization.

acute grief   the most severe stage of the grief response; usually resolved within 1–2 months and followed by a gradual return to the preloss level of functioning.

afterpains   cramplike pains due to contractions of the uterus that occur after childbirth. They are more common in multiparas, tend to be most severe during nursing, and last 2–3 days.

amniocentesis   removal of amniotic fluid by insertion of a needle into the amniotic sac. Amniotic fluid is used for assessment of fetal health or fetal maturity.

amnion   the inner of the two membranes that form the sac containing the fetus and the amniotic fluid.

amnioscopy   procedure in which the amniotic membranes are viewed via insertion of an amnioscope in the vagina.

amniotic fluid   the liquid surrounding the fetus in utero. It absorbs shocks, permits fetal movements, and helps maintain a stable environment.

amniotic fluid embolus   amniotic fluid that has leaked into the chorionic plate and entered the maternal circulation.

amniotomy   the artificial rupturing of the amniotic membranes.

ampulla   the outer two-thirds of the fallopian tube; fertilization of the ovum by a spermatozoon usually occurs here.

antepartal education   programs teaching childbirth preparation.

antepartum   time between conception and the onset of labor; usually used to describe the period during which a woman is pregnant.

Apgar score   the Apgar scoring system is used to evaluate newborns at 1 minute and 5 minutes after delivery. The total score is achieved by assessing five signs: heart rate, respiratory effort, muscle tone, reflex irritability, and color. Each of the signs is assigned a score of 0, 1, or 2. The highest score is 10.

areola   pigmented ring surrounding the nipple of the breast.

autosomes   chromosomes that are not sex chromosomes.

Barr body   deeply staining chromatin mass located against the inner surface of the cell nucleus. Found only in normal females; also called *sex chromatin*.

basal body temperature (BBT)   the lowest waking temperature.

baseline rate   the average fetal heart rate observed during a 10-minute period of monitoring.

baseline variability   changes in the fetal heart rate that result from the interplay between the sympathetic and the parasympathetic nervous systems.

biopsychosocial   an approach that recognizes the biologic, psychologic, and social factors that affect the individual.

birth center   a setting for labor and delivery that emphasizes a family-centered approach rather than for obstetric technology and treatment.

birth rate   number of live births per 1000 population.

birthing room   a room for labor and delivery with a relaxed atmosphere.

blastocyst   the inner solid mass of cells within the morula.

bloody show   pink-tinged mucous secretions resulting from rupture of small capillaries as the cervix effaces and dilates.

Bradley method   partner- or husband-coached natural childbirth.

Braxton Hicks contractions   intermittent painless contractions of the uterus. They occur more frequently toward the end of pregnancy and are sometimes mistaken for true labor pains.

Brazleton's neonatal behavioral assessment   a brief examination used to identify the infant's behavioral states and responses.

breasts mammary glands.

broad ligament ligament extending from lateral margins of uterus to pelvic wall; keeps the uterus centrally placed and provides stability within the pelvic cavity.

bronchopulmonary dysplasia chronic pulmonary disease of multifactorial etiology characterized initially by alveolar and bronchial necrosis, which results in bronchial metaplasia and interstitial fibrosis. Appears in x-ray films as generalized small, radiolucent cysts within the lungs.

brown adipose tissue (BAT) fat deposits in neonates that provide greater heat-generating activity than ordinary fat. Found around the kidneys, adrenals, and neck, between the scapulas, and behind the sternum; also called *brown fat*.

calorie amount of heat required to raise the temperature of 1 g of water 1 degree centigrade.

caput succedaneum swelling or edema occurring in or under the fetal scalp during labor.

cardinal ligaments the chief uterine supports, suspending the uterus from the side walls of the true pelvis.

cardinal movements the positional changes of the fetus as it moves through the birth canal during labor and delivery.

cardiopulmonary adaptation adaptation of the neonate's cardiovascular and respiratory systems to life outside the womb.

caudal block local anesthetic injected into the epidural space.

cephalhematoma subcutaneous swelling containing blood found under the periosteum of an infant's skull several days after delivery. Usually disappears within a few weeks to 2 months.

cervical cap a "cup-shaped" device placed over the cervix to prevent pregnancy.

cervical dilatation process in which the cervical os and the cervical canal widen from less than a centimeter to approximately 10 cm, allowing delivery of the fetus.

cervix the "neck" between the external os and the body of the uterus. The lower end of the cervix extends into the vagina.

Chadwick's sign violet bluish color of the vaginal mucous membrane caused by increased vascularity; visible from about the fourth week of pregnancy.

chloasma brownish pigmentation over the bridge of the nose and cheeks during pregnancy and in some women who are taking oral contraceptives. Also called *mask of pregnancy*.

chorion the fetal membrane closest to the intrauterine wall; it gives rise to the placenta and continues as the outer membrane surrounding the amnion.

chromosomes the threadlike structures within the nucleus of a cell that carry the genes.

chronic grief grief response involving a denial of the reality of the loss, which prevents any resolution.

circumcision surgical excision of the prepuce (foreskin) of the penis.

cleavage rapid mitotic division of the zygote; cells produced are called *blastomeres*.

client one who seeks and receives services.

client advocacy an approach to client care in which the nurse educates and supports the client and protects the client's rights.

cold stress excessive heat loss resulting in compensatory mechanisms (increased respirations and nonshivering thermogenesis) to main core body temperature.

colostrum secretion from the breast before the onset of true lactation; contains mainly serum and white blood corpuscles. It has a high protein content, provides some immune properties, and cleanses the neonate's intestinal tract of mucus and meconium.

condom a rubber sheath that covers the penis to prevent conception or disease.

conduction loss of heat to a cooler surface by direct skin contact.

contraceptive sponge a small pillow-shaped polyurethane sponge with a concave cupped area on one side, designed to fit over the cervix to prevent pregnancy.

contraction stress test (CST) a means of evaluating the respiratory function (oxygen and carbon dioxide exchange) of the placenta. Used to identify fetus at risk for intrauterine asphyxia.

conjugate vera the true conjugate, which extends from the middle of the sacral promontory to the middle of the pubic crest.

convection loss of heat from the warm body surface to cooler air currents.

cornua the elongated portions of the uterus where the fallopian tubes open.

corpus the upper two-thirds of the uterus.

corpus luteum a small yellow body that develops within a ruptured ovarian follicle; it secretes progesterone in the second half of the menstrual cycle and atrophies about 3 days before the beginning of menstrual flow. If pregnancy occurs, it continues to produce progesterone until the placenta takes over this function.

cotyledon   one of the rounded portions into which the placenta's uterine surface is divided, consisting of a mass of villi, blood vessels, and an intervillous space.

couvade   in some cultures, the male's observance of certain rituals and taboos to signify the transition to fatherhood.

crisis   any naturally occurring turning point, such as courtship, marriage, pregnancy, parenthood, and death.

crisis intervention   actions to be taken by the nurse when crisis threatens to overwhelm the client, to help the client deal with the crisis, regain his or her equilibrium, grow from the experience, and improve coping skills.

crowning   appearance of the presenting fetal part at the vaginal orifice during labor.

deceleration   periodic decrease in the baseline fetal heart rate.

decidua basalis   the part of the decidua that unites with the chorion to form the placenta. It is shed in lochial discharge after delivery.

decidua capsularis   the part of the decidua surrounding the chorionic sac.

decidua vera (parietalis)   nonplacental decidua lining the uterus.

descriptive statistics   statistics that report facts in a concise and easily retrievable way.

diagonal conjugate   distance from the lower posterior border of the symphysis pubis to the sacral promontory; may be obtained by manual measurement.

diaphragm   a flexible disk that covers the cervix to prevent pregnancy.

diastasis recti abdominis   separation of the recti abdominis muscles along the median line. In women, seen with repeated childbirths or multiple gestation. In the newborn, usually caused by incomplete development.

diploid number of chromosomes   a set of maternal and a set of paternal chromosomes. In humans the diploid number of chromosomes is 46.

drug-addicted infant   the newborn of an alcoholic or drug-addicted woman.

ductus arteriosus   a communication channel between the main pulmonary artery and the aorta of the fetus.

ductus venosus   a fetal blood vessel that carries oxygenated blood between the umbilical vein and the inferior vena cava, bypassing the liver; it becomes a ligament after birth.

duration   the time length of each contraction, measured from the beginning of the increment to the completion of the decrement.

dystocia   difficult labor due to mechanical factors produced by the fetus or the maternal pelvis or due to inadequate uterine or other muscular activity.

eclampsia   a major complication of pregnancy of unknown cause. It occurs more often in the primigravida and is accompanied by elevated blood pressure, albuminuria, oliguria, tonic and clonic convulsions, and coma. May occur during pregnancy (usually after the twentieth week of gestation) or within 48 hours after delivery.

ectoderm   outer layer of cells in the developing embryo that gives rise to the skin, nails, and hair.

effacement   thinning and shortening of the cervix that occurs late in pregnancy or during labor.

embryo   the early stage of development of the young of any organism. In humans, the period from 2–8 weeks' gestation, which is characterized by cellular differentiation and predominantly hyperplastic growth.

en face   an assumed position in which one person looks at another and maintains his or her face in the same vertical plane as that of the other.

endoderm   the inner layer of cells in the developing embryo that give rise to internal organs such as the intestines.

endometritis   infection of the endometrium.

endometrium   the mucous membrane that lines the inner surface of the uterus; the innermost layer of the corpus.

engagement   the entrance of the fetal presenting part into the true pelvis and the beginning of the descent through the pelvic canal.

engorgement   vascular congestion or distention. In obstetrics, the swelling of breast tissue brought about by an increase in blood and lymph supply to the breast, preceding true lactation.

engrossment   characteristic sense of absorption, preoccupation, and interest in the infant demonstrated by fathers during early contact with their infants.

epidural block   regional anesthesia effective through the first and second stages of labor.

episiotomy   incision of the perineum to facilitate delivery and to avoid laceration of the perineum.

Epstein's pearls   small, white blebs found along the gum margins and at the junction of the soft and hard palates; commonly seen in the newborn as a normal manifestation.

Erb-Duchenne paralysis paralysis of the upper arm due to damage to the fifth and sixth cervical nerves during delivery. The most common form of brachial palsy.

erythema toxicum innocuous pink papular rash of unknown cause with superimposed vesicles that appears within 24–48 hours after birth and resolves spontaneously within a few days.

erythroblastosis fetalis hemolytic disease of the newborn characterized by anemia, jaundice, enlargement of the liver and spleen, and generalized edema. Caused by isoimmunization due to Rh incompatibility or ABO incompatibility.

estrogens hormones estradiol and estrone, produced primarily by the ovary.

evaporation loss of heat incurred when water on the skin surface is converted to a vapor.

exchange transfusion the replacement of 70%–80% of the newborn's circulating blood by withdrawing the recipient's blood and injecting a donor's blood in equal amounts, for the purpose of preventing the accumulation of bilirubin or other byproducts of hemolysis in the blood.

external os cervical opening into the vagina.

fallopian tubes tubes that extend from the lateral angle of the uterus and terminate near the ovary; they serve as a passageway for the ovum from the ovary to the uterus and for the spermatozoa from the uterus toward the ovary. Also called *oviducts* and *uterine tubes*.

false pelvis the portion of the pelvis above the linea terminalis; its primary function is to support the weight of the enlarged pregnant uterus.

family-centered care an approach to health care based on the concept that a hospital can provide professional services to mothers, fathers, and infants in a homelike environment that would enhance the integrity of the family unit.

female reproductive cycle (FRC) the monthly rhythmic changes in sexually mature females.

ferning formulation of palm-leaf pattern by the crystallization of cervical mucus as it dries at midmenstrual cycle. Helpful in determining time of ovulation. Observed via microscopic examination of a thick layer of cervical mucus on a glass slide. This pattern is also observed when amniotic fluid is allowed to air dry on a slide and is a useful and quick test to determine whether amniotic membranes have ruptured.

fertility awareness methods natural family planning.

fertility rate number of births per 1000 women, age 15–44 in a given population per year.

fertilization impregnation of an ovum by a spermatozoon.

fetal alcohol syndrome (FAS) syndrome caused by maternal alcohol ingestion and characterized by microcephaly, intrauterine growth retardation, short palpebral fissures, and maxillary hypoplasia.

fetal attitude the relation of the fetal parts to one another.

fetal blood sampling blood sample drawn from the fetal scalp (or from the fetus in breech position) to evaluate the acid-base status of the fetus.

fetal bradycardia a fetal heart rate less than 120 beats/minute during a 10-minute period of continuous monitoring.

fetal death death of the developing fetus after 20 weeks' gestation. Also called *fetal demise*.

fetal lie relationship of the long axis of the fetus to the long axis of the mother.

fetal position relationship of the landmark on the presenting fetal part to the front, sides, or back of the maternal pelvis.

fetal presentation the fetal body part that enters the maternal pelvis first. The three possible presentations are cephalic, shoulder, or breech.

fetal tachycardia a fetal heart rate of 160 beats/minute or more during a 10-minute period of continuous monitoring.

fetoscopy a technique for directly observing the fetus and obtaining a sample of fetal blood or skin.

fetus the child in utero from about the ninth week of gestation until birth.

fimbria any structure resembling a fringe; the fringelike extremity of the fallopian tube.

folic acid an important mineral directly related to the outcome of pregnancy and to maternal and fetal health.

follicle-stimulating hormone (FSH) hormone produced by the anterior pituitary during the first half of the menstrual cycle, stimulating development of the graafian follicle.

fontanelle in the fetus, an unossified space or soft spot consisting of a strong band of connective tissue lying between the cranial bones of the skull.

foramen ovale septal opening between the atria of the fetal heart. Normally, the opening closes shortly after birth; if it remains open, it can be surgically repaired.

frequency   the time between the beginning of one contraction and the beginning of the next contraction.

fundus   the rounded uppermost portion of the uterine corpus that extends above the points of attachment of the fallopian tubes.

gametogenesis   the process by which germ cells are produced.

gestation   period of intrauterine development from conception through birth; pregnancy.

gestational age assessment tools   systems used to evaluate the newborn's external physical characteristics and neurologic and/or neuromuscular development to accurately determine gestational age. These replace or supplement the traditional calculation from the mother's last menstrual period.

Goodell's sign   softening of the cervix that occurs about the second month of pregnancy.

graafian follicle   the ovarian cyst containing the ripe ovum; it secretes estrogen.

gravida   a pregnant woman.

grief   an emotional state; a reaction to loss.

grief work   the inner process of working through or managing the bereavement.

haploid number of chromosomes   half the diploid number of chromosomes. In humans, there are 23 chromosomes, the haploid number, in each germ cell.

Hegar's sign   a softening of the lower uterine segment found upon palpation in the second or third month of pregnancy.

heterozygous   a genotypic situation in which two different genes occur at a given locus on a pair of homologous chromosomes.

homozygous   a genotypic situation in which two similar genes occur at a given locus on a pair of homologous chromosomes.

hyaline membrane disease   respiratory disease of the newborn characterized by interference with ventilation at the alveolar level, thought to be caused by the presence of fibrinoid deposits lining the alveolar ducts. Also called *respiratory distress syndrome (RDS)*.

hydramnios   an excess of amniotic fluid, leading to overdistension of the uterus. Frequently seen in diabetic pregnant women even if there is no coexisting fetal anomaly.

hydrops fetalis   a severe form of erythroblastosis fetalis presenting with marked anemia and cardiomegaly.

hyperbilirubinemia   excessive amount of bilirubin in the blood; indicative of hemolytic processes due to blood incompatibility, intrauterine infection, septicemia, neonatal renal infection, and other disorders.

hypnoreflexogenous method   a combination of hypnosis and conditioned reflexes used during childbirth.

hypocalcemia   abnormally low level of serum calcium levels.

induction of labor   the process of causing or initiating labor by use of medication or surgical rupture of membranes.

infant of a diabetic mother (IDM)   at-risk infant born to a woman previously diagnosed as diabetic or who develops symptoms of diabetes during pregnancy.

inferential statistics   statistics that allow an investigator to draw conclusions about what is happening between two or more variables in a population and to suggest or refute causal relationships between them.

infertility   diminished ability to conceive.

informed consent   a legal concept that protects a person's right to autonomy and self-determination by specifying that no action may be taken without that person's prior understanding and freely given consent.

infundibulopelvic ligament   ligament that suspends and supports the ovaries.

intensity   the strength of the uterine contraction during acme.

internal os   an inside mouth or opening; the opening between the cervix and the uterus.

intrapartum   time from the onset of true labor until the delivery of the infant and placenta.

intrauterine device (IUD)   a device inserted into the uterus that prevents pregnancy by producing a local sterile inflammatory reaction.

involution   rapid reduction in size and return of the uterus to a normal condition similar to its prepregnant state.

ischial spines   prominences that arise near the junction of the ilium and ischium and jut into the pelvic cavity; used as a reference point during labor to evaluate the descent of the fetal head into the birth canal.

isthmus   the straight and narrow part of the fallopian tube with a thick muscular wall and an opening (lumen) 2–3 mm in diameter; the site of tubal ligation. Also a constriction in the uterus that is located above the cervix and below the corpus.

karyotype   the set of chromosomes arranged in a standard order.

Kegel's exercises   perineal muscle tightening that strengthens the pubococcygeus muscle and increases its tone.

kernicterus   deposition of unconjugated bilirubin in the basal ganglia of the brain.

lacto-ovovegetarians   vegetarians who include milk, dairy products, and eggs in their diets, and occasionally fish, poultry, and liver.

lactose intolerance   a condition in which an individual has difficulty digesting milk and milk products.

lactovegetarians   vegetarians who include dairy products but no eggs in their diets.

Lamaze method   a method of childbirth preparation, also known as *psychoprophylaxis.*

lanugo   fine, downy hair found on all body parts of the fetus after 20 weeks' gestation, with the exception of the palms of the hands and the soles of the feet.

large for gestational age (LGA)   excessive growth of a fetus in relation to the gestational time period.

last menstrual period (LMP)   the last normal menstrual period experienced by the mother prior to pregnancy; sometimes used to calculate the infant's gestational age.

Leboyer method   birthing technique that eases the newborn's transition to extrauterine life; lights are dimmed in the delivery room and noise level is kept to a minimum.

lecithin/sphingomyelin (L/S) ratio   a ratio of two components of surfactant that can help determine fetal lung maturity.

Leopold's maneuvers   series of four maneuvers designed to provide a systematic approach whereby the examiner may determine fetal presentation and position.

letdown reflex   pattern of stimulation, hormone release, and resulting muscle contraction that forces milk into the lactiferous ducts, making it available to the infant; milk ejection reflex.

lightening   moving of the fetus and the uterus downward into the pelvic cavity; engagement.

local infiltration   injection of an anesthetic agent into the subcutaneous tissue in a fanlike pattern.

lochia   maternal discharge of blood, mucus, and tissue from the uterus that may last for several weeks after birth.

lochia alba   white vaginal discharge that follows lochia serosa and that lasts from about the tenth to the twenty-first day after delivery.

lochia rubra   red, blood-tinged vaginal discharge that occurs following delivery and lasts 2–4 days.

lochia serosa   pink, serous, and blood-tinged vaginal discharge that follows lochia rubra and lasts until the seventh to tenth day after delivery.

loss   a state of being deprived of, or without, something one has had.

luteinizing hormone (LH)   anterior pituitary hormone responsible for stimulating ovulation and for development of the corpus luteum.

macrosomia   condition seen in some neonates of large body size and high birth weight, as those born of prediabetic and diabetic mothers.

mastitis   inflammation of the breast.

maternal mortality   number of deaths from any cause during the pregnancy cycle per 100,000 live births.

meconium   dark green or black material present in the large intestine of a full-term infant; the first stools passed by the newborn.

meiosis   the process of cell division that occurs in the maturation of sperm and ova that decreases their number of chromosomes by one half.

Mendelian inheritance   a major category of inheritance whereby a trait is determined by a pair of genes on homologous chromosomes; also called *single gene inheritance.*

mesoderm   the intermediate layer of germ cells in the embryo that give rise to connective tissue, bone marrow, muscles, blood, lymphoid tissue, and epithelial tissue.

milia   tiny white papules appearing on the face of a neonate as a result of unopened sebaceous glands; they disappear spontaneously within a few weeks.

mitleiden   a phenomenon in which expectant fathers develop symptoms similar to those of the pregnant woman: weight gain, nausea, and various aches and pains.

mitosis   process of cell division whereby both daughter cells have the same number and pattern of chromosomes as the original cell.

modeling   the process of teaching behaviors through role playing or having the client talk with a person who has mastered a similar crisis.

molding   shaping of the fetal head by overlapping of the cranial bones to facilitate movement through the birth canal during labor.

Mongolian spot   dark flat pigmentation of the lower back and buttocks noted at birth in some infants; usually disappears by the time the child reaches school age.

mons pubis   mound of subcutaneous fatty tissue covering the anterior portion of the symphysis pubis.

Moro reflex   flexion of the newborn's thighs and knees accompanied by fingers that fan then clench as the arms are simultaneously thrown out and then brought together as though embracing something. This reflex can be elicited by startling the newborn with a sudden noise or movement; also called the *startle reflex.*

morula   developmental stage of the fertilized ovum in which there is a solid mass of cells.

multigravida   female who has been pregnant more than once.

multipara   female who has had two or more deliveries in which the fetus reached viability.

myometrium   the middle layer of the corpus of the uterus; also known as the *muscular uterine layer.*

Nägele's rule   a method of determining the estimated date of confinement (EDC): after obtaining the first day of the last menstrual period, one subtracts 3 months and adds 7 days.

neonatal mortality   number of deaths of infants in the first 28 days per 1000 live births.

neonatology   the specialty that focuses on the managment of high-risk conditions of the newborn.

newborn screening tests   tests that detect inborn errors of metabolism that, if left undiscovered, cause mental retardation and physical handicaps.

nipple   a protrusion about 0.5–1.3 cm in diameter in the center of each mature breast.

nonstress test (NST)   method of evaluating fetal status by observation of baseline variability and acceleration of the fetal heart rate with fetal movement.

nullipara   female who has not delivered a viable fetus.

nurse-midwife   a certified nurse-midwife (CNM) is an RN who has received special training and education in the care of the family during childbearing and the prenatal, intrapartal, and postpartal periods.

nursing diagnosis   a two-part statement that includes the health problem and related etiology.

nursing process   a framework of problem identification and resolution, consisting of assessment, analysis, planning, implementation, and evaluation.

obstetric conjugate   distance from the middle of the sacral promontory to an area approximately 1 cm below the pubic crest.

oligohydramnios   decreased amount of amniotic fluid.

oogenesis   process during fetal life whereby the ovary produces oogenia, cells that become primitive ovarian eggs.

oophoritis   infection of the ovaries.

oral contraceptives   "birth control pills" that work by inhibiting the release of an ovum and by maintaining a type of mucus that is hostile to sperm.

ovarian ligaments   ligaments that anchor the lower pole of the ovary to the cornua of the uterus.

ovary   female sex gland in which the ova are formed and in which estrogen and progesterone are produced. Normally there are two ovaries, located in the lower abdomen on each side of the uterus.

ovulation   normal process of discharging a mature ovum from an ovary approximately 14 days prior to the onset of menses.

ovum   female reproductive cell; egg.

oxytocin   hormone normally produced by the posterior pituitary, responsible for stimulation of uterine contractions and the release of milk into the lactiferous ducts.

para   a woman who has borne offspring who reached the age of viability.

paracervical block   a local anesthetic agent injected transvaginally adjacent to the outer rim of the cervix.

passive acquired immunity   transferral of antibodies (IgG) from the mother to the fetus in utero.

pelvic cavity   bony portion of the birth passages; a curved canal with a longer posterior than anterior wall.

pelvic cellulitis   infection involving the connective tissue of the broad ligament or, in severe cases, the connective tissue of all the pelvic structures.

pelvic diaphragm   part of the pelvic floor composed of deep fascia and the levator ani and the coccygeal muscles.

pelvic inlet   upper border of the true pelvis.

pelvic outlet   lower border of the true pelvis.

perimetrium   the outermost layer of the corpus of the uterus; also known as the *serosal layer.*

perinatal mortality   both neonatal and fetal deaths per 1000 live births.

perinatology   the medical specialty concerned with the diagnosis and treatment of high-risk conditions of the pregnant woman and her fetus.

perineal body   wedge-shaped mass of fibromuscular tissue found between the lower part of the vagina and the anal canal.

perineum   the area of tissue between the anus and scrotum in the male or between the anus and vagina in the female.

periodic breathing   sporadic episodes of apnea, not associated with cyanosis, which last for about 10 seconds and commonly occur in preterm infants.

periods of reactivity   predictable patterns of neonate behavior during the first several hours after birth.

phototherapy   the treatment of jaundice by exposure to light.

physiologic anemia of infancy   a harmless condition in which the hemoglobin level drops in the first 6–12 weeks after birth, then reverts to normal levels.

physiologic jaundice   a harmless condition caused by the normal reduction of red blood cells, occurring 48 or more hours after birth, peaking at the fifth to seventh days, and disappearing between the seventh to tenth day.

pica   the eating of substances not ordinarily considered edible or to have nutritive value.

placenta previa   abnormal implantation of the placenta in the lower uterine segment.

polar body   a small cell resulting from the meiotic division of the mature oocyte.

polycythemia   an abnormal increase in the number of total red blood cells in the body's circulation.

postpartum   period after childbirth or delivery.

postterm infant   any infant delivered after 42 weeks' gestation.

postterm labor   labor that occurs after 42 weeks of gestation.

precipitous labor   labor lasting less then 3 hours.

preeclampsia   toxemia of pregnancy, characterized by hypertension, albuminuria, and edema.

pregnancy-induced hypertension (PIH)   a hypertensive disorder including preeclampsia and eclampsia as conditions, characterized by the three cardinal signs of hypertension, edema, and proteinuria.

premature rupture of membranes (PROM)   spontaneous rupture of the membranes and leakage of amniotic fluid prior to the onset of labor.

prep   shaving of the pubic area.

presentation   the fetal body part that enters the maternal pelvis first. The three possible presentations are cephalic, shoulder, or breech.

presenting part   the fetal part present in or on the cervical os.

preterm infant   any infant born before 38 weeks' gestation.

preterm labor   labor occurring between 20–38 weeks of pregnancy.

primigravida   a woman who is pregnant for the first time.

primipara   a woman who has given birth to her first child.

problem-oriented record system   a system of charting observations and interventions in a format composed of subjective data, objective data, analysis, and plan.

progesterone   a hormone produced by the corpus luteum, adrenal cortex, and placenta whose function it is to stimulate proliferation of the endometrium to facilitate growth of the embryo.

prolactin   a hormone secreted by the anterior pituitary that stimulates and sustains lactation.

prolonged labor   labor lasting more than 24 hours.

pseudomenstruation   blood-tinged mucus from the vagina in the newborn female infant; caused by withdrawal of maternal hormones that were present during pregnancy.

ptyalism   excessive salivation.

pubis   the slightly bowed front portion of the innominate bone.

pudendal block   perineal anesthesia provided for the latter part of the first stage, the second stage of labor, delivery, and episiotomy repair.

puerperal morbidity   a maternal temperature of 100.4F (38.0C) or higher on any two of the first 10 postpartal days excluding the first 24 hours. The temperature is to be taken by mouth at least four times per day.

puerperium   the period or state of confinement after completion of the third stage of labor until involution of the uterus is complete, usually 6 weeks.

radiation   heat loss incurred when heat transfers to cooler surfaces and objects not in direct contact with the body.

Read method   natural childbirth preparation centered on eliminating the fear-tension-pain syndrome.

reciprocal inhibition   the principle that it is impossible to feel relaxed and tense at the same time; the basis for relaxation techniques.

recommended dietary allowances (RDA) government recommended allowances of various vitamins, minerals and other nutrients.

regional anesthesia injection of local anesthetic agents so that they come into direct contact with nervous tissue.

respiratory distress syndrome see *hyaline membrane disease.*

RhoGAM an anti-Rh₀(D) gamma-globulin given after delivery to an Rh-negative mother of an Rh-positive fetus or child. Prevents development of permanent active immunity to the Rh antigen.

risk factors any findings that suggest the pregnancy may have a negative outcome, either for the woman or her unborn child.

rooting reflex an infant's tendency to turn the head and open the lips to suck when one side of the mouth or the cheek is touched.

round ligaments ligaments that arise from the side of the uterus near the fallopian tube insertion to help the broad ligament keep the uterus in place.

rugae transverse ridges of mucous membranes lining the vagina, which allow the vagina to stretch during the descent of the fetal head.

rupture of membranes (ROM) refers to the rupturing of amniotic membranes; may be spontaneous or induced.

sacral promontory a projection into the pelvic cavity on the anterior upper portion of the sacrum; serves as an obstetric guide in determining pelvic measurements.

salpingitis infection of the fallopian tubes.

scarf sign the position of the elbow when the hand of a supine infant is drawn across to the other shoulder until it meets resistance.

sex chromosomes the X and Y chromosomes, which are responsible for sex determination.

single gene inheritance see *Mendelian inheritance.*

sinusoidal pattern a wave form of fetal heart rate where long-term variability is present, but there is no short-term variability.

small for gestational age (SGA) inadequate weight or growth for gestational age; birth weight below the tenth percentile.

spermatogenesis process by which mature spermatozoa are formed, during which chromosome number is reduced by half.

spermatozoa mature sperm cells of the male produced by testes.

spermicides a variety of creams, foams, jellies and suppositories, inserted into the vagina prior to intercourse, which destroy sperm or neutralize vaginal secretions and thereby immobilize sperm.

spinal block injection of a local anesthetic agent directly into the spinal fluid in the spinal canal to provide anesthesia for vaginal delivery and cesarean birth.

spinnbarkeit describes the elasticity of the cervical mucus that is present at ovulation.

station relationship of the presenting fetal part to an imaginary line drawn between the pelvic ischial spines.

sterility inability to conceive or to produce offspring.

stillbirth an infant born dead after 20 weeks of gestation.

striae gravidarum stretch marks; shiny reddish lines that appear on the abdomen, breasts, thighs, and buttocks of pregnant women as a result of stretching skin.

subinvolution failure of a part to return to its normal size after functional enlargement, such as failure of the uterus to return to normal size after pregnancy.

surfactant a surface-active mixture of lipoproteins secreted in the alveoli and air passages that reduces surface tension of pulmonary fluids and contributes to the elasticity of pulmonary tissue.

suture fibrous connection of opposed joint surfaces, as in the skull. Also, the uniting of edges of a wound.

symphysis pubis fibrocartilagenous joint between the pelvic bones and the midline.

taking-hold phase period beginning on the second or third day after delivery as the mother resumes control of her life.

taking-in phase period lasting 2–3 days after delivery characterized by maternal passivity and dependence.

telangiectatic nevi (stork bites) small clusters of pink-red spots appearing on the nape of the neck and around the eyes of infants; localized areas of capillary dilatation.

teratogens nongenetic factors that can produce malformations of the fetus.

testes the male gonads, in which sperm and testosterone are produced.

thermal neutral zone (TNZ) the environmental temperature range within which the rates of oxygen consumption and metabolism are minimal and internal body temperature is maintained.

tonic neck reflex   postural reflex seen in the newborn. When the supine infant's head is turned to one side, the arm and leg on that side extend while the extremities on the opposite side flex; also called the *fencing position.*

TORCH   acronym used to describe a group of infections that represent potentially severe problems during pregnancy. *TO* = toxoplasmosis, *R* = rubella, *C* = cytomegalovirus, *H* = herpesvirus.

transverse diameter   the largest diameter of the pelvic inlet; helps determine the shape of the inlet.

trisomy   the presence of three homologous chromosomes rather than the normal two.

trophoblast   the outer layer of the blastoderm that will eventually establish the nutrient relationship with the uterine endometrium.

true pelvis   the portion that lies below the linea terminalis, made up of the inlet, cavity, and outlet.

tubal ligation   suturing or tying shut the fallopian tubes to prevent pregnancy.

umbilical cord   the structure connecting the placenta to the umbilicus of the fetus and through which nutrients from the woman are exchanged for wastes from the fetus.

uterosacral ligaments   ligaments that provide support for the uterus and cervix at the level of the ischial spines.

uterus   hollow muscular organ in which the fertilized ovum is implanted and in which the developing fetus is nourished until birth.

vagina   the musculomembranous tube or passageway located between the external genitals and the uterus of the female.

vasectomy   surgical removal of a portion of the vas deferens (ductus deferens) to produce infertility.

vegan   a "pure" vegetarian who consumes no food from animal sources.

vena caval syndrome   symptoms of dizziness, pallor, and clamminess resulting from lowering blood pressure when the pregnant woman lies supine and the enlarging uterus presses on the vena cava; also known as *supine hypotensive syndrome.*

vernix caseosa   a protective cheeselike whitish substance made up of sebum and desquamated epithelial cells that is present on the fetal skin.

version   a change of position, usually to alter the presenting fetal part and facilitate delivery.

vulva   the external structure of the female genitals, lying below the mons pubis.

Wharton's jelly   yellow-white gelatinous material surrounding the vessels of the umbilical cord.

zona pellucida   transparent inner layer surrounding an ovum.

zygote   a fertilized egg.

Index